国际经典内科学教科书

第10版
Cecil Essentials of Medicine
希氏内科学精要
中英双语版

原　著　Edward J. Wing, MD, FACP, FIDSA
Former Dean of Medicine and Biological Sciences
Professor of Medicine
Warren Alpert Medical School of Brown University, Providence, Rhode Island

Fred J. Schiffman, MD, MACP
Sigal Family Professor of Humanistic Medicine
Vice Chair, Department of Medicine
Warren Alpert Medical School of Brown University, Providence, Rhode Island

中英双语版　编辑委员会　主任委员　王　辰

── 第3分册 ──

肾脏疾病

主　译　李雪梅　赵明辉

北京大学医学出版社

XISHI NEIKEXUE JINGYAO（DI 10 BAN） DI 3 FENCE SHENZANG JIBING（ZHONGYING SHUANGYU BAN）

图书在版编目（CIP）数据

希氏内科学精要：第 10 版 . 第 3 分册，肾脏疾病：汉、英 /（美）爱德华·温（Edward J. Wing），（美）弗雷德·谢夫曼（Fred J. Schiffman）原著；李雪梅，赵明辉主译 . -- 北京：北京大学医学出版社，2024. 11. -- ISBN 978-7-5659-3251-9

Ⅰ. R5

中国国家版本馆 CIP 数据核字第 2024YC3853 号

北京市版权局著作权合同登记号：图字：01-2024-4518

Elsevier (Singapore) Pte Ltd.
3 Killiney Road, #08-01 Winsland House I, Singapore 239519
Tel: (65) 6349-0200; Fax: (65) 6733-1817

Cecil Essentials of Medicine, Tenth Edition
Copyright © 2022 by Elsevier, Inc. All rights are reserved, including those for text and data mining, AI training, and similar technologies.
Publisher's note: Elsevier takes a neutral position with respect to territorial disputes or jurisdictional claims in its published content, including in maps and institutional affiliations.
Previous editions copyrighted 2016, 2010, 2007, 2004, 2001, 1997, 1993, 1990, and 1986.
ISBN-13: 978-0-323-72271-1

This translation of Cecil Essentials of Medicine, Tenth Edition by Edward J. Wing and Fred J. Schiffman was undertaken by Peking University Medical Press and is published by arrangement with Elsevier (Singapore) Pte Ltd.
Cecil Essentials of Medicine, Tenth Edition by Edward J. Wing and Fred J. Schiffman 由北京大学医学出版社进行翻译，并根据北京大学医学出版社与爱思唯尔（新加坡）私人有限公司的协议约定出版。

《希氏内科学精要（第 10 版） 第 3 分册 肾脏疾病（中英双语版）》（李雪梅 赵明辉 主译）
ISBN: 978-7-5659-3251-9
Copyright © 2024 by Elsevier (Singapore) Pte Ltd. and Peking University Medical Press.
All rights reserved. No part of this publication may be reproduced or transmitted in any form or by any means, electronic or mechanical, including photocopying, recording, or any information storage and retrieval system, without permission in writing from Elsevier (Singapore) Pte Ltd. and Peking University Medical Press.

注 意

本译审由北京大学医学出版社独立完成。相关从业及研究人员必须凭借其自身经验和知识对文中描述的信息数据、方法策略、搭配组合、实验操作进行评估和使用。由于医学科学发展迅速，临床诊断和给药剂量尤其需要经过独立验证。在法律允许的最大范围内，爱思唯尔、译文的原文作者、原文编辑及原文内容提供者均不对译文或因产品责任、疏忽或其他操作造成的人身及（或）财产伤害及（或）损失承担责任，亦不对由于使用文中提到的方法、产品、说明或思想而导致的人身及（或）财产伤害及（或）损失承担责任。

Published in China by Peking University Medical Press under special arrangement with Elsevier (Singapore) Pte Ltd. This edition is authorized for sale in the People's Republic of China only, excluding Hong Kong SAR, Macau SAR and Taiwan. Unauthorized export of this edition is a violation of the contract.

希氏内科学精要（第 10 版） 第 3 分册 肾脏疾病（中英双语版）

主　　译：李雪梅　赵明辉

出版发行：北京大学医学出版社

地　　址：（100191）北京市海淀区学院路 38 号　北京大学医学部院内

电　　话：发行部 010-82802230；图书邮购 010-82802495

网　　址：http://www.pumpress.com.cn

E - m a i l：booksale@bjmu.edu.cn

印　　刷：北京信彩瑞禾印刷厂

经　　销：新华书店

策划编辑：高　瑾

责任编辑：高　瑾　　责任校对：靳新强　　责任印制：李　啸

开　　本：889 mm×1194 mm　1/16　　印张：14　　字数：520 千字

版　　次：2024 年 11 月第 1 版　2024 年 11 月第 1 次印刷

书　　号：ISBN 978-7-5659-3251-9

定　　价：96.00 元

版权所有，违者必究

（凡属质量问题请与本社发行部联系退换）

中英双语版 编辑委员会

主任委员

王　辰

委　员（按姓氏笔画排序）

王　洁　　王伊龙　　王建祥　　巴　一　　代华平　　宁　光　　宁晓红　　朱　兰
任景怡　　刘海鹰　　李小鹰　　李梦涛　　李雪梅　　杨爱明　　张福杰　　郑金刚
房静远　　赵　晶　　赵明辉　　郝　伟　　姜　辉　　栗占国　　贾继东　　夏维波
黄　慧　　黄晓军　　曹　彬　　彭　斌　　潘　慧

第 1 分册　内科学概论・呼吸与危重症医学・术前和术后照护
　　　　　　主译　王　辰　代华平　赵　晶　黄　慧

第 2 分册　心血管疾病
　　　　　　主译　郑金刚　任景怡

第 3 分册　肾脏疾病
　　　　　　主译　李雪梅　赵明辉

第 4 分册　胃肠疾病・肝脏与胆道系统疾病
　　　　　　主译　房静远　杨爱明　贾继东

第 5 分册　血液疾病
　　　　　　主译　黄晓军　王建祥

第 6 分册　肿瘤疾病
　　　　　　主译　王　洁　巴　一

第 7 分册　内分泌疾病与代谢疾病・女性健康・男性健康・骨与骨矿物质代谢疾病
　　　　　　主译　宁　光　朱　兰　姜　辉　夏维波　潘　慧

第 8 分册　肌肉骨骼与结缔组织疾病
　　　　　　主译　栗占国　李梦涛

第 9 分册　感染性疾病
　　　　　　主译　刘海鹰　张福杰　曹　彬

第 10 分册　神经疾病・老年医学・缓和医疗・酒精和物质使用
　　　　　　主译　彭　斌　王伊龙　李小鹰　宁晓红　郝　伟

医学名词审定指导

任慧玲　　李晓瑛　　冀玉静　　张燕舞　　李军莲

中英双语版 序言

让我国医学生与国际医学生站在同一起跑线上的首要之事，是为其提供具有世界先进水平的标准教材。我们应争取使每一位医学生都能接触到内容经典、充分代表现代医学水平的国际权威原文教材并力求准确翻译，提供原文与中文双语对照版本，使医学生和医生在学习中形成双语医学词语、概念、概念间逻辑及由此构成的医学知识体系。在这样的思想驱动下，国际经典内科学教科书《希氏内科学精要（第10版）》中英双语版应运而生。

《希氏内科学》原著以其论述严谨准确、系统全面，被誉为"标准的内科学参考书"。自1927年首次出版以来，在内科学领域渐享世界级声誉，成为全球众多优秀医学院校，包括哈佛医学院、斯坦福大学医学院、约翰斯·霍普金斯大学医学院、牛津大学医学部、剑桥大学医学院、墨尔本大学医学院、新加坡国立大学医学院及多伦多大学医学院等普遍采用的内科学参考书。首版《希氏内科学精要》则诞生于1986年，旨在凝炼其全本的精华和要点，以最为简洁明确的方式向以医学生为主体的医学界精辟传达《希氏内科学》的核心信息，包括书中所体现出的人文精神。此后，每版精要本都力求凝炼地反映当时最新医学成果和医疗实践指南，愈来愈成为各国医学生、住院医师、专培医师及教师学习和传授内科学的主要教本，在世界医学教材体系中居引领地位。《希氏内科学》和《希氏内科学精要》两个版本不仅在英语国家被广泛使用，更被翻译为葡萄牙语、西班牙语、希腊语、意大利语、日语、简体中文版，为全球医学界广泛采用。

中国的医学生、住院医师、专培医师需要培养国际专业信息获取能力。将精要本原文引进并准确翻译，以中英文对照的形式呈现，便于读者进行双语对照阅读和学习，使之在学习理解国际标准医学内容的同时，学习好中英文医学词语，为国际医学交流打好基础。相信此举对于提高我国的医学教育水平，培养国际型医学人才至为有益。

《希氏内科学精要》精练地涵盖了内科学的所有主要领域，包括心血管疾病、呼吸疾病与危重症、消化疾病、肾脏疾病、内分泌和代谢疾病、风湿疾病、血液疾病、肿瘤、感染性疾病、神经与老年疾病等，构建了较为系统的知识体系。在翻译引进过程中，我们遵循将相关内容集中的原则，将原书按系统器官拆分为十个分册，使其更具有专科阅读的对应性，以更加灵活轻便的形式为读者提供多样化的阅读选择。

为确保译文质量，我们在译者遴选上采取了严谨的标准。从《希氏内科学（第26版）》翻译团队中择优选取责任心强、译文优质的译者，同时吸纳了临床医学专业"101"计划核心教材的编者团队。每个分册均由主译专家带领各自译者团队完成翻译、审校、交叉互审、通审四级审校工作。这些译者具备扎实的英语与专业能力，他们在翻译过程中，深入理解原文，准确阐述作者思想，并多角度审视译文的准确性、流畅性与风格一致性，确保译文的忠实性、规范性与可读性，在不同的语言和文化间架起坚实的桥梁。尤其值得称赞的是，对原著中疏漏或不够完善之处，译文中以"译者注"的形式加以适当解释和说明，使译文内容在忠实于原著的基础上更为准确。

　　本书读者定位于具有一定学习能力和基础的高等医学院校医学专业8年制、5年制学生以及相关医学专业人员，可作为医务人员的内科学参考书、住院医师规范化培训和专科医师规范化培训辅导教材、研究生入学考试辅导教材、内科学教师参考书、内科学各专科医师复习回顾其他专科知识的重要读本。

呼吸与危重症医学教授
中国医学科学院院长
北京协和医学院校长
2024年11月

对学习者教科书重要。

对学医者内科学重要。

世界上的内科学教科书，

首推《希氏内科学精要》。

中文是中国医生主要执业用语。

英文是国际医学交流的主要文字。

学习医学，当以双语对应阅读为好。

如此，可获纵横国际之效。

本书力求有助于此。

In Memoriam

Thomas E. Andreoli, MD

Dr. Thomas Andreoli, along with Drs. Lloyd Hollingsworth (Holly) Smith, Jr., Fred Plum, and Charles C.J. Carpenter, was one of the four founding editors of *Cecil Essentials of Medicine*. He served as editor for editions one through eight before he passed away on April 14, 2009. Dr. Andreoli was born in the Bronx, New York, in 1935, attended Catholic primary and high schools, and graduated from St. Vincent College and the Georgetown School of Medicine. He trained as a resident at Duke University under legendary Chair of Medicine Dr. Eugene Stead, who recognized him as a brilliant physician and scientist and encouraged his research career. Dr. Andreoli received his research training at the NIH and then in the laboratory of Dr. Tosteson at Duke. His research focused on the biochemical and biophysical properties of renal tubular cell membranes and their role in water and electrolyte transport. He made fundamental discoveries on the normal renal physiology, illuminating the way to subsequent work by many others on renal health and disease. His research was recognized with numerous awards and election to honorific societies both in the United States and in Europe. Dr. Andreoli also served as editor of *The American Journal of Physiology: Renal Physiology* and Editor in Chief of *Kidney International*.

Tom's national prominence and leadership qualities were recognized early in his career when he became head of Nephrology at the University of Alabama in Birmingham. There he helped faculty and trainees develop outstanding research, organized clinical services, and created a hemodialysis program to build one of the outstanding Divisions of Nephrology in the country. In 1979, Dr. Andreoli was appointed Chair of the Department of Internal Medicine at the University of Texas, Houston, where he assembled an outstanding faculty focused on research, clinical care, and teaching. In 1988, he accepted the position as Chairman of Internal Medicine at the University of Arkansas School of Medicine, a position he held until his death. There he again assembled a distinguished faculty who were outstanding researchers but also dedicated to outstanding clinical care and teaching. Morning report and clinical rounds with Dr. Andreoli were rigorous and riveting, focusing on the individual patient, not only their diagnoses and treatment but also on each patient's personal concerns and well-being. Dr. Andreoli was revered by medical students, his house staff, faculty, and colleagues, and I (EJW) personally can attest to what he regarded as his most cherished role—the mentorship and education of the next generation of physicians.

One of Dr. Andreoli's great interests was *Cecil Essentials of Medicine,* for which he was the editor/chief editor for eight of its ten editions, an interest that reflected his commitment to the education of students, house staff, and other physicians in the "essentials" of Internal Medicine.

Dr. Andreoli was devoted to his family. He was married to Elizabeth Berglund Andreoli from 1987 until his death. He was previously married to Dr. Kathleen Gainor Andreoli, mother of his three children and their ten grandchildren. Being of Italian ancestry and from Bronx, New York, it is not surprising that Dr. Andreoli was a passionate fan of the New York Yankees, Italian opera, which he could sing in Italian, and Frank Sinatra.

Dr. Andreoli's legacy lives on in his numerous previous students, house staff, colleagues, and in this book.

缅 怀

托马斯·安德里奥利博士

托马斯·安德里奥利（Thomas E. Andreoli）博士携手李奥德·霍灵斯沃斯·史密斯［Lloyd Hollingsworth（Holly）Smith］博士、弗雷德·普拉姆（Fred Plum）博士和查尔斯·卡彭特（Charles C.J. Carpenter）博士同为《希氏内科学精要》的创始编者。他在 2009 年 4 月 14 日去世前，曾担任该书第 1 至第 8 版的编者。安德里奥利博士于 1935 年出生于美国纽约布朗克斯区，就读于天主教小学和中学，后毕业于圣文森特学院和乔治城大学医学院。他在杜克大学医学院接受住院医师培训期间师从著名内科主任尤金·斯特德（Eugene Stead）博士，后者将其视为杰出的医生和科学家，并鼓励他投身科研事业。安德里奥利博士在美国国立卫生研究院接受科研训练后，前往杜克大学托斯特森（Tosteson）博士的实验室继续深造。他重点研究肾小管细胞膜的生化和生物物理特性及其在水和电解质转运中所发挥的作用。他在正常肾脏生理学方面的重要发现为后续关于肾脏健康和疾病的研究铺平了道路。安德里奥利博士的研究工作荣获多个学术奖项，并入选美国和欧洲的多个荣誉学会。他还担任《美国生理学杂志：肾脏生理学篇》（The American Journal of Physiology: Renal Physiology）的编辑以及《国际肾脏杂志》（Kidney International）的主编。

安德里奥利博士担任阿拉巴马大学伯明翰分校肾脏病学系主任后不久，即因其杰出领导力而赢得全美业内声誉。他帮助本校师生们取得科研突破，负责临床业务的组织实施，并因开创血液透析业务而使该科跻身全美顶级肾脏内科之列。1979 年，安德里奥利博士被任命为得克萨斯大学休斯敦分校内科系主任，他在该系组建了一支科研、临床诊疗和教学并重的优秀教职团队。自 1988 年起，他担任阿肯色大学医学院内科学系主任，直至辞世。在这里他再次组建了一支卓越的教职团队，他们不仅科研工作出色，临床诊疗和教学工作也出类拔萃。安德里奥利博士带领的晨会报告和查房非常严谨而引人入胜，不仅尽心竭力于每位患者的诊断和治疗，还关注到他们每个人的个体情况和福祉。安德里奥利博士深受医学生、住院医师、教职人员和同事的崇敬，我（EJW）可以证明，他最珍视的角色当属培养和教育下一代医生。

安德里奥利博士对《希氏内科学精要》倾注了满腔热忱，先后担任了该书 10 版中 8 版的编者/主编，践行他为医学生、住院医师和其他各科医生们传授内科学"精要"的承诺。

安德里奥利博士高度重视家庭。他与第二任妻子伊丽莎白·伯格兰德·安德里奥利（Elizabeth Berglund Andreoli）的婚姻从 1987 年延续到辞世。他与第一任妻子凯瑟琳·盖娜·安德里奥利（Kathleen Gainor Andreoli）博士育有三个子女和十个孙辈。作为意大利裔和纽约布朗克斯人，安德里奥利博士是纽约洋基队、意大利歌剧（他能用意大利语演唱）和美国著名歌手、演员、主持人弗兰克·辛纳屈（Frank Sinatra）的忠实拥趸。安德里奥利博士将永远被他的众多学生、住院医师和同事怀念，并因本书而流芳百世。

In Memoriam

Charles C.J. Carpenter, MD

Dr. Charles C.J. Carpenter joined Drs. Thomas Andreoli, Lloyd Hollingsworth Smith, Jr., and Fred Plum as a founder of *Cecil Essentials of Medicine*. He served as editor for seven editions and was followed in that role by Dr. Ivor Benjamin and then Dr. Edward Wing. Sadly, Chuck passed away on March 19, 2020, surrounded by his wife and children. He was Professor Emeritus of Medicine at The Warren Alpert Medical School of Brown University and Physician-in-Chief Emeritus at The Miriam Hospital.

Chuck was born in Savannah, Georgia, on January 5, 1931. He attended college at Princeton and medical school at Johns Hopkins where he also did his house staff training, including chief residency, and then joined the Johns Hopkins faculty. With his young family, he travelled to Calcutta, India, where he carried out landmark studies for the treatment of cholera.

Before coming to Brown in 1986, he was Chair of Medicine at Baltimore City Hospital and Case Western Reserve University.

His contributions to medical science and clinical care were many. While in Calcutta, using basic scientific evidence coupled with practical approaches, Dr. Carpenter developed "oral rehydration therapy" to address the cholera epidemic there. This treatment has saved millions of lives. While at Case, one of his innovations was to develop the nation's first Division of Geographic Medicine because of his strong belief that all physicians should be medical citizens of the world. In 1987, as he became deeply involved in the clinical management of persons living with HIV, he initiated a unique program in which Brown University faculty and trainees assumed responsibility for all HIV care in the Rhode Island State prison system.

Dr. Carpenter served as Chairman of the American Board of Internal Medicine and President of the Association of American Physicians. He has been a member of the NIH AIDS Executive Committee, the National Advisory Allergy and Infectious Diseases Council, and the USPHS AIDS Task Force. He was Chair of the Antiretroviral Treatment Panel of the International AIDS Society-USA and authored their recommendations on antiretroviral treatment. He also served as Chair of the Treatment Committee to evaluate the President's Emergency Plan for HIV/AIDS Relief. He became the director of the Brown University International Health Institute and the director of the Lifespan/Brown Center for AIDS Research with several Boston hospitals.

Throughout his career, Dr. Carpenter was the recipient of many international, national, and regional awards, accepting each with characteristic humility. With both small and large groups of learners, Chuck made certain that every member of his team was well educated, and each felt that they contributed to the well-being of their patients. His ability to sit calmly at the bedside, hold the patient's hand, comfort them, and listen in a genuinely focused way, influenced so many physicians. He was truly grateful for the opportunity to care for those less fortunate than he, and the feeling of being privileged to do so was clearly transmitted to all. Dr. Carpenter was a wonderful blend of profound compassion combined with the adherence to scholarship and teaching. Sir William Osler wrote that physicians should "Do the kind thing and do it first." Chuck lived by this precept. Vigor and insight characterized his approach to clinical and ethical challenges, always with younger colleagues at his side. In a recent tribute to him, many emphasized that Dr. Carpenter dedicated his life to his patients, many of whom were the most vulnerable members of society. We hope that we will have some of his strength and use his example as our compass as we are challenged to reduce suffering and improve the health of all for whom we are responsible.

He is survived by his wife of 61 years, Sally; three sons, Charles, Murray, and Andrew; and seven grandchildren.

缅 怀

查尔斯·卡彭特博士

查尔斯·卡彭特（Charles C.J. Carpenter）博士与 托马斯·安德里奥利（Thomas E. Andreoli）博士、李奥德·霍灵斯沃斯·史密斯（Lloyd Hollingsworth Smith）博士和弗雷德·普拉姆（Fred Plum）博士共同开创了《希氏内科学精要》。他共担任了 7 版的编者，嗣后由艾弗·本杰明（Ivor Benjamin）博士和爱德华·温（Edward Wing）博士接任。查尔斯·卡彭特博士于 2020 年 3 月 19 日在妻子和子女们的陪伴下辞世。他曾担任布朗大学沃伦·阿尔珀特医学院的内科学系名誉教授和米里亚姆医院的名誉主任医师。

查尔斯·卡彭特博士于 1931 年 1 月 5 日出生于美国佐治亚州萨凡纳市。他在普林斯顿大学获得学士学位后进入约翰斯·霍普金斯大学医学院，并完成了包括住院总医师在内的住院医师培训，随后加入了约翰斯·霍普金斯大学的教职团队。他曾携妻子和年幼的孩子前往印度加尔各答，在当地对霍乱的治疗进行了具有里程碑意义的研究工作。

在 1986 年入职布朗大学之前，他曾担任巴尔的摩市医院和凯斯西储大学医学院的内科学主任。

他在医学科学研究和临床诊疗领域建树颇多。在加尔各答期间，基于基础科学证据及临床实践，查尔斯·卡彭特博士开创了"口服补液疗法"以遏制当地的霍乱疫情。这一疗法拯救了数百万人的生命。秉承医生无国界的世界公民理念，他在凯斯西储大学做了一项开创性工作，建立了美国首个地缘医学部（研究地理环境因素对人体健康和疾病影响的学科）。1987 年，他深度参与人类免疫缺陷病毒（HIV）携带者的临床管理，并发起了一个独特的项目——由布朗大学教职团队和医学生们承担罗德岛州监狱系统内所有艾滋病相关诊疗工作。

查尔斯·卡彭特博士曾担任美国内科医师委员会主席和美国医师协会主席。他曾是美国国立卫生研究院艾滋病行政委员会、美国国家过敏与传染病咨询委员会以及公共卫生服务部艾滋病工作组的成员。他还曾担任国际艾滋病学会-美国分会抗逆转录病毒治疗组主席，并撰写了抗逆转录病毒治疗建议。他还担任过艾滋病治疗委员会主席，该委员会负责评估美国总统防治艾滋病紧急救援计划；曾担任布朗大学国际健康研究所所长，以及大学与多家波士顿当地医院合办的生命周期/布朗大学艾滋病研究中心主任。

查尔斯·卡彭特博士在职业生涯中获得过诸多国际性、全美和地区性奖项，同时展现其谦逊品格。无论学员人数多寡，查尔斯·卡彭特博士都会确保人人都能受到良好教育，并让他们感到自己也对患者的健康做出了贡献。他能够安静地坐在病床边，握住患者的手，安慰他们，并全神贯注地听取患者倾诉，这一举动深深地感染了许多医生。他十分珍视诊治不幸染病者的机会，并且能够将这种殊荣感传递给所有人。查尔斯·卡彭特博士完美地融汇了对患者的宅心仁厚与对学术和教学的坚守。威廉·奥斯勒（William Osler）爵士曾写道，医生应该"行善事，为人先"，而这正是查尔斯·卡彭特博士一生奉行的信条。他在面对临床和伦理挑战时充满活力和洞察力，始终重视提携年轻同事。许多人的悼词中都重点指出，查尔斯·卡彭特博士将毕生致力于患者福祉，其中许多人属于社会上最弱势群体。我们希望，在我们面临减少患者痛苦及改善其健康状况的挑战时，能够拥有他的力量，并以他为榜样获得指引。

查尔斯·卡彭特博士与妻子萨丽（Sally）共度了 61 年的婚姻时光，育有查尔斯（Charles）、穆雷（Murray）和安德鲁（Andrew）三子以及七个孙辈。

ABOUT THE EDITORS

Dr. Edward J. Wing was an editor of *Cecil Essentials of Medicine,* editions 8 and 9, and is the lead editor of edition 10. He graduated from Williams College in 1967 and from the Harvard Medical School in 1971. He was a resident in Internal Medicine at the Peter Bent Brigham and completed an Infectious Diseases Fellowship at Stanford University. Joining the faculty at the University of Pittsburgh in 1975, he focused his NIH-funded research on mechanisms of cell-mediated immunity as well as various clinical aspects of Infectious Diseases. From 1990 to 1998, the University and UPMC appointed him as Physician-in-Chief at Montefiore Hospital, then Chief of Infectious Diseases, and finally Interim Chair of Medicine.

In 1998, Dr. Wing became Chair of Medicine at Brown University (1998–2008) where he consolidated the department across hospitals, practice plans, and training programs. As Dean of Medicine and Biological Sciences at Brown University (2008–2013) he strengthened ties with affiliated hospitals (Lifespan and Care New England), increased research, and oversaw the construction of a new medical school building. International exchange programs with medical schools in Kenya, the Dominican Republic, and Haiti were established during his years as chairman and dean. Dr. Wing has cared for patients with HIV since the beginning of the epidemic in outpatient clinics. He continues to be active in research, clinical care, and teaching.

Dr. Fred J. Schiffman, who along with Dr. Edward Wing is editor of *Cecil Essentials of Medicine,* 10th edition, attended Wagner College and then the New York University School of Medicine, from which he graduated in 1973. He performed his early house staff training at Yale-New Haven Hospital and then spent two years at the National Cancer Institute. He returned to Yale as Chief Medical Resident followed by a hematology fellowship. He became Medical Director of Yale's Primary Care Center before coming to Brown University in 1983, where he has been a leader in the medical residency program as well as Associate Physician-in-Chief at The Miriam Hospital.

Dr. Schiffman holds The Sigal Family Professorship in Humanistic Medicine at The Warren Alpert Medical School of Brown University. His scholarly interests include the structure and function of the human spleen and the intersection of the arts and medical care. He has directed or championed many projects and programs, including those that encourage and reinforce wellness and resilience in patients, families, and caregivers. He began a novel program that places medical students and physicians with other nonmedical professionals as they share in the viewing of works of art in the Museum of the Rhode Island School of Design. Dr. Schiffman recently led a Brown University edX course entitled, "Artful Medicine: Art's Power to Enrich Patient Care," with worldwide participation. Dr. Schiffman has also edited texts on hematologic pathophysiology, consultative hematology, and the anemias.

原著主编

爱德华·温（Edward J. Wing）博士是《希氏内科学精要》第 8 版和第 9 版的编者，以及第 10 版的主编。他先后于 1967 年和 1971 年毕业于威廉姆斯学院和哈佛医学院。他曾在彼得·本特·布里格姆医院任内科住院医师，后在斯坦福大学完成了传染病学的专科医师（Fellowship）课程。自 1975 年加入匹兹堡大学医学院以来，他通过美国国立卫生研究院资助的研究项目，探索细胞介导免疫的机制以及传染病学各领域的临床诊疗工作。1990—1998 年期间，他先后被匹兹堡大学及其医学中心任命为蒙特菲奥里医院的主任医师、传染病科主任，后担任内科临聘主任。

1998 年起，温博士担任布朗大学医学院的内科主任（1998—2008 年）。在此期间，他在不同医院、实践计划和培训项目间对内科进行整合。在担任布朗大学医学与生物科学院院长（2008—2013 年）期间，他加强了与各附属医院（Lifespan 医院和 Care New England 医院）间的联系，提升了科研工作的水准，并为医学院建成了一座新楼。在担任主任和院长期间，他还建立了与肯尼亚、多米尼加共和国和海地的医学院的国际交流项目。温博士自艾滋病流行初期便在门诊诊治艾滋病患者，并始终工作在科研、临床和教学一线。

弗雷德·谢夫曼（Fred J. Schiffman）博士与爱德华·温（Edward Wing）博士共同担任《希氏内科学精要》第 10 版的主编。他就读于瓦格纳学院，随后进入纽约大学医学院，并于 1973 年毕业。他在耶鲁大学附属纽黑文医院接受早期住院医师培训，随后在美国国家癌症研究所工作了两年。回到耶鲁大学后，他担任住院总医师，然后完成了血液学专科医师课程，随后成为耶鲁初级保健中心医学主任。他于 1983 年入职布朗大学，领导医学住院医师项目并担任米里亚姆医院的副主任医师。

谢夫曼博士担任布朗大学沃伦·阿尔珀特医学院人文医学系的西格尔家庭医学教授。他的学术兴趣涵盖人体脾脏的结构和功能，以及艺术与医疗的交叉融合。他主持或参与了许多项目和计划，其中包括许多旨在鼓励和加强患者、家人和医护人员的福祉与康复能力的项目。他所创办的一个新项目可以让医学生和医生与其他非医学专业人士一起，共同欣赏罗德岛设计学院博物馆的艺术作品。谢夫曼博士近期还主持了布朗大学名为"艺术与医学：艺术赋能患者照护"的 edX 课程，此课程的参与者来自全球多个国家。谢夫曼博士还出版了有关血液病理生理学、血液科会诊和贫血的著作。

原著者名单

Jinnette Dawn Abbott, MD
Rajiv Agarwal, MD
Marwa Al-Badri, MD
Hyeon-Ju Ryoo Ali, MD
Jason M. Aliotta, MD
Khaldoun Almhanna, MD, MPH
Mohanad T. Al-Qaisi, MD
Zuhal Arzomand, MD
Akwi W. Asombang, MD, MPH
Su N. Aung, MD, MPH
Christopher G. Azzoli, MD
Christina Bandera, MD
Debasree Banerjee, MD
Mashal Batheja, MD
Jeffrey J. Bazarian, MD, MPH
Selim R. Benbadis, MD
Ivor J. Benjamin, MD, FAHA, FACC
Eric Benoit, MD
Marcie G. Berger, MD
Clemens Bergwitz, MD
Nancy Berliner, MD
Jeffrey S. Berns, MD
Pooja Bhadbhade, DO
Ratna Bhavaraju-Sanka, MD
Tanmayee Bichile, MD
Ariel E. Birnbaum, MD
Charles M. Bliss, Jr., MD
Andrew S. Blum, MD, PhD
Bryan J. Bonder, MD
Russell Bratman, MD
Glenn D. Braunstein, MD
Alma M. Guerrero Bready, MD
Richard Bungiro, PhD
Anna Marie Burgner, MD, MEHP
Jonathan Cahill, MD
Andrew Canakis, DO
Benedito A. Carneiro, MD, MS
Brian Casserly, MD
Abdullah Chahin, MD, MA, MSc
Philip A. Chan, MD
Kimberle Chapin, MD
William P. Cheshire, Jr., MD
Waihong Chung, MD, PhD
Emma Ciafaloni, MD

Joaquin E. Cigarroa, MD
Michael P. Cinquegrani, MD
Andreea Coca, MD, MPH
Harvey Jay Cohen, MD
Scott Cohen, MD, MPH
Beatrice P. Concepcion, MD, MS
Nathan T. Connell, MD, MPH
Maria Constantinou, MD
Roberto Cortez, MD
Timothy J. Counihan, MD, FRCPI
Anne Haney Cross, MD
Cheston B. Cunha, MD, FACP
Joanne S. Cunha, MD
Susan Cu-Uvin, MD
Noura M. Dabbouseh, MD
Kwame Dapaah-Afriyie, MD, MBA
Erin M. Denney-Koelsch, MD
Andre De Souza, MD
An S. De Vriese, MD, PhD
Neal D. Dharmadhikari, MD
Leah Dickstein, MD
Don Dizon, MD, FACP, FASCO
Robyn T. Domsic, MD, MPH
Kim A. Eagle, MD
Michael G. Earing, MD
Pamela Egan, MD
Wafik S. El-Deiry, MD, PhD, FACP
Mitchell S. V. Elkind, MD, MS
Tarra B. Evans, MD
Michael B. Fallon, MD
Dimitrios Farmakiotis, MD
Francis A. Farraye, MD
Ronan Farrell, MD
Panayotis Fasseas, MD, FACC
Mary Anne Fenton, MD
Fernando C. Fervenza, MD, PhD
Sean Fine, MD
Arkadiy Finn, MD
Timothy Flanigan, MD
Brisas M. Flores, MD
Andrew E. Foderaro, MD
Theodore C. Friedman, MD, PhD
Joseph Metmowlee Garland, MD, AAHIVM

Eric J. Gartman, MD
Abdallah Geara, MD
Raul Macias Gil, MD
Timothy Gilligan, MD, FASCO
Michael Raymond Goggins, MB BCh BAO, MRCPI
Geetha Gopalakrishnan, MD
Vidya Gopinath, MD
Susan L. Greenspan, MD, FACP
Osama Hamdy, MD, PhD
Johanna Hamel, MD
Sajeev Handa, MD, SFHM
Mitchell T. Heflin, MD, MHS
Robert G. Holloway, MD, MPH
Christopher S. Huang, MD
Zilla Hussain, MD
T. Alp Ikizler, MD
Iris Isufi, MD
Carlayne E. Jackson, MD
Paul G. Jacob, MD, MPH
Matthew D. Jankowich, MD
Niels V. Johnsen, MD, MPH
Jessica E. Johnson, MD
Rayford R. June, MD
Tareq Kheirbek, MD, ScM, FACS
Alok A. Khorana, MD, FACP, FASCO
Sena Kilic, MD
David Kim, MD
James Kleczka, MD
James R. Klinger, MD
Patrick Koo, MD, ScM
Pooja Koolwal, MD
Mary P. Kotlarczyk, PhD
Nicole M. Kuderer, MD
Awewura Kwara, MD
Jennifer M. Kwon, MD, MPH
Richard A. Lange, MD, MBA
Jerome Larkin, MD
Alfred I. Lee, MD, PhD
Daniel J. Levine, MD
David E. Lewandowski, MD
Kelly V. Liang, MD, MS
Kimberly P. Liang, MD, MS
David R. Lichtenstein, MD

扫描二维码了解更多信息

Douglas W. Lienesch, MD
Geoffrey S.F. Ling, MD, PhD
Ester Little, MD, FACP
Yi Liu, MD
Nicole L. Lohr, MD, PhD
John R. Lonks, MD, FACP, FIDSA, FSHEA
Gary H. Lyman, MD, MPH
Jeffrey M. Lyness, MD
Shane Lyons, MD, MRCPI, MRCP(UK)
Diana Maas, MD
Talha A. Malik, MD, MSPH
Sonia Manocha, MD
Susan Manzi, MD, MPH
Frederick J. Marshall, MD
F. Dennis McCool, MD
Russell J. McCulloh, MD
Kelly McGarry, MD, FACP
Eavan Mc Govern, MD, PhD
Robin L. McKinney, MD
Anthony Mega, MD
Shivang Mehta, MD
Douglas F. Milam, MD
Maria D. Mileno, MD
Abhinav Kumar Misra, MBBS, MD
Orson W. Moe, MD
Niveditha Mohan, MBBS
Larry W. Moreland, MD
Alan R. Morrison, MD, PhD
Steven F. Moss, MD
Christopher J. Mullin, MD, MHS
Sinéad M. Murphy, MB, BCh, MD, FRCPI
Sagarika Nallu, MD, FAAP, FAAN, FAASM
Javier A. Neyra, MD, MSCS
Ghaith Noaiseh, MD

Thomas A. Ollila, MD
Steven M. Opal, MD
Biff F. Palmer, MD
Jen Jung Pan, MD, PhD
Anna Papazoglou, MD
Aric Parnes, MD
Nayan M. Patel, DO, MPH
Ari Pelcovits, MD
Mark A. Perazella, MD
Michael F. Picco, MD, PhD
Kate E. Powers, DO
Laura A. Previll, MD, MPH
Nilum Rajora, MD
Adolfo Ramirez-Zamora, MD
John Reagan, MD
Rebecca Reece, MD
Harlan Rich, MD, AGAF, FACP
Jennifer H. Richman, MD
Lisa R. Rogers, DO
Ralph Rogers, MD
Michal G. Rose, MD
James A. Roth, MD
Sharon Rounds, MD
Jason C. Rubenstein, MD
Abbas Rupawala, MD
Jenna Sarvaideo, DO
Ramesh Saxena, MD, PhD
Fred J. Schiffman, MD, MACP
Ruth B. Schneider, MD
Kristin A. Seaborg, MD
Anil Seetharam, MD
Stuart Seropian, MD
Jigme Michael Sethi, MD
Sanjeev Sethi, MD, PhD
Elizabeth Shane, MD
Esseim Sharma, MD

Shani Shastri, MD, MPH
Barry S. Shea, MD
Lauren Shevell, MD, MPH
Joseph A. Smith, Jr., MD
Robert J. Smith, MD
Davendra P.S. Sohal, MD, MPH
Christopher Song, MD, FACC
Thomas Sperry, MD
Jeffrey M. Statland, MD
Emily M. Stein, MD
Jennifer L. Strande, MD, PhD
Rochelle Strenger, MD
Thomas R. Talbot, MD, MPH
Christopher G. Tarolli, MD, MSEd
Yael Tarshish, MD
Pushpak Taunk, MD
Philip Tsoukas, MD
Allan R. Tunkel, MD, PhD
Jeffrey M. Turner, MD
Zoe G.S. Vazquez, MD
Stacie A. F. Vela, MD
Paul M. Vespa, MD, FCCM, FAAN, FANA, FNCS
Wanpen Vongpatanasin, MD
Marcella D. Walker, MD
Eunice S. Wang, MD
Sharmeel K. Wasan, MD
Thomas J. Weber, MD
Brandon J. Wilcoxson, MD
Edward J. Wing, MD, FACP, FIDSA
Ellice Wong, MD
John J. Wysolmerski, MD
Rayan Yousefzai, MD
Thomas R. Ziegler, MD
Rebecca Zon, MD

ACKNOWLEDGMENTS

Dr. Schiffman and I wish to thank first of all, the authors of the 128 chapters that make up the tenth edition of *Cecil Essentials of Medicine.* They have worked diligently to compose the material for each chapter and apply their mastery as they added the newest information, in clear language, to the text. Their efforts are apparent in the excellence of the book, and we are immensely grateful for their work. We wish to also thank Marybeth Thiel, Jennifer Ehlers, and Dan Fitzgerald from Elsevier who guided and supported our work as editors and whose expertise has made this volume possible. Finally, we are always thankful to our wives, Dr. Rena Wing and Ms. Gerri Schiffman, without whose love, support, and especially humor, this book would not have happened.

致 谢

谢夫曼博士和我首先要致谢《希氏内科学精要》第 10 版全书 128 章的各位作者。感谢他们精益求精地撰写每一章节，并运用其专业知识，以简明的语言将前沿资讯呈现在书中。正是他们的辛勤努力确保了本书的卓越地位，对他们唯有由衷的感激。我们还要感谢爱思唯尔出版集团的玛丽贝丝·蒂尔（Marybeth Thiel）、詹妮弗·埃勒斯（Jennifer Ehlers）和丹·菲茨杰拉德（Dan Fitzgerald），他们对本书的编辑工作给予了指导和支持，其专业水准保障了本书的完稿。最后，要特别感谢我们的妻子——蕾娜·温（Rena Wing）博士和盖瑞·谢夫曼（Gerri Schiffman）女士，对她们的爱和支持，特别是积极乐观的心态始终心存感激，她们为本书的圆满完成发挥了不可或缺的作用。

总目录

第 1 分册

第 1 篇　内科学概论　Introduction to Medicine
第 2 篇　呼吸与危重症医学　Pulmonary and Critical Care Medicine
第 3 篇　术前和术后照护　Preoperative and Postoperative Care

第 2 分册

心血管疾病　Cardiovascular Disease

第 3 分册

肾脏疾病　Renal Disease

第 4 分册

第 1 篇　胃肠疾病　Gastrointestinal Disease
第 2 篇　肝脏与胆道系统疾病　Diseases of the Liver and Biliary System

第 5 分册

血液疾病　Hematologic Disease

第 6 分册

肿瘤疾病　Oncologic Disease

第 7 分册

第 1 篇　内分泌疾病与代谢疾病　Endocrine Disease and Metabolic Disease
第 2 篇　女性健康　Women's Health
第 3 篇　男性健康　Men's Health
第 4 篇　骨与骨矿物质代谢疾病　Diseases of Bone and Bone Mineral Metabolism

第 8 分册

肌肉骨骼与结缔组织疾病　Musculoskeletal and Connective Tissue Disease

第 9 分册

感染性疾病　Infectious Disease

第 10 分册

第 1 篇　神经疾病　Neurologic Disease
第 2 篇　老年医学　Geriatrics
第 3 篇　缓和医疗　Palliative Care
第 4 篇　酒精和物质使用　Alcohol and Substance Use

第 3 分册

肾脏疾病

第3分册译者名单

主　译

李雪梅　赵明辉

译　者（按姓氏笔画排序）

马　杰　中国医学科学院北京协和医院	郑　华　中国医学科学院北京协和医院
王　玉　北京大学第一医院	赵明辉　北京大学第一医院
叶文玲　中国医学科学院北京协和医院	秦　岩　中国医学科学院北京协和医院
刘立军　北京大学第一医院	黄　婧　北京大学第一医院
李明喜　中国医学科学院北京协和医院	崔　昭　北京大学第一医院
李雪梅　中国医学科学院北京协和医院	樊晓红　中国医学科学院北京协和医院
张　宏　北京大学第一医院	滕　菲　中国医学科学院北京协和医院
郑　可　中国医学科学院北京协和医院	

第 3 分册目录

肾脏疾病　Renal Disease

1. Renal Structure and Function, 4
   肾脏结构与功能，5

2. Approach to the Patient With Renal Disease, 18
   肾脏疾病患者的接诊，19

3. Fluid and Electrolyte Disorders, 38
   水和电解质紊乱，39

4. Glomerular Diseases, 66
   肾小球疾病，67

5. Major Nonglomerular Disorders of the Kidney, 98
   常见的非肾小球肾脏疾病，99

6. Vascular Disorders of the Kidney, 126
   肾脏血管疾病，127

7. Acute Kidney Injury, 150
   急性肾损伤，151

8. Chronic Kidney Disease, 170
   慢性肾脏病，171

索引 Index，186

CECIL ESSENTIALS OF MEDICINE

Renal Disease

Renal Disease

1. Renal Structure and Function, 4
2. Approach to the Patient With Renal Disease, 18
3. Fluid and Electrolyte Disorders, 38
4. Glomerular Diseases, 66
5. Major Nonglomerular Disorders of the Kidney, 98
6. Vascular Disorders of the Kidney, 126
7. Acute Kidney Injury, 150
8. Chronic Kidney Disease, 170

肾脏疾病

1 肾脏结构与功能，5

2 肾脏疾病患者的接诊，19

3 水和电解质紊乱，39

4 肾小球疾病，67

5 常见的非肾小球肾脏疾病，99

6 肾脏血管疾病，127

7 急性肾损伤，151

8 慢性肾脏病，171

Renal Structure and Function

Orson W. Moe, Javier A. Neyra

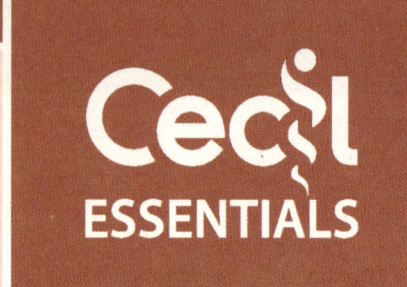

INTRODUCTION

The kidney maintains the composition and quantity of body fluids, and kidney failure is manifested by dysfunction of multiple organs. Chronic kidney disease is approaching epidemic proportions worldwide, and acute kidney injury affects a very high percentage of hospital admissions and ambulatory patients, with high rates of morbidity and mortality. The etiologies of these conditions are very diverse and often geographically specific. In addition to loss of glomerular filtration and tubular function, kidney diseases include hypertension, urolithiasis, and a host of electrolyte disorders that do not affect the glomerular filtration rate (GFR) but nonetheless cause significant morbidity and mortality. To understand these conditions, a thorough knowledge of the anatomy and function of the kidney is requisite.

Approximately 25% of the cardiac output is distributed to the kidneys, where the blood is continuously cleansed of toxins. In addition to excretion, the kidney is an important metabolic organ and a source of endocrine molecules. Renal failure represents a disruption of all of these functions. Selected aspects of renal structure and function are reviewed briefly in this chapter to set the foundation for the subsequent chapters that deal with specific renal diseases.

RENAL STRUCTURE

Macroscopic Anatomy

The kidneys are seated against the posterior wall of the abdomen in the retroperitoneal space, rendering them readily accessible for percutaneous biopsy. The lower poles may be palpable on deep inspiration in a lean individual. Each human kidney weighs about 120 to 170 g; is about 11 cm long, 6 cm wide, and 3 cm thick; and is endowed with approximately 1 million nephrons with interindividual variations. The "kidney size" commonly referred to in clinical sonographic reports is actually the cephalocaudal renal length, which is not an accurate surrogate for renal volume and mass and may be influenced by patients' body habitus. Despite this caveat, renal length is an acceptable clinical surrogate of renal volume.

The kidney is surrounded by a fibrous capsule (anteriorly, Gerota fascia and posteriorly, fascia retro renalis). The renal arteries enter the kidney and the renal vein and ureters leave the kidney in the renal pelvis. The bisected surface consists of the lighter-colored outer *cortex* and the darker inner *medulla* (Fig. 1.1A). A sample from a clinical biopsy typically originates from the cortex in the lower pole. The medulla is divided into outer and inner regions, and the outer medulla is subdivided into outer and inner stripes. The medulla has multiple conical contours, called *pyramids*, with their apices abutting on the renal pelvis as papillae. The contact points of the renal pelvis with the renal papillae are cup-like structures called *calyces*. Interpolated between the pyramids are centripetal extensions of cortical tissue called *columns of Bertin* (see Fig. 1.1A).

Renal Circulation

Each kidney receives blood from a single renal artery, although supernumerary arteries are present in up to one third of individuals. Just before or after the renal artery enters the kidney, it divides into interlobar arteries that pass between the pyramids of the kidney radially up the columns of Bertin (see Fig. 1.1A). The interlobar arteries further divide into arcuate arteries, which arch along the corticomedullary junction (see Fig. 1.1B). Arcuate arteries give rise to cortical ascending arteries, which bring blood to the glomeruli. Afferent arterioles ramify into glomerular capillaries, distributing blood to individual glomeruli. Features of the renal circulation are summarized in Table 1.1.

The glomerular capillary is the site for glomerular ultrafiltration. Even though the efferent arteriole is downstream from the glomerular capillary, it is not a venule because it has arteriolar walls and is upstream of the second capillary system surrounding the tubules. The peritubular capillaries provide oxygen and nutrients for the kidney, collect the fluid and solutes reabsorbed by tubules to return into the circulation, and deliver the solutes to be secreted by tubule into the tubule fluid. The peritubular capillaries surrounding the cortical and juxtamedullary nephrons originate from the efferent arterioles of cortical and juxtamedullary glomeruli, respectively. In certain pathologic settings, peritubular capillary flow or integrity can be disrupted, decreasing oxygenation and promoting ischemic injury.

The vessels that run parallel to loops of Henle are called *vasa recta* (see Fig. 1.1D) because of their long, straight structures. Blood from the peritubular capillaries is returned to the circulation by a venous system that mirrors the architectural structure of the arterial supply: interlobular vein, arcuate vein, interlobar vein, and renal vein. The parallel countercurrent nature of the vasculature provides the basis for the very high medullar tonicity, which allows urine concentration but also direct arteriovenous diffusion of oxygen, giving rise to the very low oxygen tension in the medulla. This low oxygen tension renders the kidney prone to ischemic injury, which is one of the most common causes of acute kidney injury (see Chapter 7).

Renal Nerves

The capsules of the kidney and the ureters have pain fibers derived from splanchnic nerves. This explains the costovertebral angle pain that occurs when the kidneys are inflamed and during renal colic during kidney stone passage. The renal parenchyma does not have pain fibers but is richly innervated with sympathetic nerves that enter the renal parenchyma with the renal artery. The sympathetic nerves

肾脏结构与功能

赵明辉 译 王玉 叶文玲 审校 赵明辉 通审

引言

肾脏负责维持机体体液的成分和量。肾衰竭表现为多个器官的功能异常。慢性肾脏病在全球范围内已接近流行病的程度，急性肾损伤可影响很高比例的住院和非住院患者，发病率和死亡率高。这些疾病病因多种多样，经常有地域特异性。除了肾小球滤过功能和肾小管功能丧失外，肾脏疾病还包括高血压、尿路结石和一系列电解质紊乱，虽不影响肾小球滤过率（GFR），但发病率和死亡率较高。要了解这些肾脏疾病，就必须全面掌握肾脏解剖和功能的知识。

大约25%的心输出量被分配给肾脏，以持续清除血液内的毒素。除了排泄功能，肾脏还是重要的代谢和内分泌器官。肾衰竭意味着所有这些功能的破坏。本章对主要肾脏结构和功能进行简要回顾，为随后肾脏疾病个论章节的介绍奠定基础。

肾脏结构

大体解剖

肾脏位于腹膜后间隙内，紧靠腹部后壁，便于经皮活检。消瘦的人深吸气时可触及肾下极。每个肾脏重约120～170 g，长11 cm，宽6 cm，厚3 cm；每个肾脏约有1百万个肾单位，有一定个体间差异。临床超声图像报告中通常提到的"肾脏大小"其实是肾脏头尾的长度，并非肾脏体积和质量的准确的替代指标，且可能受患者体型的影响。虽然有上述不足，肾脏长度仍是临床可接受的肾脏体积的替代指标。

肾脏由一层纤维囊包裹（前面称杰氏筋膜，后面称肾后筋膜）。肾动脉由肾盂处进入肾脏，而肾静脉和输尿管由肾盂处离开肾脏。肾脏纵切面上可见到外层浅颜色的皮质和内层深颜色的髓质（图1.1A）。临床肾活检的样本一般取自肾下极的皮质。髓质分为外髓和内髓，外髓又分为外条带区和内条带区。肾髓质有多个圆锥形结构，称为肾锥体，其顶端与肾盂相接称为肾乳头。肾盂和肾乳头连接处的杯状结构称为肾盏。肾锥体之间穿插的向心延伸的肾皮质组织称作肾柱（见图1.1A）。

肾脏循环

虽然有1/3的人存在不止一根肾动脉，多数人每个肾脏只有一根肾动脉接收血液。肾动脉在将要进入肾脏前或刚进入肾脏后就分成叶间动脉，穿行于肾锥体之间向上辐射到肾柱（图1.1A）。叶间动脉进一步分为弓状动脉，呈拱形走行于皮髓交界部（图1.1B）。弓状动脉分出皮质升支动脉（小叶间动脉），把血液带到肾小球。入球小动脉分支进入肾小球毛细血管，把血液供应给每个肾小球。肾脏循环的特点总结于表1.1。

肾小球毛细血管是肾小球完成滤过的部位。虽然出球小动脉位于肾小球毛细血管的下游，但它并不是小静脉，有动脉壁，并且是肾小管管周二级毛细血管网的上游。肾小管管周毛细血管为肾脏提供氧气和营养物质，收集肾小管重吸收的液体和溶质使其返回血循环，并将由肾小管分泌的溶质递送到肾小管腔。围绕皮质肾单位和髓旁肾单位的肾小管管周毛细血管分别源于皮质肾小球和髓旁肾小球的出球小动脉。在一些病理情况下，肾小管管周毛细血管的血流或完整性受损，可导致缺氧，促进缺血性损伤。

与亨利袢伴行的血管因其长、直的结构特点被称为直小血管（图1.1D）。血液从肾小管管周毛细血管回到血液循环经过的静脉系统与肾脏动脉血供结构形成镜像关系：小叶间静脉、弓状静脉、叶间静脉和肾静脉。这种血管结构的平行逆流特性为髓质的高张力提供了基础，既利于尿液浓缩，还允许氧气直接通过动静脉弥散，使肾髓质的氧气张力极低。这种低氧气张力使肾脏容易发生缺血损伤，是急性肾损伤最常见的原因之一（第7章）。

肾脏神经

肾被膜和输尿管的痛觉神经源于脾神经。这解释了肾脏炎症时的肋脊角痛以及肾结石排石时的肾绞痛。肾实质没有痛性神经纤维，但有丰富的交感神经随着肾动脉进入肾实质。交感神经毗邻肾小动脉

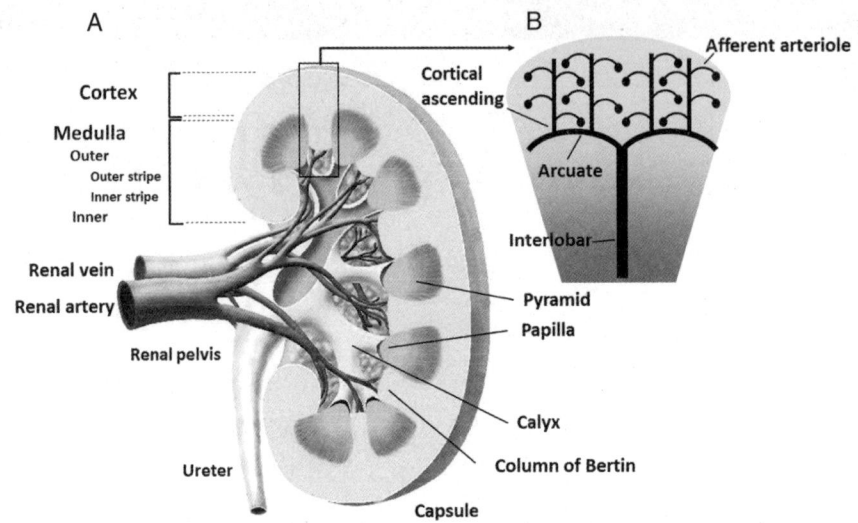

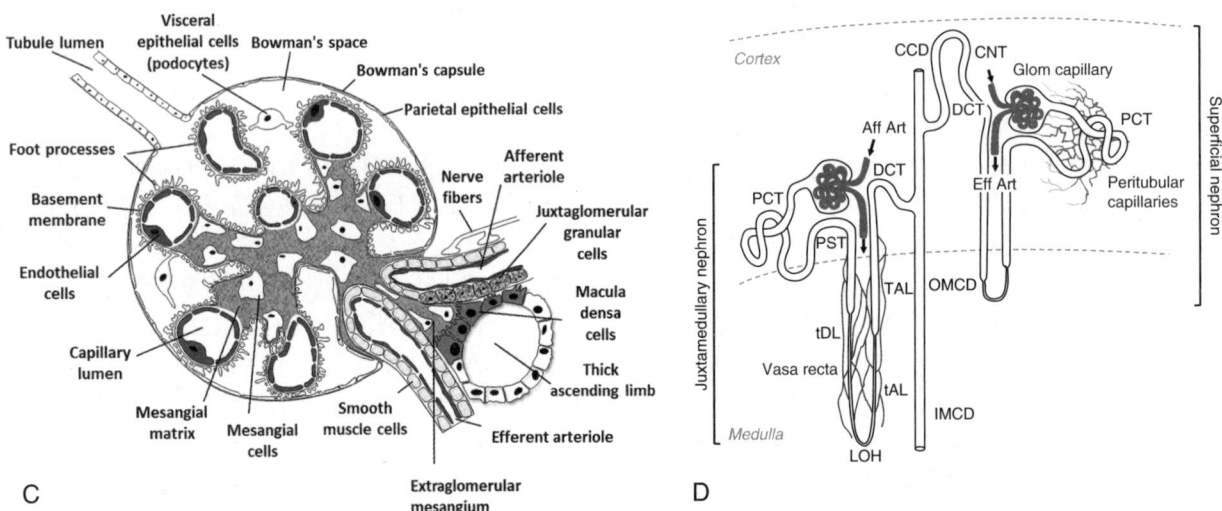

Fig. 1.1 (A) Gross anatomy of the kidney. (B) Schematic representation of the vasculature within a column of Bertin. (C) Structural components of the glomerulus. (D) Schematic representation of a superficial and a juxtamedullary nephron based on the location of their glomeruli. The tubules are intimately intertwined with the capillary system. The peritubular capillaries come off the efferent arteriole leaving the glomerular capillary. The capillaries that bathe the long descending and ascending limbs of the Henle loop are called the vasa recta due to their straight nature. The tubular segments are named axially: *CCD*, Cortical collecting duct; *CNT*, connecting tubule; *DCT*, distal convoluted tubule; *IMCD*, inner medullary collecting duct; *LOH*, loop of Henle; *OMCD*, outer medullary collecting duct; *PCT*, proximal convoluted tubule; *PST*, proximal straight tubule; *TAL*, thick ascending limb; *tAL*, thin ascending limb; *tDL*, thin descending limb.

TABLE 1.1 Characteristics of the Renal Circulation

Feature	Implications
Few or no anastomoses	Very prone to regional disruption of blood supply
Among the highest blood flow rates per gram of tissue	Lowest oxygen extraction (lowest arteriovenous O_2 difference)
Functional arteriovenous shunts	Solutes and gases (e.g., O_2) can diffuse directly from artery to vein without passing through capillaries
Two capillary systems in tandem	The two capillaries serve completely different functions, in the glomeruli and tubules in sequence

abut on the arterioles (see Fig. 1.1 C), stimulate renin release, decrease renal blood flow, and promote renal retention of sodium (Na^+). Renal sympathetic denervation has been proposed as a novel treatment of resistant hypertension using radiofrequency energy delivered via an intrarenal arterial catheter radially to disrupt the nerve fibers on the renal artery, but thus far the data have not been conclusive.

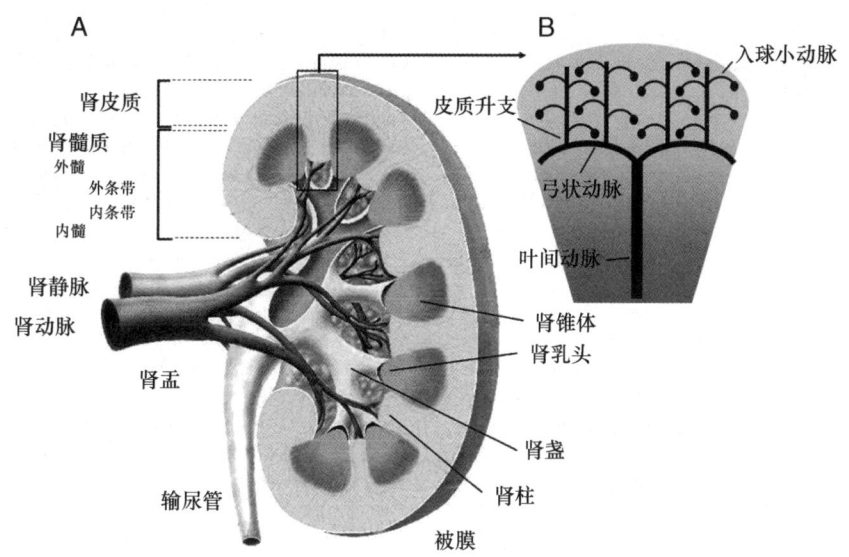

图 1.1 （A）肾脏大体解剖结构。（B）肾柱内血管结构模式图。（C）肾小球结构。（D）浅表肾单位和髓旁肾单位的模式图。肾小管与毛细血管系统紧密交织在一起。管周毛细血管源自出球小动脉。环绕在亨利袢长降支和升支的毛细血管因其笔直的性质而被称为直小血管。肾小管的节段按轴向命名；CCD，皮质集合管；CNT，连接小管；DCT，远曲小管；IMCD，近髓集合管；LOH，亨利袢；OMCD，外髓集合管；PCT，近曲小管；PST，近直小管；TAL，升支粗段；tAL，升支细段；tDL，降支细段

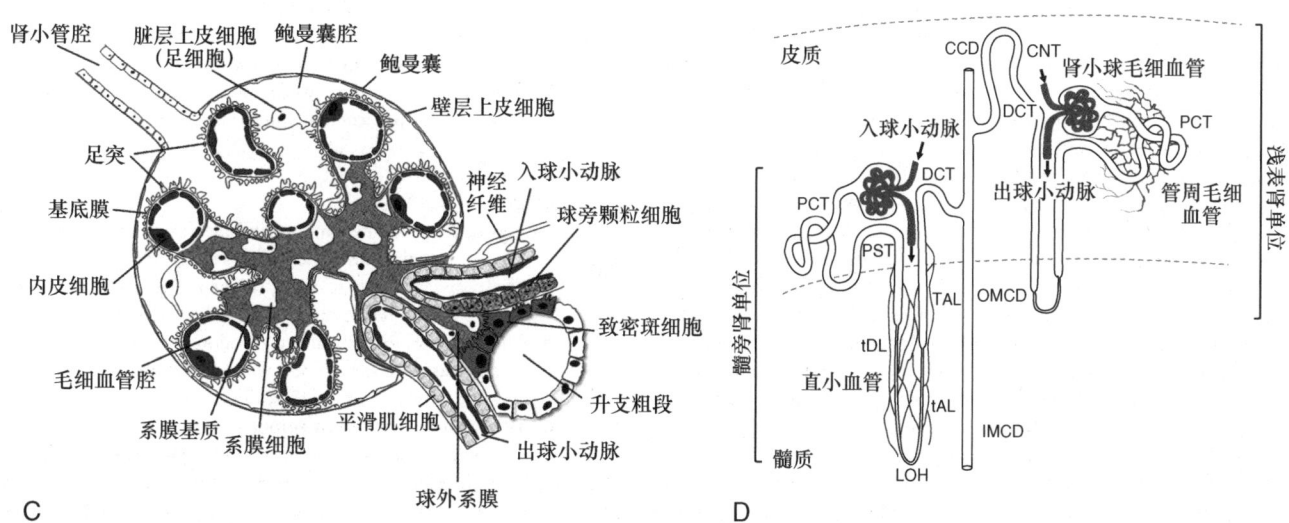

表 1.1	肾脏循环的特点
特点	意义
很少或没有交通支	易出现区域性血液供应中断
每克组织血流率最高	最低的氧气摄取率（最低的动静脉氧气差）
功能性动静脉分流	溶质和气体（例如 O_2）可以直接从动脉扩散到静脉，无需通过毛细血管
两个串联的毛细血管系统	两种毛细血管依次在肾小球和肾小管中发挥完全不同的功能

（图 1.1C），可以刺激肾素分泌，减少肾血流量，促进钠潴留。肾交感神经去除术通过肾动脉导管的射频能量消融破坏肾动脉的交感神经，被视为治疗难治性高血压的新方法，但迄今为止，数据尚无定论。

Walk the Nephron

The functional unit of the kidney is the nephron. Each human kidney has approximately 1 million nephrons. Approximately 30% of these have their glomeruli situated deep in the cortex and are referred to as *juxtamedullary nephrons*; the rest are in the outer cortex and are referred to as *superficial nephrons*. Each nephron is a glomerulus followed by a tubule that ends in the renal pelvis. The surrounding capillaries and the interstitial space are important functional components of the nephron.

Glomerulus

The glomerulus consists of the glomerular vasculature (arterioles and capillaries) supported by the mesangium (mesangial cells and matrix) inside Bowman's capsule (parietal and visceral epithelial cells) (see Fig. 1.1 C). The visceral cells of Bowman's capsule are the podocytes, so named because of their numerous "foot processes." The smooth muscle layers of the afferent and efferent arterioles are critical in determining arteriolar tone. The glomerular capillary contacts the mesangium on one side and is separated from the foot processes of the podocytes on the opposite side by the glomerular basement membrane (GBM). The glomerulus filters large volumes of water and small solutes while retaining most of the proteins and all of the cells in the blood. The glomerular filtration barrier is a tripartite structure composed of the capillary endothelium, the GBM, and the podocyte slit diaphragm.

Lining the inside of the GBM is a single layer of fenestrated endothelial cells. The fenestrations (50 to 100 nm in diameter) provide a barrier to negatively charged large molecules in the blood. The GBM contains laminin, type IV collagen, entactin (nidogen), and proteoglycans that restrict movement of large molecules (e.g., albumin) from the capillary into Bowman's space. The GBM contains dense negative charges due to glycoproteins with sialic acid residues that restrict the passage of anionic plasma solutes. It can be the site of deposition of immunocomplexes that cause glomerulonephritis (e.g., membranous glomerulonephritis, membranoproliferative glomerulonephritis, lupus nephritis). Autoantibodies against the GBM cause severe inflammation and loss of filtration. Autoantibodies against a podocyte membrane glycoprotein (M-type phospholipase A2 receptor, PLA2R) can cause antibody-mediated primary membranous nephropathy. The epithelial layer consists of podocytes and the parietal epithelium, which is flat and squamous with few organelles. At the vascular pole, the parietal epithelium is contiguous with a completely different epithelium—the proximal convoluted tubule.

On the visceral side of Bowman's space are the podocytes, which constitute part of the filtration barrier. These cells have a highly interdigitating system of foot processes that rest against the basement membrane. The podocyte cell bodies lie within the extracellular matrix. The spaces between foot processes are filtration slits of approximately 40 nm in diameter bridged by slit diaphragms, which are also negatively charged, contributing to the containment of middle-size negatively charged particles in the capillary. In the last decade, there have been momentous advances in identifying the components of the slit diaphragm complex and understanding their functions. A full discussion is not possible here, but major slit diaphragm–associated proteins include nephrin, podocin, neph-1/2/3, FAT-1, R-cadherin, catenin, CD2AP, ZO-1, and α-actinin 4. Mutations of many of these genes cause congenital proteinuric kidney disease (see Chapter 4).

Tubules

The parietal epithelium of Bowman's capsule becomes the renal tubule (see Fig. 1.1 D) as it leaves the glomerulus. The renal tubule is a prototypical polarized epithelium. Its salient characteristics are summarized in Fig. 1.2. A simple cylinder would not suffice in terms of surface area for transport. In the luminal apical membrane, surface amplification is achieved either by protrusions or by a more extensive form of protrusions called the *brush border* in the proximal tubule. Between cells are structures called *tight junctions*. Although they are called tight junctions, some are truly tight (with high resistance to solute and charge movement), whereas others are quite leaky to solutes. In addition to resistance, these complexes also regulate whether the junction is more permeable to one ion type compared with another selective permeability. On the other side of the tight junction is the intercellular space, which is contiguous with the interstitial space. The basolateral cell membrane on the interstitial-capillary side amplifies its surface area by infoldings into the cell and interdigitations between two cells.

The movement of a solute can be through a cell (transcellular transport) or around the cell (paracellular transport) (see Fig. 1.2A). Solute transport is an energy-consuming process that requires metabolic fuels. There are many kinds of transport proteins (see Fig. 1.2B). ATPases directly couple hydrolysis of adenosine triphosphate (ATP) to transport. Cotransporters (or symporters) move two solutes in the same direction, and countertransporters (antiporters) move two different solutes in opposite directions. Channels function as protein-lined "holes" that allows specific solutes to permeate. Different transporters can also be coupled together to form a new transport system. Finally, there are proteins that protrude outside the cell in the junctional area to provide a conduit for paracellular transport.

Specialized Structures
Interstitium

The space between the tubules and peritubular capillaries constitutes about 5% to 10% of renal volume and harbors interstitial fibroblasts and dendritic cells. In diseases such as interstitial nephritis (see Chapter 5), the interstitium is full of inflammatory cells, which elaborate cytokines and chemokines that profoundly affect filtration and tubular function. The resident fibroblasts are stellate cells with projections that physically contact tubules and capillaries, provide scaffold support, and secrete and maintain matrix. These cells, when stimulated by cytokines, can transform into myofibroblasts and contribute to interstitial fibrosis, a common pathobiologic feature of kidney disease. Some specialized fibroblasts in the deep cortex are sensors of oxygen and producers of circulating erythropoietin. The dendritic cells are antigen-presenting cells that express major histocompatibility complex (MHC) class II molecules. They are in intimate communication with the renal parenchyma, constantly sampling and responding to the local antigenic environment. Dendritic cells are involved with innate and adaptive immunity and are major players in immunologic homeostasis and diseases of the renal parenchyma.

Juxtaglomerular Apparatus

A unique feature of the nephron is that each thick ascending limb traverses back to and engages in physical contact with its parent glomerulus. The tubular cell at the point of contact is different from the rest of the thick ascending limb and is called the *macula densa*. The tripartite structure comprising the macula densa, the afferent and efferent glomerular arterioles, and the extraglomerular mesangium, a special part of the mesangium that protrudes outside the glomerulus, is called the *juxtaglomerular apparatus* (JGA) (see Fig. 1.1 C). The JGA is an important structure in the maintenance of GFR by tubuloglomerular feedback and regulation of afferent arteriole resistance and is the site of endocrine renin production.

Organelles Such as Mitochondria and Endoplasmic Reticulum

The kidney is second to the heart in mitochondrial content and oxygen consumption per unit mass. In addition to their role as the

肾单位

肾单位是肾脏的功能单元。人类每个肾脏约有100万个肾单位。约30%的肾单位因其肾小球位于皮质深部，称为髓旁肾单位，其余肾单位则位于皮质外带，称为表浅肾单位。每个肾单位由一个肾小球和后接的肾小管组成，肾小管末端终止于肾盂。环绕的毛细血管和肾间质也是肾单位重要的功能组成部分。

肾小球

肾小球由肾小球血管结构（微小动脉和毛细血管）组成，在鲍曼囊（壁层上皮细胞和脏层上皮细胞）内，由系膜（系膜细胞和基质）支撑（图1.1C）。鲍曼囊（肾小囊）的脏层细胞因有大量的足突被称为足细胞。入球小动脉和出球小动脉的平滑肌层对决定小动脉张力至关重要。肾小球毛细血管一侧与系膜相接，另一侧则通过肾小球基底膜（GBM）与足细胞的足突相连。肾小球可以滤过大量的水和小分子溶质，而阻留血液中绝大多数蛋白质和所有的细胞。肾小球的滤过屏障由三层结构组成，即毛细血管内皮细胞、GBM和足细胞的裂隙膜。

沿GBM内侧分布的是一层带窗孔的内皮细胞。这些直径50～100 nm的窗孔是血液中带负电荷的大分子的滤过屏障。GBM包含层粘连蛋白、Ⅳ型胶原、巢蛋白和蛋白聚糖，限制大分子（如白蛋白）从毛细血管进入鲍曼囊。由于蛋白聚糖带有唾液酸残基使GBM带有密集的负电荷，从而限制了带阴离子的血浆溶质通过。引起肾小球肾炎（如膜性肾病、膜增生性肾小球肾炎、狼疮性肾炎）的免疫复合物可以沉积在GBM。针对GBM的自身抗体可引起严重的炎症反应并造成肾小球滤过功能丧失。针对足细胞膜上糖蛋白（M型磷脂酶A2受体，PLA2R）的自身抗体可以引起抗体介导的原发性膜性肾病。上皮层包括足细胞和壁层上皮细胞，壁层上皮细胞呈扁平鳞状且细胞器很少。壁层上皮在尿极［译者注：原文（血管极）错误］与一种完全不同的上皮-近曲肾小管相接。

在鲍曼囊脏层侧的是足细胞，组成滤过屏障的一部分。足细胞的足突高度交织，覆盖在基底膜上。足细胞胞体处于细胞外基质中。足突之间的滤过间隙直径约40 nm，由带负电荷的裂隙膜桥接，限制中等大小带负电荷的颗粒由毛细血管滤出。近十年来，在确定裂隙膜组成及功能方面取得了巨大进展。这里虽不能进行详述，但主要裂隙膜相关蛋白包括肾病蛋白（nephrin）、足突蛋白（podocin）、neph-1/2/3、FAT-1、R-钙黏蛋白（cadherin）、连环蛋白（catenin）、CD2AP、ZO-1和α-肌动蛋白（actinin）4。其中许多基因的突变可引起表现为蛋白尿的先天性肾脏疾病（第4章）。

肾小管

鲍曼囊的壁层上皮在离开肾小球时成为肾小管（图1.1D）。肾小管上皮是一种典型的极化上皮。其突出的特点总结于图1.2。对于转运而言，一个简单的圆柱体的表面积是不够的。在肾小管腔面侧，通过表面凸起或更广泛的凸起形成刷状缘（近曲小管）来放大表面积。细胞间是被称作紧密连接的结构。虽被称为紧密连接，部分也确实紧密（对溶质和电荷运动有很强的阻力），但另一些则对溶质有很大的通透性。除了阻力外，这些结构还能调节连接部位对不同离子类型选择性通透性的高低。紧密连接的另一侧为细胞间隙，与间质相接。间质-毛细血管侧的基底细胞膜则通过向细胞内折叠及形成细胞间指状突起来放大其表面积。

溶质可以通过细胞（跨细胞转运）或绕细胞（细胞旁转运）转运（图1.2A）。溶质转运是一个需要代谢燃料的耗能过程。肾小管细胞有多种转运蛋白（图1.2B）。三磷酸腺苷（ATP）酶直接水解ATP为转运提供能量。协同转运蛋白（或同向转运蛋白）可以同向转运两种溶质，而逆向转运蛋白（或反向转运蛋白）则沿相反方向转运两种不同溶质。通道作为内衬蛋白质的"孔"，有允许特定溶质渗透的功能。不同的转运蛋白也可以偶联在一起形成新的转运系统。最后，有蛋白质在连接区突出到细胞外，为细胞旁转运提供通道。

特殊结构
间质

肾间质是肾小管和管周毛细血管之间的空隙，约占肾脏体积的5%～10%，驻留着间质成纤维细胞和树突状细胞。当发生间质性肾炎时（见第5章），肾间质中可有大量炎症细胞浸润，由此产生的细胞因子和趋化因子可显著影响滤过功能和肾小管功能。固有的成纤维细胞为星状细胞，其突触与肾小管和毛细血管相接，提供脚手架样支撑，并分泌/维持细胞外基质。当受到细胞因子的刺激时，这些细胞可转化为肌成纤维细胞，导致肾间质纤维化，这是肾脏疾病共有的病理生理特征。有些位于皮质深部的特殊的成纤维细胞可以感知氧分子，生成促红细胞生成素入血。树突状细胞是表达主要组织相容性复合体（MHC）Ⅱ类分子的抗原提呈细胞。它们与肾实质密接，不断采集并对周围抗原环境做出反应。树突状细胞参与天然免疫和获得性免疫，是维持免疫稳态和肾实质疾病的重要参与者。

球旁器

肾单位的一个独有特征是，每一个肾小管升支粗段均会折返并与其起始的肾小球密切接触。相接处的肾小管细胞与其他升支粗段的细胞不同，称为致密斑。球旁器（JGA）是一个由致密斑、入球和出球小动脉，以及突出肾小球外的球外系膜三部分组成的结构（见图1.1C）。JGA是一个重要结构，通过管球反馈和调节入球小动脉阻力维持肾小球滤过率，还是产生肾素的部位。

线粒体和内质网等细胞器

肾脏在单位质量线粒体含量和氧耗上仅次于心

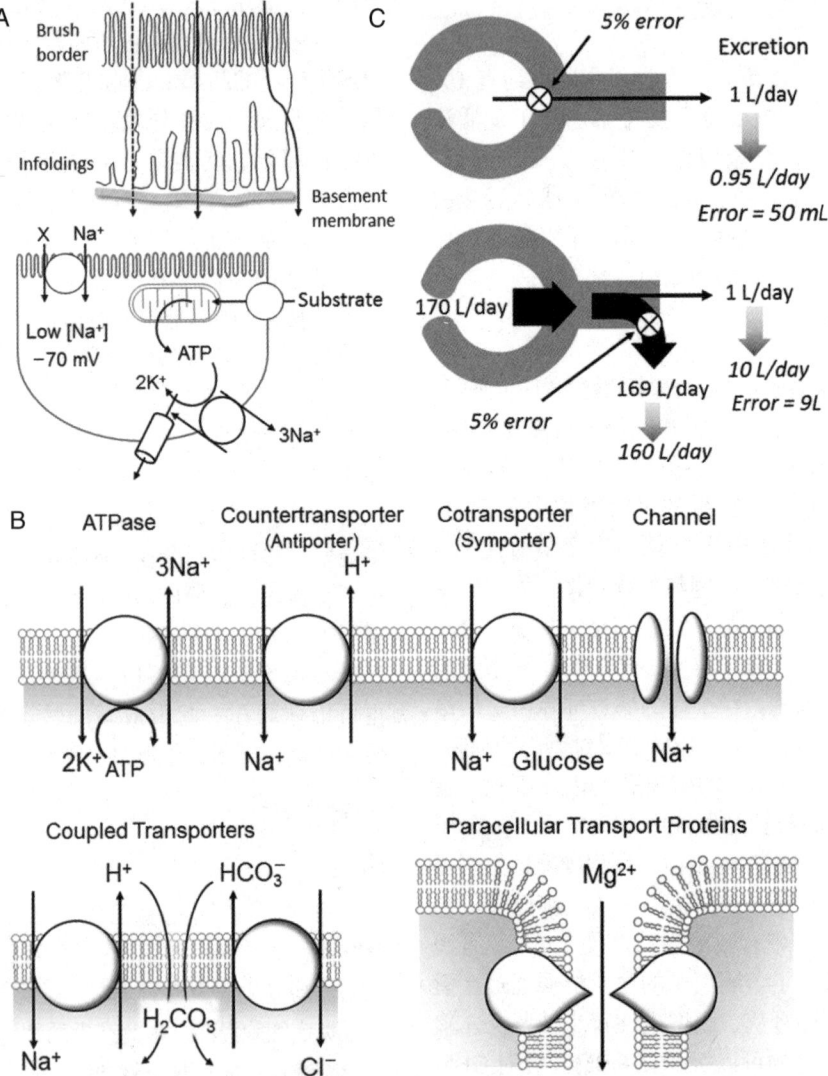

Fig. 1.2 (A) *Top,* Transcellular and paracellular transport of solutes. Solute transport is an energy-consuming process that requires metabolic fuels; a sodium cotransporter and a sodium-potassium countertransporter are shown. (B) Transport proteins. *Top,* Adenosine triphosphatases (ATPases) directly couple ATP hydrolysis to transport. Cotransporters (symporters) move two solutes in the same direction (e.g., Na^+-glucose cotransporter or sodium-glucose linked transporter [SGLT]), and countertransporters (antiporters) move two different solutes in opposite directions. Channels function as protein-lined "holes" that allow specific solutes to permeate. *Lower left,* Different transporters can be coupled together to form a new transport system. *Lower right,* Proteins that protrude outside the cell in the junctional area provide a conduit for paracellular transport. (C) Comparison of a pure filtration (or secretion) design *(top)* and a filtration-reabsorption design *(bottom).* See text for details.

power generator of a cell, mitochondria serve many roles as regulatory, synthetic, and adaptive functions in the cell. Mitochondria are under complex regulation and undergo a plethora of abnormalities in many kidney diseases. Mitochondria-targeted therapeutics are emerging with the notion that maintenance of mitochondria health can prevent pathogenesis and progression of chronic kidney disease. The endoplasmic reticulum (ER) helps maintain the quality of proteins through the unfolded protein response (UPR) pathway, and ER dysfunction with maladaptive UPR activation is named ER stress. ER stress is now known to be present in a wide variety of kidney diseases, and modulators of ER stress will assume important therapeutic roles.

RENAL FUNCTION

Excretory Function

Renal excretion of a substance can be mediated and modified by one or a combination of three processes: filtration, secretion, and reabsorption. Fig. 1.2C compares two designs—pure filtration (or secretion) and filtration-reabsorption—and their implications in terms of demands on regulation. The filtration-reabsorption mechanism allows high filtration rates to be achieved, and the coupling with reabsorption prevents loss of valuable fluid and electrolytes. This design also enables economy in transport mechanisms through adaptive targeting of key solutes while allowing the rest to be excreted. However, there is a price

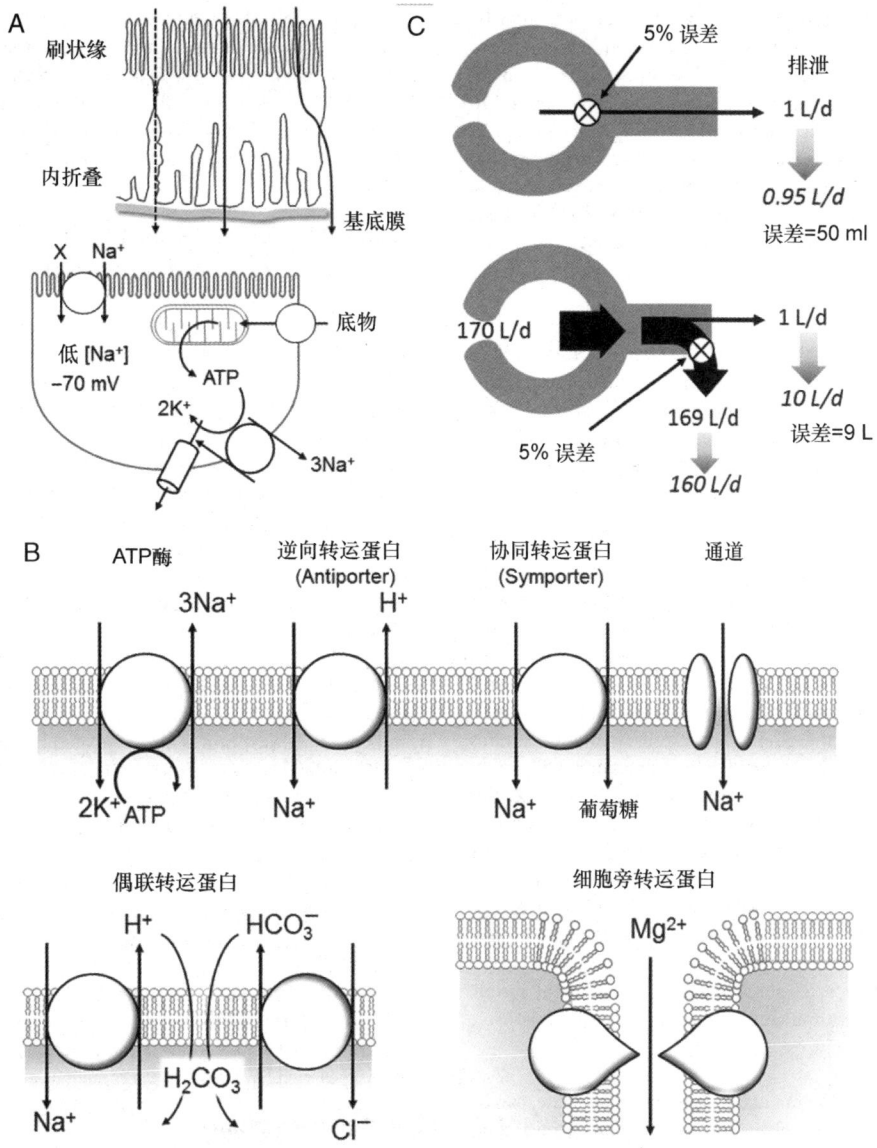

图 1.2 （A）上，溶质的跨细胞和细胞旁转运。溶质转运是需要代谢燃料的耗能过程，图中展示了钠协同转运蛋白和钠钾逆向转运蛋白。（B）转运蛋白。上，ATP 酶直接偶联 ATP 水解来进行转运。协同转运蛋白［如钠-葡萄糖协同转运蛋白（SGLT）］同向转运两种溶质，逆向转运蛋白可在相反的方向转运两种不同溶质。通道的功能就像内衬蛋白质的"孔"，允许特定溶质渗透。左下，不同转运蛋白可偶联在一起形成新的转运系统。右下，蛋白在细胞连接部位突出胞外成为细胞旁转运的通道。（C）单纯滤过（或分泌）（上）与滤过-重吸收（下）的比较。详见文中

脏。除了为细胞产能，线粒体还在细胞中发挥调节、合成和适应功能。线粒体受到复杂调控，在许多肾脏疾病中发生多种异常。因为维持线粒体的健康可预防慢性肾脏病的发生和进展，线粒体靶向治疗正不断涌现。内质网（ER）可通过未折叠蛋白反应（UPR）通路维持蛋白质的质量，UPR 异常活化导致的 ER 功能异常称为内质网应激。目前认为内质网应激存在于多种肾脏疾病中，调控内质网应激可能具有重要的治疗价值。

肾功能

排泄功能

肾脏对某种物质的排泄受到以下三个过程的一个或多个联合介导及调控：滤过、分泌和重吸收。图 1.2C 比较了两种类型：单纯滤过（或分泌）和滤过-重吸收的按需调控的场景。滤过-重吸收机制保证了高效滤过，与重吸收耦合则防止了宝贵的水和电解质的丢失。该设置通过按需锁定靶向关键溶质，同时允许其他溶质排出体外，确保了转运机制的经济性。但是这种配置也要付出一定代价。以通过单纯滤过（或分泌）模式

to be paid for this configuration. Consider the excretion of 1 L/day by pure filtration (or secretion). If there is a 5% error (reduction in filtration or secretion), only 0.95 L/day will be excreted—a difference of 50 mL. Compare this to a filtration-reabsorption mechanism wherein 170 L/day is filtered and 169 L/day is reabsorbed, resulting in the same 1 L/day excretion. A 5% error (reduction) in reabsorption would result in reabsorption of 160 L/day and excretion of 10 L/day, with an absolute error of 9 L. One consequence of a filtration-reabsorption design is that regulation has to have exquisite fidelity, and even small errors are not tolerated.

Filtration

Filtration occurs exclusively at the glomerulus. The GFR, measured as volume per unit time, has been the standard quantitative surrogate for overall kidney function, although there are many disturbances of renal function that are not associated with a decrease in GFR (e.g., nephrotic syndrome, tubulopathies, renovascular hypertension, kidney stones). Numerically, GFR can be conceptualized as an equation:

$$GFR = K_f \times (\Delta P - \Delta \Pi)$$

where the ultrafiltration coefficient, K_f, is equal to the surface area for filtration multiplied by the hydraulic permeability; the hydrostatic driving force, ΔP, is the pressure gradient between the glomerular capillary and Bowman's space, which drives fluid to go into Bowman's space to form urine; and the osmotic driving force, $\Delta \Pi$, is the osmotic pressure gradient between the glomerular capillary and Bowman's space, which holds fluid back in the capillary and slows down filtration.

Many renal diseases affect the determinants of GFR. Glomerular disease (see Chapter 4) decreases K_f by affecting both the filtration surface area and the hydraulic permeability. Changes in ΔP are commonly involved in diseases that reduce GFR. Changes in renal blood flow and more importantly in afferent and efferent arteriolar resistances can drastically affect ΔP and GFR. Functional changes in ΔP, such as prerenal failure from hypovolemia, hepatorenal syndrome (see Chapter 7), or intra-abdominal hypertension can radically lower GFR simply by hemodynamic changes without any structural glomerular lesions.

Reabsorption

High GFR, which is required to maintain a high metabolic rate, can be sustained only if there is high reclamation to maintain intravascular volume and prevent circulatory collapse. Tubular reabsorption thwarts the loss of valuable solutes and allows for finer tuning of the water and solutes not reabsorbed. The resulting tubular contents are excreted. In the mammalian kidney, tubular reabsorption assumes critical roles in the regulation of excretion of many solutes (Table 1.2). A universal mechanism of reabsorption is energy-dependent transepithelial transport, which is mostly Na^+ dependent but can be Na^+ independent. The proximal tubules participate in the reabsorption of all solutes, but some solutes are sequentially reabsorbed by the proximal and distal segments; in these cases, the generic design tends to be high-capacity reabsorption proximally and more of a high-gradient reabsorption for fine tuning distally. The axial difference can occur within the same nephron segment (e.g., early vs. late proximal tubule) or across different segments (e.g., proximal vs. distal nephron segments).

Secretion

Secretion is an ancient mode of excretion that is found in lower-order organisms. Although the human nephron is not primarily secretory in nature, a number of solutes are still handled by secretion. For example, the renal excretion of potassium (K^+), hydrogen ions (H^+), and uric acid involves secretion. Many organic cations and anions are secreted by the proximal tubule, and so are many exogenous toxins such as xenobiotics. The secretion of creatinine by organic cation transporters in the proximal tubule is the reason why creatinine clearance overestimates GFR. The secretion of furosemide by organic cation transporters in the proximal tubule is why response to this drug is attenuated in settings of renal hypoperfusion and/or proximal tubular damage such in acute kidney injury.

Integrated Models of Excretion

The modes of excretion are coordinated in a precise, complex, and concerted fashion to effect excretion with exquisite accuracy (see Table 1.2). The kidney is capable of a large range of urinary tonicity (<50 to 1200 mOsm), depending on the need of the organism to excrete or conserve electrolyte-free water. Water is filtered at the glomerulus and is handled isotonically in the proximal tubule. At the lumen of the distal convoluted tubule, urine is maximally dilute as a consequence of low water permeability throughout the thick ascending limb of Henle. The subsequent fate of the urine determines whether there is electrolyte-free water excretion (dilute urine), achieved by low water permeability of the collecting duct, or electrolyte-free water conservation (concentrated urine), effected by the action of antidiuretic hormone (ADH), which renders the collecting tubule permeable to water.

Na^+ homeostasis basically occurs via filtration-reabsorption; it is regulated by changes in effective arterial blood volume (EABV) mediated by neurohormonal afferent signals (e.g., renin-angiotensin-aldosterone system [RAAS]) that act directly on tubules. In the proximal tubule, Na^+ reabsorption is also regulated by peritubular physical factors. K^+ undergoes an interesting sequence in which the filtered load is largely reabsorbed in the proximal tubule and the thick ascending limb; the final determinant of excretion is secretion by the collecting duct, for which aldosterone and distal Na^+ delivery are major regulators.

Only Ca^{2+} that is not bound to plasma protein is filtered; it is reabsorbed largely via paracellular pathways in the proximal tubule and thick ascending limb and via transcellular pathways in the distal convoluted tubule.

A massive amount of bicarbonate (HCO_3^-) is filtered and must be reclaimed to forestall catastrophic acidosis. H^+ secretion provides the mechanism for HCO_3^- reclamation as well as acid excretion, with the H^+ being carried by urinary buffers such as ammonia.

Metabolic Function

The kidney is a major metabolic organ. It consumes a wide range of fuels, regulates plasma levels of metabolic substrates, and is a major source of gluconeogenesis. Metabolic substrates such as amino acids, glucose, organic anions, and fatty acids are converted to ATP, the universal energy unit for all cells (see Fig. 1.2A). ATP is directly hydrolyzed by proteins such as Na^+/K^+-ATPase to create a low intracellular Na^+ concentration ($[Na^+]$) and a negative interior cell voltage, thus translating the chemical energy into chemical gradients. About 80% to 90% of the oxygen consumption of the kidney can be attributed to Na^+ transport. For example, a protein such as the Na^+-glucose cotransporter (sodium-glucose linked transporter [SGLT], see Fig. 1.2B) on the proximal tubule luminal membrane, couples the movement of Na^+ ions to glucose molecule (carrying a net positive charge). The low cell $[Na^+]$ and negative voltage energize glucose uptake, allowing the proximal tubule to capture most of the filtered glucose that otherwise would be lost in the urine. In normal physiology, this glucose reclamation is beneficial to conserve calories. The pharmacologic inhibition of Na^+-coupled glucose reabsorption (SGLT-2 inhibitors) leads to low glycosuric threshold and creation of a "glucose sink" to control glycemia. Surprisingly, many additional beneficial cardiovascular and renal effects have been observed with SGLT-2 inhibitors that are not explained by glycemic control.

每天排出 1 L 为例。若有 5% 的误差（滤过或分泌），则只有 0.95 L 会被排出，差别是 50 ml。与滤过-重吸收机制相比，每天滤过 170 L 并重吸收 169 L，同样是排出 1 L。5% 重吸收的误差（减少）导致每天重吸收 160 L 而排出 10 L，则绝对误差为 9 L。因此，滤过-重吸收机制要求调节务必精准，即使是微小的误差也不能容忍。

滤过

滤过仅发生在肾小球。肾小球滤过率（GFR）是以单位时间内滤过的体积来衡量的，虽然很多肾脏功能的紊乱与 GFR 下降不相关（如肾病综合征、肾小管病、肾血管性高血压、肾结石），但 GFR 一直是标准的定量替代整体肾功能的指标。GFR 可由如下公式计算：

$$GFR = K_f \times (\Delta P - \Delta \Pi)$$

其中超滤系数 K_f 等于滤过面积乘以水通透性；静水驱动力 ΔP 指肾小球毛细血管腔和鲍曼囊腔之间的压差，这个压差驱动液体进入鲍曼囊腔形成尿液；渗透驱动力 $\Delta \Pi$ 指肾小球毛细血管腔和鲍曼囊腔之间的渗透压差，该压差使液体留在毛细血管内，减慢滤过。

很多肾脏疾病影响 GFR 的决定因素。肾小球疾病（见第 4 章）通过同时影响滤过面积和水通透性降低了 K_f。ΔP 改变常见于降低 GFR 的疾病。肾血流变化，特别是入球和出球小动脉阻力可显著影响 ΔP 和 GFR。ΔP 的功能性改变，如低血容量性肾前性肾衰竭、肝肾综合征（见第 7 章）或腹内高压，可在无任何肾小球结构性病变的情况下，仅通过血流动力学的变化即导致 GFR 显著下降。

重吸收

维持高代谢率需要高 GFR，只有在有高回收力以维持血管内容量及防止循环衰竭的情况下才能维持。肾小管重吸收可避免有价值的溶质丢失，并对水和未被重吸收的溶质进行精细的调节。最终留在肾小管内的内容物被排出体外。在哺乳动物的肾脏中，肾小管重吸收在很多溶质排出的调控中发挥重要作用（表 1.2）。一种普遍的重吸收机制是能量依赖性跨上皮细胞转运，多数是 Na^+ 依赖，但也可以是非 Na^+ 依赖。近端肾小管参与所有溶质的重吸收，但有些溶质被近端小管和远端小管序贯重吸收，在这种情况下，一般倾向于在近端小管高容量重吸收，远端小管则更多是高梯度重吸收以精细调控。轴向差异可发生在同一肾单位节段内（如近端小管起始段和末段）或横向的不同节段内（如肾单位的近端和远端节段）。

分泌

分泌是一种在低等生物中发现的古老的排泄方式。尽管人类肾单位并不以分泌为主，但仍有许多溶质通过分泌来处理。例如，肾脏对 K^+、H^+ 和尿酸的排泄仍涉及分泌机制。许多有机阳离子和阴离子，以及许多外源性毒素如异生物是通过近端肾小管分泌的。肌酐通过有机阳离子转运体在近端肾小管分泌是肌酐清除率高过 GFR 的原因。呋塞米通过近端肾小管有机阳离子转运体分泌，因此在肾脏低灌注和（或）近端肾小管损伤（如急性肾损伤）时，对这种药物的反应会减弱。

排泄的综合模式

排泄模式是一个精准、复杂且协调的过程，以达到准确无误（表 1.2）。肾脏可依据机体排出或保留自由水的需要，在较大范围内调节尿液张力（< 50 ～ 1200 mOsm）。水从肾小球滤过，在近端肾小管内保持等张力。缘于亨利襻升支粗段对水的低通透性，尿液在远曲肾小管被最大限度稀释。随后尿液的命运决定于是因集合管对水的低通透性而排出无电解质的自由水（稀释尿），还是因抗利尿激素（ADH）的作用使集合管可通透水而保留无电解质的自由水（浓缩尿）。

Na^+ 稳态主要经滤过-重吸收来维持。它受直接作用于肾小管的神经激素传入信号〔如，肾素-血管紧张素-醛固酮系统（RAAS）〕介导的有效动脉血容量（EABV）变化的调控。在近端肾小管，Na^+ 重吸收还受管周物理因素调节。K^+ 则经历了一个有趣的过程，滤过液中的 K^+ 大部分在近端小管和升支粗段重吸收；决定最终排泄的是集合管的分泌，醛固酮和远端 Na^+ 输送是其主要调控因素。

只有 Ca^{2+} 离子以非蛋白结合形式被滤过。在近端肾小管和升支粗段主要经细胞旁途径重吸收，在远曲小管则经跨细胞途径重吸收。

大量碳酸氢根（HCO_3^-）被滤过，必须回收以防止灾难性的酸中毒。由氨等尿液缓冲剂携带的 H^+ 的分泌有助于回收 HCO_3^- 和排酸。

代谢功能

肾脏是主要的代谢器官。它消耗多种能量，调节血浆中代谢底物的水平，是糖异生的主要来源。代谢底物，如氨基酸、葡萄糖、有机阴离子和脂肪酸可转化成 ATP，是各种细胞通用的能量单元（图 1.2A）。ATP 可以被 Na^+/K^+-ATP 酶等蛋白质直接水解，产生细胞内低 Na^+ 浓度和细胞内负电压，从而使化学能量转化为化学梯度。约 80% ～ 90% 的肾脏氧耗用于 Na^+ 转运。例如，位于近端肾小管管腔面的钠-葡萄糖协同转运蛋白（SGLT，见图 1.2B），偶联 Na^+ 离子和葡萄糖分子（携带正电荷）的运动。细胞内低 Na^+ 浓度和负电压为葡萄糖摄取提供了能量，使近端肾小管能捕获大部分滤过的葡萄糖，否则这些葡萄糖将随尿液流失。正常生理状态下，葡萄糖回收有益于贮存能量。药物抑制钠-偶联葡萄糖重吸收（SGLT-2 抑制剂）可以降低肾糖阈，促进肾排糖来控制血糖。令人吃惊的是，SGLT-2 抑制剂还被观察到具有仅仅用降糖难以解释的心血管和肾脏保护效果。

TABLE 1.2 Solute Excretion

Solute	Filtration	Reabsorption	Secretion	Fe (%)	Regulation
Water	Yes	Yes	No	0.3-6.0	Responds primarily to body tonicity but also EABV. ADH is the major regulator of collecting duct water permeability.
Na^+	Yes	Yes	No	0.2-2.0	Responds to EABV. Reabsorption is stimulated by sympathetic nerves, angiotensin II, aldosterone; inhibited by atrial natriuretic peptides, dopamine, uroguanylin.
K^+	Yes	Yes	Yes	5-20	Responds to total body potassium status. Secretion is controlled primarily by aldosterone and distal Na^+ delivery.
Ca^{2+}	Yes	Yes	No	2-10	Responds to serum ionized $[Ca^{2+}]$ and body need for calcium. Major calciotropic hormones include parathyroid hormone, vitamin D, and calcitonin. Renal epithelia directly respond to ionized calcium via the calcium sensing receptor.
Mg^{2+}	Yes	Yes	No	3-5	Responds to total body magnesium status and requirements. Paracrine regulation is via epidermal growth factor.
HCO_3^-	Yes	Yes	Yes	0.1-0.5	Most bicarbonate reabsorption is to reclaim the filtered load. Responds to systemic acid-base status, which can be mediated by direct sensing by the renal epithelia or via hormonal actions (e.g., angiotensin II, endothelin). Bicarbonate can also be secreted in the collecting duct when alkali excretion is required.
Phosphate	Yes	Yes	No	5-20	Responds to serum phosphate concentration and body phosphate status. Reabsorption primarily resides in the proximal tubule and is regulated by parathyroid hormone and fibroblast growth factor-23.
Glucose	Yes	Yes	No	0.2-0.5	The proximal tubule reclaims almost all filtered glucose except when the filtered load exceeds reabsorptive capacity. The cortical proximal tubule performs gluconeogenesis from other organic substrates.
Uric acid	Yes	Yes	Yes	10-50	Major routes of uric acid clearance are (1) renal excretion and (2) intestinal secretion and uricolysis. Handling of both secretion and reabsorption in the proximal tubule is complex, and regulatory mechanisms are unclear.
Creatinine	Yes	No	Yes	1.0-1.2	Filtered at the glomerulus and secreted by the proximal tubule. The contribution of the tubules to creatinine clearance increases when GFR declines.

ADH, Antidiuretic hormone; *EABV*, effective arterial blood volume; *FE*, fractional excretion under normal physiology.

TABLE 1.3 Some Endocrine Hormones Elaborated by the Kidney

Hormone	Source	Function	Drugs
Renin	JGA	Converts angiotensinogen to angiotensin I as an integral part of the renin-angiotensin-aldosterone system	Renin inhibitor ACE inhibitor Angiotensin receptor blocker Mineralocorticoid receptor blocker
1,25(OH)$_2$ vitamin D	Mostly proximal tubule	Converts the precursor 25(OH) vitamin D to its active form, 1,25(OH)$_2$ vitamin D	25-Hydroxyvitamin D 1,25-Dihydroxyvitamin D Synthetic vitamin D analogues
Erythropoietin	Renal interstitial cells	Stimulates erythropoiesis in the bone marrow	Recombinant human erythropoietin Glycosylated recombinant human erythropoietin Other "EPO mimetic" erythropoiesis-stimulating agents

ACE, Angiotensin-converting enzyme; *JGA*, juxtaglomerular apparatus.

The amount of filtered organic molecules far exceeds the metabolic consumption by the kidney. Very large amounts of organic metabolic substrates are passively filtered daily; these substrates are not meant to be excreted, but the high GFR and lack of retention at the glomerular capillaries obligate their presence in the glomerular urine. In the proximal tubule, the bulk of the filtered organic molecules are reclaimed from the urine and returned to the systemic circulation. Several thousands of millimoles of amino acids, glucose, and organic cations and anions are retrieved each day by the kidney from the urine.

Metabolic and Endocrine Function

The kidney rivals the liver as a gluconeogenic organ that sustains circulating blood glucose levels. Although there is no doubt that this is a critical physiologic function, there are no clinical examples of hypoglycemia stemming purely from lack of renal gluconeogenesis.

In addition to the prominent and more obvious roles in solute and water balance, the kidney also is an important endocrine organ. The autocrine and paracrine substances elaborated by the kidney are important for both intrarenal and systemic regulation. Although this subject is not addressed fully here, three of these substances are highlighted because they represent important pharmacologic targets (Table 1.3).

Renin

As the initiating component of the RAAS, renin is important for maintenance of the circulation. The RAAS permits the kidney to have a constant GFR in the face of low and fluctuating salt intake, a property

表 1.2	溶质排泄				
溶质	滤过	重吸收	分泌	FE（%）	调节
水	是	是	否	0.3~6.0	主要对体内张力做出反应，也受 EABV 影响 ADH 是集合管水通透性的主要调节因素
Na^+	是	是	否	0.2~2.0	对 EABV 反应 交感神经、血管紧张素Ⅱ、醛固酮可刺激重吸收；心房利钠肽、多巴胺和尿鸟苷可抑制重吸收
K^+	是	是	是	5~20	对全身钾状态做出反应 分泌主要受醛固酮和远端 Na^+ 输送的控制
Ca^{2+}	是	是	否	2~10	对血清钙离子 $[Ca^{2+}]$ 和机体钙需求做出反应 主要的钙调激素包括甲状旁腺激素、维生素 D 和降钙素 肾上皮细胞通过钙敏感受体直接对钙离子做出反应
Mg^{2+}	是	是	否	3~5	对全身镁状态和需求做出反应 旁分泌通过表皮生长因子调节
HCO_3^-	是	是	是	0.1~0.5	多数碳酸氢盐从滤过液中重吸收 对全身酸碱状态做出反应，可通过肾脏上皮细胞的直接感应或激素作用（如血管紧张素Ⅱ、内皮素）介导 需要排碱时，碳酸氢盐也可在集合管分泌
磷酸盐	是	是	否	5~20	对血清磷酸盐浓度和体内磷酸盐状态做出反应 重吸收主要存在于近端肾小管，受甲状旁腺激素和成纤维细胞生长因子-23 调节
葡萄糖	是	是	否	0.2~0.5	近端肾小管回收几乎所有滤过的葡萄糖，除非滤过负荷超过重吸收能力。 皮质近端肾小管利用其他有机底物进行糖异生
尿酸	是	是	是	10~50	尿酸清除的主要途径是①肾脏排泄及②肠道分泌和尿酸溶解 近端肾小管分泌和重吸收的过程复杂，调节机制尚不清楚
肌酐	是	否	是	1.0~1.2	肾小球滤过，近端肾小管分泌 当肾小球滤过率下降时，肾小管对肌酐清除的贡献增加

ADH，抗利尿激素；EABV，有效动脉血容量；FE，正常生理状态下的排泄分数。

表 1.3	肾脏产生的一些内分泌激素		
激素	产生部位	功能	药物
肾素	球旁器	作为肾素-血管紧张素-醛固酮系统的组成部分，将血管紧张素原转化为血管紧张素 I	肾素抑制剂 ACE 抑制剂 血管紧张素受体阻滞剂 盐皮质激素受体阻滞剂
1,25- 二羟维生素 D	近端小管为主	将前体 25（OH）维生素 D 转化为其活性形式 1,25（OH）$_2$ 维生素 D	25- 羟维生素 D 1,25- 二羟维生素 D 合成维生素 D 类似物
促红细胞生成素	肾间质细胞	刺激骨髓红细胞生成	重组人促红细胞生成素 糖基化重组人促红细胞生成素 其他"EPO 模拟物"红细胞生成刺激剂

ACE，血管紧张素转换酶。

肾脏滤过的有机分子的数量远超代谢消耗所需。每天有大量有机代谢底物被动滤过；这些底物并不需要被排泄，但高 GFR 及肾小球毛细血管滞留能力的缺乏，使它们不得不出现在肾小球尿液（原尿）中。在近端肾小管，大量滤过的有机分子从尿中回收并返回体循环。肾脏每天从尿中回收数千毫摩尔的氨基酸、葡萄糖、有机阳离子和阴离子。

代谢和内分泌功能

肾脏作为可与肝脏相媲美的糖异生器官，负责维持循环中葡萄糖水平。虽然这无疑是一个重要的生理功能，但是尚无纯粹因肾脏糖异生缺乏导致低血糖的临床案例。

除了在维持溶质和水平衡中发挥显著作用，肾脏还是一个重要的内分泌器官。肾脏自分泌和旁分泌的物质对肾脏内部和全身调节都很重要。本文未对此一一详述，但重点介绍了其中 3 个物质，因为它们是重要的药物靶点（表 1.3）。

肾素

作为 RAAS 系统的始动成分，肾素在维持循环中发挥重要作用。在盐摄入量低且波动时，RAAS 可保证肾脏 GFR 稳定。这对陆地生物的生存至关重要。如前

that is vital for terrestrial existence. Renin is produced by the JGA (see earlier discussion). Despite the benefits and importance of the RAAS in physiology, its continuous and excessive activation in many disease states appears to be maladaptive and contributes to kidney and cardiovascular injury. Pharmacologic blockade of RAAS pathways at various levels has proved beneficial in animal disease models and human clinical studies, and agents to block RAAS signaling are now in clinical use, with others under development (see Table 1.3).

Vitamin D

1α-Hydroxylase (cytochrome P-450 isoenzyme 27B1) is found primarily in the proximal tubule, where the major body defense for maintaining phosphate homeostasis is localized. The kidney is one of the most important organs for maintaining calcium and phosphate homeostasis, not just as the major controller of external balance but as an elaborator of systemic factors such as vitamin D and the Klotho protein. Conversion of the precursor 25(OH)-hydroxyvitamin D to its active form, $1,25(OH)_2$dihydroxyvitamin D, is achieved not exclusively but substantially in the kidney and is mediated by 1α-hydroxylase. Vitamin D deficiency is an important complication in chronic kidney disease. Replacement of vitamin D is efficacious in reducing the complications of chronic kidney disease.

Erythropoietin

Erythropoietin, which is produced mainly in the kidney, stimulates erythropoiesis. The erythropoietin-producing cells are strategically located in the cortical interstitium to sense the balance between oxygen delivery and consumption. The current model suggests that upregulation of renal erythropoietin production (mainly by anemia and hypoxia) occurs via an increase in the number of latent erythropoietin-producing cells. The mechanism of erythropoietin deficiency in kidney disease is not well known, although it does not simply involve destruction of erythropoietin-producing interstitial cells. One possible mechanism is decreased renal oxygen consumption as a consequence of reduced GFR; this results in higher renal tissue oxygen tension and suppression of erythropoietin production. Another theory is direct inhibition of the erythropoietin-producing cells by inflammatory cytokines. Others have proposed transdifferentiation of erythropoietin-producing cells into myofibroblasts and a decrease in the number of interstitial cells that can be recruited to produce erythropoietin.

The use of erythropoiesis-stimulating agents (ESAs) has revolutionized the treatment of anemia associated with chronic kidney disease, but because of incomplete understanding of erythropoietin and erythropoietin receptor biology, the clinical outcome is far from ideal due to inability to tailor the optimal hematocrit for individual patients and uncertainty about possible extra-erythropoietic effects of erythropoietin. The new class of hypoxia-inducible factor prolyl hydroxylase inhibitors as ESAs increases endogenous erythropoietin production.

SUGGESTED READINGS

Kaissling B, Le Hir M: The renal cortical interstitium: morphological and functional aspects, Histochem Cell Biol 130:247-262, 2008.

Maezawa Y, Cina D, Quaggin SE: Glomerular cell biology, Waltham, 2013, Academic Press, pp 721-757.

Moe OW, Giebisch G, Seldin DW: Logic of the kidney. In Lifton RP, Somio S, Glebisch GH, et al, editors: Genetic diseases of the kidney, New York, 2009, Elsevier, pp 39-73.

Reiser J, Sever S: Podocyte biology and pathogenesis of kidney disease, Annu Rev Med 64:357-366, 2013.

所述，肾素由球旁器产生。尽管生理状态下RAAS有益且重要，但在许多疾病状态下其持续和过度的活化属于适应不良，可损伤肾脏和心血管。疾病动物模型和临床研究均证实针对RAAS通路不同水平进行药理阻断是有益的，一些阻断RAAS通路的药物已经在临床应用，还有其他药物处于研发中（表1.3）。

维生素D

1α-羟化酶（细胞色素P-450同工酶17B1）主要位于近端肾小管，这里是维持磷稳态的关键部位。作为维持钙磷稳态最重要的器官之一，肾脏不仅是外部平衡的主要控制者，也是如维生素D和Klotho蛋白等系统因素的调控者。前体25-羟维生素D转化成具有活性的1,25-二羟维生素D，虽然并不完全但主要是在肾脏完成，由1α-羟化酶介导。维生素D缺乏是慢性肾脏病的一个重要并发症。补充维生素D可有效减少慢性肾脏病的并发症。

促红细胞生成素

促红细胞生成素（EPO）主要由肾脏产生，刺激红细胞生成。产EPO的细胞位于皮质的间质内以感知供氧和耗氧间的平衡。目前认为，肾脏EPO上调（主要由贫血和低氧诱发）是通过增加潜在的产EPO细胞的数量所致。罹患肾脏疾病时EPO缺乏的机制尚未阐明，可能并不简单的是因为产EPO的间质细胞毁损所致。一种可能的机制是肾氧耗因GFR下降而减少，导致肾组织氧张力升高，从而抑制EPO产生。另一种理论是炎性细胞因子直接抑制了产EPO细胞。其他原因包括产EPO细胞转分化成肌成纤维细胞，以及可被募集产生EPO的间质细胞数量减少。

红细胞生成刺激剂（ESA）的应用使慢性肾脏病相关贫血的治疗发生了革命性的变化。但由于尚未完全阐明EPO和EPO受体的生物学机制，尚不能为个体患者量身定制最佳血细胞比容（红细胞压积），以及EPO有可能的促红细胞生成之外效应的不确定性，使得EPO应用的临床结果仍欠理想。新型缺氧诱导因子脯氨酰羟化酶抑制剂可增加内源性EPO的产生。

推荐阅读

Kaissling B, Le Hir M: The renal cortical interstitium: morphological and functional aspects, Histochem Cell Biol 130:247-262, 2008.

Maezawa Y, Cina D, Quaggin SE: Glomerular cell biology, Waltham, 2013, Academic Press, pp 721-757.

Moe OW, Giebisch G, Seldin DW: Logic of the kidney. In Lifton RP, Somio S, Glebisch GH, et al, editors: Genetic diseases of the kidney, New York, 2009, Elsevier, pp 39-73.

Reiser J, Sever S: Podocyte biology and pathogenesis of kidney disease, Annu Rev Med 64:357-366, 2013.

2
Approach to the Patient With Renal Disease

Rajiv Agarwal

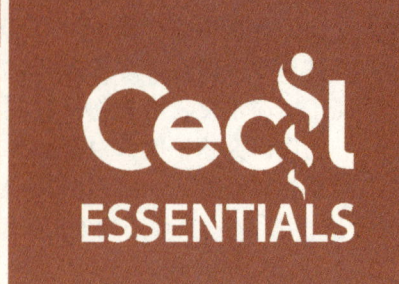

INTRODUCTION

Chronic kidney disease (CKD) is commonly defined as having an estimated glomerular filtration rate (GFR) of less than 60 mL/min/1.73 m^2 for at least 3 months. Most patients with CKD are seen in the outpatient setting, and at first consultation an important objective is to uncover the cause of CKD. In the long term the objectives of care are the preservation of kidney and cardiovascular function and the prevention of the long-term complications of CKD. Once kidney function deteriorates to the extent that it can no longer sustain an appropriate quality of life the objective of care evolves to the provision of renal replacement therapy. In some patients, discussion may be about withholding the provision of renal replacement therapy. In contrast to the clinical approach to patients with CKD, most patients with acute kidney injury (AKI) are hospitalized. The focus of their care also starts with accurate determination of the cause of AKI, but over a period of days to weeks it is important to reverse the kidney failure if possible, replace kidney function if needed, and manage the many potential adverse consequences of AKI. Thus, the approach to the care of patients with AKI and CKD are largely non-overlapping and are discussed separately.

Distinction of AKI From CKD

Because of the widespread use of automated systems for serum chemistry analysis, an elevated serum creatinine concentration is the most common initial manifestation of kidney disease. This test is performed as a screen for renal function abnormalities in most metabolic panels; in most cases, an elevated serum creatinine concentration reflects reduced filtration function of the kidney. After ensuring that intravascular volume is appropriate, the approach to the patient depends on whether kidney failure is acute or chronic. Accordingly, the initial step in evaluating an elevated serum creatinine level is to assess the time course and duration of the changes to distinguish AKI from CKD.

A careful history, physical examination, and laboratory evaluation, including imaging studies, are all fundamental to this process. The highest priority is to address acute volume depletion, bleeding, and other causes of intravascular volume loss. Evidence of chronicity may be discovered by searching the records for prior abnormalities of serum creatinine, albuminuria or proteinuria, abnormal urine sediment, or anatomic features such as the presence of multiple cysts in both kidneys discovered on an ultrasound or CT scan. Similarly, a call to the primary care doctor may provide clues to suggest the presence of kidney disease at an earlier time. In the United States, electronic medical record systems are ubiquitous and deep knowledge of this electronic record is often essential to discover the onset date of CKD.

Small kidney size, as assessed by ultrasound, can be highly suggestive of CKD. The size of the kidney depends on the height of the patient, but in general, a kidney length on ultrasound images of less than 9 cm in an adult male is considered small. The presence of normal-sized or even large kidneys does not exclude the diagnosis of CKD. In fact, it is common in patients with diabetic nephropathy for kidneys to be 11 or 12 cm long. Radiography of clavicles or hands is not commonly performed but may demonstrate renal osteodystrophy and suggest the presence of CKD.

Anemia is common in both AKI and CKD and therefore is not a differentiating feature. However, the presence of secondary hyperparathyroidism points toward CKD. Rarely, if the initial evaluation is unrevealing, a kidney biopsy may be required to distinguish AKI from CKD and to define the etiology of injury.

APPROACH TO THE PATIENT WITH CHRONIC KIDNEY DISEASE

If the elevated creatinine concentration is thought to be chronic in nature, the history and physical examination should focus initially on detection of diabetes mellitus and hypertension, the two most common causes of CKD. In all cases, the evaluation also includes laboratory testing of renal function, serum electrolytes, complete blood count, testing for albuminuria, and microscopic urine sediment analysis. Kidney ultrasound is almost always obtained early in the evaluation to eliminate ureteral or bladder obstruction, a cause of reversible renal failure. In addition, the ultrasound provides important information about kidney size, symmetry, and echogenicity. Kidney biopsy may be needed in some patients, but parenchymal scarring is common in many forms of CKD so the biopsy may not be diagnostic.

Because diabetes and hypertension are common causes of kidney disease, it is important to recognize the associated presentations. To establish a likely diagnosis of diabetic nephropathy, a long-standing history of documented diabetes mellitus is typical. An eye exam that notes diabetic retinopathy often goes hand-in-hand with diabetic nephropathy; however, the absence of diabetic retinopathy does not rule out CKD due to diabetes mellitus. Albuminuria and large kidneys on ultrasound are often seen. However, as many as a third of patients with CKD due to type 2 diabetes mellitus do not have albuminuria. In patients with diabetes mellitus or hypertension, the urinary sediment is usually unremarkable, so the presence of red blood cells (RBCs) casts or a significant number of dysmorphic erythrocytes should initiate a careful evaluation for other causes of CKD.

In cases of hypertensive nephrosclerosis, established hypertension typically antedates the diagnosis of renal failure for many years, and the presence of hypertensive retinopathy or cardiovascular disease (e.g., left ventricular hypertrophy) is common. Proteinuria is typically minimal or absent (<2 g/day), and the kidneys are symmetrically small on ultrasound.

Although hypertension and type 2 diabetes mellitus are common, among patients with CKD it is important not to assume that diabetes

肾脏疾病患者的接诊

刘立军 译　张宏　秦岩 审校　赵明辉 通审

引言

慢性肾脏病（CKD）通常定义为估算的肾小球滤过率（GFR）低于 60 ml/（min·1.73 m²）并持续至少 3 个月。多数 CKD 患者在门诊就诊时发现，首诊的重要目标是明确 CKD 的病因。CKD 的长期治疗目标是保护患者肾脏和心血管功能，预防长期并发症。一旦肾功能恶化到无法维持生活质量，治疗目标则转变为肾脏替代治疗。对于某些患者，可能还需要面临是否终止肾脏替代治疗的讨论。与 CKD 患者的临床管理方法相比，大多数急性肾损伤（AKI）患者需要住院治疗。其治疗重点同样始于准确判定 AKI 的病因，但在接下来的数日至数周内，主要目标是尽可能逆转肾衰竭，必要时进行肾脏替代支持治疗，同时处理 AKI 的潜在的诸多并发症。因 AKI 和 CKD 患者的临床管理并不一致，下面将分别讨论。

AKI 与 CKD 的鉴别

因自动化血清生化分析系统的广泛使用，且多数代谢检查的组合都将血清肌酐纳入肾功能的筛查指标，因此，化验检查发现血清肌酐升高往往是肾脏疾病最常见的始发表现。多数情况下，血清肌酐升高反映了肾脏滤过功能的减退。发现患者血清肌酐升高后，在确保血管内容量充足的情况下，患者的接诊管理取决于判定肾损伤是急性还是慢性。首要步骤是分析血清肌酐变化的时间过程和持续时长，以鉴别 AKI 和 CKD。

仔细询问病史、体格检查和实验室评估，包括影像学检查，都是鉴别诊断的基础。最先应考虑是否存在急性血管内容量不足、出血和其他原因导致的血管内容量丢失。慢性的证据可以通过回顾病历记录来发现，如既往出现血清肌酐异常、白蛋白尿或蛋白尿、尿沉渣异常，超声或 CT 发现双肾存在多发囊肿等解剖异常。同样，联系初级保健医生也可提供一些既往肾脏疾病的线索。在美国，电子病历系统无处不在，深入了解这些电子病历记录对于发现 CKD 的发病时间往往至关重要。

超声检查发现肾脏体积小高度提示 CKD。肾脏大小取决于患者身高，通常成年男性的肾脏长度在超声上小于 9 cm 即视为肾脏缩小。但肾脏大小正常或偏大并不能排除 CKD 的诊断。事实上，在糖尿病肾病患者中，肾脏长达 11 cm 或 12 cm 的情况很常见。锁骨或手部的 X 射线检查并非常规，但如显示有肾性骨营养不良则提示存在 CKD。

贫血在 AKI 和 CKD 中都很常见，因此并非鉴别要点。然而，存在继发性甲状旁腺功能亢进则指向 CKD。少数情况下，如果初步评估结果不明确，可能需要肾活检以区分 AKI 和 CKD，并确定肾损伤的病因。

慢性肾脏病患者的接诊

如果考虑血清肌酐升高为慢性的，病史和体格检查应首先明确是否存在糖尿病和高血压，这是导致慢性肾衰竭的两个最常见的原因。完整的评估还包括肾功能实验室检查、血电解质、全血细胞计数、白蛋白尿检测和显微镜下尿沉渣分析。早期评估还应包括肾脏超声检查，以排除输尿管或膀胱梗阻，这是导致可逆性肾衰竭的原因之一。此外，超声检查还提供关于肾脏大小、对称性和回声等重要信息。一些患者可能需要肾活检，但各种病因导致的 CKD 均可表现为肾实质瘢痕化，此时肾活检可能难以起到诊断作用。

糖尿病和高血压是肾脏疾病的常见病因，因此识别相关的表现非常重要。如疑诊糖尿病肾病，长期的糖尿病病史是重要依据。眼科检查发现糖尿病视网膜病变，往往与糖尿病肾病同时发生；但是，没有糖尿病视网膜病变并不能排除糖尿病导致的 CKD。白蛋白尿和超声检查中发现肾脏变大，是常见表现。但是，多达 1/3 的 2 型糖尿病导致的 CKD 患者没有白蛋白尿。糖尿病或高血压患者的尿沉渣通常无明显异常，但如果出现红细胞（RBC）管型或大量异形红细胞，则应对其他导致 CKD 的原因进行仔细评估。

在高血压性肾硬化症病例中，已确诊的高血压通常比肾衰竭的诊断早很多年，而且高血压视网膜病变或心血管疾病（如左心室肥大）也很常见。蛋白尿通常没有或很少（< 2 g/d），超声检查可见肾脏对称性变小。

虽然高血压和 2 型糖尿病常见，但并非所有 CKD 患者均为糖尿病或者高血压所致。诊断糖尿病或高血压作

and hypertension are always the cause of CKD. The diagnosis of hypertension or diabetes mellitus as the cause of CKD requires that no other identifiable cause of kidney disease is apparent after a thorough evaluation. Notably, in individuals with hypertension, genes such as *APOL1* have been identified that appear to be associated with a greater risk of renal disease, and genetic analysis may emerge as one approach to identify those most at risk so that strategies for prevention can be tested in the future.

Once a diagnosis of CKD is established, ongoing evaluation is required, because those with CKD are at increased risk for complications such as hypertension, metabolic bone disease, anemia, hyperkalemia, and metabolic acidosis. Furthermore, the initial diagnosis of CKD may be modified over time, such as by the discovery of RBC casts in a patient with diabetes mellitus. AKI may be superimposed on CKD. The assessment of hypertension requires an accurate assessment of blood pressure. Measurements of three readings after quiet rest at intervals of 1 minute using an oscillometric device is now recommended; auscultatory methods utilizing Korotkoff sounds are no longer recommended. If hypertension or volume overload becomes difficult to manage, the dietary intake of sodium can be estimated by 24-hour urine collection. The number of medications prescribed to patients with CKD is substantial, which calls for monitoring for medication adherence. The latter, for instance, may provide clues to lack of control of BP. For a more detailed approach and slightly different opinion on the measurement of the arterial blood pressure, see "Cardiovascular Disease" Chapter 11.

History and Examination

The signs and symptoms of CKD depend on the stage at presentation. Early in the clinical course, nonspecific fatigue is typical, and there may be no discernable clues to CKD on examination, highlighting the need for laboratory screening. As filtration rate declines, the signs and symptoms of CKD become more common and may include pedal edema, facial puffiness, flank pain, polyuria, nocturia, and hypertension. Symptoms referable to uremia, such as nausea, dysgeusia, and vomiting, tend to occur late and should not be relied on to make a diagnosis of early CKD.

Sometimes the manifestations of the primary disease predominate. For example, the presence of fever, arthralgia, and rash in a young woman with renal failure and active urinary sediment is highly suggestive of lupus nephritis; or intravenous drug use, cardiac murmur, vegetations on cardiac valve, and positive blood culture should alert to a possible diagnosis of endocarditis-associated glomerulonephritis. A family history of deafness, hematuria, and CKD can point to the diagnosis of Alport's syndrome; or a history of cerebral hemorrhage due to a ruptured aneurysm may suggest underlying polycystic kidney disease.

Medication history should focus on exposure to nephrotoxins, including long-term use of nonsteroidal anti-inflammatory drugs (NSAIDs), lithium, exposure to cisplatin, and recent escalation of the dose of diuretics. Some nonprescription drugs can lead to CKD (e.g., cocaine-induced glomerulonephritis, Ma Huang–induced ephedrine kidney stones).

Past medical history may clue in to possible etiologies; for example, diabetic retinopathy to diabetic nephropathy; recurrent urinary tract infection to renal calculi; and hepatitis C, infective endocarditis, or Wegner's granulomatosis to glomerulonephritis.

Physical examination can reveal the presence of anemia, skin rash (such as in endocarditis, Fabry's disease, Henoch-Schönlein purpura, or cryoglobulinemia), rales, pericardial or pleural friction rub, pedal edema, abdominal bruit, or enlarged kidneys. Retinal examination is of particular importance and may reveal diabetic retinopathy or changes associated with hypertension; in a patient with rapid deterioration of renal function, retinal examination may show cholesterol emboli or septic emboli, pointing to the existence of cholesterol emboli or bacterial endocarditis as possible causes. Rectal examination to assess prostate enlargement in men and pelvic examination in women may point to clues to urinary tract obstruction such as a tumor or neurogenic bladder. Examination of the muscle mass is important when interpreting serum creatinine concentration (see later discussion).

The assessment of blood pressure is particularly important. Often, blood pressure is elevated in the clinic but normal at home *(white coat hypertension)*. Occasionally, the blood pressure is elevated at home but not in the clinic *(masked hypertension)*. In patients who complain of orthostatic symptoms but appear to have normal or high blood pressure in the clinic, home blood pressure measurements or 24-hour ambulatory blood pressure monitoring may be required. The latter may reveal very low blood pressure with orthostatic symptoms, and antihypertensive therapy may need to be modified.

The overall condition of the patient and level of functional status is important in deciding therapies. For example, transplantation may be an option for a patient with correctable cardiovascular disease and dialysis for someone with calcified iliac arteries where kidney transplant may not be possible. However, the physician and the patient's family may share the decision to forego renal replacement in an elderly person with advanced dementia and poor functional status.

Assessment of Kidney Function

Knowledge of both the severity of renal impairment and the rate of change in renal function is important in managing CKD. Rapid deterioration of kidney function over a few weeks to a few months may not reflect native renal disease progression; rather, it may reflect superimposed volume depletion (e.g., escalation in the dose of diuretics), exposure to nephrotoxins (e.g., NSAID use), or urinary tract obstruction. Alternatively, rapid progression of kidney disease may be seen in certain disease states such as malignant hypertension, crescentic glomerulonephritis, microangiopathic hemolytic anemia (thrombotic thrombocytopenic purpura, scleroderma), vasculitides (lupus nephritis, Wegener's granulomatosis), atheroembolic renal disease, or multiple myeloma. In general, a slower progression of decline in kidney failure is anticipated in patients with CKD caused by polycystic kidney disease, hypertension, or diabetes mellitus.

Serum creatinine is the most commonly measured of kidney functions. Along with the assessment of albuminuria, it is an important component for staging CKD (Fig. 2.1). If estimated GFR is less than 60 mL/min/1.73 m^2 for 3 months or longer, kidney disease is said to be chronic.

Notably, serum creatinine concentration does not rise to above the population threshold of normal (about 1.3 mg/dL in men and 1.1 mg/dL in women) until approximately 40% of kidney function is lost. In earlier stages of kidney disease, serum creatinine is maintained in the normal range by enhanced tubular secretion of creatinine. This process of creatinine secretion requires cationic transporters, and drugs that compete with creatinine secretion (e.g., cimetidine, triamterene, trimethoprim) may cause elevation of serum creatinine without depressing true GFR. A clinical clue to an impairment in cationic transport of creatinine is the lack of rise in blood urea nitrogen despite an increase in serum creatinine concentration.

With advanced kidney failure, the magnitude of absolute changes in serum creatinine concentration may be more rapid. The relationship between serum creatinine and GFR is nonlinear, accelerating as the GFR declines. This means, for example, that an increase in serum creatinine concentration from 3 to 3.5 mg/dL is associated with a lesser decline in GFR than is a change from 1 to 1.5 mg/dL. Specific knowledge of the baseline level of serum creatinine is important; for example, change from 0.6 to 1.2 mg/dL is still within the normal range in an adult man but actually reflects an approximately 57% loss of GFR.

为 CKD 病因需要全面评估除外其他潜在病因。值得注意的是，在高血压患者中，已发现 *APOL1* 等基因与肾脏疾病的高风险有关，未来基因分析可能会成为明确高风险人群的一种方法，以便将来制定预防策略。

一旦确诊为 CKD，就需要持续进行评估，因为 CKD 患者出现高血压、代谢性骨病、贫血、高钾血症和代谢性酸中毒等并发症的风险会增加。此外，CKD 的最初诊断可能会随着时间的推移而改变，例如在糖尿病患者中发现红细胞管型。AKI 可叠加在 CKD 上。评估高血压需要准确测量血压。建议在安静休息后，使用电子血压计测量三次，每次间隔 1 min；不再建议使用柯氏音听诊法测量血压。如果高血压或容量超负荷难以控制，可通过收集 24 h 尿液来估算饮食中的钠摄入量。通常处方给 CKD 患者的药物数量较多，因此应监测服药依从性，依从性差可能为血压控制不佳的原因。有关动脉血压测量的详细方法和不同观点，请参阅《心血管疾病分册》第 11 章。

病史和检查

CKD 患者的体征和症状取决于就诊时所处的阶段。病程早期的典型症状是非特异性乏力，体格检查可能无法发现 CKD 的蛛丝马迹，因此需要进行实验室筛查。随着 GFR 下降，CKD 症状和体征会更常见，可见足部水肿、面部水肿、腰痛、多尿、夜尿和高血压。与尿毒症有关的症状，如恶心、纳差和呕吐等往往出现得较晚，不应作为早期 CKD 诊断的依据。

有时，原发疾病的表现占主导地位。例如，一名年轻女性出现发热、关节痛和皮疹，同时伴有肾衰竭和活动性尿沉渣，则高度提示狼疮性肾炎；静脉注射药物者，出现心脏杂音、心脏瓣膜赘生物以及血培养阳性，则应警惕心内膜炎相关性肾小球肾炎的可能诊断。耳聋、血尿和 CKD 的家族史提示 Alport 综合征的诊断；动脉瘤破裂导致的脑出血病史可提示多囊肾病。

用药史应重点关注肾毒性药物的暴露史，包括长期使用非甾体抗炎药（NSAID）、锂、顺铂以及近期增加利尿剂的剂量。一些非处方药可导致 CKD（如可卡因引起的肾小球肾炎、麻黄碱引起的肾结石）。

既往病史也可提示可能的病因；例如，糖尿病视网膜病变提示可能存在糖尿病肾病；反复尿路感染提示肾结石；丙型肝炎、感染性心内膜炎或韦格纳肉芽肿病提示相关的肾小球肾炎。

体格检查可发现贫血、皮疹（如心内膜炎、法布里病、过敏性紫癜或冷球蛋白血症）、啰音、心包或胸膜摩擦音、足部水肿、腹部搏动或肾脏肿大。视网膜检查尤为重要，可发现糖尿病视网膜病变或与高血压相关的改变；在肾功能急剧恶化的患者中，视网膜检查可显示胆固醇栓子或感染中毒性栓子，表明胆固醇结晶栓塞或者感染性心内膜炎是可能的病因。对男性进行直肠检查以评估前列腺肥大，对女性进行盆腔检查，可发现尿路梗阻的线索，如肿瘤或神经源性膀胱。在解释血清肌酐浓度时，检查肌肉质量非常重要（见下文讨论）。

血压评估尤为重要。患者一般在医院血压升高，但在家中血压正常（白大衣高血压）。偶尔，患者在家时血压升高，但在医院时血压并不升高（隐匿性高血压）。对于主诉有直立性症状但在诊所血压正常或偏高的患者，可能需要进行家庭血压测量或 24 h 动态血压监测。24 h 动态血压监测可能会发现血压非常低并伴有直立性症状，因此可能需要调整降压治疗。

在决定治疗方案时，患者的全身状况和功能状态的水平非常重要。例如，对于心血管疾病可以纠正的患者来说，移植可能是一种选择，而对于髂动脉钙化而无法进行肾移植的患者来说，透析可能是一种选择。然而，对于晚期痴呆和功能状况不佳的老年人，医生和患者家属可能会共同决定放弃肾脏替代治疗。

肾功能评估

了解肾功能损伤的严重程度和肾功能变化的速度对于 CKD 的管理非常重要。几周到几个月内肾功能的快速变化可能并不反映原发肾脏疾病的进展，它可能反映了叠加的容量耗竭（如利尿剂剂量的增加）、肾毒性药物暴露（如使用非甾体抗炎药）或尿路梗阻等因素。另外，在某些疾病状态下，肾病可呈现快速进展，如恶性高血压、新月体性肾小球肾炎、微血管病性溶血性贫血（血栓性血小板减少性紫癜、硬皮病）、血管炎（狼疮性肾炎、韦格纳肉芽肿病）、动脉粥样硬化性肾病及多发性骨髓瘤等。一般来说，由多囊肾病、高血压或糖尿病引起的 CKD 患者的肾功能进展较慢。

血清肌酐是最常检测的肾功能指标。它与白蛋白尿一起评估，是对 CKD 进行分期的重要组成部分（图 2.1）。如果估算的 GFR 持续 3 个月或更长时间低于 60 ml/(min·1.73 m^2)，则肾脏疾病被视为慢性的。

值得注意的是，在肾功能丧失约 40% 之前，血清肌酐不会超过正常人群的临界值（男性约为 1.3 mg/dl，女性约为 1.1 mg/dl）。在肾脏疾病的早期阶段，肾小管分泌肌酐的功能增强，因此血清肌酐会维持在正常范围内。肌酐分泌过程需要阳离子转运体，与肌酐分泌竞争的药物（如西咪替丁、氨苯蝶啶、甲氧苄啶等）可能会导致血清肌酐升高，但不会降低真正的 GFR。肌酐阳离子转运受损的一个临床表现是，尽管血清肌酐浓度升高，但血尿素氮却没有升高。

在肾衰竭晚期，血清肌酐浓度的绝对变化幅度可能会更快。血清肌酐与 GFR 之间的关系是非线性的，肌酐随着 GFR 的下降而加快上升。例如，血清肌酐浓度从 3 mg/dl 上升到 3.5 mg/dl，比从 1 mg/dl 上升到 1.5 mg/dl 时其 GFR 的下降程度要小。对血清肌酐基线水平的具体了解非常重要；例如，血清肌酐从 0.6 mg/dl 上升至 1.2 mg/dl，虽仍属于成年男性的正常范围，但实际上却反映出约 57% 的 GFR 下降。

			Persistent albuminuria categories Description and range		
Prognosis of CKD by GFR and Albuminuria Categories: KDIGO 2012			A1	A2	A3
			Normal to mildly increased	Moderately increased	Severely increased
			<30 mg/g <3 mg/mmol	30–300 mg/g 3–30 mg/mmol	>300 mg/g >30 mg/mmol
GFR categories (ml/min/1.73 m²) Description and range	G1	Normal or high	≥90		
	G2	Mildly decreased	60–89		
	G3a	Mildly to moderately decreased	45–59		
	G3b	Moderately to severely decreased	30–44		
	G4	Severely decreased	15–29		
	G5	Kidney failure	<15		

Green: Low risk (if no other markers of kidney disease, no CKD); Yellow: moderately increased risk; Orange: high risk; Red: very high risk.

Fig. 2.1 Chronic kidney disease (CKD) nomenclature used by the Kidney Disease Improving Global Outcomes (KDIGO) consortium. CKD is defined as abnormalities of kidney structure or function, present for 3 months or longer, with implications for health. CKD is classified on the bases of cause, glomerular filtration rate (GFR), and albuminuria. (From KDIGO: 2012 clinical practice guideline for the evaluation and management of chronic kidney disease, Kid Intl Suppl 3:18, 2013. Available at http://www.kdigo.org/clinical_practice_guidelines/pdf/CKD/KDIGO_2012_CKD_GL.pdf. Accessed June 1, 2014.)

The relationship between GFR and serum creatinine is best interpreted at steady state and not when the GFR is changing rapidly. For example, bilateral nephrectomy in a patient with previously normal kidney function (as might occur in a patient with renal cell carcinoma) results in a drop in GFR from 100 to 0 mL/min. However, serum creatinine would be expected to increase by only about 1 mg/dL/day, and a plateau may not be achieved before 1 week. This delay reflects the fact that the generation of creatinine is insufficient to saturate the volume of distribution of creatinine. A plateau will be reached more rapidly if the rate of creatinine generation is increased, the volume of distribution of creatinine is small, or residual renal function is substantial. Given these variables, it is important to be aware that serum creatinine may be a poor marker of GFR in non–steady-state conditions. Similarly, among patients with end-stage renal disease receiving renal replacement therapy although the laboratory may report eGFR (estimated GFR), this is a poor estimate of GFR given that the creatinine is being removed by extracorporeal means.

There also are several conditions in which serum creatinine may be falsely low in relation to the GFR. Because creatinine generation is dependent on muscle mass, low creatinine generation occurs in diseases associated with sarcopenia, such as motor neuron diseases (amyotrophic lateral sclerosis), wasting illnesses (advanced cancer, tuberculosis, cardiac cachexia), and even malnutrition. Visual examination of muscle mass (thighs, arms, temporal muscles) may therefore be important in the interpretation of serum creatinine concentrations. Other conditions associated with low creatinine generation include cirrhosis and advanced age. Creatinine generation is reduced in sepsis, and kidney function may be worse than is detectable by estimation of GFR through measurement of serum creatinine.

Among patients with severe CKD (e.g., GFR <20 mL/min), creatinine is secreted and urea is absorbed by the tubule. Tubular secretion of creatinine is fortuitously balanced by tubular reabsorption of urea, making measurements of urea clearance and creatinine clearance useful in estimating true GFR. An average of creatinine and urea clearance closely approximates true GFR in such situations.

At steady state—that is, when the patient is neither gaining nor losing weight—the 24-hour urine urea nitrogen measurement can be used to estimate dietary protein intake. In addition to its excretion in urine, nitrogen is lost through the gut, through the skin, and, as non-urea nitrogen, through the kidney in proportion to body weight. It is estimated that 31 mg/kg/day of non-urea nitrogen is excreted in this fashion. Dietary protein intake can be calculated as 6.25 g protein per gram of total daily nitrogen excretion. Accordingly, the formula for dietary protein intake in grams per day is (urine urea nitrogen + 0.031 × body weight in kg) × 6.25.

Although urea by itself is less useful to assess kidney function, it can be helpful in conjunction with the serum creatinine measurement. Urea is reabsorbed by the tubule in sodium-avid states. The normal ratio of urea to creatinine is 10:1. In states of volume depletion such as diuretic use, diarrhea, sweat losses, or third spacing (e.g., leakage of fluid outside the vascular compartment such as in peritoneal cavity [ascites] or pleural space [pleural effusion]), the urea-to-creatinine ratio may be greater than 20:1. Sometimes, ratios greater than 20:1 are also seen in catabolic states (e.g., long-bone fracture, corticosteroid use, burns, sepsis), increased gut protein load (upper gastrointestinal bleeding, high-protein diet), or obstructive uropathy. In contrast, creatinine may rise disproportionally more than urea, for example in advanced cirrhosis, low-protein diets, or states associated with the use of cationic transport inhibitors (e.g., cimetidine).

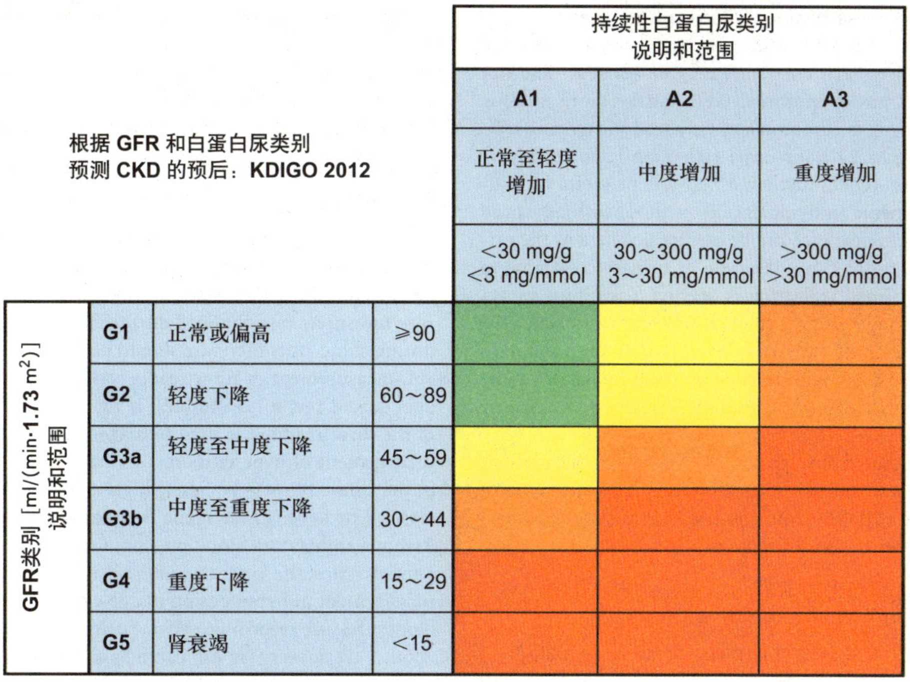

		根据 GFR 和白蛋白尿类别 预测 CKD 的预后：KDIGO 2012	持续性白蛋白尿类别 说明和范围		
			A1 正常至轻度增加	A2 中度增加	A3 重度增加
			<30 mg/g <3 mg/mmol	30~300 mg/g 3~30 mg/mmol	>300 mg/g >30 mg/mmol
GFR类别 [ml/(min·1.73 m²)] 说明和范围	G1	正常或偏高 ≥90	绿	黄	橙
	G2	轻度下降 60~89	绿	黄	橙
	G3a	轻度至中度下降 45~59	黄	橙	红
	G3b	中度至重度下降 30~44	橙	红	红
	G4	重度下降 15~29	红	红	红
	G5	肾衰竭 <15	红	红	红

绿色：低风险（如果没有其他肾病标志物，则无 CKD）；黄色：中度增加的风险
橙：高风险；红色：极高风险。

图 2.1 慢性肾脏病（CKD）采用改善全球肾脏预后联盟（KDIGO）的命名，是指肾脏结构或功能出现异常，且持续 3 个月或更长时间，并对健康产生影响。CKD 根据病因、GFR 和白蛋白尿进行分类（引自 KDIGO：2012 clinical practice guideline for the evaluation and management of chronic kidney disease，Kid Intl Suppl 3：18，2013. Available at http://www.kdigo.org/clinical_practice_guidelines/pdf/CKD/KDIGO_2012_CKD_GL.pdf. Accessed June 1，2014.）

阐释 GFR 与血清肌酐之间的关系最好在稳态下进行，而非 GFR 快速变化时。例如，肾功能正常的患者（如肾细胞癌患者）进行双侧肾切除术后，其 GFR 会从 100 ml/min 降至 0 ml/min。然而，血清肌酐预计每天仅增加约 1 mg/dl，而且在 1 周内可能不会达到高峰。这种延迟反映了肌酐生成量不足以使肌酐分布容积达到饱和这一事实。如果肌酐生成速度加快、肌酐分布容积较小或残余肾功能较强，则会更快达到稳态。考虑到这些变量，我们必须意识到，在非稳态条件下，血清肌酐并非反映 GFR 的合适指标。同样，在接受肾脏替代疗法的终末期肾病患者中，尽管实验室可能会报告 eGFR（估算的 GFR），但由于肌酐是通过体外途径清除的，因此对 GFR 的估算并不准确。

此外，在一些情况下，血清肌酐与 GFR 相比可能会假性偏低。由于肌酐生成取决于肌肉质量，肌酐生成低可见于肌肉减少症相关的疾病中，如运动神经元疾病（肌萎缩性脊髓侧索硬化症）、消耗性疾病（晚期癌症、肺结核、心脏恶病质）甚至营养不良。因此，目测肌肉质量（大腿、手臂和颞部肌肉）对于解释血清肌酐浓度可能很重要。其他与肌酐生成量低有关的情况包括肝硬化和高龄。感染中毒症时肌酐生成减少，肾功能可能比通过血清肌酐测量的 eGFR 所反映的更差。

在晚期 CKD 患者（如 GFR < 20 ml/min）中，肾小管分泌肌酐，重吸收尿素。肾小管分泌的肌酐与肾小管重吸收的尿素正好平衡，因此测量尿素清除率和肌酐清除率有助于估算真实的 GFR。在这种情况下，肌酐和尿素清除率的平均值很接近真实的 GFR。

在稳态下，即患者体重既不增加也不减少时，24 h 尿液尿素氮测量值可用于估算饮食中蛋白质的摄入量。除了通过尿液排泄外，氮还会通过肠道、皮肤排出，通过肾脏按体重比例以非尿素氮的形式流失。据估计，以这种方式排出的非尿素氮为 31 mg/(kg·d)。膳食蛋白质摄入量可按每克每日总氮排泄量 6.25 g 蛋白质计算。因此，以克为单位的每日膳食蛋白质摄入量计算公式为 [尿液尿素氮 + 0.031 × 体重（kg）] × 6.25。

虽然尿素本身对评估肾功能作用不大，但与血清肌酐结合使用会有帮助。在无钠状态下，尿素会被肾小管重吸收。尿素与肌酐的正常比为 10∶1。在容量耗竭状态下，如使用利尿剂、腹泻、汗液丢失或第三间隙 [如腹腔（腹水）或胸膜腔（胸腔积液）等向血管腔外液体渗漏]，尿素与肌酐比可能大于 20∶1。有时，在分解代谢状态（如长骨骨折、使用皮质类固醇、烧伤、感染中毒症）、肠道蛋白负荷增加（上消化道出血、高蛋白饮食）或梗阻性肾病时，尿素与肌酐比也会大于 20∶1。相反，肌酐的升高也可能会超过尿素的升高，例如在晚期肝硬化、低蛋白饮食或使用阳离子转运体抑制剂（如西咪替丁）的情况下。

For many decades, the assessment of creatinine clearance by a 24-hour urine collection has been the mainstay of assessing renal function. However, given that creatinine may be secreted (and not just filtered), this test may overestimate GFR. Furthermore, voiding outside the collection jug is common and may lead to errors in estimating GFR. Although a 24-hour urine collection is not routinely recommended to assess renal function, it may still be useful for estimating GFR in sarcopenic individuals and in those with advanced liver disease. Creatinine clearance can be easily calculated as the urinary flow rate (in mL/min) times the ratio of urinary creatinine to plasma creatinine. A timed collection is needed. Creatinine excretion approximates 15 mg/kg/day. Although this rate is variable (the coefficient of variation from day to day over 28 days on a standard diet varies from 6% to 22%) and depends on meat intake, it can be used to estimate whether urine has been grossly undercollected or overcollected.

Usually, GFR is estimated through the use of equations that account for age in years, race, sex, and serum creatinine. The Modification of Diet in Renal Disease (MDRD) equation uses a creatinine measurement (Scr) that has been calibrated to an isotope dilution mass spectrometry standard:

$$\text{GFR } [\text{in mL/min}/1.73\,\text{m}^2] = 175 \times (\text{Scr})^{-1.154} \times (\text{Age})^{-0.203} \times 0.742 \text{ [if female]} \times 1.212 \text{ [if black]}$$

A newer equation, called the Chronic Kidney Disease Epidemiology Collaboration (CKD-EPI) equation, is less likely to estimate GFR as low if the GFR is higher than 60 mL/min/1.73 m². This equation is more complicated:

$$\text{GFR } [60\,\text{ml/min}/1.73\,\text{m}^2] = 141 \times min(\text{Scr}/k, 1)^{\alpha} \times max(\text{Scr}/k, 1)^{-1.209} \times 0.993^{\text{Age}} \times 1.018 \text{ [if female]} \times 1.159 \text{ [if black]}$$

where Scr is serum creatinine (in mg/dL), κ is 0.7 for females and 0.9 for males, α is −0.329 for females and −0.411 for males, *min* indicates the minimum of Scr/κ or 1, and *max* indicates the maximum of Scr/κ or 1. Several calculators to estimate GFR using the CKD-EPI equation or the MDRD equation are available on the World Wide Web or as applications for personal devices.

Assessment of Albuminuria

The assessment of albuminuria is fundamental because it may point to the cause of the CKD. Furthermore, the severity of albuminuria is directly associated with an accelerated progression of CKD and cardiovascular disease. As a result, albuminuria is now used to stage CKD (see Fig. 2.1).

Albumin excretion rate is normally less than 10 mg/24 hr, and an excretion rate of 30 mg/24 hr or higher is considered abnormal and moderately increased. An albumin excretion rate of 300 mg/24 hr or higher is considered severely increased. Albuminuria can be more conveniently assessed by measuring the ratio of urine albumin and urine creatinine concentrations in a spontaneously voided urine specimen. Given that the creatinine excretion rate averages 1 g/day, an albumin-to-creatinine ratio of 30 mg/g creatinine or higher is considered abnormal and moderately increased; a ratio of 300 mg/g creatinine is considered severely increased.

An albumin excretion rate higher than 2200 mg/24 hr (which corresponds to approximately 3000 mg protein/24 hr) is considered nephrotic. Such a degree of albuminuria/proteinuria is often accompanied by edema, hypoalbuminemia, and hyperlipidemia. The combination of these disorders is referred to as the *nephrotic syndrome* and reflects a profound disorder of glomerular permselectivity. Common causes of nephrotic syndrome in adults are diabetic nephropathy, focal segmental glomerulosclerosis, membranous nephropathy, and amyloidosis. Among children, minimal change nephropathy and focal segmental glomerulosclerosis are important causes of nephrotic syndrome.

Assessment of Blood Pressure

Hypertension is a common accompaniment of CKD, yet the evaluation of hypertension often is performed poorly. Current management of hypertension is directed most often to management of blood pressure measurements obtained during clinic visits. Measurement of BP during clinic visits therefore should be accurately performed. At present, measurement of three readings of BP in the nondominant arm, after seated rest for 5 minutes, is the standard of care. The average of the three readings is used to make clinical decisions regarding the management of hypertension. Despite accurate measurements of BP in the clinic, BP may be falsely higher in the clinic *(white coat hypertension)* or lower in the clinic *(masked hypertension)* compared with 24-hour ambulatory blood pressure measurements. At present, in the United States, the latter technique is mostly limited to research or to management of hypertension in a few difficult cases. However, home blood pressure recordings self-measured by the patient twice daily for about 1 week every month can help diagnose and manage hypertension more effectively. Self-performance of these measurements may promote adoption of a more healthful diet and better medication adherence by the patient, as well as reducing therapeutic inertia on the part of the physician.

An important cause of poor control of BP in patients with or without CKD is poor medication adherence. Pill burden directly relates to nonadherence with medications, and patients with CKD are often prescribed multiple medications. Thus, the assessment of adherence to medications should be a routine part of assessment.

Assessment of Dietary Sodium Intake

At steady state, when body weight is neither increasing nor decreasing, the dietary sodium intake can be judged by 24-hour urine collection. To establish adequacy of urine collection, the measurement of urine creatinine in 24-hour urine sample is important. The creatinine excretion rate in an adequately collected specimen should approach 1 g/day for women and 1.5 g/day for men. Dietary potassium and protein intake can be monitored similarly. Measurement of urine urea nitrogen in the 24-hour urine sample can reveal the adequacy of dietary protein intake. Dietary sodium restriction can improve blood pressure, can enhance the biologic actions of inhibitors of the renin-angiotensin system, and may protect the heart, blood vessels, and kidneys independent of improvement in blood pressure.

Microscopic Urinalysis

Microscopic urinalysis at initial evaluation and on an ongoing basis can reveal vital information about the health of the kidney. Evaluation should be performed by centrifugation of at least 12 mL of a freshly voided specimen. Cells, casts, crystals, and other elements can corroborate the diagnosis of the cause of CKD. Examples are shown in Figs. 2.2 through 2.5.

Renal Imaging

Bladder ultrasonography is a tool that can be used to assess residual urine volume. The wide availability of this tool allows diagnosis of bladder outlet obstruction without the need to catheterize the patient.

几十年来，通过收集 24 h 尿液来评估肌酐清除率一直是评估肾功能的主要方法。然而，由于肌酐可以被分泌（而不仅仅是过滤），这种检测方法可能会高估 GFR。此外，尿液排在收集壶外的情况很常见，也会导致应用肌酐清除率来估算 GFR 出现误差。虽然 24 h 尿液收集并不是评估肾功能的常规推荐方法，但对于肌肉减少者和晚期肝病患者，24 h 尿液收集仍可用于估算 GFR。肌酐清除率可以通过尿流率（单位：ml/min）乘以尿肌酐与血浆肌酐的比值轻松计算出来。定时采集尿液标本也是需要的。肌酐排泄量约为 15 mg/（kg·d）。虽然该量是可变的（标准饮食 28 天内每天的变化系数从 6% 到 22% 不等），并且取决于肉类的摄入量，但仍可用于估计尿液收集是否严重不足或收集过量。

通常，GFR 是根据年龄、种族、性别和血清肌酐计算得出的。肾脏病饮食改良试验（MDRD）方程使用的是根据同位素稀释质谱标准校准的肌酐测量值（Scr）：

$$\text{GFR} [\text{按照 ml}/(\text{min} \cdot 1.73 \text{ m}^2)] = 175 \times (\text{Scr})^{-1.154} \times (\text{年龄})^{-0.203} \times 0.742 (\text{女性}) \times 1.212 (\text{黑人})$$

CKD 流行病学协作组（CKD-EPI）方程是一个较新的公式，如果 GFR 高于 60 ml/（min·1.73 m²），则 GFR 估计值较低的可能性较小。该方程更为复杂：

$$\text{GFR} [60 \text{ ml}/(\text{min} \cdot 1.73 \text{ m}^2)] = 141 \times \min(\text{Scr/k}, 1)^{\alpha} \times \max(\text{Scr/k}, 1)^{-1209} \times 0.993^{\text{年龄}} \times 1.018 (\text{女性}) \times 1.159 (\text{黑人})$$

其中，Scr 是血清肌酐（以 mg/dl 为单位），k 女性为 0.7，男性为 0.9，α 女性为 −0.329，男性为 −0.411，min 表示 Scr/k 的最小值或 1，max 表示 Scr/k 或 1 的最大值。在万维网（World Wide Web）或个人设备的应用程序上，有几种计算器可以使用 CKD-EPI 方程或 MDRD 方程估算 GFR。

白蛋白尿评估

白蛋白尿的评估非常重要，因为它可以提示 CKD 的病因。此外，白蛋白尿的严重程度与 CKD 和心血管疾病的加速进展直接相关。因此，白蛋白尿现在用来对 CKD 进行分期（图 2.1）。

白蛋白排泄率通常低于 10 mg/24 h，30 mg/24 h 或更高的排泄率视为异常和中度增加。300 mg/24 h 或更高的白蛋白排泄率是严重增加。通过测量自然排出的尿液标本中尿白蛋白和尿肌酐浓度的比值，可以更方便地评估白蛋白尿。鉴于肌酐排泄率平均为 1 g/d，白蛋白与肌酐的比值达到或超过 30 mg/g 肌酐为异常和中度增高；比值达到 300 mg/g 肌酐为重度增高。

白蛋白排泄率超过 2200 mg/24 h（相当于约 3000 mg 蛋白质/24 h）即为肾病范围蛋白尿，这种程度的白蛋白尿/蛋白尿通常伴有水肿、低白蛋白血症和高脂血症。这些异常被统称为肾病综合征，反映了肾小球通透性选择性的严重失调。成人肾病综合征的常见病因是糖尿病肾病、局灶节段性肾小球硬化、膜性肾病和淀粉样变性。在儿童中，微小病变肾病和局灶节段性肾小球硬化是重要原因。

血压评估

高血压是 CKD 的常见并发症，但对高血压的评估往往做得不够。目前对高血压的管理通常是针对门诊时测量的血压。因此，应在门诊期间准确测量血压。目前的标准是，在坐位休息 5 min 后，测量非惯用手臂的 3 次血压。3 次血压读数的平均值可用于对高血压的临床治疗决策。尽管诊室血压测量结果准确，但与 24 h 动态血压测量结果相比，诊室血压可能会假性升高（白大衣高血压）或假性降低（隐匿性高血压）。目前，在美国，24 h 动态血压测量大多仅限于研究或少数疑难病例的高血压治疗。然而，患者每月 1 次、每次持续 1 周、每天 2 次的家庭血压自我测量可以帮助更有效地诊断和管理高血压。自测血压可以促进患者更健康的饮食习惯，更好地坚持服药，在医生层面同时改善用药的习惯。

无论是否患有 CKD，患者血压控制不佳的一个重要原因是服药依从性差。药物负担直接导致用药的依从性差，而 CKD 患者通常会被处方多种药物。因此，对服药依从性的评估应成为常规评估的一部分。

膳食钠摄入量评估

在体重稳态下，膳食钠摄入量可通过 24 h 尿液采集来判断。要确定尿液收集是否充分，测量 24 h 尿样中的尿肌酐非常重要。在收集充分的标本中，女性的尿肌酐排泄率应接近 1 g/d，男性接近 1.5 g/d。饮食中钾和蛋白质的摄入量也可进行类似监测。通过测量 24 h 尿样中的尿素氮可以了解饮食中蛋白质摄入量是否充足。饮食限钠可改善血压，增强肾素-血管紧张素系统抑制剂的生物作用，并可保护心血管和肾脏，而该保护作用与血压改善无关。

显微镜检尿液分析

初次评估和持续的尿液显微镜检查可以揭示肾脏健康的重要信息。应通过离心至少 12 ml 的新鲜尿标本来进行检查。细胞、管型、结晶和其他成分可以证实 CKD 病因的诊断。示例参见图 2.2 至 2.5。

肾脏影像

膀胱超声检查是一种可用于评估残余尿量的工具。可广泛用于诊断膀胱出口梗阻，不再需要对患者进行插管。

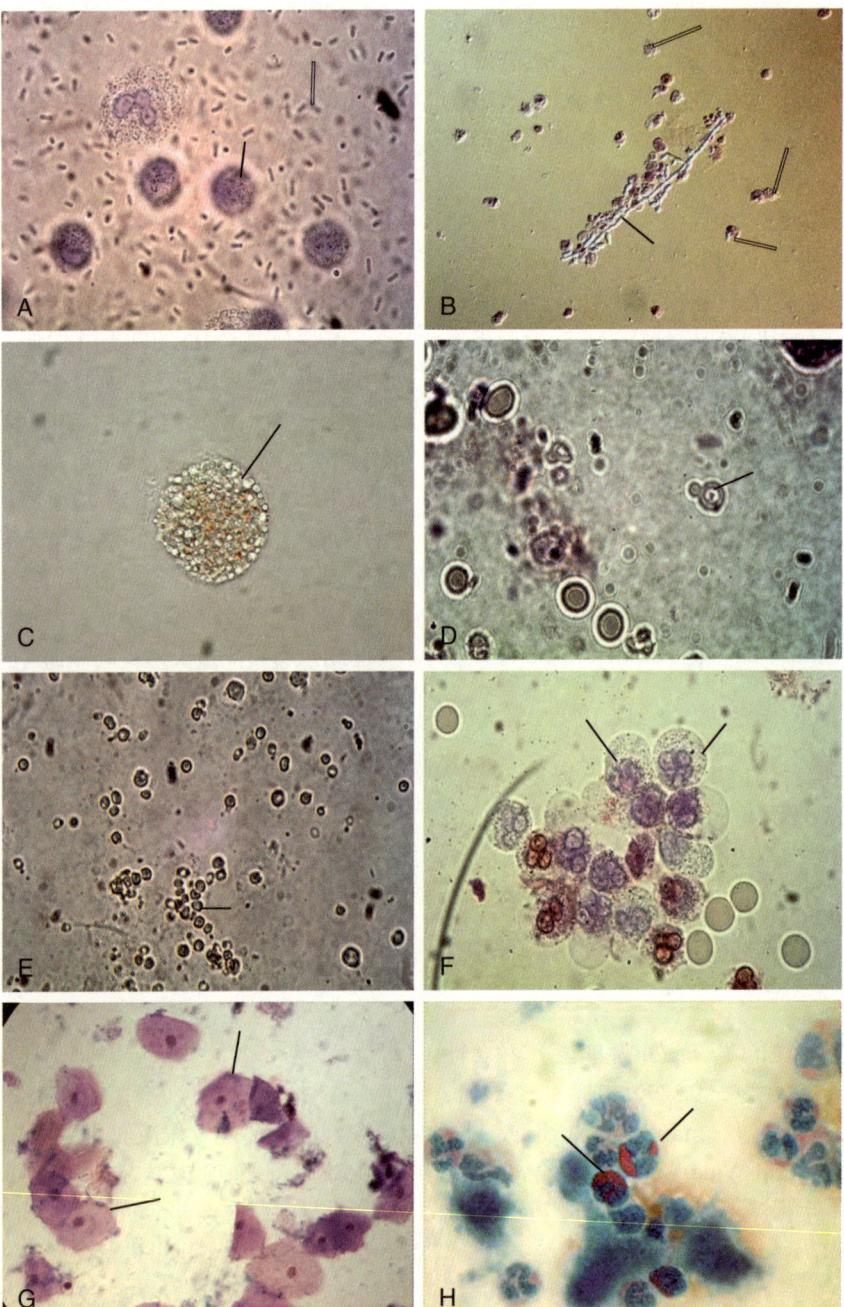

Fig. 2.2 Cells often found in urine of patients with kidney disease. (A) Sternheimer-Malbin–stained urine sediment (100× objective) in a patient with urinary tract infection. *Solid line* shows a leukocyte and *hollow line* indicates bacteria. (B) Sternheimer-Malbin–stained urine sediment (40×) in a patient with fungal urinary tract infection. *Solid line* shows a pseudohypha and *hollow lines* indicate leukocytes. (C) Unstained urine sediment (40×) shows an oval fat body in a patient with nephrotic syndrome. (D) Sternheimer-Malbin–stained urine sediment (100×) in a patient with immunoglobulin A (IgA) nephropathy. *Solid line* shows an acanthocyte characterized by outpouching of the red blood cell (RBC) membrane. (E) Sternheimer-Malbin–stained urine sediment (40×) in a patient with IgA nephropathy shows many acanthocytes *(solid line)*. When acanthocytes constitute more than 5% of the RBCs, their presence is considered significant. (F) Sternheimer-Malbin–stained urine sediment (100×) in a patient with recovering acute tubular necrosis (ATN). *Solid lines* indicate glitter cells. The granules of these leukocytes have a Brownian motion and appear to glitter under the microscope. These cells can be seen in large numbers during the recovery stage of ATN and in patients with urinary tract infection. (G) Sternheimer-Malbin–stained urine sediment (40×) shows numerous squamous cells, indicating poor collection technique. (H) Hansel-stained urine sediment (100×) shows eosinophils that can be seen in patients with allergic interstitial nephritis, cholesterol emboli, or, sometimes, urinary tract infection.

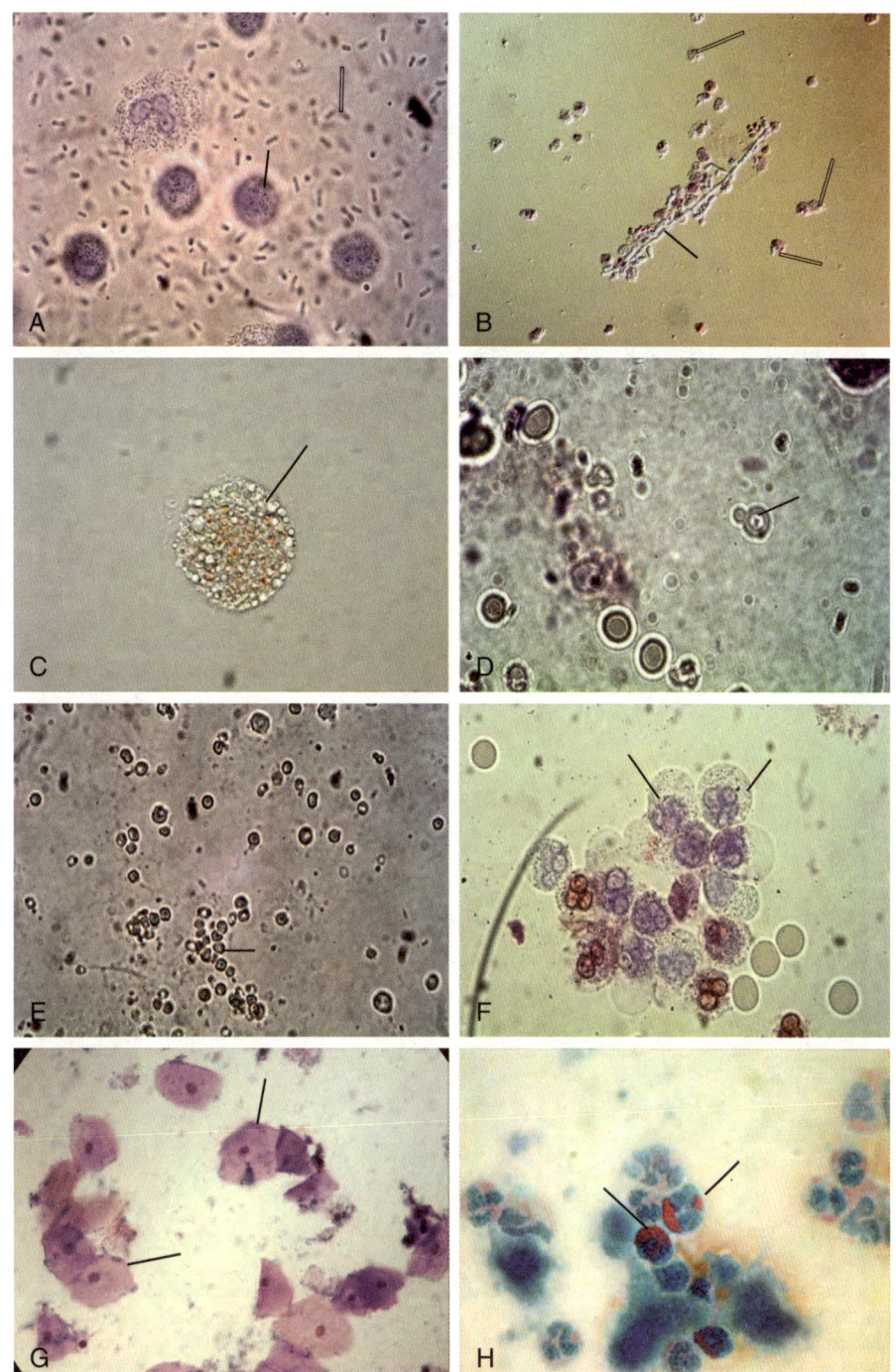

图 2.2 在肾脏疾病患者的尿液中经常可以发现的细胞。（**A**）尿路感染患者的 Sternheimer-Malbin 染色尿沉渣（100×），实线表示白细胞，空心线表示细菌。（**B**）真菌性尿路感染患者的 Sternheimer-Malbin 染色尿沉渣（40×），实线表示假菌丝，空心线表示白细胞。（**C**）肾病综合征患者未染色的尿沉渣（40×）显示有卵圆形脂肪体。（**D**）IgA 肾病患者 Sternheimer-Malbin 染色的尿沉渣（100×）。实线表示棘细胞，特点是红细胞膜外翻。（**E**）IgA 肾病患者的 Sternheimer-Malbin 染色尿沉渣（40×）显示许多棘细胞（实线）。当棘细胞占红细胞的 5% 以上时，其存在即被认为意义重大。（**F**）一名急性肾小管坏死（ATN）恢复期患者的 Sternheimer-Malbin 染色尿沉渣（100×）。实线表示闪光细胞。这些白细胞的颗粒有布朗运动，在显微镜下看起来闪闪发光。这些细胞在 ATN 恢复阶段和尿路感染患者中大量出现。（**G**）Sternheimer-Malbin 染色尿沉渣（40×）显示大量鳞状细胞，说明收集技术不佳。（**H**）Hansel 染色尿沉渣（100×）显示嗜酸性粒细胞，可见于过敏性间质性肾炎、胆固醇栓塞或偶见于尿路感染患者

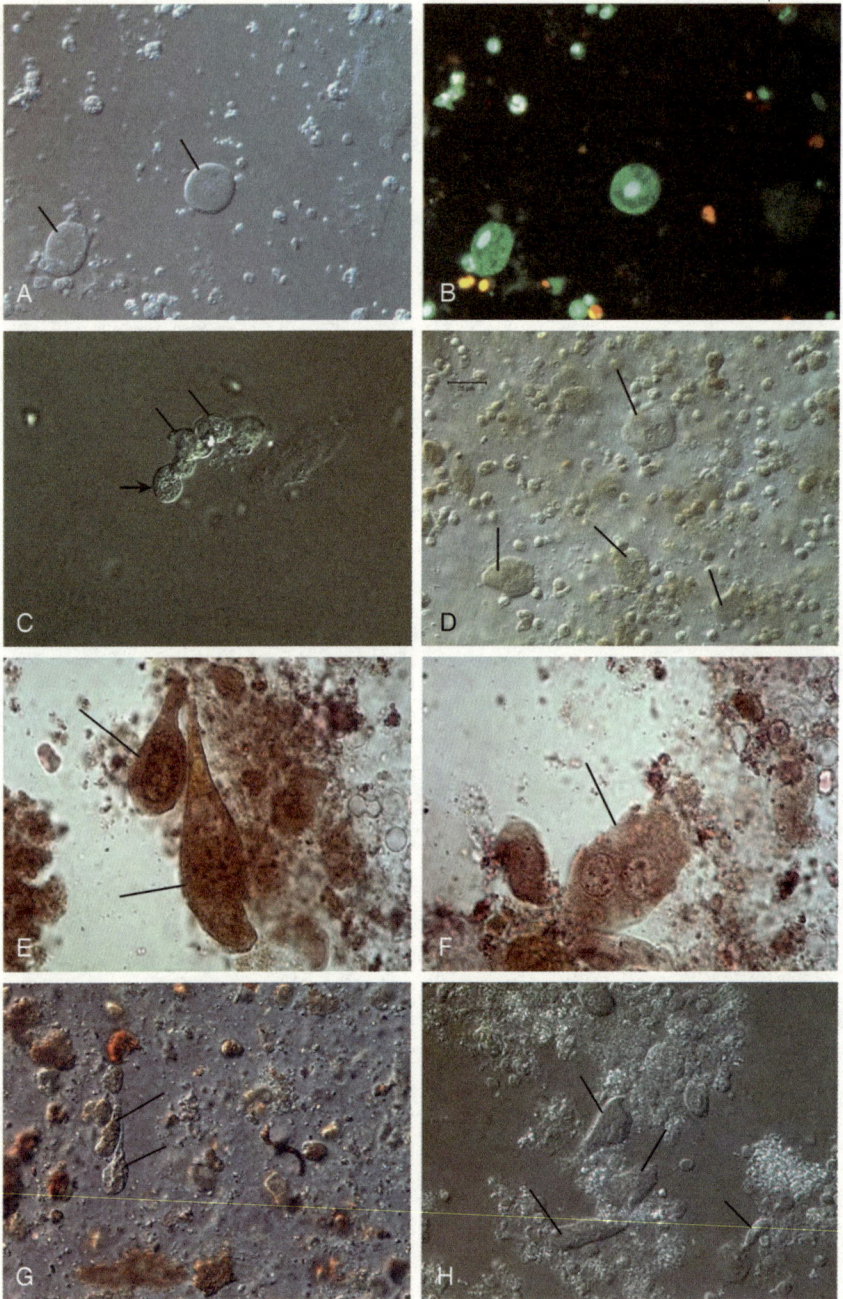

Fig. 2.3 Tubular cells often found in urine of patients with acute kidney injury. (A) Unstained urine sediment (40× objective) in a patient recovering from acute tubular necrosis (ATN). *Solid lines* show intact renal tubular epithelial cells. (B) Same specimen as in A but stained with acridine orange-propidium iodide and viewed with a triple excitation band fluorescence filter (triple-cube). Red cells are dead and green cells are live. Both tubular cells appear viable. Smaller cells are leukocytes. (C) Unstained urine sediment (40×) shows several renal tubular cells that appear monomorphic (as in images A and B), indicating acute tubular injury. The *arrow* indicates a binucleate tubular cell. (D) Unstained urine sediment (40×) shows several renal tubular cells *(solid lines)* that appear dysmorphic. Instead of being round, the cells are angular. Furthermore, these cells are multinucleated, indicating failure of the cell to divide. Large numbers of dysmorphic renal tubular cells are often seen if the acute tubular injury is substantial. (E) Unstained urine sediment (100×) shows two tear-drop-shaped dysmorphic renal tubular epithelial cells *(solid lines)*. Because the patient had jaundice, the cells appear to have a color despite lack of staining. (F) Unstained urine sediment (100×) shows one dysmorphic, binucleate renal tubular epithelial cell *(line)*. This is the same patient as in E. (G) Unstained urine sediment (40×) shows severe ATN. No dirty-brown granular casts were seen, but the tubular cells were dysmorphic *(lines)*. The large amount of granular debris and absence of casts suggests failure to form Tamm-Horsfall protein and more severe tubular injury. This patient also had jaundice, as is evident from the yellow hue. (H) Unstained urine sediment (40×) shows dysmorphic renal tubular epithelial cells (triangular, cigar-shaped, and polygonous), often multinucleated as denoted by *lines*.

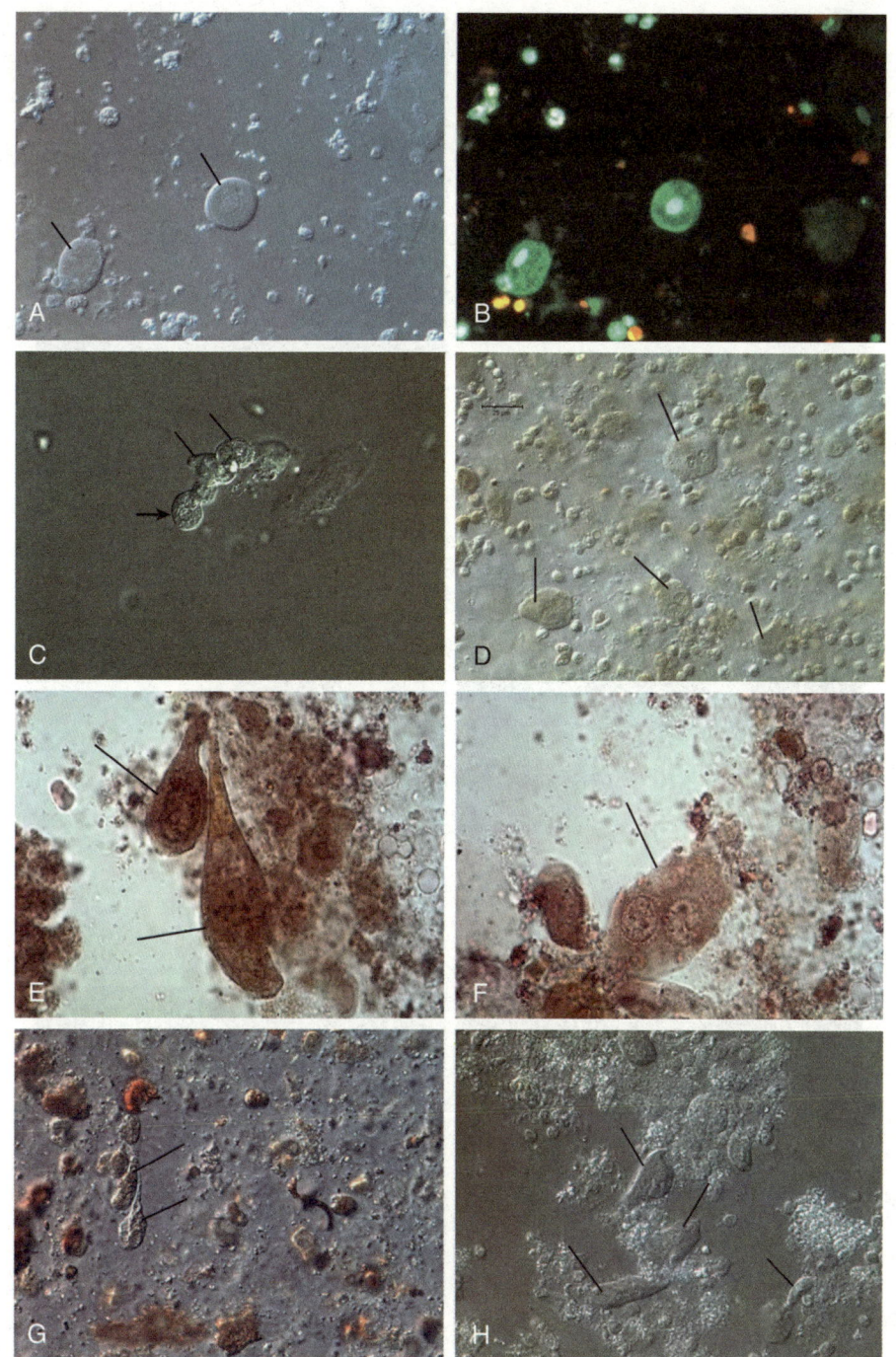

图 2.3 急性肾损伤患者尿液中常发现肾小管细胞。(A) 一名急性肾小管坏死 (ATN) 恢复期患者未染色的尿沉渣 (40×)。实线表示完整的肾小管上皮细胞。(B) 与 A 中标本相同，但用吖啶橙-碘化丙啶染色，并用三重激发带荧光滤光片 (三重立方) 观察。红色细胞为死细胞，绿色细胞为活细胞。两个肾小管细胞看起来都有活力。较小的细胞为白细胞。(C) 未染色的尿沉渣 (40×) 显示多个肾小管细胞呈单一的同一形态 (如图 A 和 B)，表明肾小管急性损伤。箭头所指为双核肾小管细胞。(D) 未染色的尿沉渣 (40×) 显示几个肾小管细胞 (实线) 出现畸形。此外，这些细胞呈多核状，表明细胞无法分裂。如果急性肾小管损伤严重，通常会出现大量形态异常的肾小管细胞。(E) 未染色的尿沉渣 (100×) 显示两个泪滴状畸形肾小管上皮细胞 (实线)。由于患者有黄疸，尽管没有染色，但细胞似乎有颜色。(F) 未染色的尿沉渣 (100×) 显示一个畸形的双核肾小管上皮细胞 (实线)。与图 E 来自同一名患者。(G) 未染色尿沉渣 (40×) 显示严重的 ATN。未见"脏"-褐色颗粒状凝集物，但肾小管细胞形态异常 (实线)。大量颗粒状碎屑和无管型表明 Tamm-Horsfall 蛋白未能形成，肾小管损伤更为严重。从黄色的色调可以看出，该患者还患有黄疸。(H) 未染色的尿沉渣 (40×) 显示肾小管上皮细胞畸形 (三角形、雪茄形和多边形)，通常呈多核状，如图中线条所示

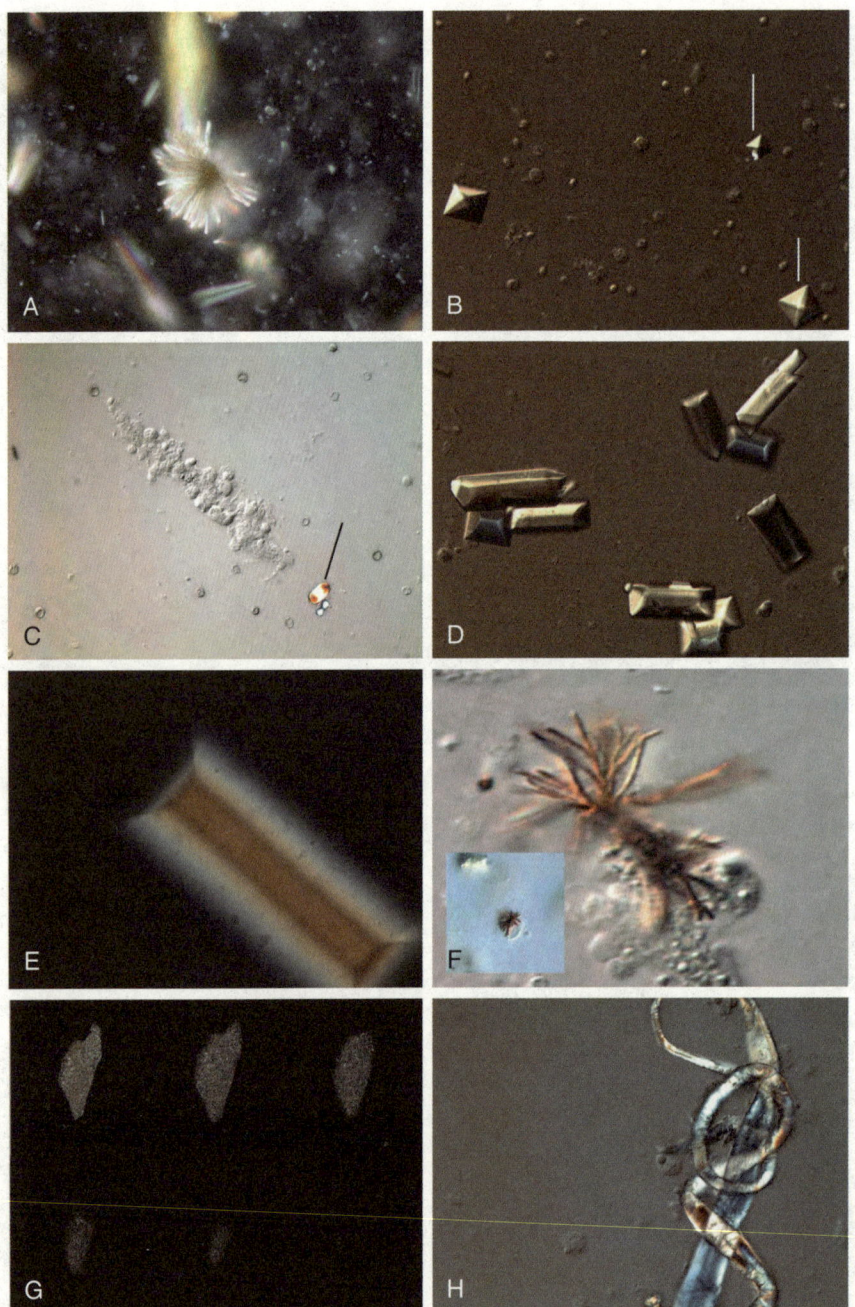

Fig. 2.4 Crystals commonly found in urine sediment. All images were made with the use of polarized light and a diffusion interference contrast microscope. (A) Uric acid crystals (40× objective). (B) Calcium oxalate dihydrate crystals *(white lines)* (40×). Large numbers are seen in patients with ethylene glycol poisoning. (C) Calcium oxalate monohydrate crystals *(solid line)* (40×). (D) Magnesium ammonium phosphate crystals, or triple phosphate crystals, are often found in patients with a complicated urinary tract infection (40×). (E) Coffin-lid appearance of magnesium ammonium phosphate crystals (100×). (F) Bilirubin crystals in a patient with acute tubular necrosis and obstructive jaundice (100×). Inset shows 40× view of the bilirubin crystals. (G) Calcium phosphate crystals (40×) in a patient with tumor lysis syndrome. Sequential images *(left to right, top to bottom)* show dissolution of the crystals within a few minutes after urine was acidified by adding 2% perchloric acid. (H) Fiber artifact in the urine is of no clinical significance.

Renal ultrasonography is the most accurate way of determining kidney size. It is commonly performed to detect renal masses, cysts, and evidence of obstruction characterized by dilatation of the pelvicalyceal system and to evaluate the size and shape of the kidneys. The presence of small kidneys (i.e., <9 cm on both sides) suggests the presence of scarring and therefore CKD. However, kidneys that are larger, typically in the range of 11 to 13 cm, are often seen in conjunction with CKD due to diabetes mellitus, amyloidosis, and multiple myeloma.

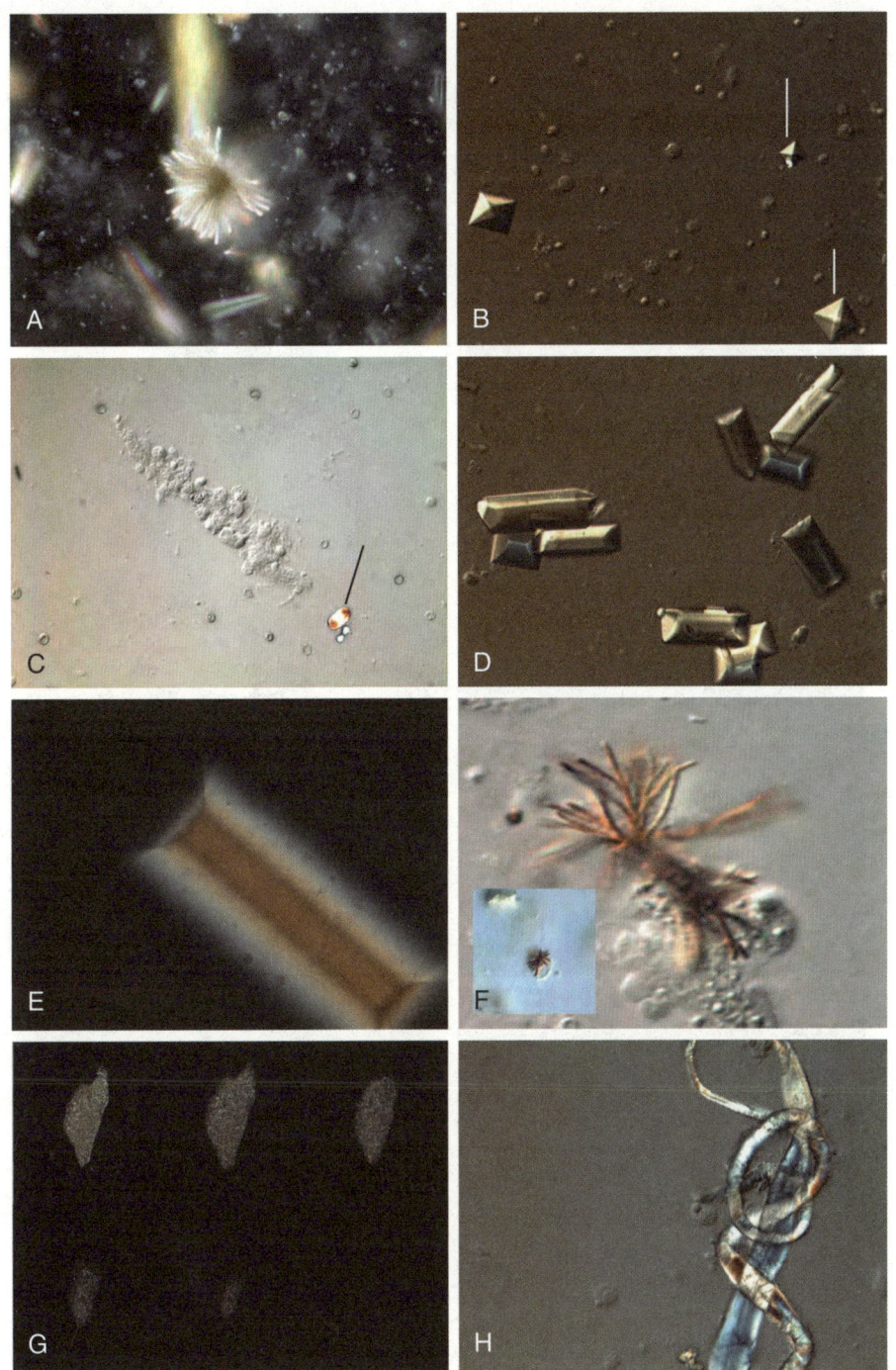

图 2.4 尿沉渣中常见的晶体。所有图像均使用偏振光和扩散干涉对比显微镜拍摄。（A）尿酸晶体（40×）。（B）草酸钙二水合物晶体（白线）（40×）。乙二醇中毒患者可见大量结晶。（C）草酸钙一水化合物晶体（实线）（40×）。（D）磷酸铵镁结晶或三磷酸结晶，常在复杂性尿路感染患者中发现（40×）。（E）磷酸铵镁晶体的棺盖外观（100×）。（F）急性肾小管坏死和阻塞性黄疸患者体内的胆红素结晶（100×）。插图为胆红素结晶的 40 倍视图。（G）肿瘤溶解综合征患者的磷酸钙结晶（40×）。序列图像（从左到右，从上到下）显示，加入 2% 高氯酸酸化尿液后，晶体在几分钟内溶解。（H）尿液中没有临床意义的纤维伪影

肾脏超声检查是确定肾脏大小最准确的方法。它通常用于检测肾脏肿块、囊肿和以肾盂肾盏系统扩张为特征的梗阻证据，以及评估肾脏的大小和形状。如果肾脏较小（即两侧肾脏均小于 9 cm），则提示存在瘢痕，因此可能是 CKD。较大的肾脏（通常在 11 cm 至 13 cm 之间）可见于糖尿病、淀粉样变性和多发性骨髓

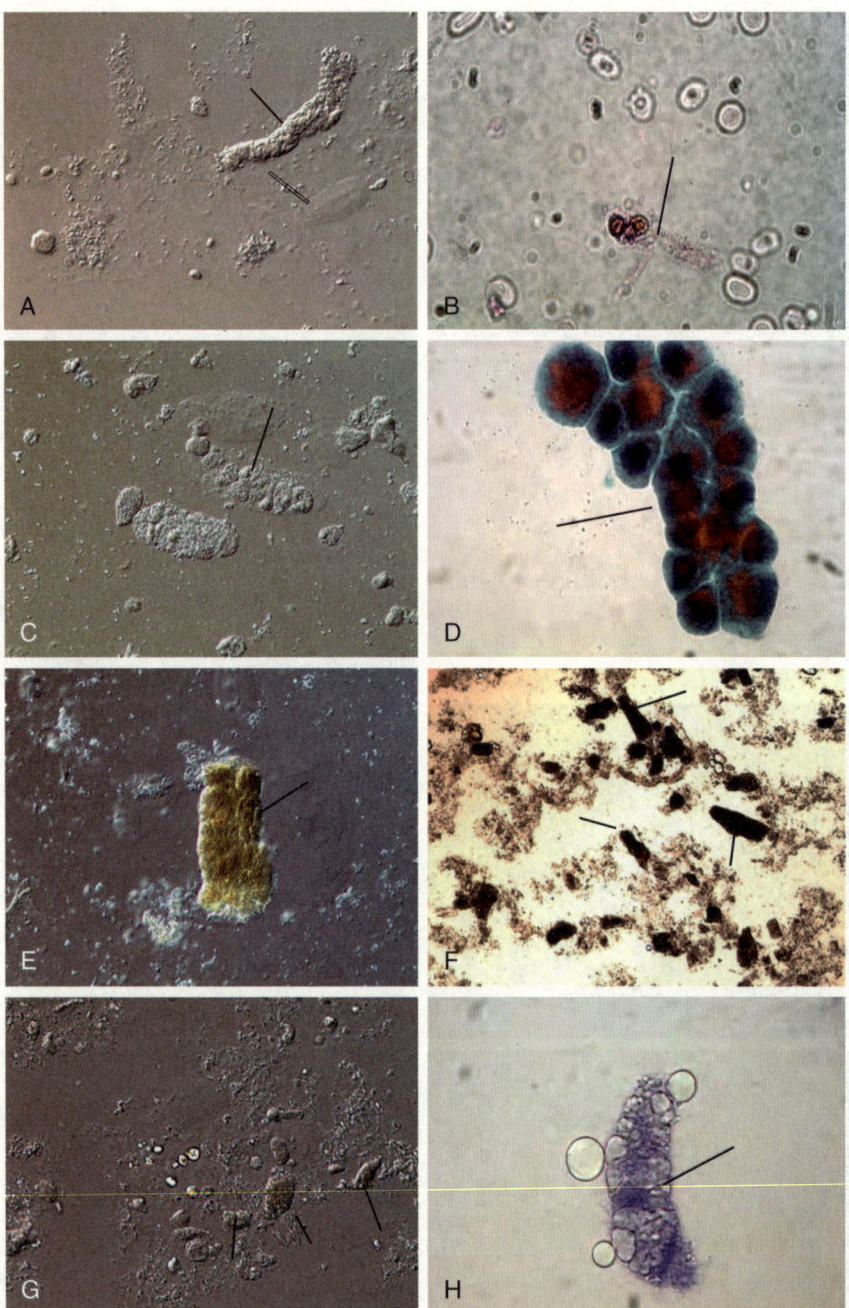

Fig. 2.5 Casts in urine. (A) Unstained urine sediment (40× objective) in a patient with glomerulonephritis. *Solid line* shows a granular cast, and *hollow line* shows a hyaline cast. (B) Sternheimer-Malbin–stained urine sediment (40×). The *solid line* points to an erythrocyte cast in a patient with immunoglobulin A nephropathy. (C) Unstained urine sediment (40×) shows several renal tubular cells and an epithelial cell cast *(solid line)* indicating acute tubular injury. (D) Papanicolaou-stained urine sediment *(solid line)* (100×) shows an epithelial cell cast in an otherwise stable patient with diabetic nephropathy. (E) Unstained urine sediment (40×) shows bilirubin-stained granular cast *(solid line)* indicating renal inflammation in a patient with liver disease. (F) Unstained urine sediment (10×) shows dirty-brown granular casts *(solid line)* indicative of acute tubular necrosis (ATN). (G) Unstained urine sediment (40×) shows severe ATN. No dirty-brown granular casts were seen, but the tubular cells *(solid lines)* were dysmorphic and multinucleated. (H) Sternheimer-Malbin–stained urine sediment (40×) shows a fatty cast *(solid line)* in a patient with nephrotic syndrome.

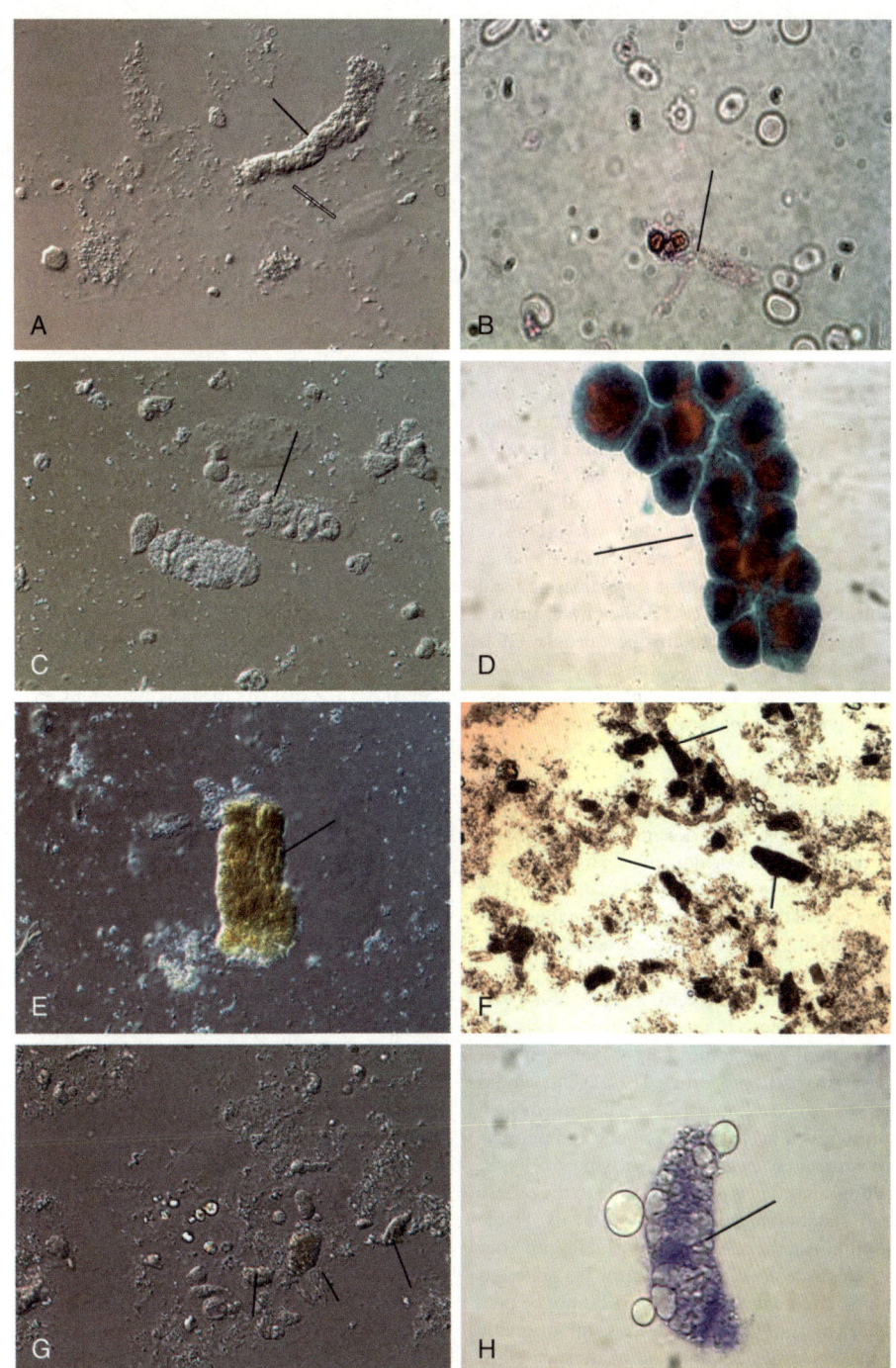

图 2.5 尿液中的管型。(**A**)一名肾小球肾炎患者未染色的尿沉渣(40 倍物镜)。实线表示颗粒状管型,空线表示透明管型。(**B**)Sternheimer-Malbin 染色尿沉渣(40×)。实线表示 IgA 肾病患者的红细胞管型。(**C**)未染色的尿沉渣(40×)显示多个肾小管细胞和上皮细胞管型(实线),表明肾小管急性损伤。(**D**)巴氏染色尿沉渣(实线)(100×)显示糖尿病肾病患者的上皮细胞管型。(**E**)未染色的尿沉渣(40×)显示胆红素染色的颗粒管型(实线),表明肝病患者的肾脏炎症。(**F**)未染色尿沉渣(10×)显示"脏"-褐色颗粒状管型(实线),表明急性肾小管坏死(ATN)。(**G**)未染色尿沉渣(40×)显示严重的 ATN。未见"脏"-褐色颗粒状结节,但肾小管细胞(实线)形态异常且多核。(**H**)Sternheimer-Malbin 染色的尿沉渣(40×)显示肾病综合征患者的脂肪管型(实线)

Therefore, the presence of small kidneys is not required to make a diagnosis of CKD.

The echogenicity of the kidneys is compared with that of liver parenchyma. Typically, the kidneys are less echogenic than the liver. Increased echogenicity of the kidneys suggests the presence of scarring and therefore CKD. Renal ultrasonography can also easily detect the presence of cysts in the kidneys and therefore is a useful technique to detect polycystic kidney disease.

Pulsed Doppler imaging is often used to calculate the resistive index by estimating the systolic and diastolic Doppler velocities in the renal cortex. A resistive index greater than 0.8 suggests that interventional procedures to revascularize the kidney would be unlikely to benefit the patient in terms of improving blood pressure or protecting the long-term decline in kidney function. If the two kidneys differ in size by 1.5 cm, it suggests the presence of renovascular disease in an adult. In children, reflux nephropathy or congenital abnormalities are more common causes of asymmetric kidney size.

Computed tomography (CT) of the kidney is often helpful to evaluate complex cysts. In contrast to simple cysts, complex cysts are suspicious for the presence of malignancy, and CT can evaluate them better than ultrasonography. Likewise, CT is important for evaluating renal masses, stones, retroperitoneal conditions (e.g., hemorrhage, tumor, abscess), and renal vein thrombosis. In morbidly obese people, CT is often used to guide kidney biopsy. The use of contrast agents to assess vascular lesions of the kidney may be not be possible if kidney function is compromised due to fear of precipitating AKI. Limiting the volume of the contrast agent and volume repletion before radiocontrast administration may minimize renal injury.

Although *intravenous pyelography* can image the structures in the kidney, contrast CT has taken the place of classic intravenous pyelography in many centers because of the risk of inducing nephrotoxicity in patients with CKD. In contrast, *retrograde pyelography* is often used by urologists to define the site and nature of obstruction within the ureter and the pelvis. In addition, during the procedure, ureteric stones can be removed with the use of a basket device.

Magnetic resonance imaging (MRI) is useful for imaging of the vasculature and therefore for the diagnosis of renal vein thrombosis and renal artery stenosis. Gadolinium-based contrast agents are often used for MRI because of their paramagnetic properties. These agents should be avoided if the GFR is less than 30 mL/min/1.73 m^2, because in such patients they have been implicated in causing a disabling and untreatable condition called *nephrogenic systemic fibrosis*. It is now believed that the risk of this disabling condition is directly related to the release of free gadolinium from gadolinium-based contrast agents. Stable macrocyclic agents that minimize the release of free gadolinium after administration such as gadoterate acid and godobutrol are preferred over the older gadolinium-based contrast agents. MRI cannot be performed in patients who have metallic implanted devices with magnetic properties such as pacemakers, artificial joints, or aneurysmal clips. Although nonferrous surgical metal can distort an MRI image, most are safe within the strong magnetic field of an MRI machine. Research now reveals that MRI examination after a total joint replacement is not only possible, but adjusting pulse sequences and parameters often can provide accurate information on soft tissue tissues and causes of joint failure.

After injection of a small amount of radioactive substance, *radionuclide imaging* can be performed to assess renal perfusion and function of the kidneys. One advantage of this technique is that it can assess kidney function and perfusion simultaneously for each kidney. It therefore allows diagnosis of renal artery stenosis, especially when it is performed before and after administration of angiotensin-converting enzyme (ACE) inhibitors.

Renal arteriography is the reference standard for the diagnosis of renal artery stenosis. It involves direct injection of a radiocontrast dye into the renal arteries. In patients with CKD, contrast injection can be limited and carbon dioxide can be injected to avoid nephrotoxicity. This technique is also useful for assessing vascular malformations in the kidney and for making a diagnosis of polyarteritis nodosa. In the latter condition, renal arteriography can detect the presence of microaneurysms.

APPROACH TO THE PATIENT WITH ACUTE KIDNEY INJURY

The initial approach to patients with AKI focuses on the following factors: (1) the evaluation of risk or susceptibility to renal injury, (2) the cause(s) of the AKI, (3) the severity of injury, and (4) the presence of distant organ effects or consequences. In all cases, it is important to evaluate and optimize intravascular volume early in the course, because this is a readily addressable factor that can prevent or minimize further injury.

Evaluation of Risk or Susceptibility to Renal Injury

The risk factors for AKI include, first and foremost, prior existence of CKD; CKD can easily be detected by a low estimated GFR or the presence of albuminuria. Other common risk factors for AKI include advanced age, diabetes mellitus, hypertension (especially when treated with inhibitors of the renin-angiotensin system), chronic liver disease or cirrhosis, and multiple myeloma.

Causes of AKI

AKI is a challenging medical problem, and a careful and stepwise approach to evaluation is essential. This approach is guided by knowledge of the causes of injury, which can be divided into five major groups: ischemia, toxins, obstruction, inflammation, and infection.

Ischemia can be caused by volume loss from the gastrointestinal system (vomiting or diarrhea), the skin (sweating, burns), or the kidneys (diuretics, Addison's disease, and solute diuresis). Comparing the body weight of the patient with those weights recorded in the medical record can be valuable. A substantial decrease in body weight may point toward volume depletion as a possible cause of AKI. Third-space fluid losses, as observed in patients with ascites, pancreatitis, or ileus, can make the diagnosis of volume depletion challenging because such patients may not have an overall loss in body weight. Ischemia is a common cause of AKI due to poor perfusion associated with significant blood loss or sepsis or both. In the setting of ischemia, glomerular hypoperfusion is aggravated when patients are taking inhibitors of the renin-angiotensin system.

Nephrotoxins can be divided into two major groups: endogenous and exogenous. The endogenous toxins include paraproteins, myoglobin, hemoglobin, uric acid (e.g., in tumor lysis syndrome), and bile acids. Exogenous toxins include contrast agents, aminoglycosides, vancomycin, chemotherapeutic agents such as cisplatin, and NSAIDs.

Inflammation can involve the glomerular, interstitial, and vascular compartments. Inflammation of these structures produces glomerulonephritis, interstitial nephritis, and vasculitis, respectively.

Infection is an important cause of injury to the nephron. Infection-associated AKI is often diagnosed in the intensive care unit, where early sepsis can manifest as a fall in urine output followed by an increase in serum creatinine, confirming AKI. The causes of AKI in the setting of sepsis are often multifactorial and include ischemia, direct tubular dysfunction due to sepsis, and concomitant administration of drugs such as nephrotoxic antibiotics (commonly, high doses of vancomycin) and procedures (radiocontrast imaging), often performed to reverse sepsis.

瘤导致的CKD。因此，肾脏小并不是诊断慢性肾衰竭的必要条件。

肾脏的回声可与肝脏实质的回声进行比较。通常情况下，肾脏的回声低于肝脏。肾脏的回声增强表明存在瘢痕，因此也表明存在CKD。肾脏超声很容易检测出肾脏中是否存在囊肿，是检测多囊肾病的有效技术。

脉冲多普勒成像通常通过估算肾皮质的收缩和舒张多普勒速度来计算阻力指数。如果阻力指数大于0.8，则表明肾脏血管再通的介入手术不太可能在改善血压或防止肾功能长期衰退方面为患者带来益处。如果两个肾脏的大小相差1.5 cm，则表明成人存在肾脏血管疾病。在儿童中，反流性肾病或先天性异常是导致肾脏大小不对称的更常见原因。

肾计算机断层成像（CT）通常有助于评估复杂性囊肿。与单纯性囊肿相比，复杂性囊肿具有恶性肿瘤的可能性，CT比超声检查能更好地对其进行评估。同样，CT对评估肾脏肿块、结石、腹膜后疾病（如出血、肿瘤、脓肿）和肾静脉血栓也很重要。对于病态肥胖者，CT通常用于引导肾活检。如果肾功能受损，担心引发AKI，可能无法使用造影剂评估肾脏血管病变。限制造影剂的用量并在使用造影剂前补充血容量可将肾损伤降至最低。

虽然静脉肾盂造影可以对肾脏结构进行成像，但在许多中心，增强CT已经取代了传统的静脉肾盂造影，因为对CKD患者来说，造影剂有诱发肾毒性的风险。与此相反，泌尿科医生通常使用逆行肾盂造影来确定输尿管和肾盂内梗阻的部位和性质。此外，在手术过程中，还可以使用网篮装置取出输尿管结石。

磁共振成像（MRI）可用于血管成像，从而诊断肾静脉血栓和肾动脉狭窄。由于钆造影剂具有顺磁性，因此常用于磁共振成像。如果患者的GFR低于30 ml/（min·1.73 m^2），则应避免使用这些造影剂，因为这些造影剂可能会导致一种无法治疗的致残性疾病——肾源性系统纤维化。目前认为，这种致残性疾病的风险与钆造影剂释放的游离钆直接相关。与老式的钆造影剂相比，钆特酸和钆布醇等稳定的大环制剂能最大限度地减少用药后游离钆的释放。对于植入具有磁性的金属装置（如心脏起搏器、人工关节或动脉瘤夹）的患者，不能进行磁共振成像。虽然外科用有色金属会使磁共振成像图像失真，但在磁共振成像仪的强磁场中，大多数金属都是安全的。现在的研究表明，全关节置换术后的磁共振成像检查不仅可行，而且调整脉冲序列和参数往往能提供有关软组织和关节故障原因的准确信息。

注射少量放射性物质后，可进行放射性核素成像，以评估肾脏的灌注和功能。这项技术的优点之一是可以同时评估每个肾脏的肾功能和灌注情况。因此，它可以用于诊断肾动脉狭窄，尤其是在比较服用血管紧张素转换酶（ACE）抑制剂前后的状态进行诊断。

肾动脉造影是诊断肾动脉狭窄的金标准。它是把造影剂直接注入肾动脉。对于患有CKD的患者，可以限制造影剂的注射量，并注射二氧化碳以避免肾毒性。这项技术还有助于评估肾脏血管畸形和诊断结节性多动脉炎。在结节性多动脉炎的情况下，肾动脉造影可以检测到微动脉瘤的存在。

急性肾损伤患者的接诊

AKI患者的初步接诊主要关注以下因素：①评估肾损伤的风险或易感性；②导致AKI的原因；③损伤的严重程度；④是否影响远隔器官及其后果。在所有病例中，在病程早期，评估和改善血管内容量重要，因为这是一个很容易解决的因素，可以防止或减少进一步的损伤。

肾损伤危险因素或易感性评估

AKI的危险因素首要是既往罹患CKD，CKD可通过估算的GFR下降或出现白蛋白尿来诊断；其他常见的AKI危险因素包括高龄、糖尿病、高血压（尤其是使用肾素-血管紧张素系统抑制剂治疗时）、慢性肝病或肝硬化以及多发性骨髓瘤。

AKI的病因

AKI是一个具有挑战性的医学问题，必须采取谨慎和循序渐进的方法进行评估。以损伤原因的分类为指导，损伤原因可分为五大类：缺血、毒素、梗阻、炎症和感染。

缺血可由胃肠道系统（呕吐或腹泻）、皮肤（出汗、烧伤）或肾脏（利尿剂、艾迪生病和溶质利尿）导致的容量损失所致。将患者的体重与医疗记录中记录的体重进行比较可能很有价值。体重大幅下降提示容量耗竭可能是导致AKI的原因。腹水、胰腺炎或回肠炎患者的第三间隙液体丢失会使容量耗竭的诊断变得困难，因为这类患者的体重可能没有下降。缺血是导致AKI的常见原因，这是因为大量失血或感染中毒症或两者同时出现会导致灌注不良。在缺血的情况下，当患者服用肾素-血管紧张素系统抑制剂时，肾小球灌注不足会加剧。

肾脏毒素可分为两大类：内源性和外源性。内源性毒素包括副蛋白、肌红蛋白、血红蛋白、尿酸（如肿瘤溶解综合征）和胆汁酸。外源性毒素包括造影剂、氨基糖苷类、万古霉素、顺铂等化疗药物和非甾体抗炎药。

炎症可累及肾小球、肾间质和血管，这些部位的炎症可分别导致肾小球肾炎、肾间质肾炎和血管炎。

感染是造成肾单位损伤的一个重要原因。感染相关性AKI常见于重症监护病房，早期败血症可表现为尿量减少，随后血清肌酐升高，从而确诊为AKI。脓毒症导致AKI的原因通常是多因素的，包括缺血、脓毒症导致的直接肾小管功能障碍以及同时服用药物，如肾毒性抗生素（常见的是大剂量万古霉素）和各种操作（使用造影剂造影），这些通常为逆转脓毒症的

Therefore, declines in urine volume, especially in the intensive care unit, should lead to a diligent search for a focus of infection.

Urinary tract obstruction is often a reversible cause of renal injury and therefore important to diagnose. Although urine output is frequently reduced with obstruction, partial obstruction may be associated with an increase in urine output. Renal ultrasound is useful to diagnose hydronephrosis; urinalysis may reveal hematuria or infection or may be bland. Left untreated, renal atrophy may ensue.

In many ways, the severity of injury is best assessed at the bedside. Oliguric renal failure (100-400 mL urine/24 hr) or anuric renal failure (<100 mL urine/24 hr) has a worse prognosis than nonoliguric renal failure (>400 mL urine/24 hr). A low fractional excretion of sodium or, if the patient is taking diuretics, a low fractional excretion of urea may suggest volume depletion as the likely cause. Fractional excretion of any substance is simply calculated as the ratio of the clearance of the analyte in question to the clearance of creatinine. However, a low fractional excretion of urea or sodium may have causes other than volume depletion. For example, because of the heterogeneous nature of nephronal injury, contrast-induced injury, sepsis, or burns often result in a low fractional excretion of sodium despite intrinsic renal failure.

Intrinsic renal injury can be detected by examining the urine sediment. The classic manifestation of acute tubular necrosis (ATN) is the presence of dirty-brown granular casts. However, in severe AKI, there may be a large amount of amorphous granular material without cast formation (see Figs. 2.3 and 2.5). This occurs because severe AKI may result in failure to produce the Tamm-Horsfall protein that is now called uromodulin, leading to no formation of casts. In the absence of dirty-brown granular casts, a diagnosis of acute tubular injury can still be made based on the presence of dysmorphic epithelial cells in the urine. These epithelial cells, under hypoxic conditions, transform from the round, fried-egg appearance of the tubular cell to angular cells taking the shape of triangles or teardrops (see Fig. 2.3). A normal sediment, on the other hand, suggests minimal or no kidney injury.

The individual elements that can be seen in the urine and may be of diagnostic importance are as follows: dysmorphic RBCs, sterile pyuria manifested by white blood cells (WBCs) in the urine without bacteria, urinary tract infection characterized by both WBCs and bacteria in the urine, dysmorphic tubular cells suggesting ATN, intact renal tubular cells suggesting recovery from AKI, bubble cells, glitter cells, and oval fat bodies (see Figs. 2.2 and 2.3).

Budding yeast in a patient with diabetes may suggest the need to remove a long-standing indwelling catheter. Uric acid crystals in large amount suggest tumor lysis syndrome, calcium oxalate crystals may suggest ethylene glycol poisoning, and magnesium ammonium phosphate (triple phosphate) crystals may suggest infection with urease-positive organisms (see Fig. 2.4).

Casts can occur in various forms, such as RBC, WBC, epithelial cell, granular, hyaline, and dirty-brown granular casts. They can also occur in various shapes, such as broad and narrow casts. Examples of these are demonstrated in Fig. 2.5.

Severity of Injury

The severity of injury needs to be assessed, as well as its relationship to the preexisting state of kidney health. Severe injury is required for AKI to be manifested when the kidney is otherwise healthy. Little damage is needed to produce a severe injury if CKD preexists. More important, however, is the response to injury. It remains unclear why certain individuals have low GFR and others with the same extent of injury do not. This likely reflects the protective nature of responses that can result in poor or better GFR.

Presence of Distant Organ Effects on Consequences

End-organ manifestations of AKI include pulmonary edema or acute respiratory distress syndrome, uremic encephalopathy as alteration of mental status or asterixis, and uremic pericarditis or pleuritis manifested as pericardial or pleural friction rub. Although pulmonary edema is still a common manifestation of uremia, uremic serositis and encephalopathy are now rare.

For a deeper discussion on this topic, see Chapter 106, "Approach to the Patient With Renal Disease," in *Goldman-Cecil Medicine*, 26th Edition.

SUGGESTED READINGS

Agarwal R, Delanaye P: Glomerular filtration rate: when to measure and in which patients?, Nephrol Dial Transplant. https://doi.org/10.1093/ndt/gfy363.

Earley A, Miskulin D, Lamb EJ: et al: Estimating equations for glomerular filtration rate in the era of creatinine standardization: a systemic review, Ann Intern Med 156:785–795, 2012.

Gansevoort RT, Matsushita K, van der Velde M, et al: Lower estimated GFR and higher albuminuria are associated with adverse kidney outcomes: a collaborative meta-analysis of general and high-risk population cohorts, Kidney Int 80:93–104, 2011.

Maroni BJ, Steinman TI, Mitch WE: A method for estimating nitrogen intake of patients with chronic renal failure, Kidney Int 27:58–65, 1985.

Perazella M, Coca S, Kanbay M, et al.: Diagnostic value of urine microscopy for differential diagnosis of acute kidney injury in hospitalized patients, Clin J Am Soc Nephrol 3:1615–1619, 2008.

Perrone RD, Madias NE, Levey AS: Serum creatinine as an index of renal function: new insights into old concepts, Clin Chem 38:1933–1953, 1992.

Pickering TG, Miller NH, Ogedegbe G, et al.: Call to action on use and reimbursement for home blood pressure monitoring: a joint scientific statement from the American Heart Association, American Society Of Hypertension, and Preventive Cardiovascular Nurses Association, Hypertension 52:10–29, 2008.

Pickering TG, Shimbo D, Haas D: Ambulatory blood-pressure monitoring, N Engl J Med 354:2368–2374, 2006.

相关治疗。因此，尿量减少，尤其是在重症监护病房，应努力寻找感染病灶。

尿路梗阻通常是肾损伤的可逆原因，因此明确诊断非常重要。虽然尿量经常会随着梗阻而减少，但部分梗阻可能会导致尿量增加。肾脏超声检查有助于诊断肾积水；尿液检查可能会发现血尿或感染，也可能无异常。如不及时治疗，可能会导致肾萎缩。

在许多方面，损伤的严重程度最好在病床边进行评估。少尿性肾衰竭（尿量100～400 ml/24 h）或无尿性肾衰竭（＜100 ml/24 h）的预后比非少尿性肾衰竭（＞400 ml/24 h）差。钠的排泄量低，或者如果患者正在服用利尿剂，尿素的排泄量低，都提示容量耗竭是可能的原因。任何物质的排泄分数都可以简单地计算为相关分析物清除与肌酐清除的比值。然而，尿素或钠的低排泄分数可能有容量耗竭以外的原因。例如，由于肾损伤的异质性，造影剂诱导的损伤、感染中毒症或烧伤，会存在肾实质性功能衰竭，但往往会导致低钠排泄分数。

肾实质损伤可检查尿沉渣。急性肾小管坏死（ATN）的典型表现是出现"脏"-褐色颗粒状管型。然而，在严重的AKI中，可能会出现大量无定形颗粒物质，但没有管型形成（见图2.3和2.5）。出现这种情况是因为严重的AKI可能会导致Tamm-Horsfall蛋白（即尿调蛋白）不能生成，从而不形成管型。在没有"脏"-褐色颗粒状管型的情况下，根据尿液中畸形上皮细胞的存在，仍可诊断为急性肾小管损伤。在缺氧条件下，这些上皮细胞会从圆形、煎蛋状的肾小管细胞转变为三角形或泪滴状的角细胞（见图2.3）。另一方面，正常的尿沉渣表明肾脏损伤极小或没有损伤。

尿液中可见到的并可能具有重要诊断意义的成分如下：形态异常的红细胞、无菌性脓尿表现为尿液中出现无细菌的白细胞、尿液中既有白细胞又有细菌的尿路感染、提示ATN的形态异常的肾小管细胞、提示从AKI恢复的完整肾小管细胞、气泡细胞、闪光细胞和卵圆形脂肪体（见图2.2和2.3）。

糖尿病患者尿检中出现酵母芽提示可能需要拔除长期留置的导尿管。大量尿酸结晶提示肿瘤溶解综合征，草酸钙结晶可能提示乙二醇中毒，磷酸铵镁（三磷酸）结晶可能提示感染了尿素酶阳性微生物（见图2.4）。

管型有多种形式，如红细胞、白细胞、上皮细胞颗粒管型、透明管型和"脏"-褐色颗粒状管型。它们还可以形成各种形状，如宽管型和窄管型。示例见图2.5。

损伤严重程度

需要评估损伤的严重程度及其与原有肾脏健康状况的关系。当肾脏健康时，需要严重损伤才能表现出AKI。如果已经存在CKD，则轻微的损伤就能产生严重损害。然而，更重要的是对损伤的反应。目前仍不清楚在相同损伤程度下为什么某些个体的GFR下降，而其他个体的却不下降。这可能反映了机体反应的保护性质，由此导致GFR较低或较高。

对远隔器官的影响和后果

AKI影响终末器官的表现包括肺水肿或急性呼吸窘迫综合征、尿毒症脑病表现为精神状态改变或眩晕、尿毒症心包炎或胸膜炎表现为心包或胸膜摩擦音。虽然肺水肿仍然是尿毒症的常见表现，但尿毒症浆膜炎和脑病现在已很少见。

有关此专题的深入讨论，请参阅 *Goldman-Cecil Medicine* 第26版第106章"肾病患者的接诊"。

推荐阅读

Agarwal R, Delanaye P: Glomerular filtration rate: when to measure and in which patients?, Nephrol Dial Transplant. https://doi.org/10.1093/ndt/gfy363.

Earley A, Miskulin D, Lamb EJ: et al: Estimating equations for glomerular filtration rate in the era of creatinine standardization: a systemic review, Ann Intern Med 156:785–795, 2012.

Gansevoort RT, Matsushita K, van der Velde M, et al: Lower estimated GFR and higher albuminuria are associated with adverse kidney outcomes: a collaborative meta-analysis of general and high-risk population cohorts, Kidney Int 80:93–104, 2011.

Maroni BJ, Steinman TI, Mitch WE: A method for estimating nitrogen intake of patients with chronic renal failure, Kidney Int 27:58–65, 1985.

Perazella M, Coca S, Kanbay M, et al.: Diagnostic value of urine microscopy for differential diagnosis of acute kidney injury in hospitalized patients, Clin J Am Soc Nephrol 3:1615–1619, 2008.

Perrone RD, Madias NE, Levey AS: Serum creatinine as an index of renal function: new insights into old concepts, Clin Chem 38:1933–1953, 1992.

Pickering TG, Miller NH, Ogedegbe G, et al.: Call to action on use and reimbursement for home blood pressure monitoring: a joint scientific statement from the American Heart Association, American Society Of Hypertension, and Preventive Cardiovascular Nurses Association, Hypertension 52:10–29, 2008.

Pickering TG, Shimbo D, Haas D: Ambulatory blood-pressure monitoring, N Engl J Med 354:2368–2374, 2006.

3

Fluid and Electrolyte Disorders

Biff F. Palmer

NORMAL VOLUME HOMEOSTASIS

In the average adult, the total body water is equal to 50% to 60% of body weight: 60% for men and 50% for women because of extra body fat, which is water free. Thus, in an average 70-kg male, total body water is 42 kg or 42 L, while in an average 70-kg female, total body water is 35 kg or L. Of the total body water, approximately two thirds is located intracellularly while one third is located extracellularly. Of the extracellular fluid (ECF) volume, only one fourth is located within the intravascular space. In a 70-kg man with a total body water of 42 L, 28 of these liters will be located intracellularly, while only 14 L are located in the ECF, and only 3.5 L are located in the extracellular intravascular compartment.

ECF volume is determined by the balance between sodium intake and excretion. Under normal circumstances, wide variations in salt intake lead to parallel changes in renal salt excretion, such that ECF volume and total body salt is maintained within narrow limits. This relative constancy of ECF volume is achieved by a series of afferent sensing systems, central integrative pathways, and both renal and extrarenal effector mechanisms acting in concert to modulate sodium excretion by the kidney (Table 3.1).

The concentration of sodium chloride (NaCl) in the plasma is regulated by renal water handling. The maintenance of plasma tonicity is achieved by sensing and effector mechanisms that differ from those that regulate volume. However, the systems that regulate volume and plasma tonicity do work in concert. For example, if the baroreceptors of the body detect that ECF volume is low, the kidney will respond by retaining NaCl. This will transiently lead to an increase in the tonicity of the ECF that will stimulate arginine vasopressin (AVP) release, causing renal water retention and expansion of the ECF volume.

Osmolality and Tonicity

Osmolality is defined as the number of particles per kilogram of solution. Plasma osmolality can be directly measured in an osmometer or can be calculated using the following equation:

$$\text{Calculated osmolality} = (\text{Na}^+ \times 2) + \text{glucose}/18 + \text{BUN}/2.8$$

where Na^+ is the sodium ion concentration and BUN is the blood urea nitrogen level.

The osmolar gap is the difference between the measured and calculated osmolality and is normally less than 10 mOsm/L. A higher value indicates the accumulation of an unmeasured substance such as ethanol, methanol, ethylene glycol, and acetone.

It is important to distinguish osmolality from tonicity. Whereas *osmolality* refers to all particles, *tonicity* describes whether the particles are effective or ineffective osmoles. Effective osmoles such as Na^+, glucose, or mannitol cannot penetrate cell membranes and thus can lead to changes in cell volume. Ineffective osmoles such as urea and alcohols are ineffective osmoles because they pass freely into and out of cells and are unable to effect changes in cell volume. As an example, chronic kidney disease patients with BUN levels greater than 100 mg/dL have no cellular shifts of fluid due to the urea. The plasma osmolality is high, but plasma tonicity is normal.

HYPONATREMIA

Hyponatremia is one of the most common electrolyte abnormalities encountered in clinical practice. Increasing age, medications, various disease states, and administration of hypotonic fluids are among the known risk factors for the disorder. Although hyponatremia is most commonly a marker of hypo-osmolality, there are three general causes of hyponatremia not associated with a hypo-osmolar state (Fig. 3.1). The first of these is pseudohyponatremia. This condition occurs in the setting of hyperglobulinemia or hypertriglyceridemia in which plasma water relative to plasma solids is decreased in blood leading to less Na^+ in a given volume of blood.

The second cause involves true hyponatremia but with elevations in the concentration of an effective osmole. Clinical examples include hyperglycemia as seen in uncontrolled diabetes or rarely hypertonic infusion of mannitol used in the treatment of cerebral edema. Increased plasma glucose concentration raises serum osmolality, which pulls water out of cells and dilutes the serum Na^+. For every 100-mg/dL rise in glucose or mannitol the serum Na^+ will quickly fall by 1.6 mEq/L. The increased tonicity will also stimulate thirst and AVP secretion, both of which contribute to further water retention. As the plasma osmolality returns towards normal, the decline in serum Na^+ will be 2.8 mEq/L for every 100-mg/dL rise in glucose. The net result is a normal plasma osmolality but a low serum Na^+.

The third cause of hyponatremia in the absence of a hypo-osmolar state is the addition of an isosmotic (or near isosmotic) non-Na^+ containing fluid to the extracellular space. This situation typically occurs during a transurethral resection of the prostate or during laparoscopic surgery when large amounts of a non-conducting flushing solution containing glycine or sorbitol are reabsorbed systemically.

The presence of hypotonic hyponatremia implies that water intake exceeds the ability of the kidney to excrete water. Because the normal kidney can excrete 20 to 30 L of water per day, the presence of hyponatremia with normal renal water excretion implies the patient is drinking at least those volumes of water. This condition is referred to as *primary polydipsia*. Urine osmolality will be less than 100 mOsm/L in this setting. Hyponatremia in association with a maximally dilute urine can also result from more moderate fluid intake combined with extremely limited solute intake, a condition often referred to as "beer potomania" syndrome.

水和电解质紊乱

王玉 译　赵明辉 李明喜 审校　赵明辉 通审

正常容量稳态

正常成人体内总水量相当于体重的50%～60%：男性为60%，女性因为体内有更多不含水分的脂肪，所以为50%。因此，对一个体重70 kg的男性而言，体内的总水量为42 kg或42 L，而对体重70 kg的女性而言，体内总水量则为35 kg或35 L。大约2/3的身体总水量位于细胞内，1/3位于细胞外。在所有细胞外液（ECF）中，只有1/4在血管内。对于一个体内总水量约为42 L、体重70 kg的男性而言，有28 L水是位于细胞内的，只有14 L位于细胞外，而其中又只有3.5 L在血管内。

ECF体积取决于钠摄入和排泄之间的平衡。正常情况下，盐摄入量的大幅变化会导致相应的肾脏排盐量的平行变化，因此ECF体积和体内总盐量维持在一个很窄的范围内。这种ECF体积的相对恒定是通过一系列传入感应系统、中枢整合通路，以及肾和肾外效应机制协同作用，调节肾脏钠排泄来实现的（表3.1）。

血浆氯化钠（NaCl）的浓度受肾脏水处理的调节。血浆张力的维持是通过与容量调节机制不同的感知和效应机制来实现的。然而，调节容量和血浆张力的系统是协同工作的。例如，如果机体的压力感受器感受到ECF减少，肾脏就会做出保留NaCl的反应。这将引起ECF张力的短暂增加，刺激精氨酸血管加压素（AVP）释放，进而导致肾脏保水和ECF体积的增加。

渗透压和张力

渗透压的定义是每千克溶液中的微粒数。血浆渗透压可以用渗透压计直接测量，也可以用下面的公式计算：

计算渗透压 =（Na^+ ×2）+ 葡萄糖/18 + BUN/2.8

其中Na^+是钠离子浓度，BUN是血尿素氮水平。

渗透压间隙是指测量的渗透压和计算的渗透压之间的差值，通常小于10 mOsm/L。该数值增高，提示有未被测量的物质如乙醇、甲醇、乙二醇及丙酮等在血液中蓄积。

区分渗透压和张力非常重要。所有微粒均可产生渗透压，而张力取决于微粒是否为有效渗透质。有效渗透溶质，如Na^+、葡萄糖或甘露醇，不能穿透细胞膜，因此可导致细胞体积变化。而无效渗透溶质，如尿素和酒精，因为可以自由进出细胞，无法影响细胞体积的变化，产生的是无效渗透压。举例来说，慢性肾脏病患者BUN水平可超过100 mg/dl，但并不会因尿素导致细胞内外水迁移。此时血浆渗透压很高，但血浆张力正常。

低钠血症

低钠血症是临床上最常见的电解质异常之一。增龄、药物、各种疾病状态，以及低张液体的使用都是导致这种异常的已知危险因素。虽然低钠血症通常是低渗状态的标志，但有三种与低渗状态无关的导致低钠血症的原因（图3.1）。第一种是假性低钠血症。这种情况见于高球蛋白血症或高甘油三酯血症，因为血浆中的水相对于血浆中的固形物是少的，导致在一定血容量中的Na^+减少。

第二种是真性低钠血症，但伴有效渗透溶质浓度升高。临床上的例子包括未控制的糖尿病中的高血糖，或相对罕见的脑水肿治疗时高张甘露醇输注。血浆葡萄糖浓度的上升会升高血清渗透压，使水移出到细胞外，从而稀释血清Na^+。葡萄糖或甘露醇浓度每升高100 mg/dl，血清Na^+会迅速降低1.6 mmol/L。张力的升高也会刺激口渴反应和AVP分泌，两者都会进一步导致机体保水。当血浆渗透压恢复正常时，葡萄糖每升高100 mg/dl，血清Na^+就会下降2.8 mmol/L。最终结果是血浆渗透压正常，但血清Na^+低。

在没有低渗情况下导致低钠血症的第三个原因是细胞外空间内加入了不含Na^+的等渗（或接近等渗）的液体。这种情况通常发生在经尿道前列腺切除术或腹腔镜手术时，因大量含有甘氨酸或山梨醇的不导电冲洗液被全身重吸收所致。

出现低张性低钠血症意味着水的摄入量超过了肾脏排水的能力。正常肾脏每天可排泄20～30 L水，因此在肾脏排水正常情况下出现低钠血症意味着患者至少饮用了多于这个容量的水。这种情况被称为原发性烦渴。在这种情况下，尿渗透压通常低于100 mOsm/L。与最大稀释尿液相关的低钠血症也可能由适度的液体摄入结合极低的溶质摄入引起，这种情况通常被称为"啤酒狂"综合征。

TABLE 3.1 Sensors and Effectors That Determine Osmoregulation and Volume Regulation

Factor	Osmoregulation	Volume Regulation
What is sensed	Plasma osmolality	Effective arterial volume (EAV)
Sensors	Hypothalamic osmoreceptors	Low and high pressure baroreceptors
Effectors	Arginine vasopressin (AVP), Thirst	Aldosterone, Angiotensin II, Sympathetic nerves
What is effected	Urine osmolality, Thirst	Urine Na^+ excretion

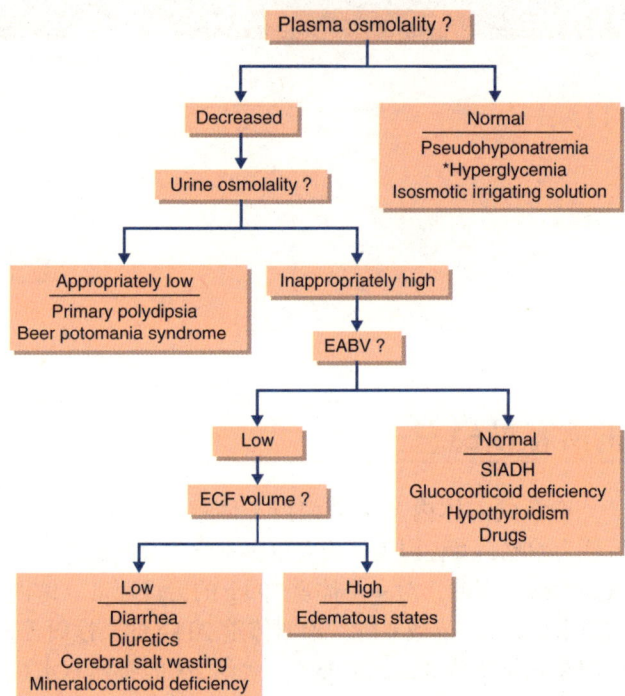

Fig. 3.1 Approach to the patient with hyponatremia. Assessment of effective arterial blood volume (EAV) is key to understanding the mechanism of renal NaCl retention and whether it is primary or in response to a low EAV. By definition, EAV is the arterial volume sensed by the kidney. Thus, if the kidney is working normally and it is retaining NaCl, EAV must be low, and if a normally functioning kidney is excreting large amounts of NaCl, the EAV is large. The physical examination is the most reliable way to assess EAV. The presence or absence of edema and orthostatic changes in blood pressure and pulse are particularly useful findings indicative of EAV. Laboratory tests are also useful in the assessment of EAV. Collection of a spot urinary sample for Na^+, Cl^-, and creatinine allows calculation of the fractional excretion of Na^+ or fractional excretion of Cl^- using the following equations: FE_{Na} (%) = [(urine Na^+ × plasma creatinine)/(plasma Na^+ × urine creatinine)] × 100 FE_{Cl} (%) = [(urine Cl^- × plasma creatinine)/(Plasma Cl^- × urine creatinine)] × 100. If these parameters are low (<0.5 to 1%), a low EAV is indicated. Other findings suggestive of a low EAV include an increase in the blood urea nitrogen (BUN)/creatinine ratio (>20:1), increased serum uric acid concentration (due to increased proximal tubular reabsorption), and increased hematocrit and serum albumin concentration secondary to hemoconcentration. *Osmolality can be normal or increased with hyperglycemia.

In the absence of primary polydipsia, hypotonic hyponatremia results when water intake exceeds the renal capacity for water excretion due to an inappropriately concentrated urine (some value >100 mOsm/L). The effective arterial blood volume (EAV) must be defined in this setting. Decreased EAV causes baroreceptor stimulation of AVP secretion and leads to decreased distal delivery of filtrate to the tip of the loop of Henle, accounting for the inability to maximally dilute the urine. If EAV is low, ECF volume can be low in the volume-depleted patient (hypovolemic hyponatremia) or can be high in the edematous patient (hypervolemic hyponatremia). A normal EAV points to euvolemic causes of hyponatremia (isovolemic hyponatremia).

Approximately two thirds of diagnosed hyponatremia cases are acquired in the hospital, where the common practices of monitoring daily fluid intake, patient weight, and Na^+ levels normally allow prompt diagnosis. Administration of hypotonic fluids in the postoperative period is a risk factor for acute iatrogenic hyponatremia, particularly because AVP levels remain increased several days after surgical procedures. Iatrogenic cases can be prevented by close monitoring of electrolytes and urine output and by fluid restriction and avoidance of solutions with low-Na^+ content; this approach applies particularly to elderly patients.

In neurosurgical patients, the syndrome of inappropriate antidiuretic hormone secretion (SIADH) and cerebral salt wasting (CSW) are two potential causes of hyponatremia. Distinguishing between these two disorders can be challenging because there is considerable overlap in the clinical presentation. The primary distinction lies in the assessment of the EAV. SIADH is a volume-expanded state due to AVP-mediated renal water retention. CSW is characterized by a contracted EAV resulting from renal salt wasting. Making an accurate diagnosis is important because the therapy of each condition is quite divergent. Vigorous salt replacement is indicated in patients with CSW, and fluid restriction is the treatment of choice in patients with SIADH.

Common causes of hyponatremia outside the hospital setting include overhydration, diarrhea, vomiting, CNS infection, extreme exercise, liver failure, renal failure, congestive heart failure, drugs, SIADH, and combinations of these and other factors. Thiazide diuretics are the most common cause of drug-induced hyponatremia. Hyponatremia typically develops in the first 2 weeks of drug initiation and is most likely to occur in elderly women and during the summer months because of the increased ingestion of hypotonic fluids when it is hot. Concomitant use of nonsteroidal anti-inflammatory drugs (NSAIDs) and selective serotonin reuptake inhibitors (SSRIs) can further increase the risk of thiazide-induced hyponatremia.

Treatment of Hyponatremia

Symptoms of hyponatremia include nausea and malaise, which can be followed by headache, lethargy, muscle cramps, disorientation, restlessness, and obtundation. When treating a patient with hyponatremia, the Na^+ concentration should be raised at the rate at which it fell. In patients with chronic hyponatremia (>48 hours duration), the serum Na^+ concentration has fallen slowly. Neurologic symptoms are generally minimal, brain size is normal, and the number of intracellular osmoles is decreased. Sudden return of ECF osmolality to normal values will lead to cell shrinkage and possibly precipitate osmotic demyelination. This complication can be avoided by limiting correction to less than 10 to 12 mEq/L in 24 hours and to less than 18 mEq/L in 48 hours. In a patient whose serum Na^+ concentration has decreased rapidly (<48 hours), neurologic symptoms are frequently present, and there is cerebral edema. In this setting, there has not been enough time to remove osmoles from the brain, and rapid return to normal ECF osmolality merely returns brain size to normal.

In general, the development of hyponatremia in the outpatient setting is more commonly chronic in duration and should be corrected slowly. By contrast, hyponatremia of short duration is more likely to be

表 3.1 决定渗透压调节和容量调节的感受器和效应器		
因素	渗透压调节	容量调节
感知对象	血浆渗透液	有效动脉血容量
感受器	下丘脑渗透压感受器	低压和高压压力感受器
效应器	精氨酸加压素，渴感	醛固酮，血管紧张素 II，交感神经系统
产生的效应	尿渗透压，口渴	尿钠排泄

如果不是原发性烦渴，不恰当的尿浓缩（渗透压 > 100 mOsm/L）使摄入的水分超过肾脏的排水能力，就会出现低张性低钠血症。在这种情况下，需要明确有效动脉血容量（EAV）。EAV 降低会引起压力感受器刺激 AVP 的分泌，导致肾小球滤液到亨利袢顶端的远距离输送减少，从而无法最大限度稀释尿液。如果 EAV 低，ECF 量在容量不足的患者中会低（低容量性低钠血症），在水肿患者中会高（高容量性低钠血症）。EAV 正常则表明等容积性原因引起的低钠血症（等容量性低钠血症）。

大约 2/3 的低钠血症病例是在医院内诊断的，常规监测患者每日液体入量、体重以及血 Na^+ 水平可及时诊断低钠血症。因为 AVP 水平在手术后数天仍保持升高状态，因此术后输注低张液体是导致急性医源性低钠血症的一个危险因素。通过密切监测电解质和尿量，限水，以及避免使用含 Na^+ 量低的溶液，可以预防医源性低钠血症的发生，这对老年患者尤其适用。

在神经外科患者中，抗利尿激素分泌失调综合征（SIADH）和脑耗盐综合征（CSW）是导致低钠血症的两个潜在原因。由于这两种疾病在临床表现上有相当多的重叠，区分具有一定的难度。主要的区别在于对 EAV 的评估。SIADH 是由 AVP 介导的肾性水潴留引起的容量扩张状态。而 CSW 是由于肾耗盐导致的 EAV 收缩状态。因为两种情况的治疗方法截然不同，因此做出准确诊断非常重要。CSW 患者应大力补盐，而 SIADH 患者则应限制液体摄入。

医院外导致低钠血症的常见原因包括过度补水、腹泻、呕吐、中枢神经系统感染、剧烈运动、肝衰竭、肾衰竭、充血性心力衰竭、药物、SIADH，以及这些因素结合其他因素。噻嗪类利尿剂是药物引起低钠血症最常见的原因。低钠血症通常发生在服药后的前两周，最容易发生在老年妇女中和夏季，这是由于炎热天气下低张液体摄入增加所致。同时服用非甾体抗炎药（NSAID）和选择性血清素再摄取抑制剂（SSRI）会进一步增加噻嗪类药物引起低钠血症的风险。

低钠血症的治疗

低钠血症的症状包括恶心和乏力，随后会出现头痛、淡漠、肌肉痉挛、定向力障碍、烦躁不安和昏迷。

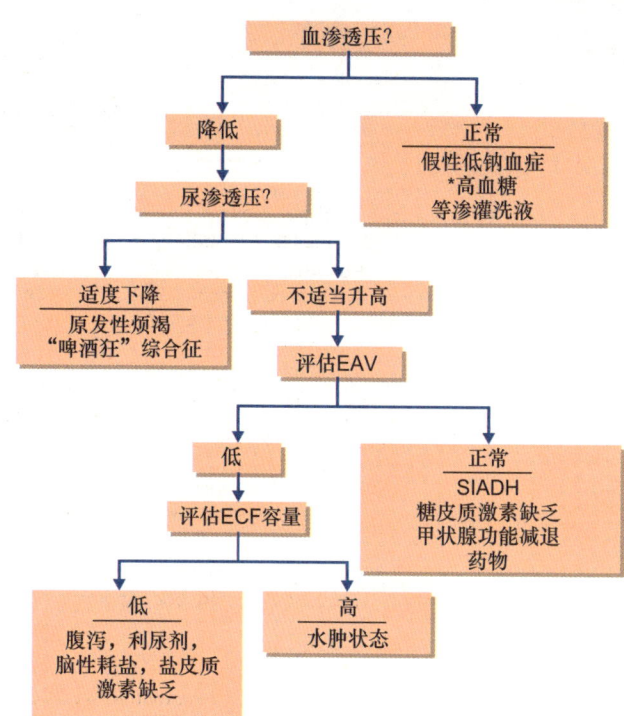

图 3.1 低钠血症诊断流程。评估有效动脉血容量（EAV）是了解肾脏潴钠机制以及肾脏潴钠是原发性还是对低 EAV 的反应的关键。根据定义，EAV 是肾脏感知到的动脉血容量。因此，如果肾脏正常工作并潴留 NaCl，则 EAV 值一定低；如果肾脏正常工作并排出大量 NaCl，则 EAV 值是高的。体格检查是评估 EAV 最可靠的方法。有无水肿以及血压和脉搏的体位性变化都是提示 EAV 高低的特别有用的指标。实验室检查也有助于评估 EAV。收集随机尿的尿 Na^+、Cl^- 和肌酐，可以通过以下公式计算 Na^+ 或 Cl^- 的排泄分数：FENa（%）= [（尿 Na^+ × 血肌酐）/（血 Na^+ × 尿肌酐）] × 100；FECl（%）= [（尿 Cl^- × 血肌酐）/（血 Cl^- × 尿肌酐）] × 100。如果这些参数较低（< 0.5% ~ 1%），则表明 EAV 值较低。其他提示低 EAV 的结果包括血尿素氮（BUN）/血肌酐比值升高（> 20 : 1）、血尿酸浓度升高（由于近端肾小管重吸收增加）、继发于血液浓缩的血细胞比容（红细胞压积）和血清白蛋白浓度升高。*渗透压可正常或因高血糖而升高

治疗低钠血症患者时，提升血 Na^+ 浓度的速度应该与其下降的速度持平。慢性低钠血症（病程超过 48 h）患者的血清 Na^+ 浓度下降缓慢。神经系统症状通常很轻微，大脑体积正常，细胞内渗透分子数量减少。ECF 渗透压突然恢复到正常值会导致细胞皱缩，并可能引发渗透性脱髓鞘。通过控制血钠纠正速度在 24 h 内升高低于 10 ~ 12 mmol/L，以及 48 h 内升高低于 18 mmol/L，可以避免这种并发症。在血清 Na^+ 浓度迅速下降（< 48 h）的患者中，通常会出现神经系统症状和脑水肿。在这种情况下，没有足够的时间来清除脑内的渗透分子，快速恢复到正常 ECF 渗透压仅会使大脑体积恢复正常。

一般来说，门诊患者的低钠血症多为慢性，应缓慢纠正。与之相对，短期发生的低钠血症更常见于接受静脉自由水输液的住院患者。使用"摇头丸"、运动

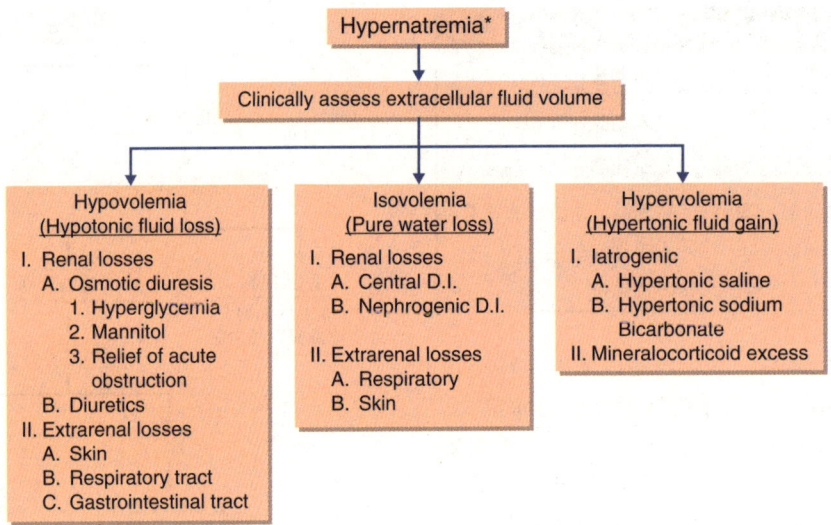

Fig. 3.2 Approach to the patient with hypernatremia.

encountered in hospitalized patients receiving intravenous free water. Use of "ecstasy," exercise-induced hyponatremia, or patients with primary polydipsia can also lead to acute hyponatremia and if symptomatic may similarly require rapid correction.

HYPERNATREMIA

Hypernatremia is a relatively common problem, particularly among the elderly and critically ill. Hypernatremia always indicates hypertonicity and shrinkage of cells. It is an independent risk factor for mortality in the ICU setting.

The initial approach to any patient with hypernatremia is to determine why there has been inadequate intake of water (Fig. 3.2). Hypernatremia is rare in conscious patients who have free access to water because of the extreme sensitivity of the thirst mechanism. Usually there is inadequate water intake due to an alteration in the level of consciousness so that patients become unaware of thirst or cannot adequately communicate the need for water or there is restricted access to water. Only rarely is there a specific lesion of the thirst center. A reduced sensation of thirst occurs in otherwise normal individuals as a feature of increasing age.

The next step is to search for the presence of accelerated water loss or increased Na^+ gain, both of which will increase the likelihood of a patient developing hypernatremia. This can be accomplished by clinical assessment of EAV. Hypovolemic hypernatremia results from fluid losses in which the Na^+ concentration is less than the plasma concentration. Hypervolemic hypernatremia can be due to iatrogenic administration of hypertonic NaCl or hypertonic $NaHCO_3$ or from mineralocorticoid excess.

Pure water loss, whether from mucocutaneous routes or from the kidneys, causes isovolemic hypernatremia. Because two thirds of pure water loss is sustained from within cells, patients will not become clinically volume depleted unless the water deficit becomes substantial. Insensible losses from the respiratory tract or skin result in concentrated urine. Inappropriate water loss by the kidney, whether from central or nephrogenic diabetes insipidus, results in dilute urine. Although renal water loss can lead to hypernatremia in patients with impaired thirst or access to water, most patients with diabetes insipidus have neither of these defects and typically present with polyuria, polydipsia, and a normal serum sodium concentration.

Evaluation of Polyuria and Polydipsia

Polyuria can be the result of an osmotic diuresis or a water diuresis. In turn, a water diuresis may result from inappropriate water loss as in either central or nephrogenic diabetes insipidus or may represent appropriate water loss as in primary polydipsia. The clinical setting and urine osmolality help to differentiate between these processes (Fig. 3.3).

Osmotic diuresis causing polyuria is often evident from the clinical setting. Poorly controlled glucose levels in a patient with diabetes mellitus, administration of mannitol to a patient with increased intracranial pressure, and high-protein enteral feedings (urea diuresis) are all examples in which polyuria is the result of osmotic diuresis. Urine osmolality greater than 300 mOsm/L in the polyuric patient is suggestive of solute or osmotic diuresis.

After excluding the presence of osmotic diuresis, one must then discriminate between the causes of water diuresis. In patients with central diabetes insipidus, the onset of symptoms is characteristically abrupt in nature, whereas patients with nephrogenic diabetes insipidus typically have a more gradual onset of symptoms. Patients with primary polydipsia are more vague in dating the onset of their symptoms. Both nephrogenic and central diabetes insipidus are characterized by severe and frequent nocturia, a feature that is typically absent in patients with primary polydipsia. Patients with central diabetes insipidus seem to have a predilection for ice water, which is not typically described in the other two conditions. A serum Na^+ concentration less than 140 mEq/L is suggestive of primary polydipsia because these patients tend to be in mild positive water balance. By contrast, a value greater than 140 mEq/L is more suggestive of either central or nephrogenic diabetes insipidus because these patients tend to be in mild negative water balance. Finally, urine osmolality will increase in response to water deprivation in primary polydipsia but show no response in diabetes insipidus. Central and nephrogenic diabetes insipidus are distinguished by the change in urine osmolality following subcutaneous administration of AVP (increased in central with no change in nephrogenic).

Treatment of Hypernatremia

Signs and symptoms of hypernatremia include lethargy, weakness, fasciculations, seizures, and coma. Increased ECF osmolality initially causes cell shrinkage within the brain. In response, cells generate

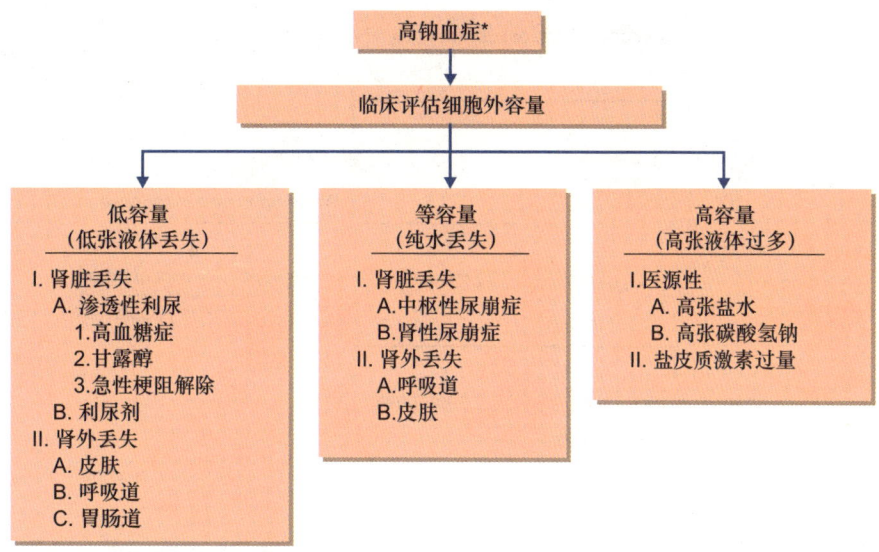

图 3.2 高钠血症诊断流程

引起的低钠血症，或患有原发性烦渴的患者也可发生急性低钠血症，如果出现症状，同样需要迅速纠正。

高钠血症

高钠血症相对常见，尤其是老年人和危重患者中。高钠血症总是表明高张和细胞皱缩。高钠血症是导致重症监护病房内死亡的一个独立危险因素。

高钠血症患者的治疗需要首先确定其水摄入不足的原因（图 3.2）。由于口渴机制极为敏感，因此在可自由获取水的清醒患者中很少出现高钠血症。通常情况下，水摄入不足是由于患者的意识状态发生了改变，无口渴意识或无法充分表达对水的需求，或者获取水的途径受到了限制。只有极少数情况下，才会有口渴中枢的特定病变。正常人随着年龄的增长，也会出现口渴感知减弱的情况。

下一步是寻找是否存在失水加速或 Na^+ 获取增加的情况，两者都会增加患者发生高钠血症的可能性。这可以通过临床评估 EAV 来实现。低容量性高钠血症是由液体流失导致的，其中 Na^+ 浓度低于血浆浓度。高容量性高钠血症可由于医源性给予高张 NaCl 或高张 $NaHCO_3$，或盐皮质激素过多所致。

纯水丢失，无论通过皮肤黏膜还是肾脏途径，都会导致等容量性高钠血症。因为 2/3 的纯水丢失来自于细胞内部，因此除非严重缺水，否则患者在临床上不会出现低容量表现。呼吸道或皮肤的不显性失水会导致尿液浓缩。而由于中枢性或肾性尿崩症导致的肾脏的不恰当失水则会导致尿液稀释。虽然在渴感感知受损或获水途径障碍的患者中肾脏失水可导致高钠血症，但大多数尿崩症患者不存在上述这些缺陷，典型表现为多尿、烦渴，而血清钠浓度正常。

多尿和烦渴的评估

多尿可能是渗透性利尿或水利尿的结果。反过来，水利尿可能是由于中枢性或肾性尿崩症造成的不恰当的失水，也可能是原发性烦渴造成相应的水丢失。临床情况和尿渗透压有助于区分这些过程（图 3.3）。

临床上导致多尿的渗透性利尿的原因通常很明显。糖尿病患者血糖水平控制不佳，颅内压增高患者使用甘露醇，以及肠内高蛋白营养（尿素性利尿）都是渗透性利尿导致多尿的例子。多尿患者尿渗透压大于 300 mOsm/L 提示存在溶质性或渗透性利尿。

除外存在渗透性利尿后，必须进一步区分导致水利尿的不同原因。中枢性尿崩症患者的特点是突然出现症状，而肾性尿崩症患者的症状通常逐渐出现。原发性烦渴患者的症状起始时间较模糊。肾性和中枢性尿崩症患者的特点均是严重而频繁的夜尿，而原发性烦渴患者通常无此表现。中枢性尿崩症患者似乎更偏好冰水，这在其他两种情况中并不常见。血清 Na^+ 浓度低于 140 mmol/L 提示原发性烦渴，因为这些患者往往处于轻度的水正平衡状态。相反，血清 Na^+ 浓度大于 140 mmol/L 更提示中枢性或肾性尿崩症，因为这些患者往往处于轻度的水负平衡状态。最后，限水会使原发性烦渴患者的尿渗透压升高，但尿崩症患者则无此反应。可通过皮下注射 AVP 后尿渗透压的变化区分中枢性和肾性尿崩症（中枢性尿崩症患者尿渗透压升高，而肾性尿崩症患者尿渗透压无变化）。

高钠血症的治疗

高钠血症的症状和体征包括淡漠、虚弱、肌肉震颤、癫痫发作和昏迷。ECF 渗透压的升高最初会导致脑细胞皱缩。细胞对此做出的反应是生成细胞内渗透

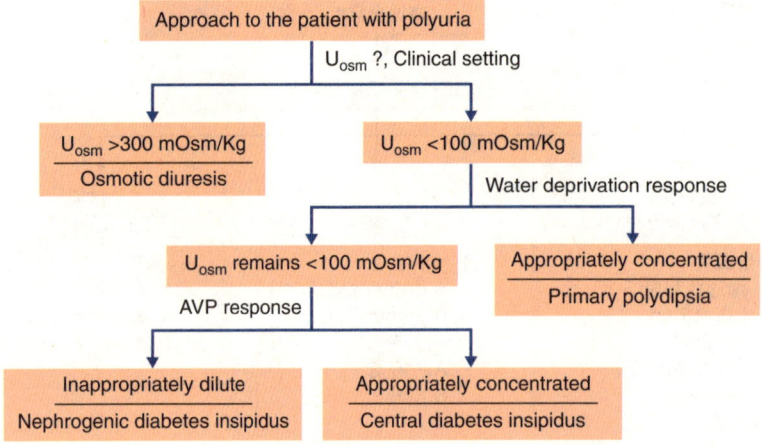

Fig. 3.3 Approach to the patient with polyuria. *AVP,* Arginine vasopressin; *U,* urine.

intracellular osmoles, which pull water back into the cells, returning brain size to normal. If extracellular osmolality is returned rapidly to normal, the extra intracellular osmoles will pull water into the brain cells, resulting in cerebral edema. Thus, in general, hypernatremia should be corrected slowly by water administration at a rate that leads to half correction in 24 hours. The water deficit can be estimated from the following formula:

$$\text{Water deficit} = \text{Current body water (0.6 in men and 0.5 in women} \times \text{body weight)} \times \left[\left([Na^+]_{plasma}/140\right) - 1\right]$$

Calculation of the amount of water to give must add insensible losses and any ongoing losses from the urinary and gastrointestinal tract. This formula also does not include the volume of isotonic saline required in those patients who may be concomitantly volume depleted. Careful monitoring of the serum Na^+ is required to ensure the rate of correction is appropriate.

HYPOKALEMIA

Hypokalemia is a common clinical disorder. Decreases in total body K^+ are usually due to gastrointestinal or renal losses whereas hypokalemia in the setting of normal total body K^+ is due to cell shift. In most cases, the cause can be determined by history, measurement of blood pressure, examination of acid-base balance, and measurement of urinary K^+ levels.

Cellular Shift With Normal Total Body Potassium

In the absence of physical and historical evidence of gastrointestinal or renal K^+ losses, either a redistribution of K^+ at the cellular level or laboratory error will account for a low serum K^+. Spurious causes of hypokalemia can be seen in leukemia patients with leukocyte counts of 100 to 250,000 $\times 10^9$/L, in which still-viable leukocytes extract K^+ from the serum in the sample tube. Interestingly, some patients with acute myeloid leukemia develop kidney K^+ wasting due to increased urinary excretion of lysozyme. This protein increases the luminal electronegativity in the collecting duct, providing a greater driving force for K^+ secretion.

The regulation of K^+ distribution between the intracellular and extracellular space is referred to as internal K^+ balance. Although the kidney is ultimately responsible for maintenance of total body K^+, factors that modulate internal balance are important in the disposal of acute K^+ loads. A large potassium meal could potentially double extracellular K^+ were it not for the rapid shift of the K^+ load into cells. The kidney cannot excrete K^+ rapidly enough in this setting to prevent life-threatening hyperkalemia. Thus, it is important that this excess K^+ be rapidly shifted and stored in cells until the kidney has successfully excreted the K^+ load. The major regulators of K^+ shift into cells are insulin and catecholamines.

Insulin excess, whether given exogenously in a patient with diabetes mellitus or endogenous secretion as seen in a normal person given a high glucose load, will lower the serum K^+. β-Adrenergic agonists used in the treatment of bronchospasm or in treating premature labor will cause similar K^+ shifts. In the setting of an acute myocardial infarction, hypokalemia may result as a sequela of high circulating epinephrine levels and might predispose to arrhythmias in this clinical setting. Other clinical disorders resulting in intracellular sequestration of K^+ are treatment of megaloblastic anemia with vitamin B_{12}, hypothermia, and barium poisoning. Hypokalemic periodic paralysis is inherited in an autosomal dominant pattern and is characterized by episodic hypokalemia resulting in muscle weakness. An acquired form of the disorder is seen in thyrotoxic patients, who are often of Japanese or Mexican descent.

Decreased Total Body Potassium

In the absence of cell shift, low serum K^+ can result from inadequate dietary intake, extrarenal losses through the gastrointestinal tract or skin, or renal losses. The urinary K^+ concentration serves as a useful guide in discerning between these possibilities. A urine K^+ concentration of less than 20 mEq/L is suggestive of extrarenal losses, whereas a urine concentration of greater than 40 mEq/L suggests renal K^+ losses. A limitation of a random value is the degree of urinary concentration. A urine K^+ concentration of 40 mEq/L may be an appropriate response in a hypokalemic patient with maximally concentrated urine due to decreased water intake. By the same token, a random urine value of less than 15 mEq/L may represent renal K^+ wasting if obtained in the setting of water diuresis.

The transtubular potassium gradient (TTKG) is a method designed to overcome the limitations of a random urine K^+ concentration in the evaluation of a dyskalemic patient:

$$TTKG = U_{potassium} \times Serum_{osmolality}/Serum_{potassium} \times U_{osmolality}$$

The formula estimates the ratio of K^+ in the lumen of the cortical collecting duct to that in the peritubular capillaries at a point where tubular fluid is isotonic relative to plasma. While still often used, the

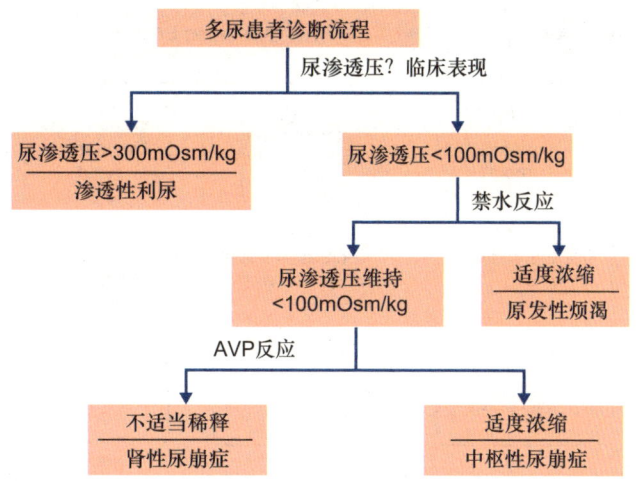

图 3.3　多尿患者临床诊断流程。AVP，精氨酸加压素

分子，将水拉回细胞内，使脑体积恢复正常。如果细胞外渗透压恢复到正常的速度过快，细胞内额外的渗透分子会将水分引入脑细胞，导致脑水肿。因此，一般来说，高钠血症应以 24 h 内纠正一半的速度补水来进行缓慢纠正。缺水量可通过以下公式估算：

缺水量＝目前身体含水量（男性：体重×0.6；女性：体重×0.5）×［（血浆钠浓度/140）－1］

计算补水量时必须加上不显性失水以及泌尿道和胃肠道的持续丢失量。该公式也不包括那些因同时存在容量不足患者所需的等张盐水量。需要密切监测血清 Na^+ 水平以确保纠正速度合适。

低钾血症

低钾血症是一种临床常见的电解质紊乱。体内总 K^+ 量的减少通常是由于胃肠道或肾脏丢失所致，而在体内总 K^+ 量正常时发生低钾血症则是由于 K^+ 向细胞内转移。在大多数情况下，低钾血症的病因可通过病史、血压测量、酸碱平衡检测，以及尿 K^+ 水平测定得以确定。

体内总钾量正常时细胞内外的 K^+ 转移

在没有胃肠道或肾性失钾证据的情况下，血清 K^+ 水平低可来自于细胞水平的 K^+ 再分布或实验室测定误差。在白细胞计数为 100～250 000×10^9/L 的白血病患者中会出现假性低钾血症，这是因为样本管中仍然存活的白细胞会从血清中摄取 K^+。有趣的是，一些急性髓性白血病患者会因尿溶菌酶排泄量增加而出现肾性失钾。这种蛋白质增加了集合管管腔的负电性，为 K^+ 在该处的分泌提供了更大的驱动力。

K^+ 在细胞内/外分布的调节被称为体内 K^+ 平衡。虽然肾脏最终负责体内 K^+ 总量的维持，但调节 K^+ 内在平衡的因素在处理急性 K^+ 负荷时也很重要。如果不能使 K^+ 负荷迅速转移到细胞内，饮食中大量的钾摄入可能会使细胞外的 K^+ 含量翻倍。这种情况下，肾脏排钾的速度无法快到足以防止出现危及生命的高钾血症。因此，在肾脏成功排出 K^+ 负荷之前，这些过多的 K^+ 能被快速转移并储存在细胞内非常重要。胰岛素和儿茶酚胺是 K^+ 转移入细胞内的主要调节者。

胰岛素过量，无论是糖尿病患者接受的外源性胰岛素，还是正常人在高糖负荷下的内源性分泌，都会降低血清 K^+。治疗支气管痉挛或早产时使用的 β 受体激动剂会导致类似的 K^+ 转移。急性心肌梗死时的低钾血症可能是高肾上腺素血症所致，并使得在这种临床情况下更易发生心律失常。还有其他一些导致细胞内 K^+ 滞留的临床情况，如使用维生素 B_{12} 治疗巨幼细胞性贫血、低体温以及钡中毒。低钾性周期性麻痹是一种常染色体显性遗传病，其特征是发作性低钾血症导致肌无力。获得性低钾性周期性麻痹可见于甲状腺功能亢进症患者，在日裔或墨西哥裔患者中更为常见。

体内总钾量减少

在没有细胞内转移的情况下，血清 K^+ 低可能是由于饮食摄入不足、通过胃肠道或皮肤等肾外途径流失，或肾性失钾所致。尿 K^+ 浓度在鉴别这些病因上非常有用。尿 K^+ 浓度低于 20 mmol/L 提示肾外失钾，而尿钾浓度高于 40 mmol/L 提示肾性失 K^+。但是随机值的局限性在于受尿液浓缩程度的影响。尿 K^+ 浓度 40 mmol/L 也可能是低钾血症患者因摄入水分减少而最大程度浓缩尿液的反应。同理，在水利尿的情况下，随机尿 K^+ 浓度低于 15 mmol/L，也可能是肾性失钾。

跨肾小管钾梯度（TTKG）的方法则可以克服随机尿液 K^+ 浓度在评估血钾异常患者时的局限性：

TTKG＝尿钾×血清渗透压/血清钾×尿渗透压

该公式估算的是皮质集合管管腔内的 K^+ 与肾小管管周毛细血管内的 K^+ 的比值，该处肾小管内液体与血浆等张。虽然仍在经常使用，但该公式所依据的假设

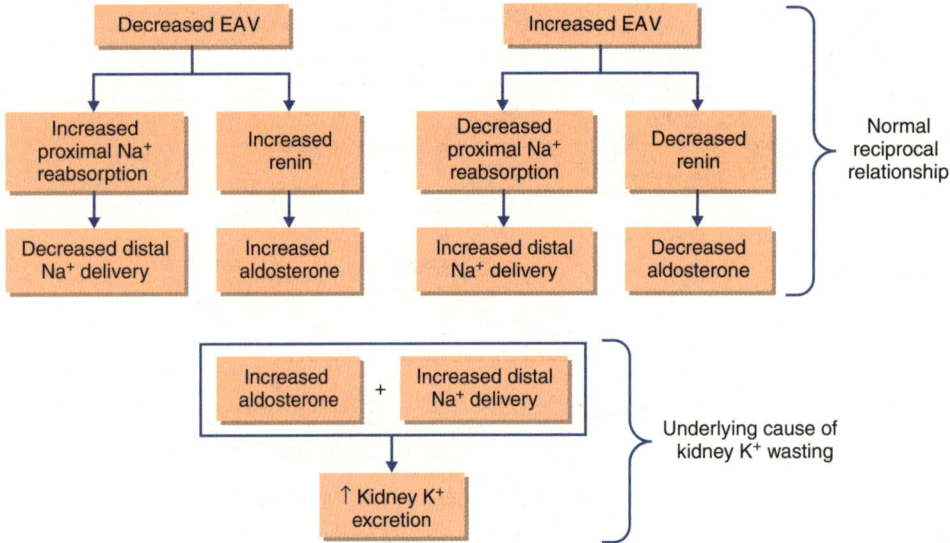

Fig. 3.4 The relationship between effective arterial volume and distal Na+ delivery in determining renal K+ excretion.

assumptions on which the formula is based have been called into question. For this reason, a urine K+ to creatinine ratio is now the preferred way to assess renal K+ handling. A ratio of less than 13 mEq K+/g creatinine or less than 2.5 mEq K+/mmol creatinine is considered an appropriate response to gastrointestinal potassium loss, remote use of diuretics, decreased dietary intake, and potassium shift into cells. Higher values suggest an inappropriate response of the kidney.

Inadequate dietary intake is an unusual cause of hypokalemia. Clinical situations associated with extreme K+-deficient diets include anorexia nervosa, crash diets, alcoholism, and intestinal malabsorption. Increased renal K+ excretion owing to magnesium deficiency (which is often present in these clinical situations) may contribute to the observed hypokalemia.

Extrarenal Potassium Losses

Sweat, with its low concentration of K+, is an unusual cause of K+ depletion. However, during physical training sweat losses can become substantial and K+ depletion may result. Gastrointestinal syndromes are the most common clinical disorders of extrarenal K+ losses. Diarrhea leads to fecal K+ wastage and is associated with a normal anion gap acidosis. Acidosis will result in K+ redistribution out of cells, leading to a degree of hypokalemia that is not as severe as the degree of total body K+ depletion.

Renal Potassium Losses

Increased distal delivery of Na+ and water and increased mineralocorticoid activity can each stimulate renal K+ secretion. Under normal physiologic conditions, these two determinants are inversely regulated by EAV (Fig. 3.4). Decreases in EAV are associated with increased aldosterone secretion but lower distal delivery of Na+ and water secondary to enhancement of reabsorption in the proximal nephron. It is for this reason that renal K+ excretion is relatively independent of volume status. It is only under pathophysiologic conditions that distal Na+ delivery and aldosterone become coupled. In this setting, renal K+ wasting will occur. This coupling can be due to a primary increase in mineralocorticoid activity or a primary increase in distal Na+ delivery. The term *primary* means that the changes are not secondary to changes in EAV. The causes of hypokalemia, grouped according to the physiologic determinants of renal K+ excretion, are given in Fig. 3.5.

Primary Increase in Mineralocorticoid Activity

Increases in mineralocorticoid activity can be due to primary increases in renin secretion, primary increases in aldosterone secretion, or increases in a non-aldosterone mineralocorticoid or increased mineralocorticoid-like effect. In all of these conditions, ECF volume is expanded and hypertension is typically present. The differential diagnosis for the patient with hypertension, hypokalemia, and metabolic alkalosis rests on the measurement of plasma renin activity and plasma aldosterone levels.

Primary Increase in Distal Sodium Delivery

Conditions that give rise to primary increases in distal Na+ delivery are characterized by normal or low ECF volume. Blood pressure is typically normal. Increases in distal Na+ delivery are most frequently due to diuretics that act proximal to the cortical collecting duct. Increased delivery can also be the result of non-reabsorbed anions such as bicarbonate as with active vomiting or a type II proximal renal tubular acidosis. Ketoanions (β-hydroxybutyrate and acetoacetate) and the Na+ salts of penicillins are other examples. The inability to reabsorb these anions in the proximal tubule results in increased delivery of Na+ to the distal nephron. Because these anions also escape reabsorption in the distal nephron, a more lumen-negative voltage develops and the driving force for K+ excretion into the tubular fluid is enhanced. Disorders of hypokalemia due to primary increases in distal Na+ delivery can best be categorized by the presence of metabolic acidosis or metabolic alkalosis.

Clinical Presentation

The most important clinical manifestations of hypokalemia occur in the neuromuscular system. Low serum K+ leads to cell hyperpolarization that impedes impulse conduction and muscle contraction. Typically, a flaccid paralysis develops in the hands and feet that moves proximally to eventually include the trunk and respiratory muscles. Death may occur from respiratory insufficiency. A myopathy may also occur that can evolve to rhabdomyolysis (muscle cell lysis) and acute kidney injury. Hypokalemia can also lead to smooth muscle dysfunction including paralytic ileus. Changes in electrocardiogram (ECG) include ST depression, T-wave flattening, and an increase in

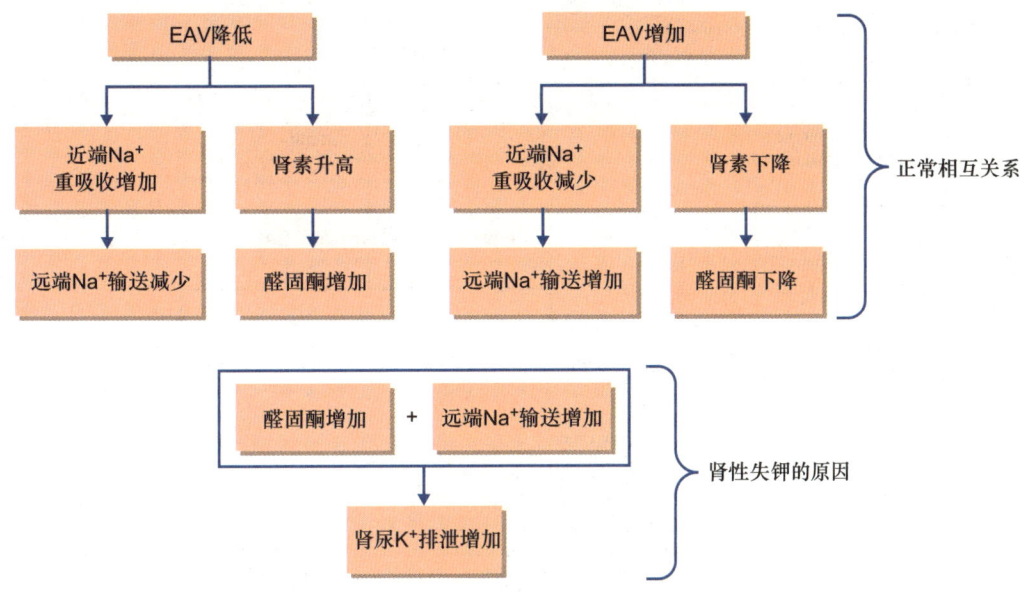

图 3.4 有效动脉血容量和远端 Na^+ 输送在决定肾脏 K^+ 排泄中的关系

已受到质疑。因此，尿 K^+ 与尿肌酐的比值现已成为评估肾脏 K^+ 处理能力的首选方法。比值低于 13 mEq K^+/g 肌酐或低于 2.5 mEq K^+/mmol 肌酐可源于胃肠道失钾、远期使用利尿剂、膳食摄入减少，以及钾转移到细胞内所致。更高的比值则提示肾性失钾。

饮食摄入不足是导致低钾血症的不常见的原因。与极度钾缺乏饮食有关的临床情况包括神经性厌食症、快速减肥饮食、酗酒和肠道吸收不良。镁缺乏（在上述临床情况下常见）导致的肾脏排 K^+ 增加可能参与了低钾血症的发生。

肾外失钾

汗液中的 K^+ 浓度低，因此出汗不是导致 K^+ 流失的一个常见原因。然而，在体育训练期间会大量出汗，可能会导致失钾。胃肠道综合征是最常见的肾外失钾临床疾病。腹泻导致 K^+ 从粪便中流失，与阴离子间隙正常性酸中毒有关。由于酸中毒会使 K^+ 重新分布到细胞外，这时发生的低钾血症不能反映全身总 K^+ 流失的严重程度。

肾性失钾

Na^+ 和水的远端输送增加以及盐皮质激素活性增加都会刺激肾脏分泌 K^+。正常生理情况下，EAV 对这两个决定因素的调节相反（图3.4）。EAV 降低与醛固酮分泌增加相关，但由于近端肾单位重吸收增强，远端 Na^+ 和水的输送减少。因此，肾脏排 K^+ 相对独立于容量状态。只有在病理生理情况下，远端 Na^+ 的输送和醛固酮的分泌才会同时发生。这种情况可能源于原发性盐皮质激素活性升高或原发性远端 Na^+ 输送增加，从而导致肾性失钾。所谓原发性是指这种变化不是继发于 EAV 的变化。图3.5 根据肾脏排 K^+ 的生理因素对低钾血症的原因进行了分类。

原发性盐皮质激素活性升高

盐皮质激素活性增高可能是由于原发性肾素分泌增加、原发性醛固酮分泌增加、非醛固酮性盐皮质激素增加或盐皮质激素样作用增高。在所有这些情况中，ECF 容量扩张，高血压是典型表现。对有高血压、低血钾和代谢性碱中毒患者的鉴别诊断依赖于血浆肾素活性和血浆醛固酮水平的测定。

原发性远端 Na^+ 输送增加

导致原发性远端 Na^+ 输送增加的情况以 ECF 容量正常或偏低为特征。血压通常正常。远端 Na^+ 输送增加最常见于使用了作用于皮质集合管近端的利尿剂。输送增加也可能来自于非重吸收性阴离子，如活动性呕吐或Ⅱ型近端肾小管酸中毒时的碳酸氢盐。酮体（β-羟基丁酸和乙酰乙酸）和青霉素 Na^+ 盐是另外的例子。由于近端肾小管无法重吸收这些阴离子，导致向远端肾单位输送的 Na^+ 增加。这些阴离子在远端肾单位也无法被重吸收，因此管腔的负电荷压增加，增强了促进 K^+ 排泄到肾小管液中的驱动力。因原发性远端 Na^+ 输送增加而导致的低钾血症可根据存在代谢性酸中毒还是代谢性碱中毒进行归类。

临床表现

低钾血症最重要的临床表现发生在神经肌肉系统。血清低 K^+ 会导致细胞超极化，进而阻碍脉冲传导和肌肉收缩。典型表现是手脚弛缓性麻痹，然后向近端蔓延，最终波及躯干和呼吸肌。患者可能会因呼吸衰竭死亡。还可能发生肌病，发展到横纹肌溶解（肌肉细胞溶解）和急性肾损伤。低钾血症还会导致包括麻痹性肠梗阻在内的平滑肌功能障碍。心电图（ECG）的变化包括 ST 段压低、T 波低平和 U 波增高。接受强心

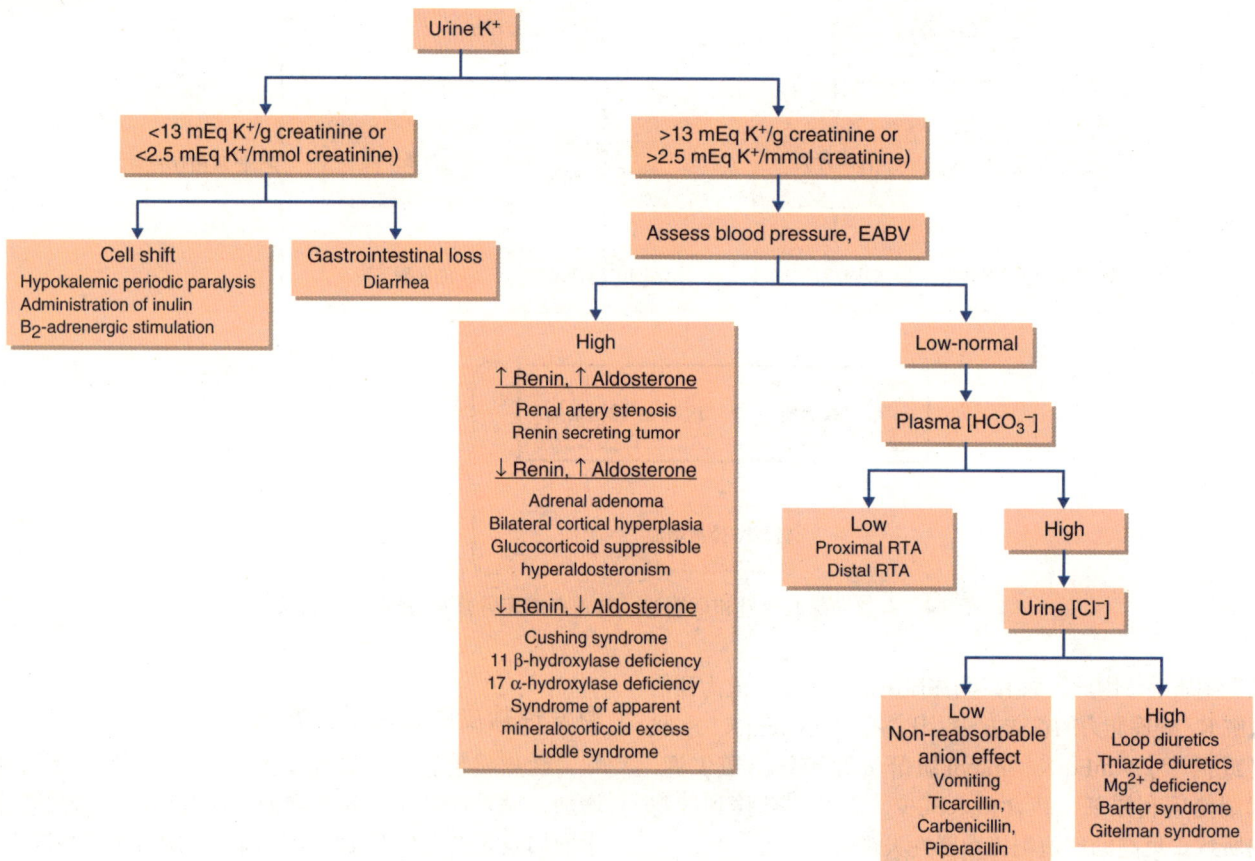

Fig. 3.5 Clinical approach to the hypokalemic patient.

the amplitude of the U wave. Patients treated with cardiac glycosides are at increased risk for premature ventricular contractions, and supraventricular and ventricular tachyarrhythmias, when hypokalemic.

Hypokalemia also causes a renal concentrating defect due both to a decrease in the medullary gradient and resistance of the cortical collecting tubule to AVP. This leads to polyuria and polydipsia. Prolonged hypokalemia can also lead to tubulointerstitial nephritis and renal failure (kaleopenic nephropathy). Because insulin release is regulated partially by serum K^+, hypokalemia can lead to glucose intolerance.

Treatment of Hypokalemia

The serum K^+ levels can at times be misleading as to the degree of deficit because a normal or even increased K^+ level can occur with significant total body K^+ depletion. In the absence of significant K^+ shifts, a decline in the serum K^+ from 4 to 3 mEq/L generally is associated with a deficit of 300 to 400 mEq intracellular K^+ per 70 kg body weight. A serum K^+ concentration of 2 mEq/L reflects a deficit of roughly 600 mEq. Despite these guidelines, the serum K^+ level should be monitored frequently during replacement therapy.

K^+ can be given orally or intravenously as the potassium chloride (KCl) salt. Potassium bicarbonate or citrate can be given if there is concomitant metabolic acidosis. The safest way to administer KCl is orally. KCl can be given in doses of 100 to 150 mEq/day. Liquid KCl is bitter tasting and, like the tablet, can be irritating to the gastric mucosa. The microencapsulated or wax-matrix forms of KCl are better tolerated.

Intravenous administration of K^+ may be necessary if the patient cannot take oral medications or if the K^+ deficit is large and is resulting in cardiac arrhythmias, respiratory paralysis, or rhabdomyolysis.

Intravenous KCl should be given at a maximum rate of 20 mEq/hour and maximum concentration of 40 mEq/L. Higher concentrations will result in phlebitis. Replacement of KCl in dextrose-containing solutions can lower the serum K^+ further secondary to insulin release. Thus, saline solutions are preferred. Depending on the specific cause, additional therapy of chronic hypokalemia involves the use of K^+-sparing diuretics such as amiloride, spironolactone or triamterene. These agents must be used cautiously in patients with renal insufficiency or in patients with other disorders that impair renal K^+ excretion.

HYPERKALEMIA

Like the hypokalemic disorders, a high serum K^+ can occur in the setting of normal or altered body stores of K^+. The body has a marked ability to protect against hyperkalemia. This includes regulatory mechanisms that will excrete excess K^+ quickly and mechanisms that will redistribute excess K^+ into cells until it is excreted. All causes of hyperkalemia therefore involve abnormalities in these mechanisms.

Pseudohyperkalemia is an in vitro phenomenon due to the mechanical release of K^+ from cells during the phlebotomy procedure, specimen processing, or in the setting of marked leukocytosis and thrombocytosis. (As noted above, with certain leukemias with high WBC counts, extraction of K^+ from the serum by cells in the sample tube can result in spurious hypokalemia.)

Excessive Dietary Intake

In the presence of normal renal and adrenal function, it is difficult to ingest enough K^+ in the diet to produce hyperkalemia. Rather, dietary

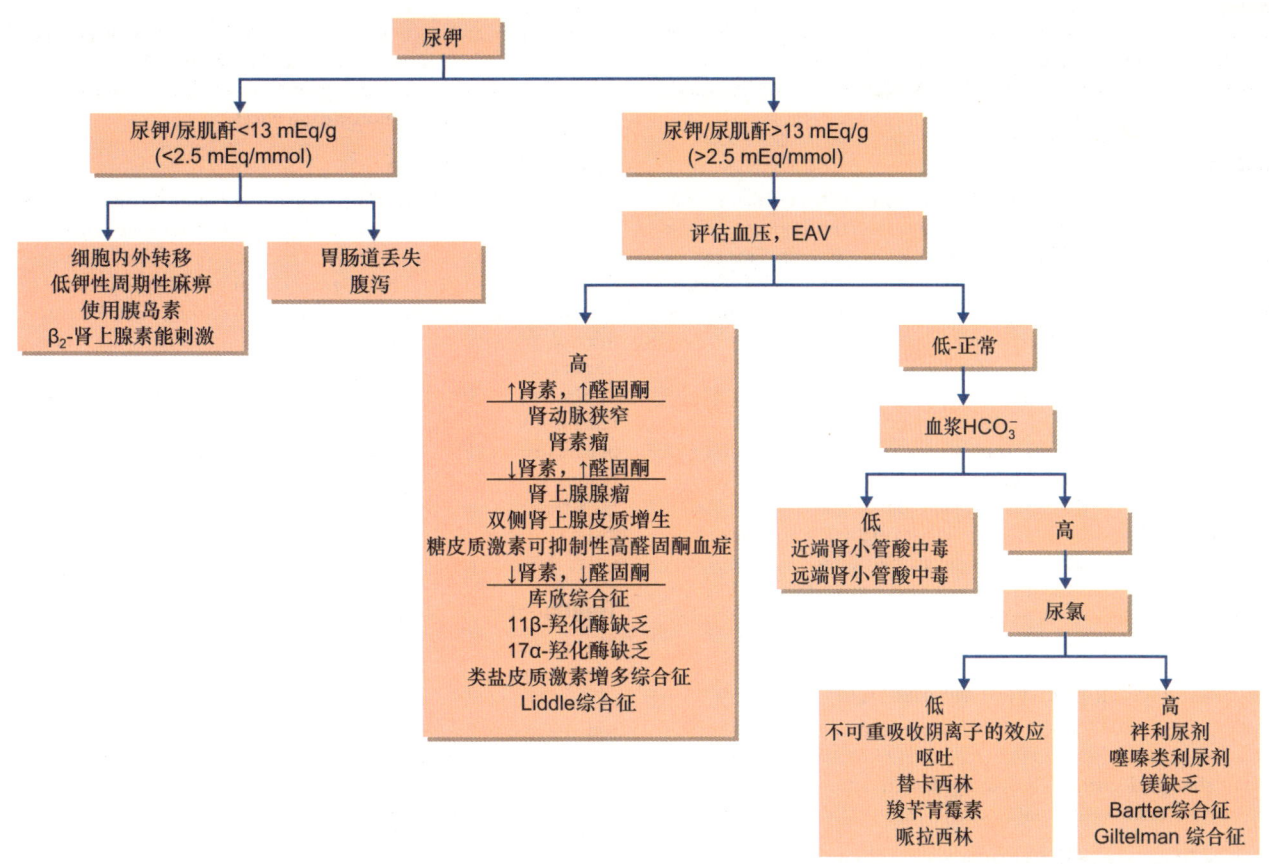

图 3.5 低钾血症患者接诊思路

苷治疗的患者如有低钾血症，发生室性早搏、室上性和室性快速性心律失常的风险增加。

由于髓质浓度梯度降低和皮质集合管对 AVP 的抵抗，低钾血症还会导致肾脏浓缩功能障碍，引起多尿和烦渴。长期低钾血症还会导致肾小管间质肾病和肾衰竭（低钾血症肾病）。由于胰岛素的释放部分受血清 K^+ 的调节，低钾血症可导致糖耐量异常。

低钾血症的治疗

在全身总 K^+ 量显著缺乏的情况下，血清 K^+ 的水平可能正常或甚至增高，因此血清 K^+ 的水平有时会误导对缺钾程度的判断。在没有明显的细胞内外 K^+ 转移的情况下，血清 K^+ 从 4 mmol/L 下降到 3 mmol/L 通常意味着每 70 kg 体重存在 300～400 mmol 的细胞内 K^+ 缺乏。2 mmol/L 的血清 K^+ 浓度反映大约 600 mEq 的 K^+ 缺乏。虽然有这些指导原则，在补钾治疗期间仍应经常监测血清 K^+ 水平。

K^+ 可以以氯化钾（KCl）盐的形式口服或静脉给药。如果同时伴有代谢性酸中毒，可给予碳酸氢钾或柠檬酸钾。氯化钾最安全的给药方式是口服。剂量为 100～150 mmol/d。液体氯化钾味道苦涩，与片剂一样，会刺激胃黏膜。微胶囊或蜡基形式的氯化钾耐受性更好。

如果患者不能口服药物，或 K^+ 的缺失量大并导致心律失常、呼吸肌麻痹或横纹肌溶解，则需静脉补 K^+。静脉氯化钾的最大给药速度为 20 mEq/h，最大浓度为 40 mmol/L。更高浓度会导致静脉炎。用含葡萄糖的溶液补充 KCl 会因胰岛素释放而进一步降低血清 K^+。因此，首选生理盐水补钾。根据具体病因，慢性低钾血症的其他治疗还包括使用保钾利尿剂，如阿米洛利、螺内酯或氨苯蝶啶。肾功能不全或患有其他影响肾脏排 K^+ 疾病的患者应慎用这些药物。

高钾血症

与低钾血症一样，高钾血症也可能发生在体内 K^+ 储备正常或改变的情况下。机体有强大的功能防止高钾血症。这包括快速排出体内过量 K^+ 的调节机制和将过量 K^+ 重新分配到细胞内直至排出体外的机制。所有导致高钾血症的病因都涉及这些机制的异常。

假性高钾血症是一种体外现象，是由于在抽血以及标本处理过程中，或在白细胞和血小板明显增多的情况下，K^+ 从细胞中机械性释放所致。（如前文所述，一些白细胞计数高的白血病样本，样本管中的细胞可摄取血清中的 K^+，导致假性低钾血症）。

饮食摄入过量

在肾脏和肾上腺功能正常的情况下，很难因为从饮食中摄入了大量的 K^+ 而产生高钾血症。饮食摄入 K^+ 参与高钾血症的发生通常见于肾功能受损时。富 K^+ 饮食包括甜瓜类水果、柑橘类果汁和含 K^+ 的低钠盐。

intake of K^+ as a contributor to hyperkalemia is usually observed in the setting of impaired kidney function. Dietary sources particularly enriched with K^+ include melons, citrus juice, and commercial salt substitutes containing K^+.

Cellular Redistribution

Cellular redistribution is a more important cause of hyperkalemia than of hypokalemia. Tissue damage is probably the most important cause of hyperkalemia due to redistribution of K^+ out of cells. This can be due to rhabdomyolysis, trauma, burns, massive intravascular coagulation, and tumor lysis (either spontaneous or following treatment). The effect of metabolic acidosis to cause K^+ exit from cells is dependent upon the type of acid present. Mineral acidosis (NH_4Cl or HCl) by virtue of the relative impermeability of the chloride anion results in the greatest efflux of K^+ from cells. By contrast, organic acidosis (lactic or β-hydroxybutyric) results in no significant efflux of K^+. Increased osmolality as in uncontrolled diabetes causes K^+ to move out of cells. In fact, it is the hypertonic state as well as insulin deficiency that accounts for hyperkalemia often seen in patients with diabetic ketoacidosis who are total body K^+ depleted. β-Adrenergic blocking agents can interfere with the disposal of acute K^+ loads. Other drugs that can result in hyperkalemia include the depolarizing muscle relaxant succinylcholine and severe digitalis poisoning.

Decreased Renal Excretion of Potassium

Decreased renal excretion of K^+ can occur because of one or more of three abnormalities: a primary decrease in distal delivery of salt and water, abnormal cortical collecting duct function, and a primary decrease in mineralocorticoid levels.

Primary Decrease in Distal Delivery (Acute and Chronic Kidney Disease)

Acute decreases in glomerular filtration rate (GFR), as occur in acute kidney injury, lead to marked decreases in distal delivery of salt and water that may secondarily decrease distal K^+ secretion. When acute kidney injury is oliguric, distal delivery of NaCl and volume are low and hyperkalemia is a frequent problem. When kidney injury is nonoliguric, however, distal delivery is usually sufficient and hyperkalemia is unusual. Decreased distal Na^+ delivery is a risk factor for hyperkalemia in patients with decompensated congestive heart failure. In chronic kidney disease patients, hyperkalemia is unusual until the GFR falls to less than 10-20 mL/min. The occurrence of hyperkalemia with a GFR of greater than 10 mL/min should raise the question of decreased aldosterone levels or a specific lesion of the cortical collecting duct.

Primary Decrease in Mineralocorticoid Activity

Decreased mineralocorticoid activity can result from disturbances that originate at any point along the renin-angiotensin-aldosterone system. Such disturbances can be the result of a disease state or be due to effects of various drugs. Hyperkalemia most commonly develops when one or more of these drugs are administered in a setting where the renin-angiotensin-aldosterone system is already impaired. One common example is the use of angiotensin-converting enzyme inhibitors (ACEI) or angiotensin-receptor blockers (ARB) in patients with diabetes mellitus with hyporeninemic hypoaldosteronism.

Distal Tubular Defects

Certain interstitial renal diseases can affect the distal nephron specifically and lead to hyperkalemia in the presence of only mild decreases in GFR and normal aldosterone levels. Amiloride and triamterene inhibit Na^+ transport, which makes the luminal potential more positive and secondarily inhibits K^+ secretion. A similar effect occurs with trimethoprim and accounts for the development of hyperkalemia following the administration of the antibiotic trimethoprim-sulfamethoxazole. Spironolactone and eplerenone compete with aldosterone and thus block the mineralocorticoid effect.

Clinical Presentation

Hyperkalemia leads to depolarization of the resting membrane because the potential across cell membranes is in part determined by the ratio of intracellular to extracellular K^+. The heart is particularly sensitive to this depolarizing effect. The progressive changes of hyperkalemia on the electrocardiogram are peaking of T waves, widening of the PR and QRS interval, development of a sine wave pattern, and eventually ventricular fibrillation and asystole. In general, ECG changes appear at a serum K^+ of 6 mEq/L with acute onset of hyperkalemia, whereas the ECG may remain normal up to a concentration of 8 to 9 mEq/L with chronic hyperkalemia. Hyperkalemia can also cause neuromuscular manifestations such as ascending paralysis and eventual flaccid quadriplegia. Hyperkalemia also decreases ammonia availability to act as a buffer for distal H^+ secretion. This effect impairs bicarbonate regeneration, leading to the development of a normal anion gap metabolic acidosis.

Treatment of Acute Hyperkalemia

The immediate treatment of life-threatening hyperkalemia is the administration of calcium, usually in the form of calcium gluconate or calcium chloride. ECG changes such as increasing PR interval or a widening QRS complex warrant treatment with calcium. Glucose and insulin therapy will shift K^+ into cells. Acute administration of glucose without insulin can potentially worsen hyperkalemia in patients with diabetes mellitus by raising extracellular osmolality and causing K^+ to shift into the extracellular space. $NaHCO_3$ administration through expansion of the ECF space results in dilution of the serum K^+. Additionally, K^+ is shifted into cells whenever concomitant metabolic acidosis is corrected. Inhalation of $β_2$-agonists such as albuterol or parenteral use of salbutamol can cause significant K^+ shifts into cells.

The effects of calcium, bicarbonate, glucose and insulin, and $β_2$-agonist therapy will provide immediate relief of acute toxicity but will not decrease total body K^+. Measures to reduce total body K^+ include the administration of K^+ binding drugs and dialysis.

Treatment of Chronic Hyperkalemia

After review of the patient's medication profile, drugs that can impair renal K^+ excretion should be discontinued if possible. Nonsteroidal anti-inflammatory drugs, either prescribed or those over-the-counter, are common offenders in this regard. Patients should be placed on a low K^+ diet with specific counseling against the use of K^+-containing salt substitutes. Diuretics are particularly effective in minimizing hyperkalemia. In patients with an eGFR less than 30 mL/min, thiazide diuretics can be used, but loop diuretics are required with more severe renal insufficiency. In chronic kidney disease patients with metabolic acidosis (bicarbonate concentration < 22 mEq/L), $NaHCO_3$ should be given. K^+-binding drugs can be utilized when hyperkalemia is refractory to the approaches outlined above. Sodium polystyrene sulfonate (Kayexalate) has been available for over 50 years but is poorly tolerated and has been linked to gastrointestinal toxicity. Patiromer and sodium zirconium cyclosilicate (ZS-9) are new K^+-binding drugs that are well tolerated when used chronically and can maintain normokalemia in the setting of renin-angiotensin-aldosterone system inhibitors.

METABOLIC ACIDOSIS

Metabolic acidosis is diagnosed by a low pH, a reduced HCO_3^- concentration, and respiratory compensation resulting in a decrease in the

细胞内外再分布

与低钾血症相比，细胞内外再分布是导致高钾血症的更重要的原因。由于 K^+ 可从细胞内释放再分布，因此组织损伤可能是造成高钾血症的最重要原因。可见于横纹肌溶解、创伤、烧伤、弥散性血管内凝血，以及肿瘤溶解（自发或治疗后）。代谢性酸中毒导致的 K^+ 从细胞中外流的效果取决于存在的酸的类型。由于细胞膜对带负电荷的氯离子的通透性差，矿物性酸中毒（NH_4Cl 或 HCl）可导致最大程度的 K^+ 从细胞内外流。相比之下，有机酸酸中毒（乳酸或 β-羟丁酸）就不会导致明显的 K^+ 外流。糖尿病控制不佳时高血糖造成的高渗导致 K^+ 从细胞中流出。实际上，正是由于高张状态和胰岛素缺乏导致了糖尿病酮症酸中毒患者在全身 K^+ 缺乏的情况下出现高钾血症。β 受体阻滞剂可干扰急性 K^+ 负荷时的排钾机制。其他可导致高钾血症的药物包括去极化肌松剂琥珀酰胆碱和严重洋地黄中毒。

肾脏排钾减少

肾脏排 K^+ 减少可能由以下三种异常中的一种或多种所致：原发性盐和水的远端输送减少、皮质集合管功能异常以及原发性盐皮质激素水平降低。

原发性远端输送减少（急性和慢性肾脏病）

急性肾损伤时肾小球滤过率（GFR）急剧下降，导致向远端输送的盐和水明显减少，继发远端泌 K^+ 减少。当急性肾损伤为少尿型时，NaCl 和水的远端输送量低，高钾血症是常见的问题。然而，当肾损伤为非少尿型时，远端盐和水的输送通常充足，因而高钾血症并不常见。远端 Na^+ 输送减少也是失代偿性充血性心力衰竭患者出现高钾血症的一个危险因素。在慢性肾脏病患者中，在 GFR 降至低于 10~20 ml/min 之前，高钾血症并不常见。在 GFR 大于 10 ml/min 时出现高钾血症，需要考虑有无醛固酮水平下降或皮质集合管有特殊病变。

原发性盐皮质激素活性降低

肾素-血管紧张素-醛固酮系统的任何一个环节出现问题，都可导致盐皮质激素活性降低。这种问题可以是疾病所致，也可以是不同药物作用的结果。在肾素-血管紧张素-醛固酮系统已经受损的情况下使用一种或多种此类药物时更易出现高钾血症。一个常见的例子是，在有低肾素性低醛固酮血症的糖尿病患者中使用血管紧张素转换酶抑制剂（ACEI）或血管紧张素受体阻滞剂（ARB）。

远端肾小管功能缺陷

某些间质性肾病可特异性影响远端肾单位，可在 GFR 仅轻度下降且醛固酮水平正常的情况下导致高钾血症。阿米洛利和氨苯蝶啶可抑制 Na^+ 转运，从而使管腔内正电荷增加，进而抑制 K^+ 分泌。甲氧苄啶有类似的作用，这也是使用甲氧磺胺嘧啶后出现高钾血症的原因。螺内酯和依普利酮会与醛固酮竞争，从而阻断盐皮质激素的作用。

临床表现

由于细胞膜的跨膜电位部分取决于细胞内外 K^+ 的比例，因此高钾血症可导致静息状态下细胞膜去极化。心脏对这种去极化效应尤为敏感。高钾血症在心电图上的渐进变化是高尖 T 波、PR 间期和 QRS 间期增宽、出现正弦波，最终心室颤动和停搏。一般来说，急性高钾血症时，血清 K^+ 浓度达到 6 mmol/L 时心电图出现变化；而慢性高钾血症时，血清 K^+ 浓度达到 8~9 mmol/L 时，心电图也可保持正常。高钾血症还可导致如上行性麻痹和最终四肢弛缓性瘫痪等神经肌肉表现。高钾血症还会减少作为远端泌 H^+ 的缓冲剂的氨的可用性。这会影响碳酸氢盐的再生，导致阴离子间隙正常的代谢性酸中毒。

急性高钾血症的治疗

治疗危及生命的高钾血症可使用钙剂，通常以葡萄糖酸钙或氯化钙的形式给药。心电图的变化，如 PR 间期延长或 QRS 波群增宽，是使用钙剂治疗的指征。葡萄糖和胰岛素治疗会将 K^+ 转移到细胞内。糖尿病患者在不使用胰岛素的情况下使用葡萄糖，可能会因为提高细胞外渗透压，导致 K^+ 转移到细胞外而加重高钾血症。应用 $NaHCO_3$ 可通过扩张 ECF 稀释血清 K^+。此外，当同时存在的代谢性酸中毒被纠正时，K^+ 可转移到细胞内。吸入 β2-激动剂（如沙丁胺醇）或胃肠外使用沙丁胺醇可导致显著的 K^+ 细胞内流。

钙剂、碳酸氢盐、葡萄糖和胰岛素，以及 β2-激动剂的治疗可立即缓解高钾血症的急性毒性，但不会减少体内 K^+ 总量。减少体内 K^+ 总量的措施包括使用 K^+ 结合剂和透析。

慢性高钾血症的治疗

检查患者的用药情况，尽可能停用会影响肾脏 K^+ 排泄的药物。非甾体抗炎药，无论是处方开具还是非处方购买的，也是引起高钾血症的常见药物。患者应注意低 K^+ 饮食，尤其应建议患者不要使用含 K^+ 的低钠盐。利尿剂对减少高钾血症尤为有用。eGFR 高于 30 ml/min〔译者注：原文（小于 30 ml/min）错误〕的患者可以使用噻嗪类利尿剂，但对于肾功能不全更严重的患者，则需要使用袢利尿剂。对于有代谢性酸中毒（碳酸氢盐浓度 < 22 mmol/L）的慢性肾脏病患者，应给予 $NaHCO_3$。当上述治疗方法对高钾血症无效时，可使用 K^+ 结合剂。聚苯乙烯磺酸钠（kayexalate）已上市 50 多年，但耐受性差，且与胃肠道毒性有关。Patiromer 和环硅酸锆钠（ZS-9）是新型 K^+ 结合药物，长期使用耐受性良好，可在使用肾素-血管紧张素-醛固酮系统抑制剂的情况下维持血钾正常。

代谢性酸中毒

代谢性酸中毒的诊断依据是血 pH 值低，HCO_3^- 浓度降低，以及由于呼吸代偿导致二氧化碳分压（P_{CO_2}）下降。

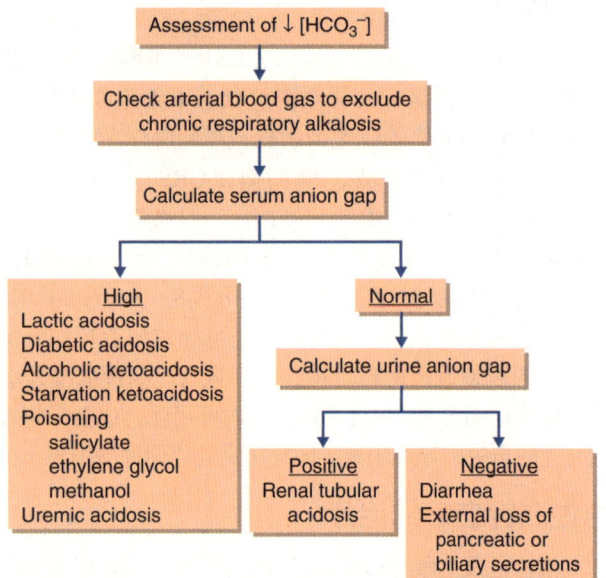

Fig. 3.6 Approach to the patient with a reduced serum HCO_3^- concentration.

partial pressure of carbon dioxide (Pco_2). A low HCO_3^- concentration alone is not diagnostic of metabolic acidosis because it also results from the renal compensation to chronic respiratory alkalosis. Measurement of the arterial pH differentiates between these two possibilities. The pH is low in hyperchloremic metabolic acidosis and high in chronic respiratory alkalosis. The clinical approach to a patient with a low serum HCO_3^- concentration is given in Fig. 3.6.

After confirming the presence of metabolic acidosis, calculation of the serum anion gap is a useful step in determining the differential diagnosis of the disorder. The anion gap is equal to the difference between the plasma concentrations of the major cation (Na^+) and the major measured anions (Cl^- + HCO_3^-).

$$\text{Anion gap} = (Na^+) - (Cl^-) - (HCO_3^-)$$

The normal value of the anion gap is approximately 12 ± 2 mEq/L. Most of the unmeasured anions consist of albumin; therefore, the normal anion gap changes in the setting of hypoalbuminemia (normal anion gap is approximately three times the serum albumin in g/dL). Because the total number of cations must equal the total number of anions, a fall in the serum HCO_3^- concentration must be offset by a rise in the concentration of other anions. If the anion accompanying excess H^+ is Cl^-, the fall in the serum HCO_3^- concentration is matched by an equal rise in the serum Cl^- concentration. The acidosis is classified as a normal gap or hyperchloremic metabolic acidosis. By contrast, if excess H^+ is accompanied by an anion other than Cl^-, the fall in HCO_3^- is balanced by a rise in the concentration of the unmeasured anion. The Cl^- concentration remains the same. In this setting, the acidosis is said to be a high anion gap metabolic acidosis.

A useful method for differentiating extrarenal from renal causes of metabolic acidosis is to measure urinary NH_4^+ excretion. Extrarenal causes of metabolic acidosis are associated with an appropriate increase in net acid excretion, primarily reflected by high levels of urinary NH_4^+ excretion. By contrast, net acid excretion and urinary NH_4^+ levels are low in metabolic acidosis of renal origin. Unfortunately, measurement of urinary NH_4^+ is not a test that is commonly available in clinical medicine. However, the amount of urinary NH_4^+ can be indirectly assessed by calculating the urinary anion gap (UAG).

$$UAG = (UNa^+ + UK^+) - UCl^-$$

Under normal circumstances, the UAG is positive, with values ranging from 30 to 50. Metabolic acidosis of extrarenal origin is associated with a marked increase in urinary NH_4^+ excretion and, therefore, a large negative value will be obtained for the UAG. If the acidosis is of renal origin, urinary NH_4^+ excretion will be minimal and the UAG will usually be positive.

The UAG can be misleading when other unmeasured ions are excreted. For example, increased urinary excretion of sodium keto acid salts in diabetic and alcoholic ketoacidosis and urinary excretion of sodium hippurate and sodium benzoate in toluene exposure can keep the UAG positive despite an appropriate increase in urinary ammonium excretion. Increased urinary excretion will also be missed when NH_4^+ is excreted with an anion other than Cl^- such as β-hydroxybutyrate or hippurate. In these settings, calculation of the urine osmolal gap is used as an indirect measure of ammonium excretion. The urine osmolal gap is the difference between the measured and the calculated urine osmolality:

$$\text{Urine osmolal gap} = \text{calculated urine osmolality (mOsmol/kg)}$$
$$= (2 \times [Na^+ + K^+]) + [\text{urea nitrogen in mg/dL}]/2.8 + [\text{glucose in mg/dL}]/18$$

The urine osmolal gap normally ranges from approximately 10 to 100 mOsmol/kg. Because NH_4^+ salts are generally the only other major urinary solute that contribute significantly to the urine osmolality, values appreciably greater than 100 mOsmol/kg reflect increased excretion of NH_4^+ salts.

Urine pH cannot reliably differentiate acidosis of renal origin from that of extrarenal origin. For example, an acid urine pH does not necessarily indicate an appropriate increase in net acid excretion. With a significant reduction in the availability of NH_4^+ to serve as a buffer, only a small amount of distal H^+ secretion will lead to a maximal reduction in urine pH. In this setting, the pH of the urine is acid but the quantity of H^+ secretion is insufficient to meet daily acid production. By contrast, alkaline urine does not necessarily imply a renal acidification defect. In conditions where availability of NH_4^+ is not limiting, distal H^+ secretion can be massive and yet the urine remains relatively alkaline because of the buffering effects of NH_4^+.

Hyperchloremic or Normal Anion Gap Metabolic Acidosis

Hyperchloremic (normal anion gap metabolic) acidosis can be of renal or extrarenal origin. Metabolic acidosis of renal origin is the result of abnormalities in tubular H^+ transport. Metabolic acidosis of extrarenal origin is most commonly caused by gastrointestinal losses of HCO_3^-. Other causes include the external loss of biliary and pancreatic secretions and ureteral diversion procedures. Fig. 3.7 provides a clinical approach to metabolic acidosis of renal origin.

Renal Origin

Proximal renal tubular acidosis (type II). The diagnosis of proximal RTA is suspected in a patient with a normal anion gap acidosis, hypokalemia, and an intact ability to acidify the urine to a pH of less than 5.5 while in a steady state. In the steady state, the serum HCO_3^- concentration is usually in the range of 16 to 18 mmol/L. Proximal RTA can be an isolated finding but most commonly is accompanied by generalized dysfunction of the proximal tubule (Fanconi syndrome). The urine anion gap is positive because proximal tubular dysfunction also impairs ammoniagenesis.

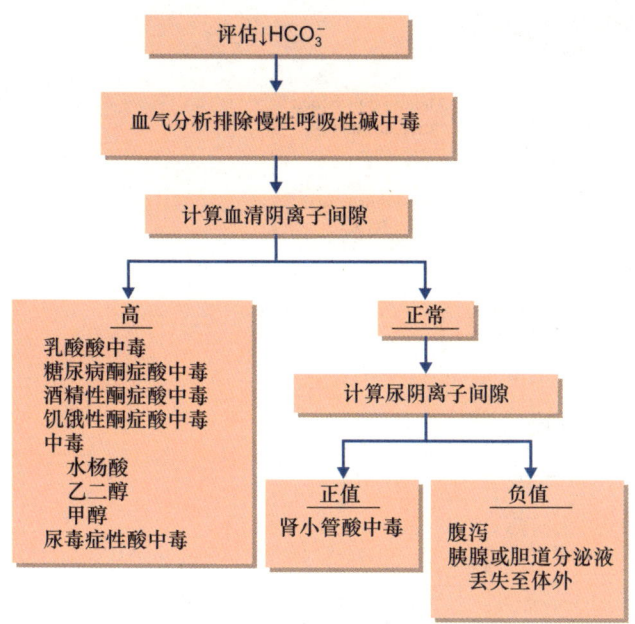

图 3.6　低血清 HCO_3^- 浓度患者的临床接诊思路

单纯 HCO_3^- 浓度降低并不能诊断为代谢性酸中毒，因为这种情况也可能见于肾脏对慢性呼吸性碱中毒的代偿。测量动脉血 pH 值可区分这两种可能性。高氯性代谢性酸中毒的血 pH 值低，而慢性呼吸性碱中毒的血 pH 值高。低血清 HCO_3^- 浓度患者的临床接诊思路见图 3.6。

确认存在代谢性酸中毒后，计算血清阴离子间隙有助于鉴别诊断。阴离子间隙等于血浆中主要阳离子（Na^+）和主要测定阴离子（$Cl^- + HCO_3^-$）的浓度差。

$$阴离子间隙 = Na^+ - (Cl^-) - (HCO_3^-)$$

阴离子间隙的正常值约为（12±2）mmol/L。绝大多数未测定的阴离子由白蛋白构成；因此，在低白蛋白血症时，正常阴离子间隙会发生变化（正常阴离子间隙约为血清白蛋白的 3 倍，血清白蛋白的单位为 g/dl）。由于阳离子总数必须等于阴离子总数，因此血清 HCO_3^- 浓度的下降必须由其他阴离子浓度的上升来抵消。如果伴随过量 H^+ 的阴离子是 Cl^-，则血清 HCO_3^- 浓度的下降必然匹配同等程度 Cl^- 浓度的升高。这种酸中毒被归类为阴离子间隙正常或高氯性代谢性酸中毒。相反，如果伴随过量 H^+ 的是 Cl^- 以外的阴离子，则 HCO_3^- 浓度的下降由未测定的阴离子浓度的升高来平衡，Cl^- 浓度保持不变。这种情况下的酸中毒被称为高阴离子间隙性代谢性酸中毒。

测定尿液 NH_4^+ 的排泄量是区分肾外源性和肾源性代谢性酸中毒的一种有用方法。肾外源性代谢性酸中毒伴有净酸排泄量的适度增加，主要反映在尿 $NH4^+$ 排泄的增多。与之相反，肾源性代谢性酸中毒时净酸排泄量和尿 NH_4^+ 水平均低。遗憾的是，尿 NH_4^+ 的测定并不是临床普遍开展的检测。不过，尿 NH_4^+ 含量可以通过计算尿阴离子间隙（UAG）来间接评估。

$$尿阴离子间隙 = 尿 Na^+ + 尿 K^+ - 尿 Cl^-$$

正常情况下，UAG 为正值，范围在 30 到 50 之间。肾外原因引起的代谢性酸中毒尿 NH_4^+ 排泄量明显增加，因此 UAG 会出现较大的负值。如果酸中毒是由肾脏原因引起的，尿 NH_4^+ 的排泄量会很少，UAG 通常会为正值。

当有其他未测定的离子排出时，UAG 可能会产生误导。例如，糖尿病和酒精性酮症酸中毒患者尿中酮酸钠盐排泄量增加，以及甲苯暴露患者尿中马尿酸钠和苯甲酸钠的排泄量增加时，虽然尿氨排泄量有适度增加，UAG 仍保持正值。当 NH_4^+ 与 Cl^- 以外的阴离子（如 β- 羟丁酸或马尿酸）一起排泄时，增加的尿排泄量也会被漏掉。在这些情况下，计算尿渗透压间隙可用来间接估算氨排泄。尿渗透压间隙是测量的尿渗透压与计算的尿渗透压之差：

$$尿渗透压间隙 = 测量的尿渗透压 - 计算的尿渗透压$$
$$计算的尿渗透压（mOsmol/kg）= [2 \times (Na^+ + K^+)] + (尿素氮\ mg/dl)/2.8 + (葡萄糖\ mg/dl)/18$$

（译者注：原文有误，公式中漏了测量的尿渗透压）。

尿渗透压间隙通常介于 10 至 100 mOsmol/kg 之间。由于 NH_4^+ 盐通常是对尿液渗透压有显著影响的唯一的其他主要尿液溶质，因此显著高于 100 mOsmol/kg 的数值提示 NH_4^+ 盐排泄增加。

尿 pH 值不能区分肾性和肾外源性酸中毒。例如，酸性尿 pH 值并不一定表明净酸排泄量的增加。当作为缓冲剂的 NH_4^+ 大量减少时，即使只有少量的远端的 H^+ 分泌也会导致尿液 pH 值大幅降低。在这种情况下，尿液的 pH 值虽然是酸性的，但 H^+ 的分泌量却不足以满足机体每日产酸的排出需要。与之相对，碱性尿液也并不一定意味着存在肾脏酸化功能缺陷。在 NH_4^+ 足够多时，远端 H^+ 的分泌量可以很大，但由于 NH_4^+ 的缓冲作用，尿液仍保持相对碱性。

高氯性或阴离子间隙正常性代谢性酸中毒

高氯性（阴离子间隙正常性代谢）酸中毒可由肾源性或肾外源性因素所致。肾源性代谢性酸中毒是肾小管 H^+ 转运异常的结果。肾外源性代谢性酸中毒最常见的原因是胃肠道丢失 HCO_3^-。其他原因包括胆汁和胰液的外部流失以及输尿管改道术。图 3.7 给出了肾源性代谢性酸中毒的临床接诊思路。

肾源性代谢性酸中毒

近端肾小管酸中毒（Ⅱ型）　如果患者有阴离子间隙正常性酸中毒、低钾血症以及在稳态时可将尿液酸化到 pH 值低于 5.5 的完整能力，则疑诊近端肾小管酸中毒（RTA）。稳态时，血清 HCO_3^- 浓度通常在 16～18 mmol/L。近端 RTA 可单独存在，但更常见的是伴有广泛的近端肾小管功能障碍（范科尼综合征）。由于近端肾小管功能障碍也会影响氨生成，所以尿阴离子间隙呈正值。

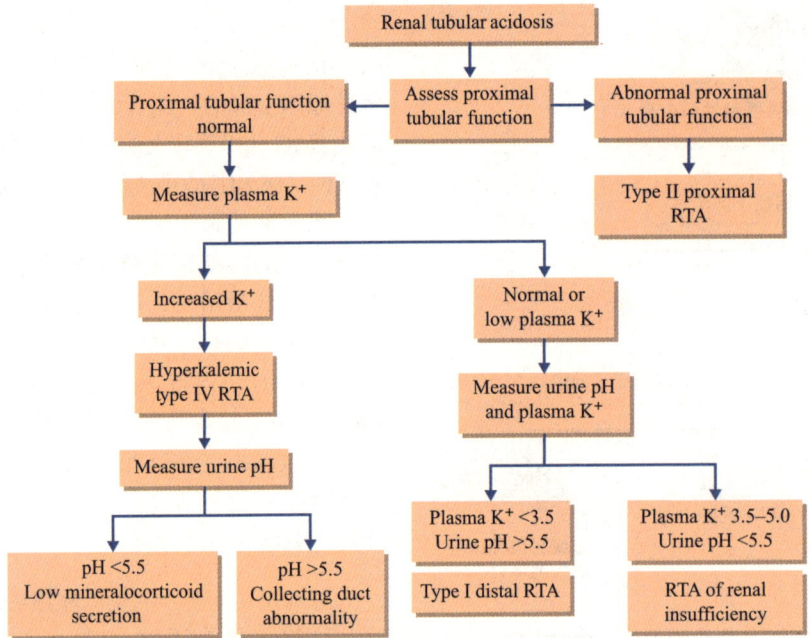

Fig. 3.7 Approach to the patient with acidosis of renal origin.

Proximal RTA is not associated with nephrolithiasis or nephrocalcinosis. However, osteomalacia can develop because of chronic hypophosphatemia and/or deficiency in the active form of vitamin D. Osteopenia may also be present because of acidosis-induced demineralization of bone. The treatment of patients with proximal RTA is difficult. Correction of the acidosis is often not possible even with large amounts of HCO_3^- (3 to 5 mmol/kg daily) because exogenous alkali is rapidly excreted in the urine. In addition, such therapy leads to accelerated renal K^+ losses. Use of a thiazide diuretic to induce enough volume depletion to lower the GFR and thus decrease the filtered load of HCO_3^- may increase the effectiveness of alkali therapy. Potassium-sparing diuretics may limit the degree of renal K^+ wasting. Once therapy is initiated, close monitoring is required to guard against severe electrolyte derangements. Acetazolamide and topiramate can cause metabolic acidosis due to inhibitory effects on carbonic anhydrase.

Hypokalemic distal renal tubular acidosis (type I). The diagnosis of distal RTA should be considered in a patient with hyperchloremic normal gap acidosis, hypokalemia, and an inability to lower the urine pH maximally. A urine pH greater than 5.5 in the setting of systemic acidosis is consistent with distal RTA. The urinary anion gap is positive. The systemic acidosis tends to be more severe than in patients with a proximal RTA with serum HCO_3^- concentrations as low as 10 mmol/L. Hypokalemia can also be severe and cause musculoskeletal weakness and symptoms of nephrogenic diabetes insipidus. Patients frequently manifest nephrolithiasis and nephrocalcinosis. This predisposition to renal calcification results from the combined effects of increased urinary Ca^{2+} excretion due to acidosis-induced bone mineral dissolution, a persistently alkaline urine pH, and low urinary citrate excretion.

Correction of the metabolic acidosis in distal RTA can be achieved by administration of alkali in an amount equal to daily acid production (usually 1 to 2 mmol/kg per day). In patients with severe K^+ deficits, correction of the acidosis with HCO_3^- can transiently cause further lowering of the extracellular K^+ concentration and result in symptomatic hypokalemia. In this setting, the K^+ deficit should be corrected prior to correcting the acidosis. Potassium citrate is the preferred form of alkali for those patients with persistent hypokalemia or with calcium stone disease.

Hyperkalemic distal renal tubular acidosis (type IV). A type IV RTA should be suspected in a patient with a hyperchloremic normal gap metabolic acidosis associated with hyperkalemia. The urinary anion gap is slightly positive, indicating little to no NH_4^+ excretion in the urine. Patients in which the disorder is caused by a defect in mineralocorticoid activity typically have a urine pH of less than 5.5, reflecting a more severe defect in NH_3 availability than in H^+ secretion. In patients with structural damage to the collecting duct, the urine pH may be alkaline, reflecting both impaired H^+ secretion and decreased urinary NH_4^+ excretion. The syndrome occurs most often in association with mild-to-moderate renal insufficiency; however, the magnitude of hyperkalemia and acidosis are disproportionately severe for the observed degree of renal insufficiency (Table 3.2). The primary goal of therapy is to correct the hyperkalemia. In many instances, lowering the serum K^+ will simultaneously correct the acidosis by restoring renal NH_4^+ production, thereby increasing the buffer supply for distal acidification.

Renal tubular acidosis of renal insufficiency. Patients with chronic kidney disease initially develop a hyperchloremic normal gap metabolic acidosis associated with normokalemia as the GFR falls below 30 mL/min. With more advanced chronic kidney disease (GFR < 15 mL/min), the acidosis changes to predominately an anion gap metabolic acidosis reflecting a progressive inability to excrete phosphate, sulfate, and the Na^+ salts of various organic acids. At this stage, the acidosis is commonly referred to as *uremic acidosis*.

Correction of the metabolic acidosis in patients with chronic kidney disease is achieved by treatment with $NaHCO_3$ 0.5 to 1.5 mmol/kg/day beginning when the HCO_3^- level is less than 22 mmol/L. Metabolic acidosis needs to be aggressively treated because it can contribute to metabolic bone disease, increase catabolism, and contribute to the progressive loss of kidney function.

Extrarenal Origin of Metabolic Acidosis

Diarrhea. Loss of HCO_3^- in intestinal secretions beyond the stomach leads to the development of metabolic acidosis. Volume loss signals the kidney to increase the reabsorption of salt. Renal retention of NaCl

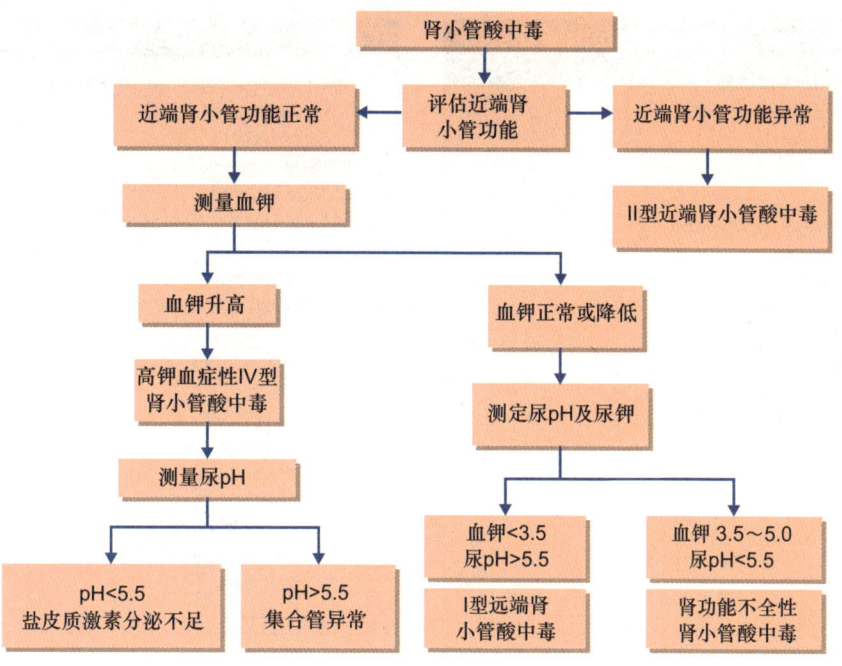

图 3.7　肾源性酸中毒患者的临床接诊思路

近端 RTA 与肾结石或肾钙化症无关。不过，由于慢性低磷血症和（或）活性维生素 D 缺乏，会出现骨软化症。酸中毒引起的骨质脱钙也可能导致骨量减少。近端 RTA 患者的治疗比较困难。由于外源性补充的碱会迅速随尿排出体外，因此即使使用大量 HCO_3^-（每天 3～5 mmol/kg 体重）也无法纠正酸中毒。此外，这种治疗还会加速肾脏 K^+ 的流失。使用噻嗪类利尿剂诱导足够的容量消耗以降低 GFR，从而降低 HCO_3^- 的滤过负荷，可能会提高补碱治疗的效果。保钾利尿剂可限制肾脏 K^+ 流失的程度。一旦开始治疗，就需要密切监测，以防发生严重的电解质紊乱。乙酰唑胺和托吡酯对碳酸酐酶有抑制作用，可导致代谢性酸中毒。

低钾血症性远端肾小管酸中毒（Ⅰ型）　如果患者有高氯性阴离子间隙正常性酸中毒、低钾血症，且无法最大限度地降低尿液 pH 值，则应考虑远端 RTA 的诊断。在全身酸中毒的情况下，尿液 pH 值仍大于 5.5 符合远端 RTA。尿阴离子间隙呈正值。全身性酸中毒的情况往往比近端 RTA 严重，血清 HCO_3^- 浓度可低至 10 mmol/L。低钾血症也可以很严重，导致肌肉骨骼无力和肾性尿崩症的症状。患者经常会有肾结石和肾钙化症表现。这种肾脏钙化的易感性是酸中毒导致的骨矿物质溶解造成尿 Ca^{2+} 排泄增加、持续碱性尿以及尿枸橼酸排泄低综合作用的结果。

纠正远端 RTA 的代谢性酸中毒可通过给予与每日产酸量（通常为每日 1～2 mmol/kg 体重）等量的碱剂来实现。对严重缺 K^+ 的患者，使用 HCO_3^- 纠正酸中毒会一过性引起细胞外 K^+ 浓度进一步降低，导致症状性低钾血症。这种情况下，应在纠正酸中毒之前先纠正 K^+ 缺乏。对持续低钾或有含钙结石的患者，枸橼酸钾是首选的碱剂。

高钾血症性远端肾小管酸中毒（Ⅳ型）　如果患者有高氯性、阴离子间隙正常的代谢性酸中毒并伴有高钾血症，应怀疑有Ⅳ型 RTA。尿阴离子间隙略呈正值，提示尿中几乎没有 NH_4^+ 排泄。因盐皮质激素活性缺陷导致者，其尿液 pH 值通常低于 5.5，反映出 NH_3 可用性缺陷比 H^+ 的分泌缺陷更为严重。在集合管结构受损的患者中，尿液 pH 值可能呈碱性，反映同时存在 H^+ 分泌受损和尿 NH_4^+ 排泄减少。该综合征最常见于轻至中度肾功能不全的患者；但是，高钾血症和酸中毒的严重程度与观察到的肾功能不全的程度不成比例（表 3.2）。治疗的首要目标是纠正高钾血症。在许多情况下，降 K^+ 治疗可通过恢复肾脏的 NH_4^+ 生成，从而增加远端酸化的缓冲供应而同时纠正酸中毒。

肾功能不全性肾小管酸中毒　慢性肾脏病患者当 GFR 低于 30 ml/min 时，最初会出现高氯性、阴离子间隙正常的代谢性酸中毒伴血钾正常。随着慢性肾脏病进展（GFR ＜ 15 ml/min），酸中毒的类型转变为高阴离子间隙性代谢性酸中毒，反映出肾脏逐渐丧失将磷酸盐、硫酸盐以及各种有机酸的 Na^+ 盐排出体外的能力。这一阶段的酸中毒通常被称为尿毒症性酸中毒。

当 HCO_3^- 水平低于 22 mmol/L 时，针对慢性肾脏病患者应启动代谢性酸中毒的治疗，每天给予 0.5～1.5 mmol/kg 体重的 $NaHCO_3$。由于代谢性酸中毒可导致代谢性骨病，增加分解代谢，并促进肾功能进行性丢失，因此需要积极治疗。

肾外源性代谢性酸中毒

腹泻　胃以外的肠道分泌物中 HCO_3^- 的丢失可导致代谢性酸中毒。容量的丢失促使肾脏增加对盐的重吸收。肾脏潴留 NaCl 加上肠道丢失 $NaHCO_3$，会产生高

TABLE 3.2 Causes of Hyperkalemic Distal (Type IV) Renal Tubular Acidosis

I. Mineralocorticoid deficiency
   A. Low renin, low aldosterone
      1. Diabetes mellitus
      2. Drugs
         a. Nonsteroidal antiinflammatory agents
         b. Cyclosporin, tacrolimus
         c. β-blockers
   B. High renin, low aldosterone
      1. Adrenal destruction
      2. Congenital enzyme defects
      3. Drugs
         a. Angiotensin-converting enzyme inhibitors
         b. Angiotensin II receptor blockers
         c. Heparin
         d. Ketoconazole
II. Abnormal cortical collecting duct
   A. Absence or defective mineralocorticoid receptor
   B. Drugs
      1. Spironolactone, eplerenone
      2. Triamterene
      3. Amiloride
      4. Trimethoprim
      5. Pentamidine
   C. Chronic tubulointerstitial disease

TABLE 3.3 Causes of Lactic Acidosis

I. Type A (tissue underperfusion and or hypoxia)
   A. Cardiogenic shock
   B. Septic shock
   C. Hemorrhagic shock
   D. Acute hypoxia
   E. Carbon monoxide poisoning
   F. Anemia
II. Type B (absence of hypotension and hypoxia)
   A. Hereditary enzyme deficiency (glucose 6-phosphatase)
   B. Drugs or toxins
      1. Phenformin, metformin
      2. Cyanide
      3. Salicylate, ethylene glycol, methanol
      4. Propylene glycol
      5. Linezolid
      6. Propofol
      7. Nucleoside reverse transcriptase inhibitors: stavudine, didanosine
   C. Systemic disease
      1. Liver failure
      2. Malignancy

---

combined with the intestinal loss of $NaHCO_3$ generates a hyperchloremic normal gap metabolic acidosis. Net acid excretion markedly increases due to increases in urinary excretion of NH_4^+. Hypokalemia due to gastrointestinal losses and the low serum pH both stimulate the synthesis of NH_3 in the proximal tubule. The increase in availability of NH_3 to act as a urinary buffer allows for a maximal increase in H^+ secretion by the distal nephron. Urine pH during chronic diarrheal states may be persistently greater than 6.0 due to the large increase in buffer capacity.

A patient who presents with hypokalemic hyperchloremic metabolic acidosis with a urine pH greater than 5.5 could have either a diarrheal state or a hypokalemic (type I) distal RTA. Although the clinical history would be the easiest way to distinguish between these two possibilities, in a patient with surreptitious laxative abuse this may not be helpful. Determination of the urinary anion gap is the best way to distinguish between them. In diarrhea, urine pH is high because of the large amount of NH_4^+ in the urine. This would be reflected by a negative urinary anion gap because most of the NH_4^+ is excreted in the urine as NH_4Cl. In hypokalemic distal RTA the urine pH is high because of the inability to secrete H^+ in the distal nephron. Urinary excretion of NH_3 is very low and the urinary anion gap is positive.

Ileal conduits. Surgical diversion of the ureter into the intestine may lead to the development of a hyperchloremic normal gap metabolic acidosis due to systemic reabsorption of NH_4^+ and Cl^- from the urinary fluid and exchange of Cl^- for HCO_3^- through activation of the Cl^-/HCO_3^- exchanger on the intestinal lumen. The main determinants for this complication are the length of time the urine is in contact with the bowel and the total surface area of bowel exposed to urine.

Anion Gap Metabolic Acidosis
Lactic Acidosis

Lactic acidosis is generated whenever an imbalance develops between the production and utilization of lactic acid. The accumulation of a nonchloride anion accounts for the increase in anion gap. Severe exercise and grand mal seizures are examples in which lactic acidosis can develop because of increased production. The short-lived nature of the acidosis in these conditions suggests that a concomitant defect in lactic acid utilization is present in most conditions of sustained and severe lactic acidosis. Type A lactic acidosis is characterized by disorders in which there is underperfusion of tissue or acute hypoxia. Such disorders include patients with cardiopulmonary failure, severe anemia, hemorrhage, hypotension, sepsis, and carbon monoxide poisoning. Type B lactic acidosis occurs in patients with a variety of disorders that have in common the development of lactic acidosis in the absence of overt hypoperfusion or hypoxia (Table 3.3).

D-Lactic Acidosis

D-Lactic acidosis is a unique form of metabolic acidosis that can occur in the setting of small bowel resections or in patients with a jejunoileal bypass. These short bowel syndromes create a situation in which carbohydrates that are normally reabsorbed in the small intestine are delivered in large amounts to the colon. In the presence of colonic bacterial overgrowth, these substrates are metabolized into D-lactate and absorbed into the systemic circulation. Accumulation of D-lactate produces an anion gap metabolic acidosis in which the serum lactate is normal because the standard test for lactate is specific for L-lactate. These patients typically present after ingestion of a large carbohydrate meal with neurologic abnormalities consisting of confusion, slurred speech, and ataxia. Ingestion of low-carbohydrate meals and antimicrobial agents to decrease the degree of bacterial overgrowth are the principal treatments.

Diabetic Ketoacidosis

Diabetic ketoacidosis is a metabolic condition characterized by the accumulation of acetoacetic acid and β-hydroxybutyric acid resulting from insulin deficiency and a relative or absolute increase in glucagon concentration. The degree to which the anion gap is elevated will depend on the rapidity, severity, and duration of the ketoacidosis as well as the status of the ECF volume. Although an anion gap acidosis is the dominant disturbance in diabetic ketoacidosis, a hyperchloremic normal gap acidosis is often present in the earliest stages of ketoacidosis when extracellular volume is near normal.

表3.2 高钾血症性远端（Ⅳ型）肾小管酸中毒的原因

Ⅰ. 盐皮质激素缺乏
　A. 低肾素，低醛固酮
　　1. 糖尿病
　　2. 药物
　　　a. 非甾体抗炎药
　　　b. 环孢素，他克莫司
　　　c. β 受体阻滞剂
　B. 高肾素，低醛固酮
　　1. 肾上腺破坏
　　2. 先天性酶缺乏
　　3. 药物
　　　a. 血管紧张素转换酶抑制剂
　　　b. 血管紧张素Ⅱ受体阻滞剂
　　　c. 肝素
　　　d. 酮康唑
Ⅱ. 皮质集合管异常
　A. 盐皮质激素受体缺失或缺陷
　B. 药物
　　1. 螺内酯，依普利酮
　　2. 氨苯蝶啶
　　3. 阿米洛利
　　4. 甲氧苄啶
　　5. 联苯胺
　C. 慢性肾小管间质病

表3.3 乳酸酸中毒的原因

Ⅰ. A型［组织低灌注和（或）缺氧］
　A. 心源性休克
　B. 感染中毒性休克
　C. 出血性休克
　D. 急性缺氧
　E. 一氧化碳中毒
　F. 贫血
Ⅱ. B型（无低血压和低氧）
　A. 遗传性酶（葡萄糖-6-磷酸酶）缺乏
　B. 药物或毒物
　　1. 苯乙双胍，二甲双胍
　　2. 氰化物
　　3. 水杨酸，乙二醇，甲醇
　　4. 丙二醇
　　5. 利奈唑胺
　　6. 丙泊酚
　　7. 核苷类逆转录酶抑制剂：司他夫定、地达诺新
　C. 系统性疾病
　　1. 肝衰竭
　　2. 恶性肿瘤

氯性阴离子间隙正常性代谢性酸中毒。由于尿 NH_4^+ 排泄增加，净酸排泄量显著增加。胃肠道损失导致的低钾血症和低血清 pH 值都会刺激近端肾小管的 NH_3 合成。作为尿液缓冲剂的 NH_3 的增加，使得远端肾单位的 H^+ 分泌最大限度增加。由于缓冲能力的大幅增加，慢性腹泻状态下的尿液 pH 值可持续高于 6.0。

尿 pH 值大于 5.5 的低钾性高氯性代谢性酸中毒患者可能是腹泻导致，也可能是有低钾性（Ⅰ型）远端 RTA。虽然临床病史是区分这两种可能性的最简单方法，但对于私下滥用泻药的患者来说则没有帮助。测定尿液阴离子间隙是区分这两种情况的最佳方法。腹泻时由于尿液中含有大量 NH_4^+，因此尿液 pH 值是高的。因为大部分 NH_4^+ 以 NH_4Cl 的形式从尿液中排出，反映在尿阴离子间隙上就是负值。在低钾性远端 RTA 时，由于远端肾单位无法泌 H^+，因此尿液 pH 值高。但尿液中 NH_3 的排泄量非常低，因此尿液阴离子间隙为正值。

回肠流出道术　将输尿管转接入肠道的外科手术可能会导致高氯性阴离子间隙正常性代谢性酸中毒，这是由于尿液中的 NH_4^+ 和 Cl^- 在肠腔被全身重吸收，以及通过激活肠腔中的 Cl^-/HCO_3^- 交换子进行了 Cl^- 与 HCO_3^- 的交换。这种并发症发生的主要决定因素是尿液与肠道接触的时间长短以及暴露于尿液的肠道总面积。

高阴离子间隙性代谢性酸中毒

乳酸酸中毒

只要乳酸的生成和利用之间出现失衡，就会产生乳酸酸中毒。非氯阴离子的蓄积导致阴离子间隙增高。剧烈运动和癫痫大发作是乳酸生成增加导致乳酸酸中毒的例子。这些情况下酸中毒持续时间短是其特点，提示大多数持续且严重的乳酸酸中毒都同时存在乳酸利用缺陷。A 型乳酸酸中毒的特点是见于组织灌注不足或急性缺氧类疾病。这些疾病包括心肺功能衰竭、严重贫血、出血、低血压、感染中毒症和一氧化碳中毒。B 型乳酸酸中毒可见于多种疾病，这些疾病的共同点是乳酸酸中毒发生在没有明显灌注不足或缺氧的情况下（表3.3）。

D-乳酸酸中毒

D-乳酸酸中毒是一种独特的代谢性酸中毒，可发生于小肠切除术或空肠回肠旁路术患者。这些短肠综合征会导致通常在小肠中被重吸收的碳水化合物大量进入结肠。在结肠细菌过度生长的情况下，这些底物会被代谢成 D-乳酸盐，并被吸收进入全身循环。D-乳酸盐的蓄积会导致高阴离子间隙性代谢性酸中毒，在这种情况下，因为乳酸盐的标准检测法特异性针对 L-乳酸盐，因此血清乳酸盐测定是正常的。这些患者通常在进食大量碳水化合物后出现神经系统异常表现，包括意识模糊、言语不清以及共济失调。主要的治疗方法是摄入低碳水化合物膳食以及使用抗生素降低细菌过度生长。

糖尿病酮症酸中毒

糖尿病酮症酸中毒是一种由于胰岛素缺乏和葡萄糖浓度相对或绝对增高导致乙酰乙酸和 β-羟丁酸蓄积为特点的代谢性异常。阴离子间隙升高的程度取决于酮症酸中毒发生的速度、严重程度和持续时间以及 ECF 容量状态。虽然高阴离子间隙性酸中毒是糖尿病酮症酸中毒的主要形式，但在酮症酸中毒最早期阶段，当细胞外液容量接近正常时，通常发生高氯性阴离子间隙正常性酸中毒。

Confirmation of the presence of ketoacids can be achieved with use of nitroprusside tablets or reagent strips. However, this test can be misleading in assessing the severity of ketoacidosis because it only detects the presence of acetone and acetoacetate and does not permit reaction with β-hydroxybutyrate. Treatment of diabetic ketoacidosis involves the use of insulin and intravenous fluids to correct volume depletion. Deficiencies in K^+, Mg^{2+}, and phosphate are common and, therefore, these electrolytes are typically added to intravenous solutions.

Alcoholic Ketoacidosis

Ketoacidosis develops in patients with a history of chronic ethanol abuse, decreased food intake, and often a history of nausea and vomiting. The presence of alcohol withdrawal, volume depletion, and starvation markedly increases the levels of circulating catecholamines and results in the peripheral mobilization of fatty acids that is much larger in magnitude than that typically found with starvation alone. The metabolism of alcohol leads to an increase in the $NADH:NAD^+$ ratio causing a higher β-hydroxybutyrate to acetoacetate ratio. The nitroprusside reaction may be diminished by this redox shift despite the presence of severe ketoacidosis. Glucose administration leads to the rapid resolution of the acidosis because stimulation of insulin release leads to diminished fatty acid mobilization from adipose tissue as well as decreased hepatic output of ketoacids.

Ethylene Glycol and Methanol Poisoning

Ethylene glycol and methanol poisoning are characteristically associated with the development of a severe anion gap metabolic acidosis. Together with the appearance of the anion gap, an osmolar gap also becomes manifest and is an important clue to the diagnosis of ethylene glycol and methanol poisoning. Metabolism of ethylene glycol by alcohol dehydrogenase generates various acids, including glycolic, oxalic, and formic acids. Ethylene glycol is a component of antifreeze and solvents and is ingested by accident or as a suicide attempt. The initial effects of intoxication are neurologic and begin with drunkenness but can quickly progress to seizures and coma. If left untreated, cardiopulmonary symptoms such as tachypnea, noncardiogenic pulmonary edema, and cardiovascular collapse may appear. Twenty-four to 48 hours after ingestion, patients may develop flank pain and acute kidney injury, which are often accompanied by abundant calcium oxalate crystals in the urine.

Methanol is also metabolized by alcohol dehydrogenase and forms formaldehyde, which is then converted to formic acid. Methanol is found in a variety of commercial preparations such as shellac, varnish, and de-icing solutions. As with ethylene glycol ingestion, methanol is ingested by accident or as a suicide attempt. Clinically, methanol ingestion is associated with an acute inebriation followed by an asymptomatic period lasting 24 to 36 hours. At this point, abdominal pain caused by pancreatitis, seizures, blindness, and coma may develop. The blindness is due to direct toxicity of formic acid on the retina. Methanol intoxication is also associated with hemorrhage in the white matter and putamen that can lead to the delayed onset of a Parkinson-like syndrome. Lactic acidosis is also a feature of methanol and ethylene glycol poisoning and contributes to the elevated anion gap.

In addition to supportive measures, the therapy for ethylene glycol and methanol poisoning is centered on reducing the metabolism of the parent compound and accelerating the removal of the alcohol from the body. Fomepizole (4-methylpyrazole) is now the agent of choice to inhibit the enzyme alcohol dehydrogenase and prevent formation of toxic metabolites.

Salicylate Poisoning

Aspirin (acetylsalicylic acid) poisoning leads to increased lactic acid production. The accumulation of lactic, salicylic, keto, and other organic acids account for the development of an anion gap metabolic acidosis. At the same time, salicylate has a direct stimulatory effect on the respiratory center. Increased ventilation lowers the Pco_2, contributing to the development of a respiratory alkalosis. Children primarily manifest an anion gap metabolic acidosis with toxic salicylate levels, whereas a respiratory alkalosis is most evident in adults.

In addition to conservative management, the initial goal of therapy is to correct systemic acidemia and to increase the urine pH. By increasing systemic pH, the ionized fraction of salicylic acid will increase and as a result, there will be less accumulation of the drug in the central nervous system. Similarly, an alkaline urine pH will favor increased urinary excretion because the ionized fraction of the drug is poorly reabsorbed by the tubule. At serum concentrations of greater than 80 mg/dL or in the setting of severe clinical toxicity, hemodialysis can be used to accelerate the removal of the drug from the body.

Pyroglutamic Acidosis

Pyroglutamic acidosis is a cause of anion gap metabolic acidosis accompanied by alterations in mental status ranging from confusion to coma. Reported cases occur in critically ill patients receiving therapeutic doses of acetaminophen, a setting in which glutathione levels are reduced because of acetaminophen metabolism and oxidative stress associated with critical illness. The diagnosis of pyroglutamic acidosis should be considered in patients with unexplained anion gap metabolic acidosis and recent acetaminophen ingestion.

METABOLIC ALKALOSIS

The pathogenesis of metabolic alkalosis involves both the generation and maintenance of this disorder. The generation of metabolic alkalosis refers to the addition of new HCO_3^- to the blood because of either loss of acid or gain of alkali. New HCO_3^- may be generated by either renal or extrarenal mechanisms. Because the kidneys have an enormous capacity to excrete HCO_3^-, even vigorous HCO_3^- generation may not be enough to produce sustained metabolic alkalosis. To maintain a metabolic alkalosis, the capacity of the kidney to correct the alkalosis must be impaired or the capacity to reclaim HCO_3^- must be enhanced.

Clinical Consequences of Metabolic Alkalosis

Metabolic alkalosis is generally considered a benign condition; however, a high blood pH can result in a number of effects that decrease tissue perfusion. Increases in blood pH (alkalemia) cause respiratory depression and decrease tissue oxygen delivery through the Bohr effect and vasoconstriction. Alkalosis should be aggressively corrected in critically ill patients in whom perfusion of the heart and brain is essential.

Approach and Treatment of Metabolic Alkalosis

Metabolic alkalosis is best approached according to the mechanism of maintenance because correction of the maintenance mechanism leads to correction of the metabolic alkalosis. If EAV can be restored with saline, the metabolic alkalosis is easily corrected. Several conditions are poorly responsive to the administration of NaCl. Metabolic alkalosis in these conditions is generally maintained by a combination of increased mineralocorticoid levels along with high distal Na^+ delivery and hypokalemia. The distinction between these entities relies on assessment of EAV (Table 3.4).

Decreased EAV: Saline Responsive

Gastrointestinal acid loss. Loss of acid, as occurs with vomiting or nasogastric suction, is a common cause of metabolic alkalosis maintained by volume contraction. The loss of gastric acid generates a metabolic alkalosis, while the loss of NaCl in the gastric fluid leads

使用硝普钠片剂或试纸条可以确认酮酸的存在。不过因为只能检测到丙酮和乙酰乙酸的存在，而不能与β-羟丁酸发生反应，这种检测方法在评估酮症酸中毒的严重程度时可能会出现误导。糖尿病酮症酸中毒的治疗包括使用胰岛素和静脉输液以纠正容量不足。K^+、Mg^{2+}和磷酸盐的缺乏很常见，因此通常会在静脉输液中添加这些电解质。

酒精性酮症酸中毒

酮症酸中毒可发生于长期酗酒、进食减少以及经常恶心呕吐的患者。酒精戒断、容量耗竭，以及饥饿会显著增加循环中儿茶酚胺的水平，导致程度远大于单纯饥饿时的外周脂肪酸动员。酒精的代谢会导致$NADH:NAD^+$比值增加，引起β-羟丁酸与乙酰乙酸的比值升高。虽然存在严重的酮症酸中毒，但硝普钠反应可能会因这种氧化还原的转变而减弱。给予葡萄糖刺激胰岛素释放可以减少脂肪组织脂肪酸动员并减少肝脏酮酸输出，因此可迅速缓解酸中毒。

乙二醇和甲醇中毒

乙二醇和甲醇中毒的特征是出现严重的高阴离子间隙性代谢性酸中毒。随着阴离子间隙的增高，还会出现渗透压间隙增高，这是诊断乙二醇和甲醇中毒的重要线索。乙二醇在乙醇脱氢酶的作用下可代谢生成包括乙醇酸、草酸和甲酸在内的多种酸。乙二醇是防冻液和溶媒的一种常见成分，通常因意外或自杀企图而摄入。中毒最初会影响神经系统，表现为醉酒，但很快就会发展为抽搐和昏迷。如不及时治疗，可能会出现呼吸急促、非心源性肺水肿和心血管衰竭等心肺症状。摄入24～48 h后，患者可能会出现腰腹痛和急性肾损伤，尿中常可见到大量草酸钙结晶。

甲醇也会被乙醇脱氢酶代谢成甲醛，然后转化为甲酸。甲醇存在于如虫胶、清漆和除冰液等多种商业制剂中。与摄入乙二醇一样，甲醇摄入也可能是由于误食或企图自杀。临床上，甲醇摄入会引起急性醉酒，随后有持续24～36 h的无症状期。在此期间，可能会出现由胰腺炎引起的腹痛、抽搐、失明和昏迷。失明是由于甲酸对视网膜有直接毒性。甲醇中毒还可引起脑白质和丘脑出血，导致迟发帕金森样综合征。乳酸酸中毒也是甲醇和乙二醇中毒的表现之一，导致阴离子间隙增高。

除支持治疗外，乙二醇和甲醇中毒的治疗重点是减少母体化合物的代谢，加速酒精从体内排出。目前，福美匹唑（4-甲基吡唑）是抑制乙醇脱氢酶、防止有毒代谢物形成的首选药物。

水杨酸中毒

阿司匹林（乙酰水杨酸）中毒会导致乳酸生成增加。乳酸、水杨酸、酮酸和其他有机酸的蓄积导致高阴离子间隙性代谢性酸中毒的发生。同时，水杨酸对呼吸中枢有直接刺激作用。通气量增加会降低P_{CO_2}，导致呼吸性碱中毒。儿童主要表现为高阴离子间隙性代谢性酸中毒伴中毒性水杨酸水平，而呼吸性碱中毒在成人中更为明显。

除保守措施外，治疗的最初目标是纠正全身酸血症及提高尿液pH值。通过提高全身pH值，增加水杨酸的离子化，从而减少药物在中枢神经系统中的蓄积。同样，碱性尿液pH值抑制离子化药物在肾小管重吸收，有利于增加其从尿液的排出。当血清浓度超过80 mg/dl或出现严重的中毒临床表现时，可采用血液透析加速药物排出体外。

焦谷氨酸酸中毒

焦谷氨酸酸中毒是引起高阴离子间隙性代谢性酸中毒的一种原因，伴有从意识模糊到昏迷的精神状态改变。已报道的病例发生在接受治疗量对乙酰氨基酚的危重患者身上，由于对乙酰氨基酚的代谢和危重症时的氧化应激，造成谷胱甘肽水平下降。对于有原因不明的高阴离子间隙性代谢性酸中毒且近期应用对乙酰氨基酚的患者，应考虑焦谷氨酸酸中毒的诊断。

代谢性碱中毒

代谢性碱中毒的发病涉及该疾病的产生和维持两方面。代谢性碱中毒的产生是指由于酸的丢失或碱的获得使血液中增加了新的HCO_3^-。新的HCO_3^-可由肾脏或肾外机制产生。由于肾脏有强大的排泄HCO_3^-的能力，因此即使有大量HCO_3^-生成也不足以产生持续的代谢性碱中毒。要维持代谢性碱中毒，必须有肾脏纠正碱中毒能力受损或重吸收HCO_3^-能力增强。

代谢性碱中毒的临床后果

代谢性碱中毒通常是一种良性情况；但是，血液pH值升高会减少多个组织的灌注。血pH值升高（碱血症）会抑制呼吸，并通过玻尔效应和血管收缩减少组织氧供。对维持心脑灌注至关重要的危重患者而言应积极纠正碱中毒。

代谢性碱中毒的处理和治疗

因为纠正维持机制就可以纠正代谢性碱中毒，因此代谢性碱中毒最好根据维持机制来处理。如果EAV可以通过生理盐水恢复，则代谢性碱中毒很容易得到纠正。有几种情况对输注氯化钠的反应很差。这些情况下的代谢性碱中毒通常是由盐皮质激素水平升高、远端Na^+输送量高和低钾血症共同作用维持的。这些情况通过评估EAV加以区分（表3.4）。

EAV减少：生理盐水反应性

胃肠道酸丢失 呕吐或胃管引流导致胃酸丢失，是引起通过容量收缩维持代谢性碱中毒的一个常见原

TABLE 3.4 Classification of Metabolic Alkalosis According to Mechanism, Cause, and Response to Administration of Saline

Effective Arterial Volume (EAV)	Low	Low	High
Urine Cl⁻ concentration (mEq/L)	<15	>15	>15
Response to saline	Corrects (saline responsive)	No correction (saline resistant)	No correction (saline resistant)
Maintenance	Low EAV	Low EAV + high distal Na$^+$ delivery and mineralocorticoid effect	High distal Na$^+$ delivery and mineralocorticoid effect

Etiology	Gastrointestinal acid loss
	  Vomiting/nasogastric suction
	  Congenital chloridorrhea
	  Villous adenoma
	Post-hypercapneic alkalosis
	Diuretics
	Non-reabsorbable anions
		Primary increase in distal delivery of Na$^+$
		Active diuretic use (loop and thiazide)
		Mg^{2+} deficiency
		Bartter syndrome
		Gitelman syndrome
			Primary increase in mineralocorticoid or mineralocorticoid like effect
			Conn's syndrome
			Liddle syndrome
			Glucocorticoid-suppressible hyperaldosteronism

TABLE 3.5 Treatment of Various Saline-Resistant Causes of Metabolic Alkalosis

DECREASED EAV		INCREASED EAV	
Cause	Treatment	Cause	Treatment
Thiazide and loop diuretics	Discontinue drug, replete EAV	Renin secreting tumor	Remove tumor
Mg^{2+} deficiency	Replete Mg^{2+} deficit	Primary hyperaldosteronism	Remove tumor, spironolactone for BAH
Gitelman syndrome	Amiloride, triamterene, or spironolactone, K$^+$ supplements, Mg^{2+} supplements	Glucocorticoid suppressible hyperaldosteronism	Dexamethasone
Bartter syndrome	Amiloride, triamterene, or spironolactone, K$^+$ supplements, Mg^{2+} supplements in some	Liddle syndrome	Amiloride or triamterene

BAH, Bilateral adrenal hyperplasia; *EAV*, effective arterial blood volume.

to volume contraction. During active vomiting, the plasma HCO$_3^-$ concentration tends to be higher than the threshold for reabsorption in the proximal nephron. The resultant bicarbonaturia leads to increased excretion of NaHCO$_3$ and KHCO$_3$, resulting in further total body Na$^+$ depletion and development of K$^+$ depletion. During this active phase, urine Cl$^-$ is less than 15 mEq/L, in the presence of high urine Na$^+$, high urine K$^+$, and a urine pH of 7 to 8. When the patient stops vomiting, equilibrium is established such that bicarbonaturia stops but a metabolic alkalosis is maintained by the volume contraction, K$^+$ depletion, and reduction in GFR. Of these factors, decreased EAV is clearly the main factor in maintenance of metabolic alkalosis. At this time, urine Na$^+$ and Cl$^-$ are both low. Administration of NaCl results in bicarbonaturia and the metabolic alkalosis is corrected.

Diuretics. Thiazide and loop diuretics are another common cause of metabolic alkalosis. These diuretics lead to metabolic alkalosis generated in the distal nephron by the combination of high aldosterone levels and enhanced distal delivery of Na$^+$. If diuretics are stopped and the patient is maintained on a low-salt diet, the alkalosis will be maintained despite the fact that distal delivery is no longer increased. In this setting, patients tend to be volume contracted and K$^+$ deficient. Once again, the contraction of EAV is the major factor leading to the maintenance of metabolic alkalosis. Saline infusion in this setting corrects the metabolic alkalosis.

Decreased EAV: Saline Resistant

In some forms of metabolic alkalosis, the alkalosis is maintained by decreased EAV, but because other maintenance factors are also present, the alkalosis is not completely saline responsive. In these patients, saline infusions may improve the metabolic alkalosis but will not completely correct it. In general, these patients may have a low EAV but typically do not have a low urine Cl$^-$. Continued use of thiazide or loop diuretics, magnesium deficiency, Gitelman syndrome, and Barrter syndrome are examples of this condition. The treatment of various causes of metabolic alkalosis is summarized in Table 3.5.

Increased EAV: Saline Resistant

The last type of metabolic alkalosis is not maintained by decreased EAV, but rather is maintained by high mineralocorticoid levels (in the presence of maintained distal delivery of Na$^+$) and K$^+$ deficiency. The most common cause of this saline-resistant alkalosis is a primary increase in mineralocorticoid levels not related to volume contraction. The mechanism of the generation of the alkalosis described above, enhanced Na$^+$ delivery with high mineralocorticoid activity, is also responsible for maintenance of the metabolic alkalosis in this setting. In addition, K$^+$ deficiency, which also occurs in this setting, exacerbates the tendency to alkalosis.

The preferred treatment of metabolic alkalosis in patients with volume expansion and primary mineralocorticoid excess is to remove the underlying cause of the persistent mineralocorticoid activity. When this is not possible, therapy is directed at blocking the actions of the mineralocorticoid at the level of the kidney.

RESPIRATORY ALKALOSIS

Primary respiratory alkalosis results from hypocapnia and is defined by an arterial partial pressure of carbon dioxide (Paco$_2$) of less than 35

表 3.4　根据机制、原因和对生理盐水的反应对代谢性碱中毒进行分类

有效动脉血容量（EAV）	低	低	高
尿氯浓度（mmol/L）	<15	>15	>15
对盐水的反应	可纠正（对盐水反应）	无法纠正（对盐水抵抗）	无法纠正（对盐水抵抗）
维持因素	低有效动脉血容量	低有效动脉血容量+高远端 Na^+ 输送及盐皮质激素效应	高远端 Na^+ 输送及盐皮质激素效应
原因	胃肠道酸丢失 呕吐/胃管抽吸 先天性氯腹泻 绒毛状腺瘤 过度换气后碱中毒 利尿剂 不可吸收的阴离子	原发性远端 Na^+ 输送增加 使用利尿剂（袢利尿剂和噻嗪类利尿剂） 镁缺乏 Batter 综合征 Gitelman 综合征	原发性盐皮质激素增多或盐皮质激素样效应 Conn 综合征 Liddle 综合征 糖皮质激素可抑制性醛固酮增多症

表 3.5　各种对生理盐水抵抗性代谢性碱中毒的治疗

有效动脉血容量减少		有效动脉血容量增多	
原因	治疗	原因	治疗
噻嗪类和袢利尿剂	停药，补充容量	肾素瘤	切除肿瘤
镁缺乏	补镁	原发性醛固酮增多症	切除肿瘤，双侧肾上腺增生使用螺内酯
Gitelman 综合征	阿米洛利，氨苯蝶啶，或螺内酯，补钾，补镁	糖皮质激素可抑制性醛固酮增多症	地塞米松
Bartter 综合征	阿米洛利，氨苯蝶啶，或螺内酯，补钾，部分需要补镁	Liddle 综合征	阿米洛利或氨苯蝶啶

因。胃酸丢失导致代谢性碱中毒，而胃液中氯化钠的丢失则会导致容量收缩。在持续呕吐时，血浆 HCO_3^- 浓度往往高于近端肾单位重吸收的阈值。由此产生的碳酸氢盐尿增加了 $NaHCO_3$ 和 $KHCO_3$ 的排泄，导致体内 Na^+ 的进一步减少并出现 K^+ 的丢失。在此期间，尿 Cl^- 低于 15 mmol/L，可见高尿 Na^+、高尿 K^+，尿液 pH 值为 7～8。当患者停止呕吐后，平衡重建，尿碳酸氢盐排泄停止，但代谢性碱中毒会因容量收缩、K^+ 消耗和 GFR 下降得以维持。在这些因素中，EAV 的减少显然是维持代谢性碱中毒的主要因素。此时，尿 Na^+ 和尿 Cl^- 都低。使用氯化钠可以纠正碳酸氢盐尿和代谢性碱中毒。

利尿剂　噻嗪类和袢利尿剂是导致代谢性碱中毒的另一个常见原因。这些利尿剂会因高醛固酮水平和远端 Na^+ 输送增加的联合作用在远端肾单位产生代谢性碱中毒。如果停用利尿剂，但患者仍维持低盐饮食，尽管远端 Na^+ 输送不再增加，但碱中毒仍会持续。这时患者一般处于容量收缩和 K^+ 缺乏状态。EAV 的减少再一次是导致代谢性碱中毒持续的主要原因。输注生理盐水可纠正代谢性碱中毒。

EAV 减少：生理盐水抵抗性

有些形式的代谢性碱中毒，虽然是通过 EAV 减少来维持的，但由于其他一些维持因素的存在，碱中毒并不完全对生理盐水有反应。这些患者输注生理盐水可改善但不能完全纠正代谢性碱中毒。一般而言，这些患者可能有低 EAV，但尿 Cl^- 通常不低。持续使用噻嗪类或袢利尿剂、缺镁、吉特曼（Gitelman）综合征和巴特（Bartter）综合征都属于这种情况。表 3.5 总结了各种原因引起的生理盐水抵抗性代谢性碱中毒的治疗方法。

EAV 增加：生理盐水抵抗性

最后一种形式的代谢性碱中毒不是通过 EAV 减少来维持的，而是通过高盐皮质激素水平（在维持远端 Na^+ 输送的情况下）和 K^+ 缺乏来维持的。这种生理盐水抵抗性碱中毒最常见的原因是与容量减少无关的原发性盐皮质激素水平升高。远端 Na^+ 输送增加伴高盐皮质激素活性，既是如上所述的碱中毒的产生机制，同时也是这种情况下代谢性碱中毒得以维持的原因。此外，这种情况下发生的 K^+ 缺乏也会加剧碱中毒。

对容量扩张和原发性盐皮质激素过多的代谢性碱中毒患者，首选的治疗方法是去除导致持续盐皮质激素活性的病因。如果无法做到这一点，则应在肾脏层面阻断盐皮质激素的作用。

呼吸性碱中毒

原发性呼吸性碱中毒是由低碳酸血症引起的，其定义是动脉二氧化碳分压（$PaCO_2$）低于 35 mmHg。原

TABLE 3.6 Compensation in Acid-Base Disorders

Disorder	Compensatory Changes
Acute respiratory acidosis	For every 10 mm Hg rise in P_{CO_2} the HCO_3^- increases by 1 mEq/L
Chronic respiratory acidosis	For every 10 mm Hg rise in P_{CO_2} the HCO_3^- increases by 3.5 mEq/L
Acute respiratory alkalosis	For every 10 mm Hg fall in P_{CO_2} the HCO_3^- decreases by 2 mEq/L
Chronic respiratory alkalosis	For every 10 mm Hg decrease in P_{CO_2} the HCO_3^- decreases by 5 mEq/L
Metabolic acidosis	1.2 mm Hg decrease in P_{CO_2} for each 1 mEq/L fall in HCO_3^- $P_{CO_2} = HCO_3^- + 15$ P_{CO_2} = last digits of pH
Metabolic alkalosis	P_{CO_2} increases by 0.7 for each mEq/L HCO_3^-

mm Hg in the setting of alkalemia. Primary respiratory alkalosis must be differentiated from secondary hypocapnia, which is a compensatory mechanism in the setting of primary metabolic acidosis.

Etiology

Respiratory alkalosis is the most frequent acid-base disturbance encountered. It is particularly common in hospitalized patients, where it can be the initial clue to the presence of gram-negative sepsis. Hepatic failure is a common and important cause of primary hypocapnia. The severity of hypocapnia correlates with the level of blood ammonia and has prognostic significance. The presence of respiratory alkalosis can be an important clue to the presence of salicylate intoxication. High progesterone levels (pregnancy) can also cause respiratory alkalosis.

Clinical Manifestation of Respiratory Alkalosis

Mild respiratory alkalosis causes lightheadedness, palpitations, and paresthesias of the extremities and the circumoral area. Acute hypocapnia decreases cerebral blood flow and causes binding of free calcium to albumin in the blood. Thus, patients with acute respiratory alkalosis might present clinically in a similar way to patients with hypocalcemia, manifesting positive Chvostek and Trousseau signs. Patients with ischemic heart disease might occasionally develop cardiac arrhythmias, ischemic electrocardiographic changes, and even angina pectoris during acute hypocapnia.

Diagnosis

The diagnosis of respiratory alkalosis is made by evaluating the patient's history, performing a physical exam, and obtaining laboratory data including a blood gas analysis. Tachypnea or Kussmaul breathing can be detected on physical exam and may be the first clue to the presence of a primary respiratory alkalosis or a compensatory respiratory mechanism in the setting of a primary metabolic acidosis. Changes in serum electrolytes can aid in the diagnosis of respiratory alkalosis. An acute fall in P_{CO_2} causes a HCO_3^--Cl^- shift in red blood cells and accounts for the small initial compensatory response in acute respiratory alkalosis in which the HCO_3^- concentration falls by 2 mEq/L for every 10 mm Hg decrease in P_{CO_2}. Table 3.6 provides the expected compensatory responses for acid-base disorders.

In chronic respiratory alkalosis, the renal HCO_3^- reabsorptive capacity decreases and there is a transient HCO_3^- diuresis. This process takes 2 to 3 days to become fully manifest. Once a new steady state is achieved, the HCO_3^- concentration will have decreased by 5 mEq/L for each 10 mm Hg fall in P_{CO_2}. A higher or lower value for the plasma HCO_3^- concentration suggests the presence of an additional metabolic disorder.

To defend ECF volume in the setting of increased urinary loss of $NaHCO_3$, the kidney retains NaCl. These changes are reflected in the serum electrolytes of patients with chronic respiratory alkalosis in which the Cl^- is typically increased with respect to the serum Na^+ concentration. Another characteristic finding is an increase of 3 to 5 mEq/L in the serum anion gap. The increased gap is due to the greater fixed negative charge on serum albumin as well as an increase in serum lactate concentration. Lactate production is increased due to a stimulatory effect of high pH on phosphofructokinase, the rate-limiting step in the glycolytic pathway.

Treatment

Primary respiratory alkalosis is treated by correcting the underlying cause. A patient with anxiety-hyperventilation syndrome should be treated by providing reassurance. Rebreathing into a paper bag or any other closed system will cause the P_{CO_2} to increase with each breath taken and lead to a partial correction of hypocapnia and improvement of symptoms. In the rare case where there is no response to conservative management, sedatives can be used. In mechanically ventilated patients, the P_{CO_2} can be increased by either raising the inspired CO_2 tension or by increasing the dead space of the ventilator circuit. Correction of respiratory alkalosis may prove helpful in correcting arrhythmias in patients with underlying coronary disease. In contrast, caution is warranted in raising the P_{CO_2} in patients with brain injury because cerebral perfusion may increase and cause further worsening of intracranial pressure. Respiratory alkalosis frequently develops as a complication of hypoxia. Administration of oxygen or return to lower altitudes can reverse the respiratory alkalosis that develops in this setting.

RESPIRATORY ACIDOSIS

Respiratory acidosis develops because of ineffective alveolar ventilation. This acid-base disorder, which is also called primary hypercapnia, needs to be differentiated from secondary hypercapnia, which develops as a compensatory mechanism in the setting of primary metabolic alkalosis. Primary hypercapnia is clinically recognized by the presence of $Paco_2$ levels of greater than 45 mm Hg on arterial blood gas analysis. However, $Paco_2$ levels of less than 45 mm Hg might still be indicative of respiratory acidosis if a primary metabolic acidosis is not adequately compensated by alveolar ventilation.

Etiology of Respiratory Acidosis

The development of respiratory acidosis is usually multifactorial. Major causes of CO_2 retention include diseases or malfunction within any element of the respiratory system, including the central and peripheral nervous systems, the respiratory muscles, the thoracic cage, the pleural space, the airways, and the lung parenchyma. The following six factors should be considered in the differential diagnosis of acute and chronic respiratory acidosis: inhibition of the medullary respiratory center, disorders of the chest wall and the respiratory muscles, airway obstruction, disorders affecting gas exchange across the pulmonary capillary, increased CO_2 production, and mechanical ventilation.

Clinical Manifestations of Respiratory Acidosis

Hypercapnic encephalopathy is a clinical syndrome that usually starts with irritability, headache, mental cloudiness, apathy, confusion, anxiety, restlessness, and can progress to asterixis, transient psychosis, delirium, somnolence, and coma. Papilledema and other manifestations of

表3.6 酸碱失衡的代偿	
失衡状态	代偿改变
急性呼吸性酸中毒	PCO_2 每升高 10 mmHg，HCO_3^- 增高 1 mmol/L
慢性呼吸性酸中毒	PCO_2 每升高 10 mmHg，HCO_3^- 增高 3.5 mmol/L
急性呼吸性碱中毒	PCO_2 每降低 10 mmHg，HCO_3^- 降低 2 mmol/L
慢性呼吸性碱中毒	PCO_2 每降低 10 mmHg，HCO_3^- 降低 5 mmol/L
代谢性酸中毒	HCO_3^- 每降低 1 mmol/L，PCO_2 降低 1.2 mmHg $PCO_2 = HCO_3^- + 15$ $PCO_2 = $ pH 值的尾数
代谢性碱中毒	HCO_3^- 每升高 1 mmol/L，PCO_2 升高 0.7 mmHg

发性呼吸性碱中毒必须与继发性低碳酸血症区分开来，后者是原发性代谢性酸中毒时的一种代偿机制。

病因

呼吸性碱中毒是最常见的酸碱紊乱。在住院患者中尤为常见，可以是革兰氏阴性菌感染中毒症的最初线索。肝衰竭是导致原发性低碳酸血症的常见且重要的原因。低碳酸血症的严重程度与血氨水平相关，并有预后意义。呼吸性碱中毒可以是水杨酸中毒的重要线索。高孕酮水平（妊娠）也会导致呼吸性碱中毒。

呼吸性碱中毒的临床表现

轻度呼吸性碱中毒会导致头晕、心悸、肢端和口周发麻。急性低碳酸血症会降低脑血流量，使血中游离钙与白蛋白结合。因此，急性呼吸性碱中毒患者的临床表现可能与低钙血症患者相似，表现为 Chvostek 和 Trousseau 征阳性。有缺血性心脏病的患者偶尔会在急性低碳酸血症时出现心律失常、缺血性心电图改变，甚至心绞痛。

诊断

呼吸性碱中毒的诊断通过评估患者的病史、进行体格检查和获取实验室检查数据（包括血气分析）来实现。体格检查时可见到呼吸过速或库斯莫尔（Kussmaul）呼吸，这可能是提示原发性呼吸性碱中毒或在原发性代谢性酸中毒情况下呼吸代偿的第一个线索。血清电解质的变化有助于呼吸性碱中毒的诊断。PCO_2 的急剧下降会导致红细胞中的 HCO_3^--Cl^- 发生转移，是急性呼吸性碱中毒的小的初始代偿反应，PCO_2 每下降 10 mmHg，HCO_3^- 浓度降低 2 mmol/L。表 3.6 列出了酸碱失衡时预期的代偿反应。

慢性呼吸性碱中毒时，肾脏对 HCO_3^- 的重吸收能力下降，出现短暂的 HCO_3^- 利尿。这个过程需要 2～3 天来完全显现。一旦达成新的稳态，PCO_2 每下降 10 mmHg，HCO_3^- 浓度将下降 5 mmol/L。血浆 HCO_3^- 浓度值高于或低于预期值都表明存在额外的代谢紊乱。

为了在尿 $NaHCO_3$ 丢失增加的情况下维持 ECF 容量，肾脏会保留 NaCl。这些变化反映在慢性呼吸性碱中毒患者的血清电解质上，表现为血清 Cl^- 的浓度相较血清 Na^+ 的浓度增高。另一特征性的表现是血清阴离子间隙增加 3～5 mmol/L。间隙增大的原因是血清白蛋白固定的负电荷增加以及血清乳酸浓度增加。由于高 pH 值对磷酸果糖激酶（糖酵解过程中的限速步骤）有刺激作用，导致乳酸生成增加。

治疗

原发性呼吸性碱中毒的治疗是纠正潜在的病因。焦虑-过度通气综合征患者应通过安抚来治疗。使用纸袋或任何其他封闭系统进行再呼吸可以使 PCO_2 随着每次呼吸升高，从而部分纠正低碳酸血症并改善症状。在极少数保守治疗无效的情况下，可以使用镇静剂。对于机械通气的患者，可通过提高吸入 CO_2 的张力或增加通气回路的无效腔（死腔）来提高 PCO_2。纠正呼吸性碱中毒可能有助于纠正冠心病患者的心律失常。相反，对脑损伤患者提高 PCO_2 时应慎重，因为可能会增加脑灌注并导致颅内压进一步恶化。呼吸性碱中毒常常是缺氧的并发症之一。吸氧或返回低海拔地区可逆转这种情况下出现的呼吸性碱中毒。

呼吸性酸中毒

呼吸性酸中毒是由无效的肺泡通气引起的。这种酸碱紊乱也被称为原发性高碳酸血症，需要与继发性高碳酸血症进行区分，后者是在原发性代谢性碱中毒的情况下的一种代偿机制。原发性高碳酸血症临床表现为动脉血气分析中 $PaCO_2$ 水平高于 45 mmHg。然而，如果原发性代谢性酸中毒不能被肺泡通气充分代偿，则 $PaCO_2$ 水平低于 45 mmHg 仍可能提示呼吸性酸中毒。

呼吸性酸中毒的病因

呼吸性酸中毒的发生通常是多因素所致。二氧化碳潴留的主要原因包括呼吸系统各个部分的疾病或功能障碍，包括中枢和周围神经系统、呼吸肌、胸廓、胸膜腔、气道，以及肺实质。急性和慢性呼吸性酸中毒的鉴别诊断应考虑以下六个因素：延髓呼吸中枢抑制、胸壁和呼吸肌异常、气道阻塞、肺毛细血管气体交换障碍、二氧化碳生成增加和机械通气。

呼吸性酸中毒的临床表现

高碳酸血症脑病是一种临床综合征，通常开始时表现为烦躁、头痛、精神混乱、淡漠、意识模糊、焦虑、烦躁不安，并可发展为癫病、一过性精神病、谵妄、嗜睡和昏迷。视乳头水肿及其他表现颅内压增高的症状，

increased intracranial pressure that are collectively named *pseudotumor cerebri* are occasionally observed in patients with either acute or chronic hypercapnia. The increase in intracranial pressure is in part due to cerebral vasodilation resulting from acidemia. Acute respiratory acidosis is typically more symptomatic than acute metabolic acidosis because CO_2 diffuses and equilibrates across the blood-brain barrier much more rapidly than does HCO_3^-, resulting in a more rapid fall in cerebral spinal fluid and cerebral interstitial pH. Severe hypercapnia can also lead to decreased myocardial contractility, arrhythmias, and peripheral vasodilatation, particularly when the blood pH falls to less than 7.1.

Diagnosis

The diagnosis of primary respiratory acidosis is made by the presence of acidemia and hypercapnia on arterial blood gas analysis. Changes in the serum chemistries can aid in the diagnosis of respiratory acidosis. Acute hypercapnia is associated with a shift of HCO_3^- out of red blood cells in exchange for Cl^-; a process termed the *red cell HCO_3^--C^- shift*. Acutely, the plasma HCO_3^- concentration increases by 1 mmol/L for each 10 mm Hg elevation in $Paco_2$. After 24 to 48 hours of hypercapnia proximal tubular cells increase H^+ secretion, resulting in accelerated HCO_3^- reabsorption. The retention of $NaHCO_3$ leads to slight expansion of the ECF compartment and causes increased renal excretion of NaCl to return volume back to normal. The net effect is increased serum HCO_3^- and decreased Cl^- concentration. In chronic respiratory acidosis, there is a 3.5 mEq/L increase in HCO_3^- for each 10 mm Hg elevation in $Paco_2$. Higher or lower plasma HCO_3^- concentrations suggest the presence of mixed respiratory and metabolic acid-base disorders.

Treatment of Respiratory Acidosis

The mainstay of treatment in respiratory acidosis is to recognize and treat the underlying cause whenever possible. Patients with acute respiratory acidosis are primarily at risk of hypoxemia rather than hypercapnia or acidemia. Thus, immediate therapeutic efforts should focus on establishing and securing a patent airway to provide adequate oxygenation. In patients with status asthmaticus, a lower ventilatory rate and peak inspiratory pressure may be required to minimize barotrauma to the lung but at the expense of a persistently higher Pco_2. Small amounts of $NaHCO_3$ can help prevent excessive falls in blood pH in this setting. The downside of such therapy is that infusion of $NaHCO_3$ can result in increased CO_2 production, causing a further increase in Pco_2 when ventilation cannot be increased.

Excessive oxygen should be avoided in patients with chronic respiratory acidosis because it may lead to worsening hypoventilation. When mechanical ventilation is required, care should be taken to lower the $Paco_2$ carefully and slowly because there is the risk of overshoot alkalemia due to the presence of a high HCO_3^- (post-hypercapneic metabolic alkalosis). The kidneys must excrete the HCO_3^- in order to normalize the acid-base status. This excretion will not occur when EAV is reduced either because of salt depletion owing to restricted intake or diuretic therapy or a salt retentive state such as heart failure and cirrhosis. Correction of the superimposed metabolic alkalosis can usually be achieved with saline and discontinuation of loop diuretics if they are being utilized. In edematous patients with heart failure, this may not be possible, and acetazolamide may be needed to correct the alkalosis.

SUGGESTED READINGS

Palmer BF: Approach to fluid and electrolyte disorders and acid-base problems, Primary Care 35:195–213, 2008.

Palmer BF: Diagnostic approach and management of inpatient hyponatremia, J Hospital Med 5:S1–S5, 2010.

Palmer BF: Managing hyperkalemia caused by inhibitors of the renin-angiotensin-aldosterone system, N Engl J Med 351:585–592, 2004.

Palmer BF: Metabolic acidosis. In Feehally J, Floege J, Tonelli M, Johnson RJ, editors: Comprehensive clinical nephrology, ed 6, Philadelphia, 2019, Elsevier, pp 149–159.

Palmer BF: A physiologic based approach to the evaluation of a patient with hyperkalemia, Am J Kidney Ds 56(2):387–393, 2010.

Palmer BF: A physiologic-based approach to the evaluation of a patient with hypokalemia, Am J Kidney Ds 56:1184–1190, 2010.

Palmer BF: Respiratory acid-base disorders. In Mount D, Sayegh M, Singh Ajay, editors: Core concepts in the disorders of fluid, electrolytes and acid-base balance, New York, 2013, Springer, pp 297–306.

Palmer BF: Respiratory alkalosis, Am J Kidney Ds 60:834–838, 2012.

Palmer BF, Alpern RJ: Metabolic alkalosis, J Am Soc Nephrol 8:1462–1469, 1997.

Palmer BF, Clegg DJ: Electrolyte and acid-base disorders in patients with diabetes mellitus, N Engl J Med 373:548–559, 2015.

Palmer BF, Clegg DJ: Electrolyte disturbances in patients with chronic alcohol-use disorder, N Engl J Med 377:1368–1377, 2017.

Palmer BF, Clegg DJ: Physiology and Pathophysiology of Potassium Homeostasis: Core Curriculum 2019; Am J Kidney Ds 74:682–695, 2019.

Palmer BF, Clegg DJ: Salicylate toxicity, N Engl J Med 382:2544–2555, 2020.

Palmer BF, Clegg DJ: The use of selected urine chemistries in the diagnosis of kidney disorders, Clin J Am Soc Nephrol 14:306–316, 2019.

统称为假性脑瘤，偶可见于急性或慢性高碳酸血症患者。颅内压升高部分是由于酸中毒导致的脑血管扩张。因为 CO_2 比 HCO_3^- 更快地扩散并在血脑屏障两侧平衡，导致脑脊液和脑间质 pH 值下降更快，因此急性呼吸性酸中毒通常比急性代谢性酸中毒更易出现症状。严重的高碳酸血症，尤其是当血 pH 值降至 7.1 以下时，还会导致心肌收缩力下降、心律失常和外周血管扩张。

诊断

原发性呼吸性酸中毒的诊断依据是动脉血气分析中的酸中毒和高碳酸血症。血清生化的改变可帮助呼吸性酸中毒的诊断。急性高碳酸血症时红细胞中 HCO_3^- 通过与 Cl^- 交换溢出；这一过程被称为红细胞 HCO_3^--Cl^- 转移。急性期，$PaCO_2$ 每升高 10 mmHg，血浆 HCO_3^- 浓度升高 1 mmol/L。高碳酸血症 24～48 h 后，近端肾小管细胞泌 H^+ 增加，导致 HCO_3^- 重吸收加速。$NaHCO_3$ 的潴留导致 ECF 轻度扩张，使肾脏排出更多的 NaCl 以恢复正常容量。最终结果是血清 HCO_3^- 浓度升高而 Cl^- 浓度降低。在慢性呼吸性酸中毒时，$PaCO_2$ 每升高 10 mmHg，血浆 HCO_3^- 浓度就会升高 3.5 mmol/L。更高或更低的血浆 HCO_3^- 浓度提示存在混合性的呼吸性和代谢性酸碱失衡。

呼吸性酸中毒的治疗

呼吸性酸中毒的主要治疗是尽可能识别并治疗基础病因。急性呼吸性酸中毒患者面临的主要风险是低氧血症，而不是高碳酸血症或酸中毒。因此，即刻治疗的重点应集中在建立和保障气道畅通以提供充分的氧合。对哮喘持续状态的患者，可能需要降低通气频率和吸气峰压以尽量减少肺部的气压伤，其代价是持续高的 PCO_2。在这种情况下，少量的 $NaHCO_3$ 有助于防止血液 pH 值过度下降。这种治疗的缺点是，$NaHCO_3$ 输注可能会导致 CO_2 生成增加，从而在通气量无法增加的情况下导致 PCO_2 进一步升高。

慢性呼吸性酸中毒患者应避免过量给氧，因为这会导致通气不足恶化。当需要机械通气时应小心缓慢地降低 $PaCO_2$，因为存在由于高 HCO_3^-（高碳酸血症后代谢性碱中毒）导致的碱中毒过度的风险。肾脏必须排出 HCO_3^- 以使酸碱状态恢复正常。当 EAV 减少时，无论是由于限制入量或使用利尿剂导致的盐缺乏，还是心力衰竭和肝硬化导致盐潴留时，肾脏无法排出 HCO_3^-。使用生理盐水和停用正在使用的袢利尿剂通常可以纠正叠加的代谢性碱中毒。在心力衰竭水肿患者中，这可能不可行，此时可能需要使用乙酰唑胺来纠正碱中毒。

推荐阅读

Palmer BF: Approach to fluid and electrolyte disorders and acid-base problems, Primary Care 35:195–213, 2008.

Palmer BF: Diagnostic approach and management of inpatient hyponatremia, J Hospital Med 5:S1–S5, 2010.

Palmer BF: Managing hyperkalemia caused by inhibitors of the renin-angiotensin-aldosterone system, N Engl J Med 351:585–592, 2004.

Palmer BF: Metabolic acidosis. In Feehally J, Floege J, Tonelli M, Johnson RJ, editors: Comprehensive clinical nephrology, ed 6, Philadelphia, 2019, Elsevier, pp 149–159.

Palmer BF: A physiologic based approach to the evaluation of a patient with hyperkalemia, Am J Kidney Ds 56(2):387–393, 2010.

Palmer BF: A physiologic-based approach to the evaluation of a patient with hypokalemia, Am J Kidney Ds 56:1184–1190, 2010.

Palmer BF: Respiratory acid-base disorders. In Mount D, Sayegh M, Singh Ajay, editors: Core concepts in the disorders of fluid, electrolytes and acid-base balance, New York, 2013, Springer, pp 297–306.

Palmer BF: Respiratory alkalosis, Am J Kidney Ds 60:834–838, 2012.

Palmer BF, Alpern RJ: Metabolic alkalosis, J Am Soc Nephrol 8:1462–1469, 1997.

Palmer BF, Clegg DJ: Electrolyte and acid-base disorders in patients with diabetes mellitus, N Engl J Med 373:548–559, 2015.

Palmer BF, Clegg DJ: Electrolyte disturbances in patients with chronic alcohol-use disorder, N Engl J Med 377:1368–1377, 2017.

Palmer BF, Clegg DJ: Physiology and Pathophysiology of Potassium Homeostasis: Core Curriculum 2019; Am J Kidney Ds 74:682–695, 2019.

Palmer BF, Clegg DJ: Salicylate toxicity, N Engl J Med 382:2544–2555, 2020.

Palmer BF, Clegg DJ: The use of selected urine chemistries in the diagnosis of kidney disorders, Clin J Am Soc Nephrol 14:306–316, 2019.

4

Glomerular Diseases

Sanjeev Sethi, An S. De Vriese, Fernando C. Fervenza

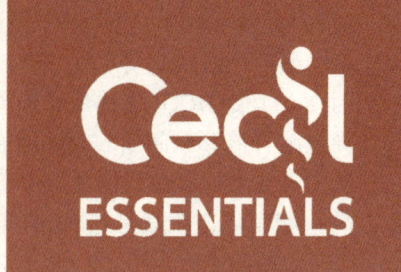

INTRODUCTION

Glomerular injury or disease can manifest as hematuria, proteinuria, hypertension, fluid retention, and a reduction in the glomerular filtration rate. Traditionally, glomerular diseases have been grouped according to clinical presentation, including asymptomatic microscopic hematuria, the nephritic syndrome, the nephrotic syndrome, rapidly progressive glomerulonephritis (RPGN), and chronic glomerulonephritis. An alternative classification of glomerular diseases is according to the histologic pattern on kidney biopsy, such as minimal change disease (MCD), membranoproliferative glomerulonephritis (MPGN), membranous nephropathy, and focal segmented glomerulosclerosis (FSGS). However, many glomerular diseases can manifest with more than one constellation of signs and symptoms and show more than one histologic pattern on renal biopsy. In addition, a particular clinical presentation or histologic pattern can be caused by different underlying disease processes. Great progress has been made in unraveling the molecular causes of glomerular diseases. For instance, autoantibodies against the phospholipase A_2 receptor or thrombospondin-7A receptor have been associated with membranous nephropathy. In the future, the etiologic approach to the classification of glomerular diseases will undoubtedly be expanded. As such, a condition can be more accurately described by combining the different approaches (e.g., antiphospholipase A_2 receptor antibody–associated membranous nephropathy presenting with nephrotic syndrome).

CLINICAL PRESENTATION

A detailed history and careful physical examination, with particular attention to the time of symptom onset, help to clarify the differential diagnosis of suspected glomerular disease. Blood pressure and fluid status should be recorded. Urine microscopy is a critical element of this assessment, and it may reveal hematuria, typically with dysmorphic red blood cells and casts. Hematuria due to glomerular disease is painless and the urine is often brown or cola-colored rather than bright red; clots are rare. The differential diagnosis should be made with other causes of brown urine, including hemoglobinuria, myoglobinuria, and specific foods or drug dyes (e.g., beetroot). Normal red blood cell excretion is 3 or fewer red blood cells per high power field or less than 8000 red blood cells per milliliter of uncentrifuged urine. To distinguish glomerular from nonglomerular hematuria, a freshly voided urinary sediment can be examined microscopically. With nonglomerular hematuria, the erythrocytes are normocytic, have a biconcave appearance, and a regular shape. In glomerular hematuria, the erythrocytes are microcytic, lack a biconcave disc appearance, and are irregularly shaped (dysmorphic). Usually 50% or more of the erythrocytes are dysmorphic and red blood cell casts may also be seen (active urinary sediment). Glomerular hematuria is generally seen throughout the voiding process and can be increased by vigorous exercise or fever. Terminal hematuria (hematuria confined to the last few milliliters of a void) is a feature of bladder disease.

Quantitative evaluation of the degree of urinary protein excretion is essential. In adults, urinary total protein excretion is less than 150 mg/24 h, and urinary albumin excretion is less than 20 mg/24 h. Persistent albumin excretion of 30 to 300 mg/24 h is termed microalbuminuria. Albumin excretion above 300 mg/24 h, the level at which the standard dipstick becomes positive, reflects overt proteinuria. Levels above 3.5 g/24 h are considered to be nephrotic-range proteinuria. It should be recognized that nephrotic-range proteinuria (>3.5 g/24 h) and nephrotic syndrome (>3.5 g/24 h and serum albumin <3.5 g/dL by bromocresol green method or <3.0 g/dL by bromocresol purple method) are not synonymous. This distinction is particularly important when the kidney biopsy reveals FSGS. Patients with full-blown nephrotic syndrome most likely have primary FSGS, whereas patients with nephrotic-range proteinuria often have FSGS due to a secondary process.

A 24-hour urine collection remains the gold standard, but it is cumbersome to perform, is often collected incorrectly, and does not provide a rapid result. The accuracy of the urine collection should be assessed by simultaneously quantifying urinary total protein and creatinine excretion. If urinary creatinine excretion is within 15% of the expected value (expected creatinine excretion in 24 hours = [140 − age in years] × weight in kg × 0.2 [× 0.85 if female]), the collection can generally be regarded as accurate. A protein-to-creatinine ratio measured on a 24-hour urine collection is a useful alternative. Using the protein and creatinine concentration available from the readings on the 24-hour urine collection, calculate the urine protein to creatinine ratio (UPCR). Then, multiply the calculated UPCR by the expected 24-hour urine creatinine excretion (as per the above-mentioned formula) to estimate the magnitude of protein in the collection.

The above-mentioned approach assumes that the patient's 24-hour urine creatinine excretion is appropriate for their body size. If this relationship is altered by malnutrition, muscle wasting, limb-loss, body-building or unusual habitus, then as carefully as possible a complete and accurate 24-hour urine collection must be obtained. For vegetarians, the expected 24-hour urine creatinine excretion should be reduced by about one third. Random "spot" or first morning UPCR should not be used to estimate proteinuria. Such values are inherently highly variable due to variation in protein excretion during the day and differences in urinary creatinine excretion based on age, gender, and lean body (muscle) mass.

Glomerular proteinuria can be classified as transient or hemodynamic (functional) (e.g., fever, exercise induced, orthostatic) or as persistent (fixed). Although functional proteinuria is benign, fixed nephrotic-range proteinuria usually results from glomerular diseases. Total proteinuria greater than 1 g/24 h in a patient with a negative

肾小球疾病

黄婧 译 崔昭 郑可 审校 赵明辉 通审

引言

肾小球损伤或疾病可表现为血尿、蛋白尿、高血压、体液潴留和肾小球滤过率降低。传统上，将肾小球疾病按照临床表现分组，包括无症状性镜下血尿、肾炎综合征、肾病综合征、急进性肾小球肾炎（RPGN）和慢性肾小球肾炎。肾小球疾病的另一种分类方法是根据肾活检的组织学形态，如微小病变（MCD）、膜增生性肾小球肾炎（MPGN）、膜性肾病和局灶节段性肾小球硬化（FSGS）。然而，许多肾小球疾病可表现出不止一组症状和体征，肾活检也可出现不止一种组织学形态。此外，特定的临床表现或组织学形态可由不同的潜在疾病引起。目前已在肾小球疾病的分子病因方面取得了很大进展。例如，已证实磷脂酶 A2 受体或血小板反应蛋白 -7A 受体的自身抗体与膜性肾病有关。未来，肾小球疾病的病因学分类方法无疑将进一步扩展。如是，将不同的方式结合起来（例如，抗磷脂酶 A2 受体抗体相关的膜性肾病伴肾病综合征）可以更准确地描述病情。

临床表现

详细的病史（尤其要注意症状出现的时间）和仔细的体格检查，有助于肾小球疾病的鉴别诊断。同时应记录血压和容量状况。尿液镜检是评估病情的重要因素，可发现血尿，典型表现是变形红细胞和管型。肾小球疾病引起的血尿是无痛性的，尿液通常呈棕色或可乐色，而不是鲜红色，血块很少见。在进行鉴别诊断时，应考虑导致棕色尿液的其他原因，包括血红蛋白尿、肌红蛋白尿和特定食物或药物染料（如甜菜根）。正常红细胞排泄量为尿沉渣镜检≤3个红细胞每高倍视野，或每毫升未离心尿液少于 8000 个红细胞。为了区分肾小球性血尿和非肾小球性血尿，可对新鲜尿液的尿沉渣进行显微镜检查。非肾小球性血尿的红细胞为正常红细胞，外观呈双凹圆盘状，形状规则。在肾小球性血尿中，红细胞为小红细胞，缺乏双凹圆盘外观，且形状不规则（异形），异形红细胞通常≥50%，还可能出现红细胞管型（活动性尿沉渣）。肾小球性血尿通常为全程血尿，剧烈运动或发热都会加重血尿。终末血尿（血尿仅限于排尿最后几毫升）是膀胱疾病的一个特征。

对尿蛋白排泄进行定量评估至关重要。在成人，尿总蛋白排泄量低于 150 mg/24 h，尿白蛋白排泄量低于 20 mg/24 h。持续的尿白蛋白排泄量在 30～300 mg/24 h 称为微量白蛋白尿。尿白蛋白排泄量大于 300 mg/24 h，即标准试纸检测呈阳性，则称为显性蛋白尿。尿蛋白排泄量大于 3.5 g/24 h 即为肾病范围蛋白尿。应注意的是，肾病范围蛋白尿（＞ 3.5 g/24 h）和肾病综合征（＞ 3.5 g/24 h，用溴甲酚绿法测得的血清白蛋白＜ 3.5 g/dl，或用溴甲酚紫法测得的血清白蛋白＜ 3.0 g/dl）不是同义词。特别是当肾活检显示 FSGS 时，这一区别尤为重要。患者呈完全的肾病综合征表现则很可能是原发性 FSGS，而肾病范围蛋白尿患者通常是继发性 FSGS。

24 h 尿液收集仍是金标准，但其操作繁琐，常收集不正确，且不能提供快速结果。应通过同步测量尿液总蛋白和肌酐排泄量来评估尿液收集的准确性。如果尿肌酐排泄量在预期值（24 h 内预期肌酐排泄量=［140－年龄（岁）］×体重（kg）×0.2［女性×0.85］）上下浮动 15% 范围内，则通常认为尿液收集是准确的。根据 24 h 尿液测定蛋白质与肌酐比值是一种有效的替代方法。使用从 24 h 尿液中测得的蛋白质和肌酐浓度数值，计算尿蛋白与肌酐比值（UPCR）。然后，用计算出的 UPCR 乘以预期的 24 h 尿肌酐排泄量（根据上述公式），即可估算出收集的 24 h 尿液蛋白质的含量。

上述方法假定患者的 24 h 尿肌酐排泄量与其体型相符。如果因营养不良、肌肉萎缩、肢体缺失、健身或特殊生活习惯导致二者不匹配，则必须尽可能仔细地采集完整且准确的 24 h 尿液。对于素食者，预期的 24 h 尿肌酐排泄量应减少约 1/3。由于尿液蛋白质在一天中的排泄量不同，以及基于年龄、性别和瘦体重（肌肉）的尿肌酐排泄量差异，因此不应使用随机尿或清晨第一次尿的 UPCR 来估算蛋白尿。

肾小球性蛋白尿可分为短暂性或血流动力学性（功能性）（如发热、运动诱发、直立性）或持续性（固定性）蛋白尿。功能性蛋白尿是良性的，但持续的肾病范围蛋白尿通常是由肾小球疾病引起的。当患者尿蛋白总量超过 1 g/24 h 而尿液检测试纸为阴性（只能

urine dipstick (which detects only albumin) suggests that the proteinuria is caused by light chains or low-molecular-weight proteins (e.g., retinol-binding protein, α_1-microglobulin).

CLINICAL SYNDROMES

Asymptomatic Microscopic Hematuria

Glomerular hematuria can occur with or without subnephrotic range proteinuria. Renal function parameters and blood pressure are typically normal.

Glomerular diseases commonly presenting with asymptomatic hematuria include IgA nephropathy, Alport syndrome, and thin glomerular basement disease.

Nephrotic Syndrome

Nephrotic syndrome is defined as persistent urinary total protein excretion greater than 3.5 g/24 h, accompanied by a serum albumin concentration less than 3.5 g/dL. Edema, hyperlipidemia, and lipiduria (i.e., doubly refractile fat bodies) are common but are not required for the diagnosis.

Complications of the nephrotic syndrome include hypogammaglobulinemia, vitamin D deficiency due to loss of vitamin D–binding protein, and iron deficiency anemia due to hypotransferrinemia. Thrombotic complications from loss of antithrombin III such as renal vein thrombosis may occur, especially in patients with greater protein loss (>10 g/24 h) and serum albumin levels less than 2 g/dL. Patients with severe nephrotic syndrome are particularly susceptible for acute renal failure when there is superimposed volume depletion, sepsis or use of nephrotoxic agents such as nonsteroidal anti-inflammatory drugs (NSAIDs).

Management of patients with nephrotic syndrome includes diuretics to control edema, regulation of blood pressure (angiotensin-converting enzyme inhibitors [ACEIs] and angiotensin-receptor blockers [ARBs] are preferred), limitation of the intake of protein to between 0.8 and 1 g/kg/day and sodium to less than 4 g/day, and control of lipid levels. Anticoagulation should be considered for patients at increased risk, especially if the nephrotic syndrome is caused by membranous nephropathy or amyloidosis.

Glomerular diseases commonly presenting with nephrotic syndrome include MCD, FSGS, membranous nephropathy, HIV-associated nephropathy, amyloidosis and diabetic nephropathy.

Nephritic Syndrome

The nephritic syndrome is defined by oliguria, edema, hypertension, proteinuria (usually <3.5 g/24 hr), and abnormal urinalysis with dysmorphic red blood cells or red blood cell casts. Glomerular diseases commonly presenting with nephritic syndrome include infection-related glomerulonephritis, IgA nephropathy, and C3 glomerulopathy.

Rapidly Progressive Glomerulonephritis

RPGN is a clinical syndrome characterized by progressive loss of kidney function with a time course of days to months in a patient with active urinary sediment (see Chapter 2 and Table 7.3). Patients may have oliguria. Most of the pulmonary-renal syndromes manifest in this fashion, and the pathologic corollary is often a focal, necrotizing, crescentic glomerulonephritis. When RPGN is suspected, renal biopsy with immunofluorescence studies is extremely helpful.

Linear deposition of immunoglobulin G (IgG) points to Goodpasture disease or anti–glomerular basement membrane (anti-GBM)–mediated glomerulonephritis. Immunoglobulins and complement suggest systemic lupus erythematosus (SLE), cryoglobulinemia, immunoglobulin A (IgA) nephropathy, or postinfectious glomerulonephritis. Negative or weak immunofluorescence (pauci-immune) findings usually indicate an antineutrophil cytoplasmic autoantibody (ANCA) vasculitis (Fig. 4.1).

Chronic Glomerulonephritis

Patients can be presumed to have chronic glomerulonephritis in the setting of a slowly progressive loss of renal function over the course of months or years, accompanied by persistent glomerular hematuria. Proteinuria is usually in the subnephrotic range. Hypertension is nearly always present. Renal ultrasound usually shows small kidneys with increased echogenicity.

Glomerular diseases often presenting as chronic glomerulonephritis include IgA nephropathy, C3 glomerulopathy, and Alport syndrome.

PRIMARY PODOCYTOPATHIES

Minimal Change Disease

MCD is defined by a renal biopsy with no significant glomerular abnormalities on light microscopy, negative immunoglobulin and complement deposition on immunofluorescence, and widespread foot

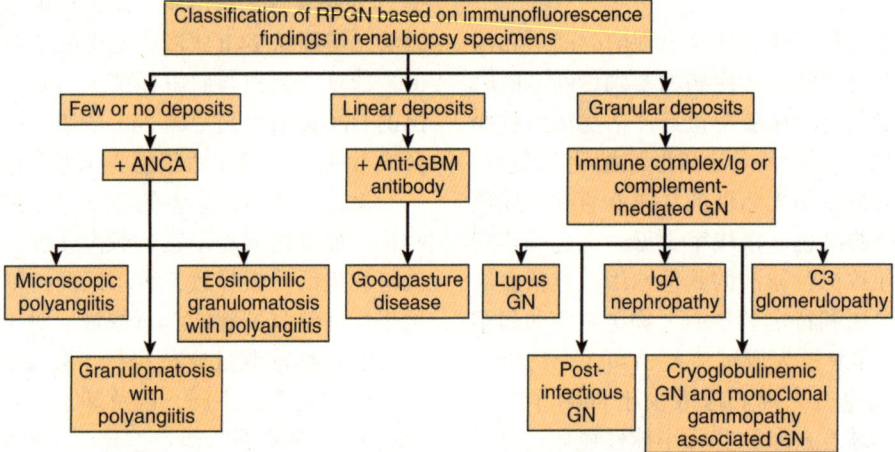

Fig. 4.1 Rapidly progressive glomerulonephritis (RPGN) is classified according to immunofluorescence microscopy findings in renal biopsy specimens. *ANCA*, Antineutrophil cytoplasmic autoantibody; *GBM*, glomerular basement membrane; *GN*, glomerulonephritis; *IgA*, immunoglobulin A.

检测到白蛋白），则提示蛋白尿由轻链或小分子量蛋白（如视黄醇结合蛋白、α1-微球蛋白）引起。

临床综合征

无症状镜下血尿

肾小球性血尿可伴或不伴非肾病范围蛋白尿。肾功能指标和血压通常正常。

通常表现为无症状血尿的肾小球疾病包括 IgA 肾病、Alport 综合征和薄基底膜肾病。

肾病综合征

肾病综合征的定义是持续尿总蛋白排泄量大于 3.5 g/24 h，伴血清白蛋白浓度低于 3.5 g/dl（译者注：如溴甲酚紫法测得的血清白蛋白应为 < 3.0 g/dl）。水肿、高脂血症和脂肪尿（即双折射脂肪体）常见，但并非诊断的必要条件。

肾病综合征的并发症包括低丙种球蛋白血症、维生素 D 结合蛋白丢失导致的维生素 D 缺乏症以及低转铁蛋白血症导致的缺铁性贫血。由于抗凝血酶Ⅲ的丢失可能出现血栓性并发症，如肾静脉血栓形成，尤其是在蛋白质丢失较多（> 10 g/24 h）和血清白蛋白水平低于 2 g/dl 的患者中。当严重的肾病综合征患者叠加出现容量耗竭、感染中毒症或使用非甾体抗炎药（NSAID）等肾毒性药物时，尤其容易发生急性肾衰竭。

肾病综合征患者的治疗包括使用利尿剂控制水肿，调节血压[首选血管紧张素转换酶抑制剂（ACEI）和血管紧张素受体阻滞剂（ARB）]，蛋白质摄入量限制于 0.8 ～ 1 g/（kg·d），钠的摄入量低于 4 g/d，并控制血脂。对于血栓高风险的患者，尤其是由膜性肾病或淀粉样变性引起的肾病综合征患者，应考虑进行抗凝治疗。

通常表现为肾病综合征的肾小球疾病包括 MCD、FSGS、膜性肾病、HIV 相关性肾病、淀粉样变性和糖尿病肾病。

肾炎综合征

肾炎综合征定义为少尿、水肿、高血压、蛋白尿（通常小于 3.5 g/24 h），以及尿检异常包括异形红细胞或红细胞管型。通常表现为肾炎综合征的肾小球疾病包括感染相关性肾小球肾炎、IgA 肾病和 C3 肾小球病。

急进性肾小球肾炎（RPGN）

RPGN 是一种临床综合征，其特征为具有活动性尿沉渣（见第 2 章和表 7.3）的患者在数天至数月时间内出现肾功能进行性丧失。患者可能出现少尿。大多数肺出血-肾炎综合征都表现为 RPGN，相应的病理为局灶性、坏死性、新月体性肾小球肾炎。当怀疑 RPGN 时，进行肾组织活检和活检组织的免疫荧光检查非常有帮助。

免疫球蛋白 G（IgG）的线样沉积提示 Goodpasture 病或抗肾小球基底膜（anti-GBM）抗体介导的肾小球肾炎。免疫球蛋白和补体沉积提示系统性红斑狼疮（SLE）、冷球蛋白血症、免疫球蛋白 A（IgA）肾病或感染后肾小球肾炎。免疫荧光阴性或弱（寡免疫）通常提示抗中性粒细胞胞质抗体（ANCA）相关血管炎（图 4.1）。

慢性肾小球肾炎

如果患者的肾功能在数月或数年内缓慢逐渐丧失、伴有持续的肾小球性血尿，则可推测其患有慢性肾小球肾炎。蛋白尿通常在肾病范围以下。几乎所有患者都有高血压。肾脏超声常显示双肾变小、回声增强。

通常表现为慢性肾小球肾炎的肾小球疾病包括 IgA 肾病、C3 肾小球病和 Alport 综合征。

原发性足细胞病

微小病变（MCD）

MCD 定义为肾活检光镜下无明显肾小球异常，免疫荧光下无免疫球蛋白和补体沉积，而电子显微镜下

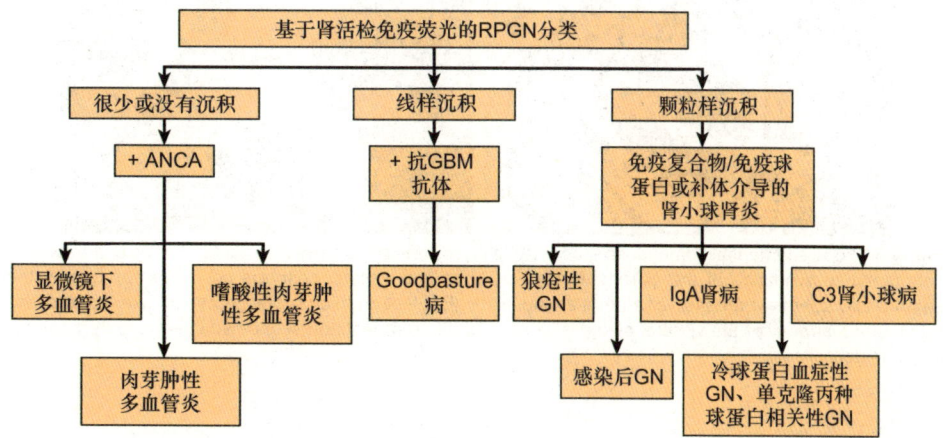

图 4.1 根据肾活检免疫荧光检查结果对急进性肾小球肾炎（RPGN）进行分类。ANCA，抗中性粒细胞胞质抗体；GBM，肾小球基底膜；GN，肾小球肾炎；IgA，免疫球蛋白 A

process effacement on electron microscopy (Fig. 4.2). MCD is the most common cause of nephrotic syndrome in children and accounts for up to 20% of adults with primary nephrotic syndrome.

The pathogenesis of MCD is unknown. The association with Hodgkin lymphoma suggests that MCD may be a consequence of T-lymphocyte abnormalities, with T cells producing a lymphokine that is toxic to glomerular epithelial cells. Most cases of MCD are idiopathic, although drugs (e.g., NSAIDs), hematologic malignancies (mainly Hodgkin lymphoma), and thymoma are well-recognized causes of secondary MCD. Concomitant interstitial nephritis suggests drugs (e.g., NSAIDs) as the likely cause of MCD.

In children, MCD usually manifests with nephrotic syndrome of acute onset. Hematuria, hypertension, or impaired renal function is unusual and suggests another diagnosis. When nephrotic syndrome occurs in a child with normal urinalysis results, the diagnosis is MCD until proven otherwise, and treatment with high-dose corticosteroid therapy can be started, often without the need of a renal biopsy.

More than 90% of children achieve complete remission after 4 to 8 weeks of treatment. Children who do not respond to corticosteroid therapy should undergo a renal biopsy. Adolescents and adults also respond to high-dose corticosteroids (>80%), but the response is slower, and treatment for 16 weeks or more may be required to achieve remission. Therapy usually is continued for 4 to 8 weeks after remission.

Among patients who have a response to corticosteroids, about 25% have a long-term remission. However, up to 25% of the patients have frequent relapses, and up to 30% become steroid dependent. For these patients, alternative therapies aiming to minimize corticosteroid toxicity include alkylating agents, antimetabolites, calcineurin inhibitors (cyclosporine or tacrolimus), and rituximab (a chimeric human-murine monoclonal antibody that targets the CD20 antigen expressed on B cells). Although these agents may allow a lower corticosteroid dose, some patients respond poorly or not at all, and their use may be complicated by significant side effects. Noncompliance is always a concern, especially in young patients.

Focal Segmental Glomerulosclerosis

FSGS is not a specific disease entity, but a lesion, caused by a wide variety of conditions. The common pathophysiologic element is podocyte injury and depletion leading to glomerular scarring (Fig. 4.3). FSGS accounts for less than 15% of cases of idiopathic nephrotic syndrome in children and up to 25% in adults. In African Americans, FSGS is often associated with the presence of the G1 and G2 polymorphisms in the *APOL1* gene. Hypertension is found in 30% to 50% of patients with FSGS, and microscopic hematuria occurs in 25% to 75% of cases. Up to 30% of those with FSGS have impaired renal function.

The pathogenesis of idiopathic or primary FSGS is unknown. A circulating permeability factor has been demonstrated in some patients. The soluble urokinase-type plasminogen activator receptor (suPAR) has been identified as a potential marker because levels are elevated in two thirds of cases of primary FSGS and levels are higher in renal transplant recipients with recurrent FSGS. However, suPAR levels do not distinguish primary from secondary FSGS, and serum levels increase with reductions in the glomerular filtration rate. Further research is needed to define the role of serum suPAR in primary FSGS.

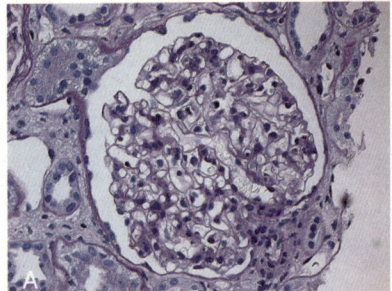 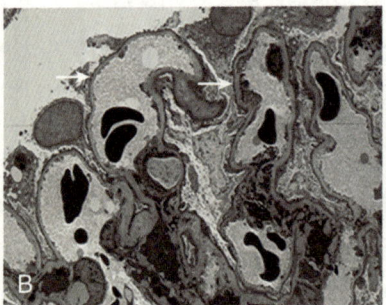 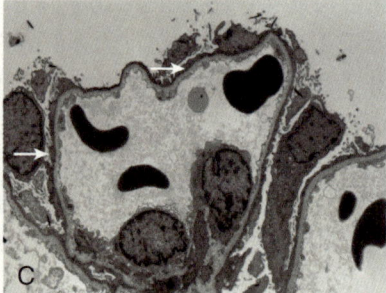

Fig. 4.2 Minimal change disease. (A) Light microscopy shows a normal-appearing glomerulus (periodic acid–Schiff, ×40). (B and C) Electron microscopy shows diffuse foot process effacement *(arrows)* (B, ×2500; C, ×4200). Immunofluorescence studies were negative for immune deposits.

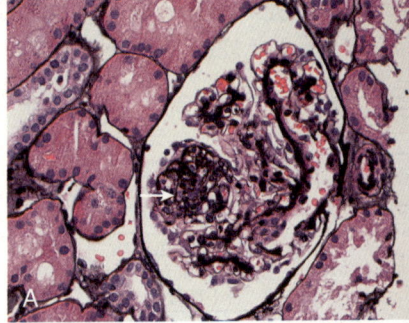 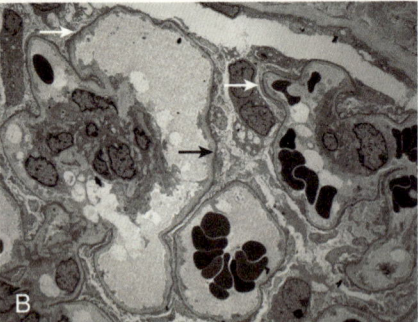

Fig. 4.3 Focal segmental glomerulosclerosis. (A) Light microscopy shows segmental sclerosis *(arrow)* with segmental consolidation of the glomerular capillary tufts and visceral epithelial cell hypertrophy over the segmentally sclerosed tufts (silver methenamine, ×40). (B) Electron microscopy shows diffuse foot process effacement *(arrows)* of the visceral epithelial cells (×1850). Immunofluorescence studies were negative for immune deposits.

可看到足突广泛融合（图 4.2）。MCD 是儿童肾病综合征最常见的病因，占成人原发性肾病综合征的 20%。

MCD 的发病机制尚不清楚。其与霍奇金淋巴瘤的关联提示 MCD 可能是 T 淋巴细胞异常的结果，T 细胞产生的淋巴因子对肾小球上皮细胞具有毒性。尽管药物（如非甾体抗炎药）、血液恶性肿瘤（主要是霍奇金淋巴瘤）和胸腺瘤是公认的继发性 MCD 的病因，大多数 MCD 仍是特发性的。合并间质性肾炎提示药物（如非甾体抗炎药）可能是 MCD 的病因。

在儿童中，MCD 常表现为急性起病的肾病综合征。血尿、高血压或肾功能受损并不常见，如有这些表现则提示 MCD 以外的其他诊断。当儿童患者出现肾病综合征且尿沉渣检查结果正常，即可诊断为 MCD，除非另有诊断，此时可开始大剂量皮质类固醇治疗，通常无需进行肾活检。

90% 以上的患儿在治疗 4～8 周后病情完全缓解。对皮质类固醇治疗无反应的儿童应进行肾活检。青少年和成人对大剂量皮质类固醇也有反应（＞80%），但反应较慢，可能需要治疗 16 周或更长时间才能达到缓解。缓解后通常需继续治疗 4～8 周。

在对皮质类固醇有反应的患者中，约 25% 的患者获得长期缓解。但是高达 25% 的患者会频繁复发，多达 30% 的患者会对类固醇产生依赖。对于这些患者，旨在减少皮质类固醇的毒副作用的替代疗法包括烷化剂、抗代谢药物、钙调磷酸酶抑制剂（环孢素或他克莫司）和利妥昔单抗（一种针对 B 细胞上表达的 CD20 抗原的人鼠嵌合单克隆抗体）。虽然这些药物可以降低皮质类固醇的剂量，但有些患者反应不佳或根本没有反应，而且这些药物的使用可能会带来严重的副作用。依从性差始终是一个令人担忧的问题，尤其是年轻患者。

局灶节段性肾小球硬化（FSGS）

FSGS 不是一种特定的疾病实体，而是一种由多种病因引起的损伤。共同的病理生理要素是足细胞损伤和耗竭导致肾小球瘢痕形成（图 4.3）。FSGS 在儿童特发性肾病综合征中占比不到 15%，在成人中则高达 25%。在非裔美国人中，FSGS 通常与 APOL1 基因的 G1 和 G2 多态性有关。30%～50% 的 FSGS 患者存在高血压，25%～75% 的患者出现镜下血尿。多达 30% 的 FSGS 患者肾功能受损。

特发性或原发性 FSGS 的发病机制尚不清楚。在一些患者中发现了循环渗透因子。可溶性尿激酶型纤溶酶原激活物受体（suPAR）是一种潜在的标志物，因为在 2/3 的原发性 FSGS 病例中血清 suPAR 水平升高，且肾移植后复发的 FSGS 患者中 suPAR 水平更高。然而，suPAR 水平并不能区分原发性和继发性 FSGS，而且血清 suAPR 水平会随着肾小球滤过率的降低而升高。目前，还需要进一步的研究以确定血清 suPAR 在原发性 FSGS 中的作用。

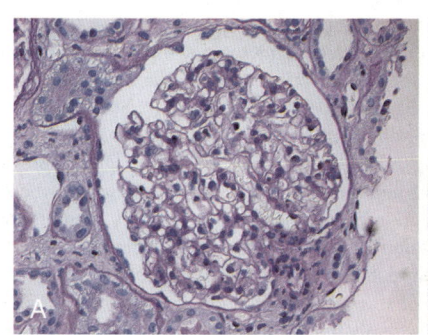 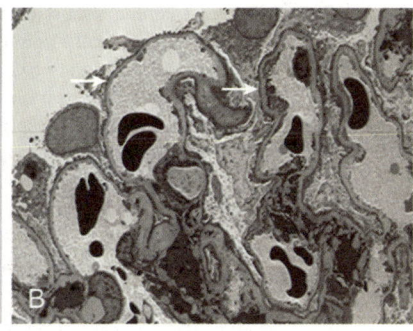 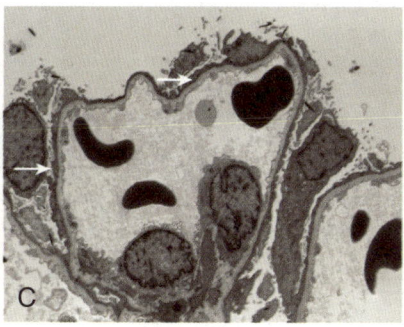

图 4.2 微小病变。（A）光镜下显示肾小球外观正常（PAS，×40）。（B 和 C）电镜显示弥漫足突融合（箭头）（B，×2500；C，×4200）。免疫荧光检查的免疫沉积为阴性

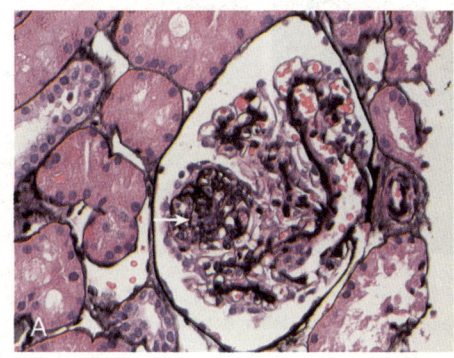 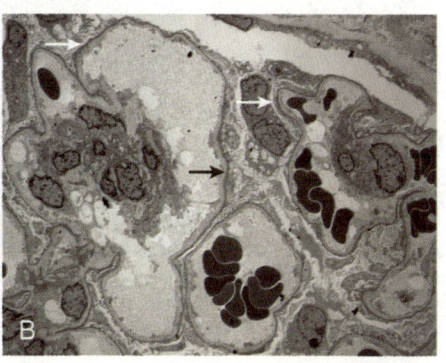

图 4.3 局灶节段性肾小球硬化。（A）光镜下显示节段性硬化（箭头），肾小球毛细血管袢节段性硬化，节段性硬化的毛细血管袢上的脏层上皮细胞增生（氨基甲酸银，×40）。（B）电镜显示脏层上皮细胞弥漫性足突融合（箭头）（×1850）。免疫荧光检查中免疫沉积为阴性

Secondary causes of FSGS include genetic mutations in podocyte genes, human immunodeficiency virus (HIV) infection, drugs, sickle cell disease, vesicoureteral reflux, obesity, unilateral renal agenesis, remnant kidneys, and aging (Table 4.1). Five histologic variants of FSGS have been described according to the Columbia classification: classic (or Not Otherwise Specified), perihilar, cellular, tip, and collapsing. However, this classification is based on LM examination only and does not take into account the degree of foot process effacement on EM. This classification has potential prognostic significance, but it should not be used as a tool to differentiate the different pathophysiologic forms of FSGS. The collapsing variant, which has the worst prognosis, is more common in African Americans and patients with HIV infection.

Spontaneous remission of proteinuria is uncommon (<5% of cases). Treatment of the primary forms consists of prolonged (>4 months) high-dose corticosteroid therapy (prednisone, 1 mg/kg/day), but there is no study comparing this approach with other forms of therapy. However, if patients are going to respond to corticosteroids, proteinuria starts to decrease soon after the start of treatment, and those who show no significant reduction (>30%) in proteinuria after 2 to 3 months of prednisone at 1 mg/kg/day (maximum 80 mg/day) are unlikely to respond, and corticosteroid therapy should be tapered and discontinued. For patients who respond to corticosteroids but undergo relapse, alternative therapy includes the use of cytotoxic drugs alone or in combination with corticosteroids, calcineurin inhibitors, and possibly rituximab. Patients with limiting side effects or contraindications to corticosteroids (e.g., obesity) can be treated with a calcineurin inhibitor as first-line therapy. Similarly to treatment with corticosteroids, if patients are going to respond to a calcineurin inhibitor, proteinuria starts to decrease soon after the start of treatment. For patients with secondary forms of FSGS, treatment should target the cause.

In all patients, treatment with an ACEI or ARB, alone or in combination, may substantially reduce proteinuria and prolong renal survival. Patients who have a non–nephrotic-range proteinuria have the best renal survival (>80% at 10 years). In patients who continue to have a high degree of proteinuria (>10 g/day), end-stage renal disease (ESRD) typically develops over 5 to 20 years. Idiopathic FSGS may recur in a transplanted kidney.

Membranous Nephropathy

Membranous nephropathy is the leading cause of nephrotic syndrome in white individuals. It occurs in persons of all ages and races but is most often diagnosed in middle age, with the incidence peaking during the fourth and fifth decades of life. The male-to-female ratio is about 2:1. Most patients have nephrotic syndrome, normal renal function, and no hypertension. Microscopic hematuria may be detected in about one third of patients.

Autoantibodies against the phospholipase A_2 receptor (PLA_2R) and thrombospondin-7A in podocytes are found in about 70% and less than 5% of patients with the primary form of the disease, respectively. Recently, three new antigens have been discovered in primary membranous nephropathy. These include neural epidermal growth factor-like 1 protein (NELL-1), semaphorin 3B (Sema3B), and protocadherin 7 (PCDH7). Secondary membranous nephropathy is caused by autoimmune diseases (e.g., SLE, autoimmune thyroiditis), infection (e.g., hepatitis B virus [HBV], hepatitis C virus [HCV]), drugs (e.g., penicillamine, NSAIDs), and solid malignancies (e.g., colon cancer, lung cancer). A subset of patients with membranous nephropathy is associated with accumulation of exostosin 1 (EXT1) and exostosin 2 (EXT2) in the glomerular basement membrane. Autoimmune disease is common in this group of patients, and EXT1/EXT2 may represent the target antigen in secondary (autoimmune) membranous nephropathy.

On light microscopy, capillary walls may appear thickened, and methenamine silver stain shows subepithelial projections ("spikes") along the capillary walls. Immunofluorescence microscopy shows marked granular deposition of IgG and C3 along the capillary walls, and subepithelial deposits are seen on electron microscopy (Fig. 4.4). Staining for IgG subclasses may help to differentiate primary from secondary membranous nephropathy. IgG1, IgG2 and IgG3 tend to be highly expressed in lupus membranous nephropathy (class V lupus nephritis), whereas IgG1 and IgG4 tend to be highly expressed in primary membranous nephropathy. IgG4 staining tends to be absent in the immune deposits of membranous nephropathy secondary to malignancy.

Up to one third of the patients with membranous nephropathy undergo spontaneous remission, and another one third of patients

TABLE 4.1 Causes of Focal Segmental Glomerulosclerosis

Primary (Idiopathic) FSGS
- Attributed to a circulating permeability factor

Secondary FSGS
- Genetic mutations in podocyte genes
- Viral: HIV-associated nephropathy, parvovirus B19, simian virus 40, cytomegalovirus
- Drug induced: heroin, interferon (α, β, γ), pamidronate, sirolimus, calcineurin inhibitors
- Adaptive: reduced nephron mass or glomerular adaptation, unilateral renal agenesis, obesity-related glomerulopathy, basement membrane defects healing phase of focal proliferative glomerulonephritis, body building, sickle cell anemia, hypertensive nephrosclerosis, thrombotic microangiopathy, aging kidney
- Other causes: hemophagocytic syndrome

FSGS, Focal segmental glomerulosclerosis; *HIV*, human immunodeficiency virus.

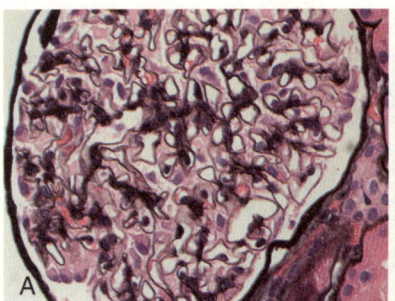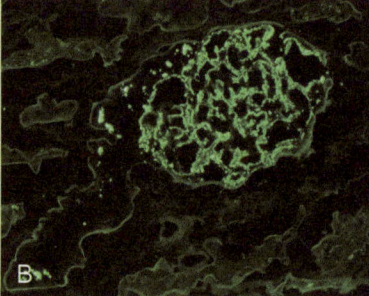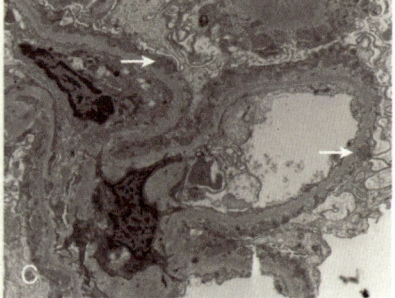

Fig. 4.4 Membranous nephropathy. (A) Light microscopy shows thickened glomerular basement membranes (×60). (B) Immunofluorescence study shows granular immunoglobulin G deposition along the capillary walls (×20). (C) Electron microscopy shows subepithelial electron-dense deposits (arrows) (×15,000).

FSGS 的继发性病因包括足细胞基因突变、人类免疫缺陷病毒（HIV）感染、药物、镰状细胞病、膀胱输尿管反流、肥胖、单侧肾发育不全、残余肾和衰老（表 4.1）。根据哥伦比亚（Columbia）分型，FSGS 有五种组织学亚型：经典型（或非特殊型）、门部型、细胞型、顶端型和塌陷型。然而，这种分类方法仅以光镜检查为基础，并没有考虑到电镜检查中足突融合的程度。虽然这种分类具有潜在的预后意义，但不能作为区分 FSGS 不同病理生理形式的工具。预后最差的塌陷型在非裔美国人和 HIV 感染者中更为常见。

蛋白尿的自发缓解不常见（< 5% 的病例）。原发性 FSGS 的治疗包括长期（> 4 个月）大剂量皮质类固醇治疗［泼尼松，1 mg/（kg·d）］，但目前还没有将这种方法与其他治疗方法进行比较的研究。如果患者对皮质类固醇治疗有反应，则蛋白尿会在开始治疗后不久就减少，应用 1 mg/（kg·d）（最多 80 mg/d）泼尼松 2~3 个月后蛋白尿仍无明显减少（> 30%）的患者，则可能不会对治疗有反应，应逐渐减量并停用皮质类固醇。而对皮质类固醇治疗有反应但复发的患者，替代疗法包括单独使用细胞毒性药物或与皮质类固醇、钙调磷酸酶抑制剂，还可考虑与利妥昔单抗联用。有皮质类固醇显著副作用或禁忌证（如肥胖）的患者，可应用钙调磷酸酶抑制剂作为一线治疗。与皮质类固醇治疗类似，如果患者对钙调磷酸酶抑制剂有反应，则蛋白尿就会在开始治疗后不久减少。对于继发性 FSGS 患者，应针对病因治疗。

对于所有患者，单独或联合使用 ACEI 或 ARB 治疗可大幅减少尿蛋白，延长肾脏存活时间。非肾病范围蛋白尿患者的肾脏存活率最高（10 年时大于 80%）。持续大量蛋白尿（> 10 g/d）的患者通常会在 5~20 年后发展为终末期肾病（ESRD）。特发性 FSGS 可能会在移植肾中复发。

膜性肾病

膜性肾病是白人肾病综合征的首要病因。其可发生于所有年龄和种族，但最好发于中年人，发病高峰年龄为 40~50 岁，男女发病比例约为 2∶1。大多数患者表现为肾病综合征，肾功能正常，无高血压。约 1/3 的患者可有镜下血尿。

原发性膜性肾病患者中约 70% 可检出针对足细胞中磷脂酶 A2 受体（PLA2R）的自身抗体，不到 5% 的患者存在针对足细胞血小板相关蛋白 -7A 的自身抗体。最近，在原发性膜性肾病中又发现了三种新的抗原，包括神经表皮生长因子样 1 蛋白（NELL-1）、脑信号蛋白 3B（Sema3B）和原钙黏蛋白 7（PCDH7）。继发性膜性肾病可由自身免疫性疾病（如系统性红斑狼疮、自身免疫性甲状腺炎）、感染［如乙型肝炎病毒（HBV）、丙型肝炎病毒（HCV）感染］、药物（如青霉胺、非甾体抗炎药）和实体恶性肿瘤（如结肠癌、肺癌）引起。一部分膜性肾病与肾小球基底膜中外骨素 1（EXT1）和外骨素 2（EXT2）的积聚有关。自身免疫性疾病在这部分患者中很常见，EXT1/EXT2 可能代表继发性（自身免疫性）膜性肾病的靶抗原。

光镜下，毛细血管壁增厚，六胺银染色显示沿毛细血管壁的上皮下突起（"钉突"）。免疫荧光可见明显的 IgG 和 C3 沿毛细血管壁颗粒状沉积，电镜下可见上皮下沉积物（图 4.4）。IgG 亚型染色有助于区分原发性和继发性膜性肾病。IgG1、IgG2 和 IgG3 倾向于在狼疮引起的膜性肾病（V 型狼疮性肾炎）中高表达，而 IgG1 和 IgG4 倾向于在原发性膜性肾病中高表达。继发于恶性肿瘤的膜性肾病 IgG4 常为阴性。

高达 1/3 的膜性肾病患者会自发缓解，另外 1/3 的患者获得部分缓解。初始治疗应包括血管紧张素 II 受

表 4.1　局灶节段性肾小球硬化的病因

原发性（特发性）FSGS
- 循环渗透因子

继发性 FSGS
- 足细胞基因的遗传变异
- 病毒：HIV 相关性肾病、细小病毒 B19、猿猴病毒 40、巨细胞病毒
- 药物诱导：海洛因、干扰素（α、β、γ）、帕米膦酸盐、西罗莫司、钙调磷酸酶抑制剂
- 适应性：肾单位数量减少或肾小球适应性降低、单侧肾发育不全、肥胖相关性肾小球病、基底膜缺陷、局灶增生性肾小球肾炎愈合期、健身、镰状细胞贫血、高血压性肾小球硬化、血栓性微血管病、肾脏老化
- 其他原因：噬血细胞综合征

FSGS：局灶节段性肾小球硬化；HIV：人类免疫缺陷病毒。

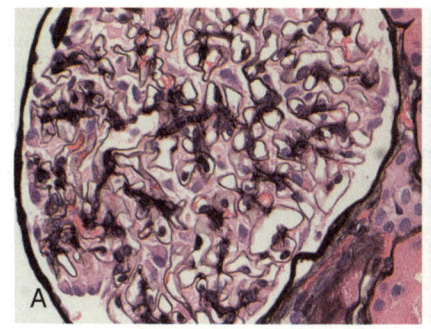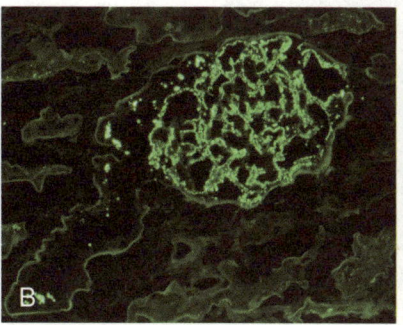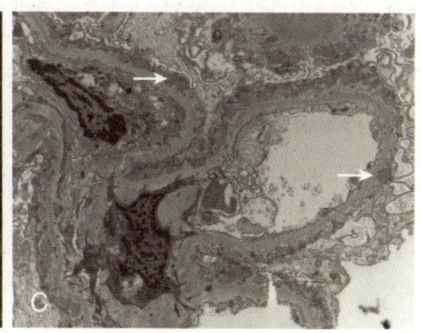

图 4.4　膜性肾病。（A）光镜下显示肾小球基底膜增厚（×60）。（B）免疫荧光检查显示 IgG 沿毛细血管壁颗粒状沉积（×20）。（C）电镜显示上皮下电子致密沉积物（箭头）（×15 000）

undergo partial remission. Initial therapy should include angiotensin II receptor blockade, a low-salt diet (<4 g/day), a low-protein diet (0.8 to 1 g/kg/day), and lipid control. If spontaneous remission occurs, it usually does so within the first 12 to 24 months.

Early treatment should be given to patients with severe nephrotic syndrome (e.g., proteinuria >10 g/24 h) and high or increasing anti-PLA_2R antibody titers, while conservative therapy is continued in asymptomatic patients, who maintain proteinuria at less than 4 g/24 h and have low or decreasing anti-PLA_2R antibody titers.

Rituximab has recently garnered attention as a potential breakthrough in the treatment of membranous nephropathy. A recent multicenter randomized controlled trial of rituximab versus cyclosporine in patients with severe membranous nephropathy (MENTOR) revealed that rituximab is not inferior to cyclosporine in inducing complete or partial remission of proteinuria but is superior in maintaining long-term remission of proteinuria and will likely become the first-line therapy for the treatment of membranous nephropathy.

The probability of renal survival is more than 80% at 5 years and about 60% at 15 years. Patients with an accelerated course should be evaluated for superimposed anti-GBM disease, acute interstitial nephritis, or renal vein thrombosis.

IMMUNE-COMPLEX GLOMERULONEPHRITIS

Infection-Related Glomerulonephritis

Poststreptococcal glomerulonephritis (PSGN) is a classic form of acute glomerulonephritis that develops 1 to 4 weeks after a pharyngitis or skin infection with specific (nephritogenic) strains of group A β-hemolytic streptococci. It typically occurs in children and usually has a benign course. More recently, however, infection-related glomerulonephritis has been recognized to have a broader spectrum, affecting elderly and immunocompromised patients and associated with different bacteria, particularly staphylococci. Unlike classic PSGN, the variant occurs when the infection is still active and has an unfavorable prognosis. The term *infection-related GN* is often used to include both PSGN and GN occurring in the setting of a concurrent infection.

Infection-related glomerulonephritis manifests clinically with the abrupt onset of nephritic syndrome. In patients with PSGN, cultures are usually negative, but elevated titers of antistreptolysin O (ASO), antistreptokinase, antihyaluronidase, and anti-deoxyribonuclease (anti-DNAse B) antibodies may provide evidence of recent streptococcal infection. Activation of the alternative complement pathway is reflected by low C3 complement levels. C4 levels are usually normal or mildly decreased. Other nephrologic conditions associated with low complement are C3 glomerulopathy, lupus nephritis, cryoglobulinemic glomerulonephritis, fibrillary glomerulonephritis, IgG4-mediated renal disease, and cholesterol emboli (Table 4.2).

Renal biopsy typically shows diffuse glomerular hypercellularity and infiltration of polymorphonuclear leukocytes, monocytes, or macrophages on light microscopy. Immunofluorescence shows granular deposition of IgG, C3, and occasionally immunoglobulin M (IgM). On electron microscopy, characteristic dome-shaped subepithelial deposits ("humps") can be seen along the GBM (Fig. 4.5).

Treatment is supportive and aims to minimize fluid overload, optimize blood pressure control, and eradicate ongoing infection. For children, the prognosis is excellent, with most patients recovering renal function in 1 to 2 months. Some patients have persistent microscopic hematuria, proteinuria, hypertension, and renal dysfunction and are said to have *atypical*, *persistent*, or *resolving* PSGN. Some of these patients have mutations or autoantibodies to proteins in the alternative complement cascade and as such represent patients with C3 glomerulopathy.

Immunoglobulin A (IgA) Nephropathy

IgA nephropathy (formerly called Berger disease) is the most common form of primary glomerulopathy. On light microscopy, mesangial proliferation is seen, along with mesangial deposition of IgA on immunofluorescence and electron-dense deposits in the mesangium on electron microscopy (Fig. 4.6).

Patients may have episodes of macroscopic hematuria accompanying an intercurrent upper respiratory tract infection (synpharyngitic) or have asymptomatic hematuria, with or without proteinuria, detected on routine urinalysis. Proteinuria is common, but nephrotic syndrome occurs in less than 10% of cases and raises the possibility of a primary podocytopathy (e.g., MCD) superimposed on the IgA nephropathy.

The pathogenesis of IgA nephropathy has been linked to galactose-deficient IgA1 (GD-IgA1) molecules and increased formation of anti–GD-IgA1 autoantibodies, with deposition of IgG or IgA anti–GD-IgA1 immune complexes in the mesangium, resulting in activation of complement and cytokine cascades. Secondary causes of IgA nephropathy include chronic liver disease, celiac disease, dermatitis herpetiformis, and ankylosing spondylitis.

In up to 60% of the patients, IgA nephropathy has a benign clinical course, and patients maintain proteinuria of less than 500 mg/24 h and preserved renal function. However, progression to ESRD occurs in up to 40% of patients over 10 to 25 years. Clinical predictors of progression include proteinuria greater than 1 g/24 h, hypertension, presence of crescents on renal biopsy, and impaired renal function at diagnosis. Any degree of proteinuria carries a worse prognosis for a patient with IgA nephropathy. IgA nephropathy frequently recurs after renal transplantation, but loss of the allograft from recurrent disease is uncommon.

The use of angiotensin II system blockade and high-dose corticosteroids has been beneficial in slowing or halting progression of renal disease. Henoch-Schönlein purpura is the systemic form of IgA nephropathy. The prognosis is generally good for children but varies in adults.

In patients with normal renal function, treatment is supportive only. Patients with persistent proteinuria greater than 1 g/24 h and/or progressive renal failure should be considered for treatment with high-dose corticosteroids with or without cytotoxic medication.

Membranoproliferative Glomerulonephritis

MPGN is not a specific disease entity but a pattern of glomerular injury resulting from predominantly subendothelial and mesangial deposition of immune complexes or complement factors and their products. On light microscopy, mesangial hypercellularity, endocapillary proliferation, and capillary wall remodeling with double-contour formation are characteristic, and they result in a lobular accentuation of the glomerular tufts. Immunofluorescence microscopy shows immunoglobulins or complement factors, depending on the underlying cause of MPGN. Electron microscopy typically shows mesangial and subendothelial deposits, and, less commonly, intramembranous and subepithelial deposits (Fig. 4.7).

Based on a recent proposal, MPGN can be classified as immune complex mediated or complement mediated. Immune complex–mediated MPGN shows immunoglobulin and complement factors on immunofluorescence

TABLE 4.2 Glomerular Diseases Associated With Hypocomplementemia
Acute lupus nephritis
C3 glomerulopathy (C3 glomerulonephritis and dense deposit disease)
Cholesterol emboli
Cryoglobulinemic glomerulonephritis
Postinfectious glomerulonephritis
IgG4-related nephropathy
Fibrillary glomerulonephritis

体阻滞剂、低盐饮食（＜4 g/d）、低蛋白饮食[0.8～1 g/（kg·d）]和控制血脂。自发缓解通常在最初的12～24个月内发生。

对于严重肾病综合征（如蛋白尿大于10 g/24 h）和抗PLA2R抗体滴度高或持续升高的患者，应及早治疗；而对于无症状的患者，若蛋白尿持续在4 g/24 h以下且抗PLA2R抗体滴度较低或不断降低，则应继续保守治疗。

最近，利妥昔单抗作为膜性肾病治疗的潜在突破点引起了人们的关注。近期的一项针对严重膜性肾病患者的多中心随机对照研究（MENTOR）显示，在诱导蛋白尿完全或部分缓解方面，利妥昔单抗不劣于环孢素，在维持蛋白尿长期缓解上则更胜一筹，因此有可能成为治疗膜性肾病的一线疗法。

膜性肾病的5年肾脏存活率超过80%，15年肾脏存活率约为60%。对于病程快速进展的患者，应评估是否合并抗GBM病、急性间质性肾炎或肾静脉血栓。

免疫复合物介导的肾小球肾炎

感染相关性肾小球肾炎

链球菌感染后肾小球肾炎（PSGN）是急性肾小球肾炎的一种典型形式，在特定的A组β-溶血性链球菌（致肾炎）菌株引起的咽炎或皮肤感染后1～4周发病。常见于儿童，病程多为良性。然而，最近人们认识到感染相关性肾小球肾炎具有更广泛的谱系，影响老年人和免疫功能低下的患者，并与不同的细菌有关，尤其是葡萄球菌。与典型的PSGN不同，该变异表型发生于感染活动期且预后不良。感染相关性肾小球肾炎这一术语通常包括PSGN和与感染同时发生的肾小球肾炎。

感染相关性肾小球肾炎的临床表现为急性发作的肾炎综合征。在PSGN患者中，培养结果通常为阴性，但抗链球菌溶解素O（ASO）、抗链球菌激酶、抗透明质酸酶和抗脱氧核糖核酸酶（抗DNAse B）抗体滴度升高，这些可提供近期链球菌感染的证据。低C3水平反映了补体替代途径的激活。C4水平通常正常或轻度降低。与低补体相关的其他肾病包括C3肾小球病、狼疮性肾炎、冷球蛋白血症性肾小球肾炎、纤维样肾小球肾炎、IgG4相关性肾病和胆固醇栓塞（表4.2）。

肾活检光镜下可见弥漫性肾小球细胞增生，以及多形核白细胞、单核细胞或巨噬细胞浸润。免疫荧光显示IgG和C3颗粒样沉积，偶见IgM。电镜下的特征性表现为沿着肾小球基底膜上皮下圆顶状沉积（"驼峰"）（图4.5）。

治疗以支持为主，旨在尽量减少体液超负荷、优化血压控制和根除持续感染。对于儿童来说，预后良好，大多数患者可在1～2个月内恢复肾功能。有些患者会出现持续性镜下血尿、蛋白尿、高血压和肾功能障碍，称为非典型、持续性或缓解中PSGN。这些患者中部分患者存在补体替代途径中蛋白的突变或自身抗体，因此认为是C3肾小球病的患者。

免疫球蛋白A（IgA）肾病

IgA肾病（以前称为Berger病）是最常见的原发性肾小球病。光镜下可见系膜增生，免疫荧光可见IgA在系膜区沉积，电镜下可见系膜区电子致密物沉积（图4.6）。

患者可在上呼吸道感染（咽炎）期间出现发作性肉眼血尿，或在常规尿检中发现无症状血尿，伴或不伴蛋白尿。蛋白尿很常见，但肾病综合征仅见于不到10%的患者，这时提示IgA肾病可能合并了原发性足细胞病（如MCD）。

IgA肾病的发病机制与半乳糖缺陷的IgA1（GD-IgA1）分子和抗GD-IgA1的自身抗体形成增加有关，IgG型或IgA型抗体与GD-IgA1形成免疫复合物沉积在系膜区，导致补体活化和细胞因子级联反应。IgA肾病的继发性原因包括慢性肝病、乳糜泻、疱疹样皮炎和强直性脊柱炎。

接近60%的IgA肾病患者的临床病程是良性的，蛋白尿维持在500 mg/24 h以下，肾功能稳定。然而，高达40%的患者会在10～25年内发展为ESRD。预测疾病进展的临床指标包括蛋白尿超过1 g/24 h、高血压、肾活检发现新月体以及确诊时即存在肾功能受损。任何程度的蛋白尿都会导致IgA肾病患者的预后更差。IgA肾病经常在肾移植后复发，但因复发而导致移植肾失功的情况并不常见。

使用血管紧张素Ⅱ系统阻滞剂和大剂量皮质类固醇能够减缓或阻止疾病进展。过敏性紫癜是IgA肾病的系统性表型，儿童的预后一般较好，成人的预后则不尽相同。

对于肾功能正常的患者，仅需要支持性治疗。对于蛋白尿持续超过1 g/24 h和（或）进行性肾功能衰竭的患者应考虑使用大剂量皮质类固醇治疗，联合或不联合细胞毒药物。

膜增生性肾小球肾炎（MPGN）

MPGN并不是一种特定的疾病实体，是主要由内皮下和系膜区免疫复合物沉积或补体因子及其产物导致的肾小球损伤模式。在光镜下，其特征为系膜细胞增生、毛细血管内增生、毛细血管壁重塑伴双轨征形成，导致肾小球毛细血管袢呈分叶状。免疫荧光可见免疫球蛋白或补体沉积，取决于MPGN的不同潜在病因。电子显微镜的典型表现是系膜区和内皮下电子致密沉积物，基底膜内和上皮下沉积物较少见（图4.7）。

根据最近的一项提议，MPGN可分为免疫复合物介

表4.2 低补体血症相关的肾小球疾病
急性狼疮性肾炎
C3肾小球病（C3肾小球肾炎和致密沉积病）
胆固醇栓塞
冷球蛋白血症性肾小球肾炎
链球菌感染后肾小球肾炎
IgG4相关性肾病
纤维样肾小球肾炎

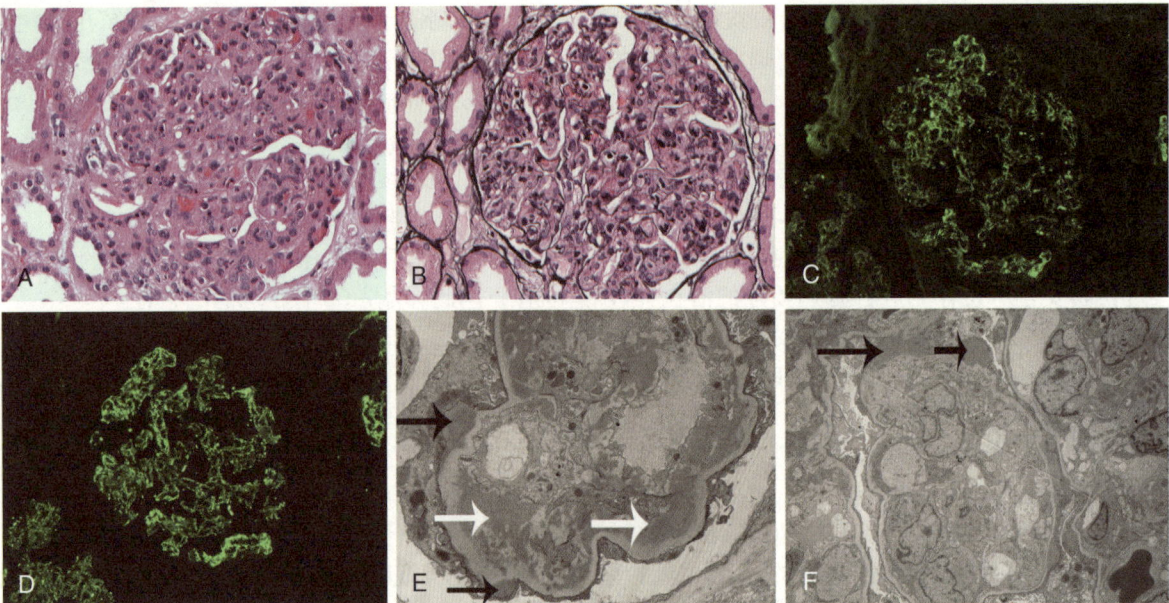

Fig. 4.5 Postinfectious glomerulonephritis. (A and B) Light microscopy shows diffuse endocapillary proliferative glomerulonephritis. Notice the prominent neutrophil infiltration in the glomerular capillaries (A, hematoxylin and eosin; B, silver methenamine; both ×40). (C and D) Immunofluorescence studies show granular immunoglobulin G and C3 deposition along the capillary walls (both ×20). (E and F) Electron microscopy shows subendothelial deposits *(white arrows)* and subepithelial humplike deposits *(black arrows)*. The subendothelial deposits likely result from circulating immune complexes that are deposited along the glomerular capillary walls and drive the inflammatory response (E, ×5800). The subepithelial deposits likely represent in situ immune complex formation (F, ×2850).

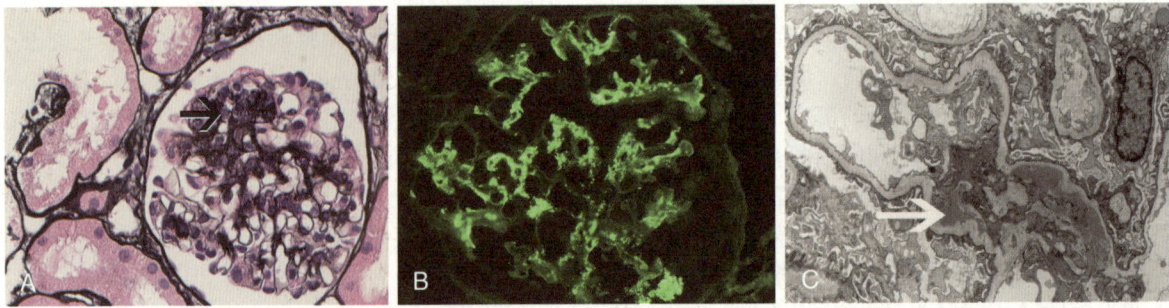

Fig. 4.6 Immunoglobulin A (IgA) nephropathy. (A) Light microscopy shows mesangial hypercellularity *(black arrow)* (silver methenamine, ×40). (B) Immunofluorescence microscopy shows bright mesangial IgA staining. (C) Electron microscopy shows large mesangial electron-dense deposits *(arrow)* (×7860).

microscopy. Complement-mediated MPGN shows complement factors and a lack of significant immunoglobulin on immunofluorescence microscopy (Fig. 4.8). Immune complex/Ig–mediated MPGN results from chronic infections, autoimmune diseases, and monoclonal gammopathies. Complement-mediated MPGN is caused by genetic or acquired dysregulation of the alternative pathway of complement (C3 glomerulopathy) and can be further subclassified as C3 glomerulonephritis and dense deposit disease (DDD) based on electron microscopy examination.

Immune complex–mediated MPGN precipitated by an infection is most commonly caused by HCV (i.e., cryoglobulinemic glomerulonephritis). The clinical presentation varies and can include nephrotic and nephritic features. In patients with cryoglobulinemic MPGN, the levels of C3, C4, and CH50 are persistently low, reflecting activation of classical complement pathway. Patients with C3 glomerulonephritis or DDD may have a persistently low level of C3 but a normal level of C4. A C3 nephritic factor is found in many cases. C3 nephritic factor is an autoantibody to alternative pathway C3 convertase, resulting in persistent breakdown of C3.

The absence of well-designed studies based on the current insights in the pathogenesis of MPGN make it impossible to give strong treatment recommendations. From a practical point of view, patients with MPGN due to chronic infections (e.g., HCV, endocarditis), autoimmune disease, and plasma cell dyscrasias (monoclonal gammopathy) should undergo treatment of the underling disease. Patients with normal kidney function, no active urinary sediment, and non–nephrotic-range proteinuria can be treated conservatively with angiotensin II blockade to control blood pressure and reduce proteinuria, because the long-term outcome is relatively benign in this setting. Follow-up is required to detect early deterioration in kidney function. Patients with C3 glomerulonephritis or DDD with proteinuria greater than 1000 mg/24 h and/or abnormal kidney function but not rapidly progressive disease, and who do not have a genetic mutation leading to factor H deficiency, can be considered for additional treatment

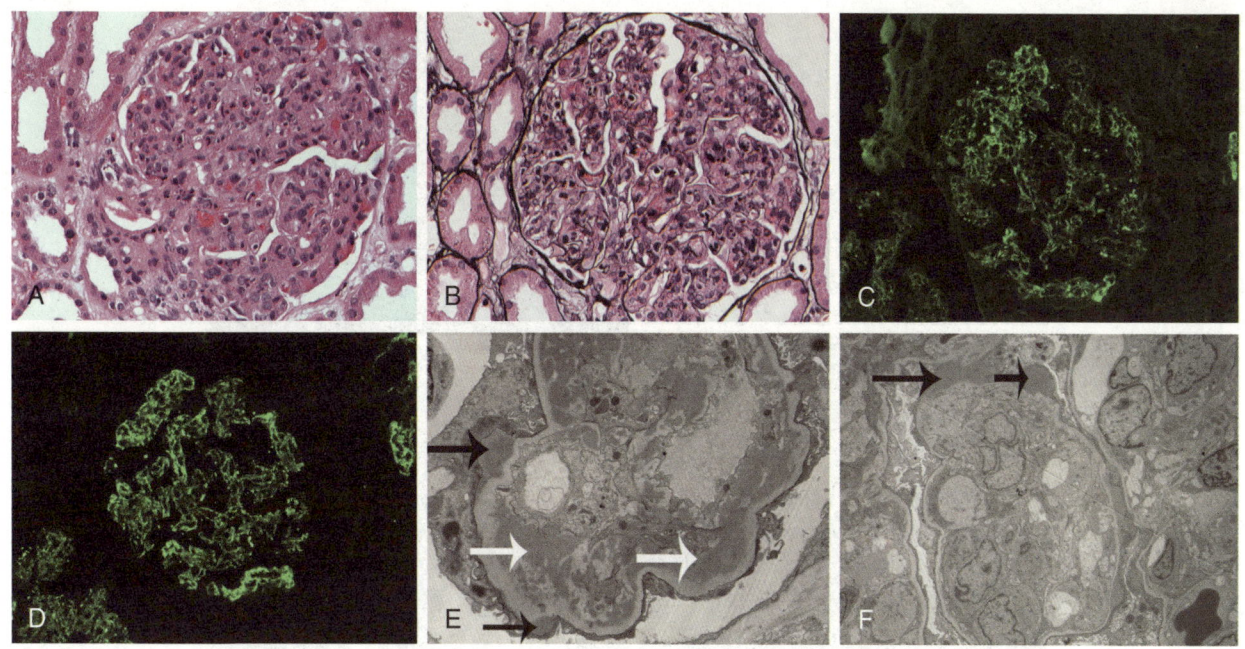

图 4.5 感染后肾小球肾炎。（**A** 和 **B**）光镜下显示弥漫性毛细血管内增生性肾小球肾炎。肾小球毛细血管袢可见明显的中性粒细胞浸润（A，HE；B，六胺银；均为 ×40）。（**C** 和 **D**）免疫荧光显示 IgG 和 C3 沿毛细血管壁颗粒状沉积（均为 ×20）。（**E** 和 **F**）电镜显示内皮下沉积物（白色箭头）和上皮下驼峰状沉积物（黑色箭头）。内皮下沉积物可能是循环免疫复合物沿肾小球毛细血管壁沉积并诱发炎症反应的结果（E，×5800）。上皮下沉积物可能是原位免疫复合物形成（F，×2850）

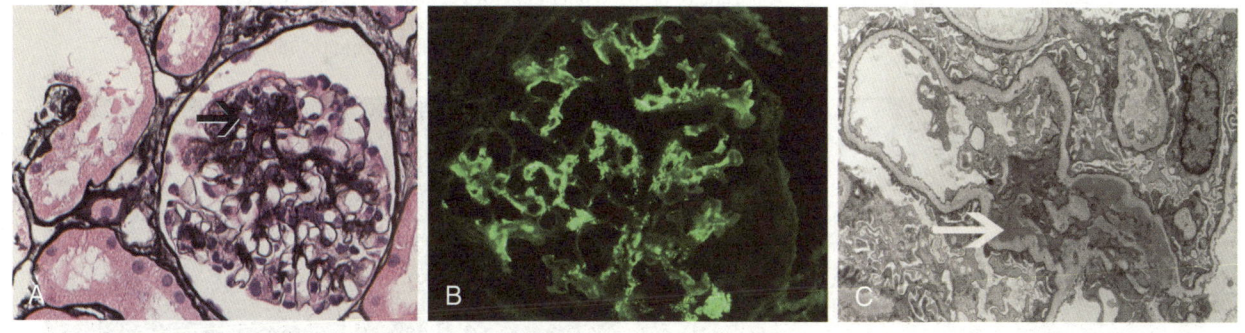

图 4.6 IgA 肾病。（**A**）光镜显示系膜细胞增生（黑色箭头）（六胺银，×40）。（**B**）免疫荧光显示明亮的系膜区 IgA 染色。（**C**）电镜显示系膜区大块电子致密物沉积（箭头）（×7860）

导型或补体介导型。免疫复合物介导的 MPGN 在免疫荧光上显示免疫球蛋白和补体沉积。补体介导的 MPGN 免疫荧光显示补体沉积，缺乏显著的免疫球蛋白沉积（图 4.8）。慢性感染、自身免疫性疾病和单克隆丙种球蛋白病会导致免疫复合物/免疫球蛋白介导的 MPGN。补体介导的 MPGN 是由基因变异或获得性补体替代途径失调（C3 肾小球病）引起的，根据电镜检查可进一步将其分为 C3 肾小球肾炎和致密物沉积病（DDD）。

由感染诱发的免疫复合物介导的 MPGN 最常见的病因是丙型肝炎病毒（HCV）感染（即冷球蛋白血症性肾小球肾炎）。其临床表现多样，可包括肾病和肾炎特征。在冷球蛋白血症性肾小球肾炎患者中，C3、C4 和 CH50 水平持续偏低，反映补体经典途径活化。C3 肾小球肾炎或 DDD 患者的 C3 水平可能持续偏低，但 C4 水平正常。在许多病例中可发现 C3 肾炎因子，是一种针对补体旁路途径 C3 转化酶的自身抗体，导致 C3 的持续裂解。

由于缺乏基于目前对 MPGN 发病机制的了解而设计完善的研究，无法给出肯定的治疗建议。从临床实践的角度，慢性感染（如 HCV 感染、心内膜炎）、自身免疫性疾病和浆细胞异常（单克隆丙种球蛋白病）引起的 MPGN 患者应接受基础疾病的治疗。对于肾功能正常、无活动性尿沉渣和非肾病范围蛋白尿的患者，可采用血管紧张素 II 受体阻滞剂进行保守治疗，以控制血压和减少蛋白尿，因为这种情况下的长期预后相对较好。需要进行随访以早期及时发现肾功能恶化。C3 肾小球肾炎或 DDD 患者，如果蛋白尿超过 1000 mg/24 h 和（或）肾功能异常但病情没有迅速进展，且没有导

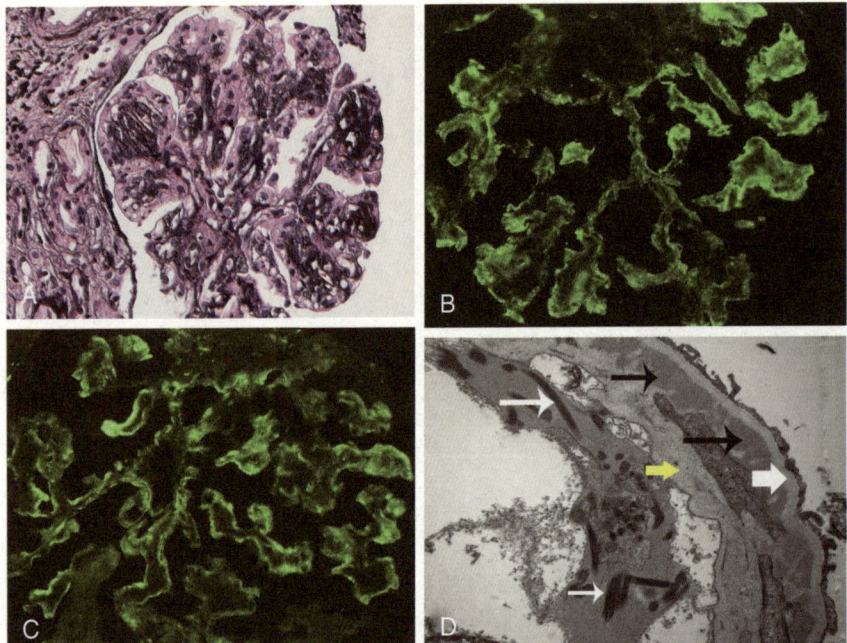

Fig. 4.7 Immune complex–mediated membranoproliferative glomerulonephritis due to hepatitis C virus infection. (A) Light microscopy shows a membranoproliferative pattern of injury with mesangial expansion, endocapillary proliferation, double-contour formation along the capillary walls, and lobular accentuation of the glomerular tufts (silver methenamine, ×40). (B and C) Immunofluorescence microscopy shows bright capillary wall staining for immunoglobulin M (B, ×40) and for C3 (C, ×40). (D) Electron microscopy shows capillary wall thickening and a double-contour formation due to accumulation of subendothelial electron-dense deposits *(black arrows)*, cellular elements, and new basement membrane formation (i.e., duplication) *(yellow arrow)* that produces the double contour. The *thick white arrow* indicates the old basement membrane, and fibrin tactoids *(white arrows)* in glomerular capillary loops indicate a prothrombotic state (×1350).

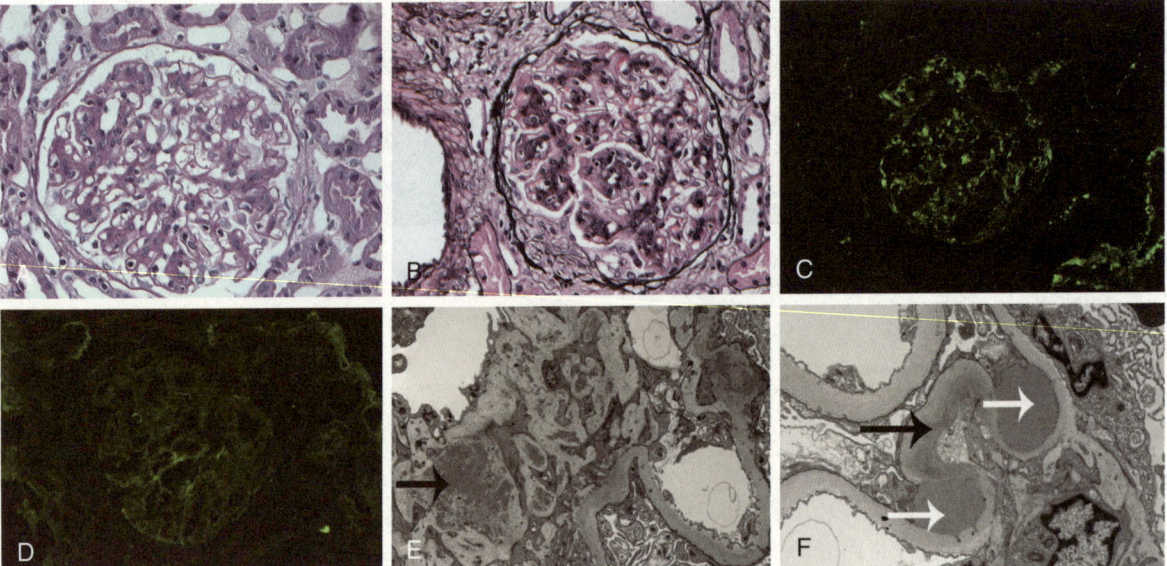

Fig. 4.8 C3 glomerulonephritis. Light microscopy shows features of mesangial proliferative glomerulonephritis (A, periodic acid–Schiff, ×40) and membranoproliferative glomerulonephritis (B, silver methenamine stain, ×40) in the same biopsy. Immunofluorescence microscopy shows bright granular mesangial and capillary wall staining for C3 (C) and negative staining for immunoglobulin G (D). (E) Electron microscopy shows a large accumulation of smudgy mesangial deposits *(arrow)* (×10,000). (F) Electron microscopy shows subendothelial deposits *(black arrow)* and subepithelial humplike deposits *(white arrows)* (×150,000). The subepithelial deposits sometimes make it difficult to distinguish C3 glomerulonephritis from postinfectious glomerulonephritis. However, C3 glomerulonephritis may not show Ig (as in this case), and the term *atypical postinfectious glomerulonephritis* sometimes is applied in cases of C3 glomerulonephritis with subepithelial humplike deposits.

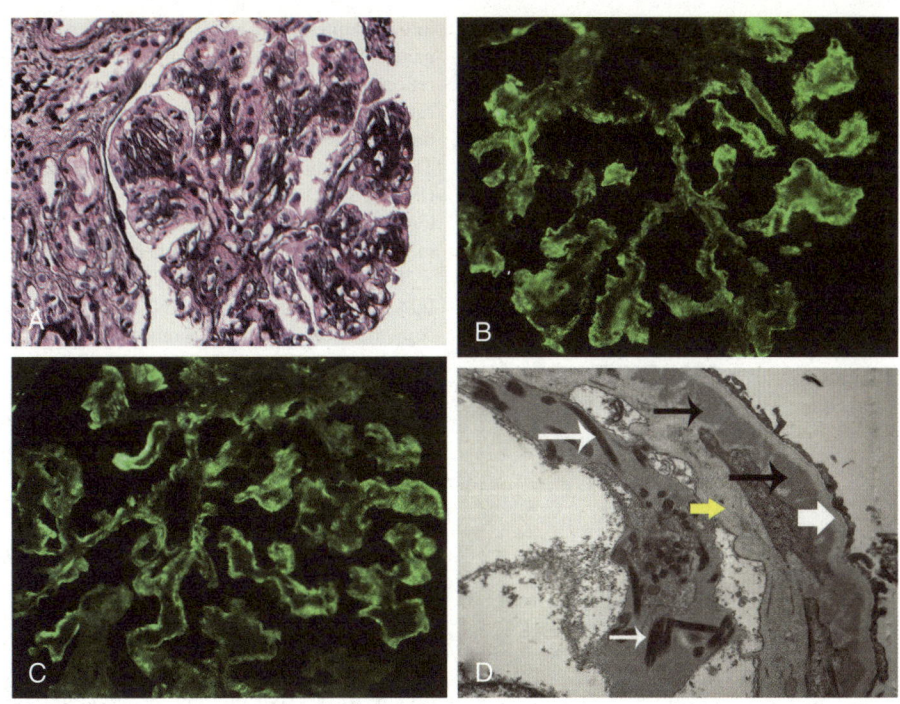

图 4.7 丙型肝炎病毒感染引起的免疫复合物介导的膜增生性肾小球肾炎。（A）光镜下显示膜增生样损伤，包含系膜扩张、毛细血管内增生、沿毛细血管壁形成双轨征、肾小球血管袢呈分叶状（六胺银，×40）。（B 和 C）免疫荧光显示毛细血管壁 IgM（B，×40）和 C3（C，×40）的明亮染色。（D）电镜显示毛细血管壁增厚和双轨征形成，双轨征由内皮下电子致密物沉积（黑色箭头）、细胞成分和新基底膜成分（即双层）（黄色箭头）所形成。白色粗箭头指示原有基底膜，肾小球毛细血管袢中的纤维蛋白簇（白色箭头）提示血栓前状态（×1350）

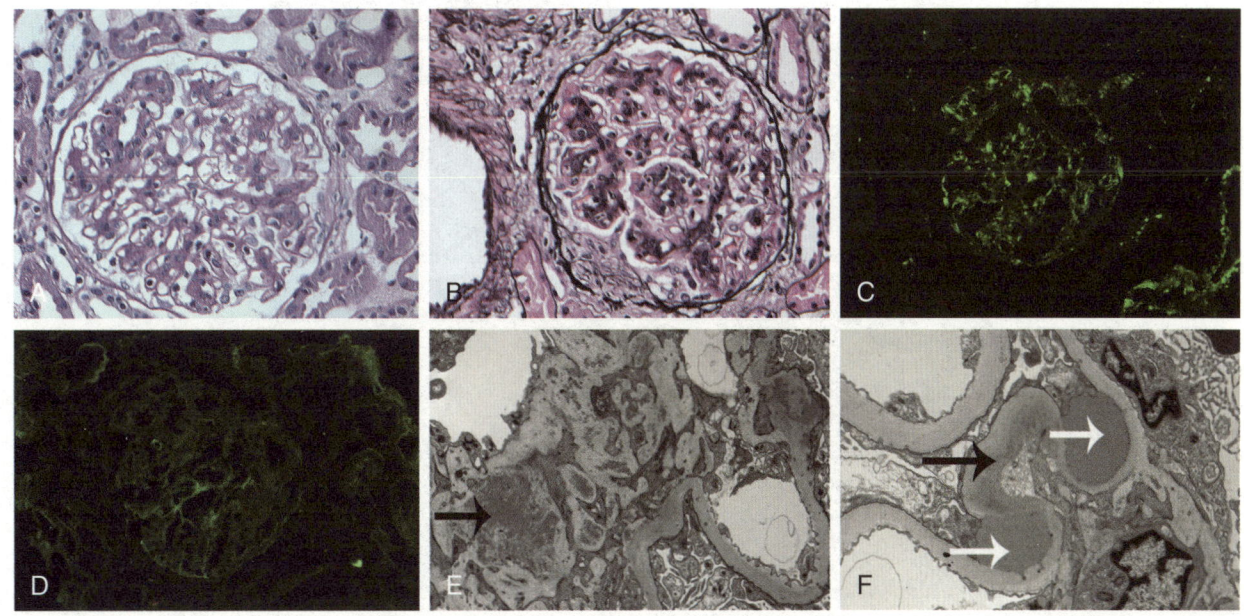

图 4.8 C3 肾小球肾炎。光镜下显示在同一肾活检标本中存在系膜增生性肾小球肾炎（A，PAS，×40）和膜增生性肾小球肾炎（B，六胺银 ×40）。免疫荧光显示系膜区和毛细血管壁的明亮颗粒状 C3 染色（C），IgG 阴性（D）。（E）电镜显示系膜区大量污泥样沉积（箭头）（×10 000）。（F）电镜显示内皮下沉积物（黑色箭头）和上皮下驼峰状沉积物（白色箭头）（×150 000）。上皮下沉积物有时使得 C3 肾小球肾炎与感染后肾小球肾炎难以区分。然而，C3 肾小球肾炎没有免疫球蛋白（如本病例所示），且非典型感染后肾小球肾炎有时即指存在上皮下驼峰样沉积的 C3 肾小球肾炎

with mycophenolate mofetil plus oral corticosteroids. Patients who have advanced renal insufficiency and severe tubulointerstitial fibrosis of renal biopsy are unlikely to benefit from immunosuppressive therapy.

Lupus Nephritis

Lupus nephritis occurs in up to 50% to 70% of patients with SLE and is associated with a poor prognosis. Proteinuria is the most common initial manifestation, and it is often in the nephrotic range and accompanied by a decline in renal function. Urinalysis does not always reflect the severity of the glomerular lesion, and kidney biopsy is indicated in those with proteinuria or active urinary sediment, or both, because the type of renal lesion influences the therapeutic decisions. The International Society of Nephrology/Renal Pathology Society (ISN/RPS) classification of lupus nephritis recognizes six morphologic classes of renal involvement (Table 4.3). However, patients may migrate from one class to another spontaneously or after treatment.

Immunofluorescence typically shows glomerular deposition of IgG, IgM, IgA, C1q, and C3 (i.e., full-house pattern). On electron microscopy, tubuloreticular inclusions are common within glomerular and vascular endothelial cells. Electron-dense deposits sometimes show fingerprint-like substructures) (Fig 4.9). Histologic lesions correlate with the prognosis; classes III and IV have the worst prognosis (see Fig. 4.9). Other manifestations of SLE include acute and chronic tubulointerstitial nephritis and glomerular capillary thrombi in patients with antiphospholipid antibodies.

Three guidelines for the management of lupus nephritis have been published recently by the American College of Rheumatology, the Kidney Disease-Improving Global Outcomes (KDIGO) working group, and the Joint European League Against Rheumatism and European Renal Association–European Dialysis and Transplant Association (EULAR/ERA-EDTA). For class I lupus nephritis, the prognosis is excellent, and no immunosuppression is required. Patients with class II lupus nephritis and proteinuria less than 1 g/24 h should be treated as dictated by the extrarenal clinical manifestations of lupus. Patients with class II lupus nephritis and proteinuria greater than 3 g/24 h should be treated with corticosteroids or calcineurin inhibitors.

TABLE 4.3 Abbreviated International Society of Nephrology/Renal Pathology Society 2003 Classification of Lupus Nephritis

Type	Morphologic Class	Renal Manifestation
I	Minimal mesangial lupus nephritis	Normal urinary sediment
II	Mesangial proliferative lupus nephritis	Low-grade hematuria and/or proteinuria Normal renal function
III	Focal lupus nephritis	Active sediment, proteinuria <3 g/1.73 m²/day
IV	Diffuse lupus nephritis	Nephritic and nephrotic syndromes Hypertension; progressive renal failure
V	Membranous lupus nephritis	Nephrotic syndrome
VI	Advanced sclerosing lupus nephritis	Inactive urinary sediment Chronic renal failure

Modified from Weening JJ, D'Agati VD, Schwartz MM, et al: The classification of glomerulonephritis in systemic lupus erythematosus revisited, J Am Soc Nephrol 15:241-250, 2004.

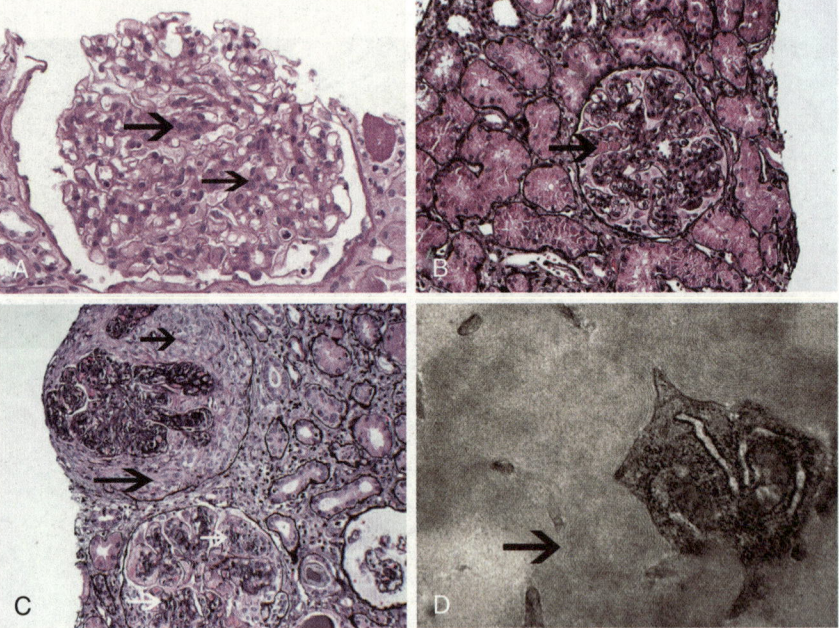

Fig. 4.9 Light microscopy (A to C) and electron microscopy (D) are used to identify lupus nephritis. (A) Mild mesangial proliferative glomerulonephritis (International Society of Nephrology/Renal Pathology Society [ISN/RPS] class II) has mesangial hypercellularity (arrows) (periodic acid–Schiff, ×40). (B) Diffuse endocapillary proliferation with cryoglobulins in the glomerular capillaries, identified as pale, silver-negative material (arrow) (silver methenamine, ×20). (C) In diffuse proliferative glomerulonephritis (ISN/RPS class IV), the glomerulus on top shows a large cellular crescent (black arrows), and the glomerulus at the bottom shows diffuse endocapillary proliferation (white arrows) (silver methenamine, ×20). (D) Electron-dense deposits have fingerprint substructures (arrow) (×46,000).

致H因子缺乏的基因突变，则可考虑接受吗替麦考酚酯联合口服皮质类固醇的额外治疗。晚期肾功能不全和肾活检发现严重肾小管间质纤维化的患者不太可能从免疫抑制治疗中获益。

狼疮性肾炎

在系统性红斑狼疮患者中，50%～70%发生狼疮性肾炎，其与不良预后相关。蛋白尿是最常见的肾脏疾病的首发表现，通常是肾病范围蛋白尿，伴有肾功能下降。尿液分析并不总能反映肾小球病变的严重程度，因为肾脏病变的类型会影响治疗决策，因此对于蛋白尿和（或）活动性尿沉渣的患者应进行肾活检。国际肾脏病学会/肾脏病理学会（ISN/RPS）将狼疮性肾炎的肾脏病理分成六种类型（表4.3）。然而，患者可能会自发或在接受治疗后从一种类型转换为另一种类型。

免疫荧光的典型表现为IgG、IgM、IgA、C1q和C3在肾小球沉积（即"满堂亮"）。在电镜下，肾小球和血管内皮细胞内常见管网状包涵体。电子致密物有时呈指纹样亚结构（图4.9）。组织学病变与预后相关；Ⅲ型和Ⅳ型预后最差（见图4.9）。系统性红斑狼疮的其他肾脏受累表现还包括急性和慢性肾小管间质性肾炎以及抗磷脂抗体阳性患者的肾小球毛细血管血栓形成。

最近，美国风湿病学会（American College of Rheumatology）、改善全球肾脏预后联盟（KDIGO）工作组以及欧洲抗风湿病联盟和欧洲肾脏协会-欧洲透析与移植协会（EULAR/ERA-EDTA）发布了三项狼疮性肾炎管理指南。Ⅰ型狼疮性肾炎的预后很好，无需使用免疫抑制剂。尿蛋白少于1 g/24 h的Ⅱ型狼疮性肾炎患者，应根据狼疮的肾外临床表现进行治疗。对于蛋白尿超过3 g/24 h的Ⅱ型狼疮性肾炎患者，应使用皮质类固醇或钙调磷酸酶抑制剂进行治疗。

表4.3 国际肾脏病学会/肾脏病理学会2003年狼疮性肾炎分类简表

分型	病理分型	肾脏表现
Ⅰ	轻度系膜性狼疮性肾炎	尿沉渣正常
Ⅱ	系膜增生性狼疮性肾炎	轻度血尿和（或）蛋白尿，肾功能正常
Ⅲ	局灶性狼疮性肾炎	活动性尿沉渣，蛋白尿＜3 g/（1.73 m^2·d）
Ⅳ	弥漫性狼疮性肾炎	肾炎和肾病综合征，高血压；进行性肾衰竭
Ⅴ	膜性狼疮性肾炎	肾病综合征
Ⅵ	晚期硬化性狼疮性肾炎	非活动性尿沉渣，慢性肾衰竭

改编自Weening JJ, D'Agati VD, Schwartz MM, et al: The classification of glomerulonephritis in systemic lupus erythematosus revisited, J Am Soc Nephrol 15：241-250，2004.

［译者注：原文表4.3有误，分型（Type）列第二行原文Ⅰ应为Ⅱ］

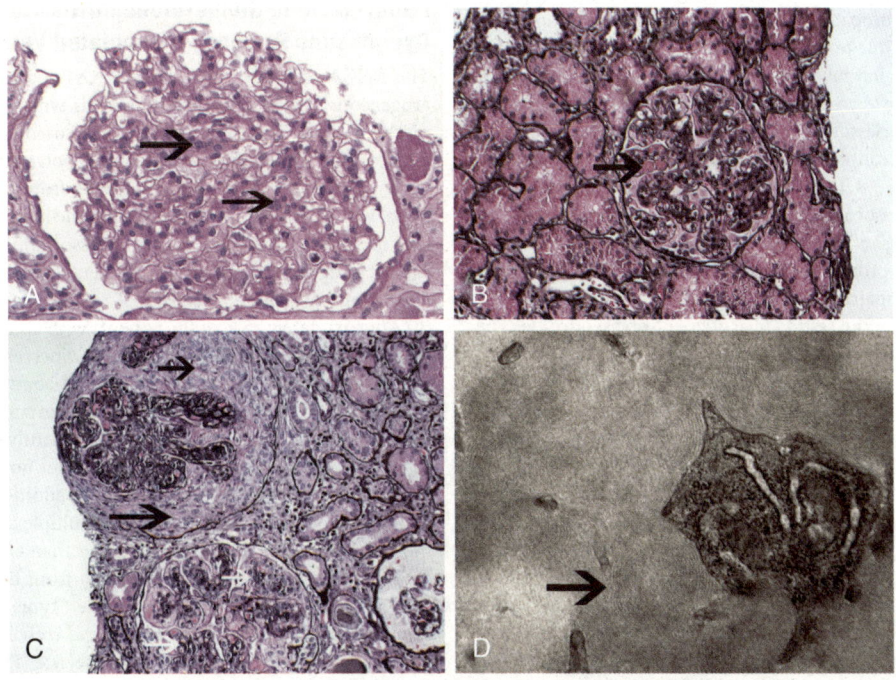

图4.9 狼疮性肾炎的光镜（A至C）和电镜（D）表现。（A）轻度系膜增生性肾小球肾炎（ISN/RPSⅡ型）可见系膜细胞增生（箭头）（PAS，×40）。（B）肾小球毛细血管内弥漫性增生伴冷球蛋白沉积，表现为淡染的非嗜银物质（箭头）（六胺银，×20）。（C）在弥漫增生性肾小球肾炎（ISN/RPSⅣ型）中，上面的肾小球显示了一个大细胞性新月体（黑色箭头），下面的肾小球显示弥漫性毛细血管内增生（白色箭头）（六胺银，×20）。（D）电子致密物具有指纹样亚结构（箭头）（×46 000）

TABLE 4.4	Cryoglobulins and Associated Diseases	
Cryoglobulinemia Type	Immunoglobulin Class	Associated Diseases
I. Monoclonal immunoglobulins	M > G > A > BJP	Myeloma, Waldenström macroglobulinemia
II. Mixed cryoglobulins with monoclonal immunoglobulins	M/G >> G/G	Sjögren syndrome, Waldenström macroglobulinemia, lymphoma, essential cryoglobulinemia
III. Mixed polyclonal immunoglobulins	M/G	Infection, SLE, vasculitis, neoplasia, essential cryoglobulinemia

A, IgA; *BJP*, Bence Jones protein (κ light chain); *G*, IgG; *M*, IgM; *SLE*, systemic lupus erythematosus.

Patients with class III or IV lupus nephritis should undergo induction therapy with corticosteroids plus cyclophosphamide or mycophenolate mofetil because both are considered equivalent. Pure class V (membranous) lupus nephritis usually has a benign prognosis, and initial therapy should be supportive. However, patients with progressive or persistent nephrotic-range proteinuria should be treated with corticosteroids plus an additional immunosuppressive agent (e.g., cyclosporine, tacrolimus, mycophenolate mofetil or rituximab). Patients with ESRD should be considered for renal transplantation because there is a low rate of recurrence in the transplanted kidney.

Cryoglobulinemic Glomerulonephritis

Cryoglobulins are immunoglobulins that precipitate at low temperatures and redissolve on rewarming. Cryoglobulinemia usually leads to a systemic inflammatory syndrome with weakness, arthralgias or arthritis, palpable purpura, peripheral neuropathy, and glomerulonephritis. Serum levels of C4 are typically low due to activation of complement by the classical pathway. The disease mainly involves small to medium-sized blood vessels and causes vasculitis due to cryoglobulin-containing immune complexes.

Cryoglobulinemia is classified as type I, II, or III on the basis of immunoglobulin composition. It can be idiopathic or occur in association with autoimmune diseases (see Fig. 4.11B), malignancy, or infection (Table 4.4). HCV infection is the most common cause of cryoglobulinemia.

Renal disease occurs in 20% to 60% of patients with cryoglobulinemia and manifests as proteinuria, microscopic hematuria, nephrotic syndrome, or renal impairment. Hypertension is common and may be severe, particularly in the setting of acute nephritic syndrome. The cryocrit values correlate poorly with disease activity. On light microscopy, renal biopsy specimens show an immune complex–mediated membranoproliferative pattern of injury, and on electron microscopy, diffuse, dense subendothelial deposits with a microtubular or crystalline appearance may be seen occluding the capillary loops.

Treatment targets the underlying pathologic process to minimize or eliminate the associated cryoglobulinemia. Patients with active HCV infection, for example, should receive antiviral therapy when possible, and those with a monoclonal gammopathy should receive appropriate antimyeloma therapy. Immunosuppressive therapy (including the use of rituximab) with or without plasmapheresis should be considered for patients with a rapidly progressive, organ- or life-threatening course, regardless of the cause of the mixed cryoglobulinemia. Overall, the renal prognosis is usually good, with few patients progressing to ESRD. The long-term outcome reflects the underlying process.

Fibrillary Glomerulonephritis and Immunotactoid Glomerulopathy

Fibrillary glomerulonephritis and immunotactoid glomerulopathy are uncommon disorders, being present in 0.5 to 1% of native kidney biopsies. Fibrillary glomerulonephritis is by far more common, accounting for approximately 85% to 90% of cases. The identification of the protein DnaJ heat shock protein family (Hsp40) member B9 (DNAJB9) in the glomeruli of patients with fibrillary glomerulonephritis but not in those with immunotactoid glomerulopathy has established that the two are distinct, pathogenically unrelated disease entities (Fig. 4.10). In approximately one third of patients with fibrillary glomerulonephritis a history of malignancy, monoclonal gammopathy or autoimmune disease can be documented. By contrast, immunotactoid glomerulopathy is more frequently associated with chronic lymphocytic leukemia and related B-cell lymphomas or multiple myeloma.

In fibrillary glomerulonephritis, light microscopic findings are nondiagnostic and variable, showing patterns that may be seen in other glomerulonephritides. Immunofluorescence microscopy is positive for IgG, C3, and usually both kappa and lambda (i.e., polyclonal) light chains. Electron microscopy shows random fibrillar deposits in the mesangium and glomerular capillary walls that are clearly distinct from those seen in amyloidosis. The fibrils are larger than those in amyloidosis (16 to 24 nm in fibrillary glomerulonephritis and 30 to 50 nm in immunotactoid glomerulopathy (with microtubular formation) versus 10 nm in diameter in amyloidosis).

The presenting clinical features of fibrillary glomerulonephritis and immunotactoid glomerulopathy are similar to those in other forms of glomerular disease, including hypertension, hematuria, proteinuria, and abnormal renal function.

No therapies have been clearly shown to be beneficial for either fibrillary glomerulonephritis or immunotactoid glomerulopathy. Patients with an associated malignancy, monoclonal gammopathy or autoimmune disease, may benefit from treatment of the underlying disorder.

Pauci-Immune Glomerulonephritis: Antineutrophil Cytoplasmic Antibody–Associated Vasculitides

The ANCA-associated vasculitides (AAVs) are a group of three heterogeneous syndromes: granulomatosis with polyangiitis (GPA, formerly Wegener's granulomatosis), microscopic polyangiitis (MPA), and eosinophilic granulomatosis with polyangiitis (EGPA, formerly Churg-Strauss syndrome). The unifying feature is a necrotizing small vessel vasculitis with a predilection for the kidneys, lungs, and peripheral nervous system that occurs in association with autoantibodies against antigens in the cytoplasm of neutrophils (i.e., myeloperoxidase [MPO] and proteinase 3 [PR3]).

Approximately 75% of the patients with GPA are PR3-ANCA positive, and 20% are MPO-ANCA positive, whereas about 50% of patients with MPA are MPO-ANCA positive and about 40% are PR3-ANCA positive. Necrotizing granulomatous inflammation, which affects the upper and lower respiratory tract and frequently precedes other disease manifestations, is characteristic of GPA but not MPA. EGPA is characterized by asthma and eosinophilia in addition to features of small vessel vasculitis such as mononeuritis multiplex. AAV is the most common cause of a RPGN in patients older than 60 years. AAV is associated with signs and symptoms ranging from limited renal disease to RPGN and pulmonary-renal syndrome (Table 4.5). Renal biopsy is characterized by a focal, necrotizing, and crescentic glomerulonephritis with pauci-immune immunofluorescence (Fig. 4.11).

Patients with newly diagnosed severe AAV vasculitis can be treated with a combination of high-dose corticosteroids and cyclophosphamide or high-dose corticosteroids and rituximab. The PEXIVAS trial

表 4.4　冷球蛋白与相关疾病		
冷球蛋白血症分型	冷球蛋白类别	相关疾病
Ⅰ. 单克隆免疫球蛋白	M > G > A > BJP	骨髓瘤，华氏巨球蛋白血症
Ⅱ. 混合性冷球蛋白伴单克隆免疫球蛋白	M/G >> G/G	干燥综合征，华氏巨球蛋白血症淋巴瘤，原发性冷球蛋白血症
Ⅲ. 混合性多克隆免疫球蛋白	M/G	感染，SLE，血管炎，肿瘤，原发性冷球蛋白血症

A，IgA；BJP，本周蛋白（κ 轻链）；G，IgG；M，IgM；SLE，系统性红斑狼疮。

Ⅲ型或Ⅳ型狼疮性肾炎患者应接受皮质类固醇联合环磷酰胺或吗替麦考酚酯的诱导治疗，因为这两种药物具有同等疗效。纯Ⅴ型（膜性）狼疮性肾炎通常预后良好，初始治疗应为支持性治疗。但是，如果患者出现蛋白尿进展或持续性肾病范围蛋白尿，则应使用皮质类固醇联合另一种免疫抑制剂（如环孢素、他克莫司、吗替麦考酚酯或利妥昔单抗）进行治疗。由于移植肾狼疮性肾炎复发率较低，ESRD 患者应考虑进行肾移植。

冷球蛋白血症性肾小球肾炎

冷球蛋白是在低温下沉淀并在复温时重新再溶解的免疫球蛋白。冷球蛋白血症通常会导致系统性炎症综合征，表现为乏力、关节痛或关节炎、可触及的紫癜、周围神经病变和肾小球肾炎。由于补体经典途径激活，血清 C4 水平通常较低。该病主要累及小到中等血管，并由含有冷球蛋白的免疫复合物介导引起血管炎。

根据免疫球蛋白的组成。冷球蛋白血症分为Ⅰ型、Ⅱ型和Ⅲ型。其可以是特发性的，也可以与自身免疫性疾病（见图 4.11B）、恶性肿瘤或感染（表 4.4）相关。丙型肝炎病毒感染是引发冷球蛋白血症的最常见原因。

20% ~ 60% 的冷球蛋白血症患者出现肾脏疾病，表现为蛋白尿、镜下血尿、肾病综合征或肾功能损害。高血压常见，尤其是在急性肾炎综合征的情况下可能很严重。冷沉淀的量与疾病活动度的相关性较差。光镜下，肾活检病理显示免疫复合物介导的膜增生样病变；电镜下，可见弥漫性、致密的微管样或结晶样物质沉积在内皮下，堵塞毛细血管袢。

治疗目标应针对潜在的病理过程，以尽量减少或消除相关的冷球蛋白血症。例如，活动性丙型肝炎病毒感染的患者应尽可能接受抗病毒治疗，单克隆丙种球蛋白病患者应接受适当的抗骨髓瘤治疗。对于病程进展迅速、危及器官或生命的患者，无论混合型冷球蛋白血症的病因如何，都应进行免疫抑制治疗（包括使用利妥昔单抗），可联合血浆置换。总体而言，肾脏预后通常良好，很少有患者进展为 ESRD。长期预后与潜在病理过程相关。

纤维性肾小球肾炎和免疫触须样肾小球病

纤维性肾小球肾炎和免疫触须样肾小球病都是少见病，在自体肾活检中仅占 0.5% ~ 1%。其中纤维性肾小球肾炎相对较多，约占这些病例中的 85% ~ 90%。在纤维性肾小球肾炎患者的肾小球中可鉴定到 DnaJ 热休克蛋白家族（Hsp40）成员 B9（DNAJB9），而在免疫触须样肾小球病患者的肾小球中却为阴性，说明二者是两个独立的疾病，致病机制不同（图 4.10）。约有 1/3 的纤维性肾小球肾炎患者有恶性肿瘤、单克隆丙种球蛋白病或自身免疫性疾病的病史。相反，免疫触须样肾小球病更常见于慢性淋巴细胞白血病和 B 细胞淋巴瘤或多发性骨髓瘤。

光镜下，纤维性肾小球肾炎的表现不具有诊断意义且多变，可以出现其他肾小球肾炎的表现。免疫荧光可见 IgG、C3 阳性，通常 kappa（κ）和 lambda（λ）轻链均阳性（即多克隆性）。电镜显示系膜和肾小球毛细血管壁上无规则原纤维沉积，与淀粉样变性所见的沉积物明显不同。这些纤维比淀粉样变性的纤维更粗［纤维性肾小球肾炎中的纤维直径为 16 ~ 24 nm，免疫触须样肾小球病中的纤维直径为 30 ~ 50 nm（伴微管形成），而淀粉样变性的纤维直径为 10 nm］。

纤维性肾小球肾炎和免疫触须样肾小球病的临床表现特点与其他形式的肾小球疾病相似，包括高血压、血尿、蛋白尿和肾功能异常。

目前尚无对纤维性肾小球肾炎或免疫触须样肾小球病有明确疗效的治疗方法。伴有恶性肿瘤、单克隆丙种球蛋白病或自身免疫性疾病的患者，可能从针对原发病的治疗中获益。

寡免疫性肾小球肾炎：抗中性粒细胞胞质抗体相关血管炎

ANCA 相关血管炎（AAV）是包括三种不同类型的综合征：肉芽肿性多血管炎（GPA，既往称为韦格纳肉芽肿）、显微镜下多血管炎（MPA）和嗜酸性肉芽肿性多血管炎（EGPA，既往称为 Churg-Strauss 综合征）。其共同特征是坏死性小血管炎，好发于肾、肺和周围神经系统，且与针对中性粒细胞胞质中抗原［即髓过氧化物酶（MPO）和蛋白酶 3（PR3）］的自身抗体有关。

GPA 患者中 PR3-ANCA 阳性约占 75%、MPO-ANCA 阳性占 20%；而 MPA 患者中 MPO-ANCA 阳性约占 50%、PR3-ANCA 阳性约占 40%。GPA 的特征是坏死性肉芽肿炎症，通常首先累及上呼吸道和下呼吸道，而 MPA 不具有该特征。EGPA 的特征是哮喘、嗜酸性粒细胞增多和小血管炎特征如多发性单神经炎。AAV 是 60 岁以上患者发生 RPGN 的最常见原因。AAV 临床体征和症状谱从局限性肾脏病到 RPGN 和肺肾综合征（表 4.5）。肾活检病理的特点为局灶性、坏死性、新月体性肾小球肾炎伴寡免疫荧光沉积（图 4.11）。

新诊断的重症 AAV 患者可使用大剂量皮质类固醇

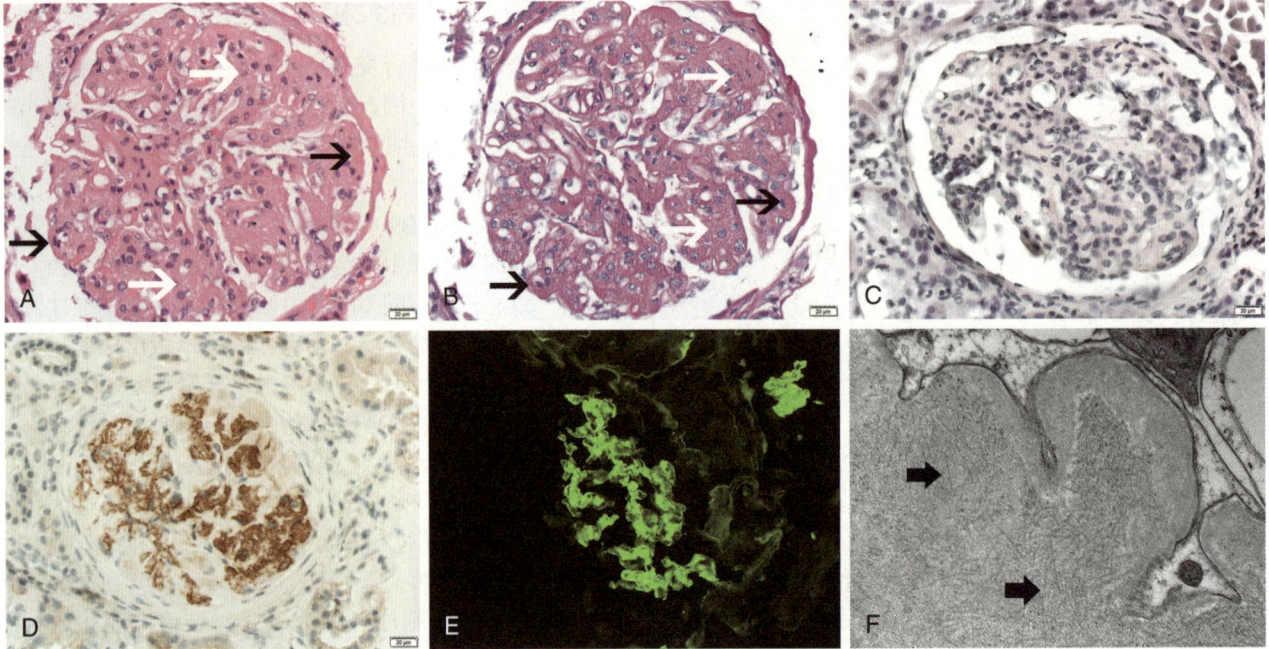

Fig. 4.10 Fibrillary glomerulonephritis. (A-B) Light microscopy showing mesangial expansion with increase in cellularity *(white arrow)* and thickened capillary walls *(black arrow)* (A, hematoxylin and eosin ×40; B, periodic acid–Schiff stain ×40). (C) Congo red stain is negative (×40). (D) Immunohistochemistry for DNAJB9 is positive. (E) Immunofluorescence studies show IgG staining in the mesangium and along capillary walls, and (F) electron microscopy shows fibrillary deposits *(thick arrows)* along the capillary walls (×30000).

TABLE 4.5 Signs and Symptoms of Antineutrophil Cytoplasmic Autoantibody Vasculitis
Abdominal pain and gastrointestinal bleeding
Cutaneous purpura, petechiae, nodules, ulcerations, and necrosis
Facial pain, necrotizing (hemorrhagic) sinusitis, and septal perforation
Hematuria, proteinuria, and renal failure
Hemoptysis and pulmonary infiltrates or nodules
Muscle and pancreatic enzymes in blood
Myalgias and arthralgias
Peripheral neuropathy (mononeuritis multiplex)

showed that addition of plasma exchange in patients with pulmonary hemorrhage, respiratory compromise, or severe renal failure (i.e., serum creatinine >5.5 mg/dL) is of no benefit. The prognosis for AAV varies. Those with severe renal failure have the worst prognosis, and even after successful therapy AAVs have a relapse rate of 30% to 50% in the first 5 years. In patients with renal involvement, rising ANCA titers are predictors of relapse. Patients with GPA or who are PR3-ANCA positive or presenting with relapsing disease are at higher risk for future relapses.

Anti–Glomerular Basement Membrane Antibody–Mediated Glomerulonephritis

Anti-GBM antibody–mediated glomerulonephritis (anti-GBM GN, formerly called Goodpasture disease) is a pulmonary-renal syndrome caused by circulating anti-GBM antibodies. On immunofluorescence staining of biopsy specimens, a linear pattern of IgG staining is seen along the GBM and alveolar basement membrane (Fig. 4.12) using antibodies directed against the α3 chain of type IV collagen (COL4A3 protein). Patients usually have RPGN and various degrees of pulmonary hemorrhage.

The treatment of anti-GBM GN is based on high-dose pulse methylprednisolone (1 g/day for 1 to 3 days) followed by corticosteroids (prednisone, 1 mg/kg/day up to 80 mg daily) in combination with oral cyclophosphamide (2 to 3 mg/kg/day up to 200 mg daily, adjusted for age and creatinine level) and plasma exchange. The prognosis is predicted in part by the percentage of circumferential crescents on the renal biopsy specimen, oliguria, and the need for dialysis. Those with an initial serum creatinine level less than 5.0 mg/dL have a 90% probability of renal survival at 5 years; but those with 100% circumferential crescents and on dialysis do not recover renal function, and immunosuppressive regimens should be avoided except in the case of pulmonary hemorrhage.

Anti-GBM GN rarely recurs. Patients with ESRD are candidates for renal transplantation after the antibody has disappeared (6 to 12 months).

GLOMERULAR DISEASES CAUSED BY PLASMA CELL DYSCRASIAS

Amyloidosis

Amyloidosis is characterized by systemic extracellular deposition of randomly arranged fibrils 8 to 12 nm in diameter that stain positive with Congo red (i.e., orange-green birefringence with polarized light) or thioflavin T. Several processes, including malignancy, genetic mutations, and aging, can produce at least 24 amyloidogenic proteins. With renal deposition, amyloid in biopsy specimens appears as pale, amorphous, extracellular deposits that are periodic acid–Schiff (PAS) and methenamine silver stain negative (Fig. 4.13).

The affinity for kidney compared with other target organs varies according to the type of amyloid protein. Renal manifestations include proteinuria, nephrotic syndrome, and renal failure. Affected patients typically have large kidneys on ultrasound, but the diagnosis depends

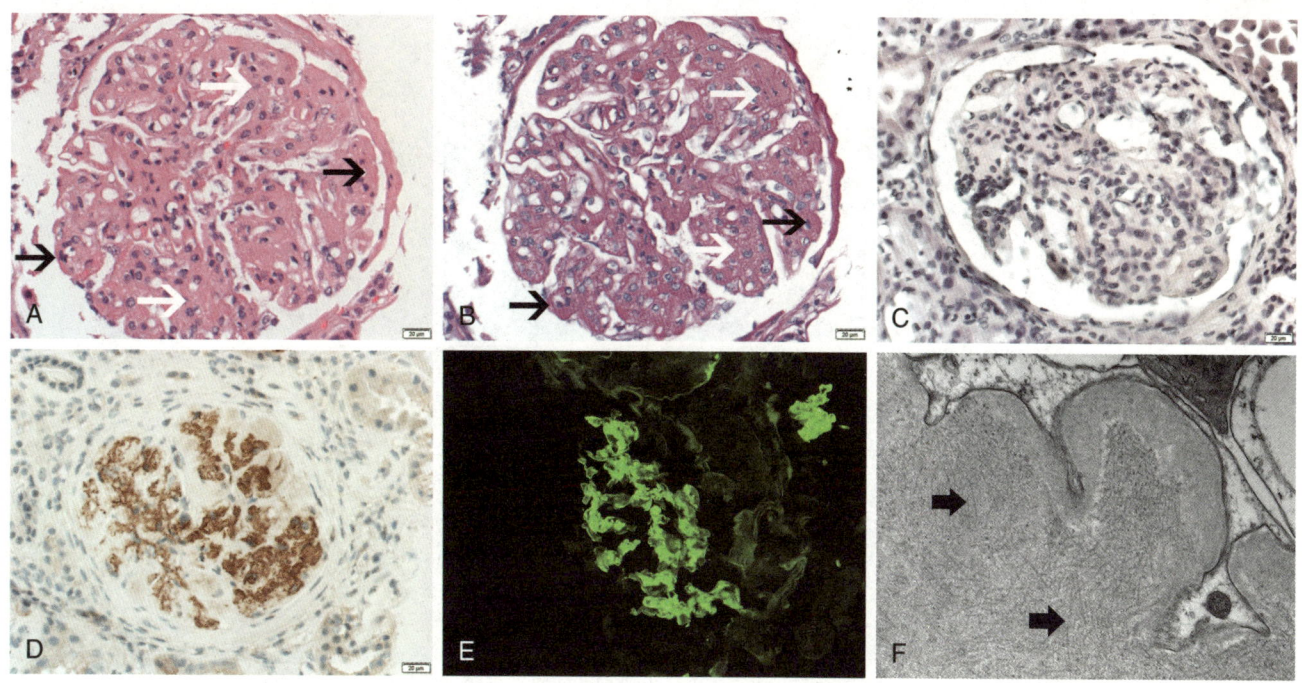

图 4.10 纤维性肾小球肾炎。（A-B）光镜下显示伴细胞增多的系膜扩张（白色箭头）和毛细血管壁增厚（黑色箭头）（A，HE×40；B，PAS×40）。（C）刚果红染色阴性（×40）。（D）DNAJB9 免疫组化阳性。（E）免疫荧光染色显示系膜区和毛细血管壁的 IgG 染色，以及（F）电镜显示沿毛细血管壁的原纤维沉积（粗箭头）（×30 000）

表 4.5 抗中性粒细胞胞质（自身）抗体相关血管炎的症状和体征
腹痛和消化道出血
皮肤紫癜、瘀斑、结节、溃疡和坏死
面部疼痛、坏死性（出血性）鼻窦炎和鼻中隔穿孔
血尿、蛋白尿和肾衰竭
咯血和肺部浸润或结节
血液中的肌肉和胰腺相关的酶升高
肌痛和关节痛
周围神经病（多发性单神经炎）

联合环磷酰胺或大剂量皮质类固醇联合利妥昔单抗治疗。PEXIVAS 研究表明，对肺出血、呼吸系统受损或严重肾衰竭（即血清肌酐大于 5.5 mg/dl）的患者额外使用血浆置换并无获益。AAV 的预后差异很大。严重肾衰竭患者的预后最差，即使初始治疗成功的患者，5 年内的 AAV 复发率也高达 30%～50%。在肾脏受累的患者中，ANCA 滴度升高是复发的预测因子。GPA 或 PR3-ANCA 阳性或出现过复发的患者，将来复发的风险更高。

抗肾小球基底膜（GBM）抗体介导的肾小球肾炎

抗 GBM 抗体介导的肾小球肾炎（anti-GBM GN，既往称为 Goodpasture 病）是一种由循环抗 GBM 抗体引起的肺-肾综合征。在肾活检标本免疫荧光染色中，使用针对Ⅳ型胶原蛋白 α3 链（COL4A3）的抗体，可见沿肾小球基底膜和肺泡基底膜的 IgG 线样沉积（图 4.12）。患者常有 RPGN，伴不同程度的肺出血。

抗 GBM 抗体介导的肾小球肾炎的基础治疗是大剂量甲泼尼龙（1 g/d，持续 1～3 天）冲击治疗，续贯皮质类固醇［泼尼松，1 mg/（kg·d），最多 80 mg/g］，联合口服环磷酰胺［2～3 mg/（kg·d），最多 200 mg/d，根据年龄和肌酐水平调整剂量］和血浆置换。肾活检标本中环状新月体比例、少尿和是否需要透析在一定程度上与预后相关。起病时血清肌酐水平低于 5.0 mg/dl 的患者，5 年肾脏存活率约 90%；但 100% 环状新月体且接受透析者的肾功能无法恢复，除非发生肺出血，否则应避免使用免疫抑制疗法。

抗 GBM 抗体介导的肾小球肾炎很少复发。ESRD 患者可在抗体消失后（6～12 个月）进行肾移植。

浆细胞病引起的肾小球疾病

淀粉样变性

淀粉样变性的特征是刚果红（即偏振光下的橙-绿双折射）或硫黄素 T 染色阳性的直径为 8～12 nm 的随机排列的纤维丝在全身细胞外沉积。包括肿瘤、基因突变、衰老在内的多种情况可以产生至少 24 种淀粉样蛋白。当淀粉样蛋白沉积于肾脏时，其在肾活检标本中呈现淡染的细胞外无定形沉积物，PAS 和六胺银染色阴性（图 4.13）。

与其他靶器官相比，不同类型的淀粉样蛋白对肾脏的亲和力也不一样。肾脏表现包括蛋白尿、肾病综合征和肾衰竭。受累患者在超声检查中通常表现为肾

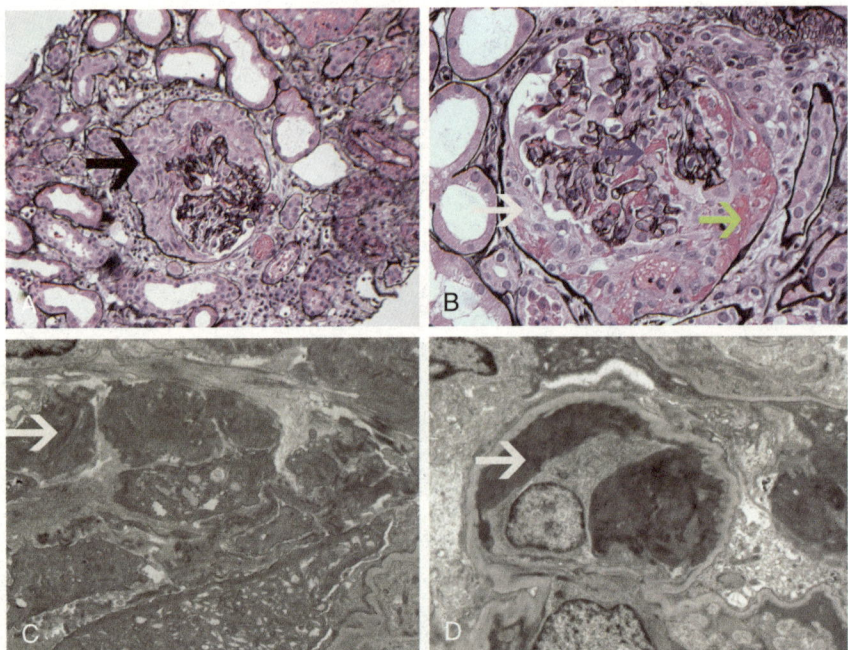

Fig. 4.11 Crescentic glomerulonephritis in a patient with MPO-ANCA associated vasculitis. (A and B) Light microscopy and silver methenamine staining show a large cellular crescent *(black arrow)* with fibrinoid necrosis *(blue arrow)*, hemorrhage into the Bowman capsule *(yellow arrow)*, and collapse of capillary tufts (A, ×20; B, ×40). (C and D) Electron microscopy shows fibrinoid necrosis (i.e., necrotizing lesion) in the Bowman space *(white arrow)* and capillary loops *(short white arrow)* (both, ×11100).

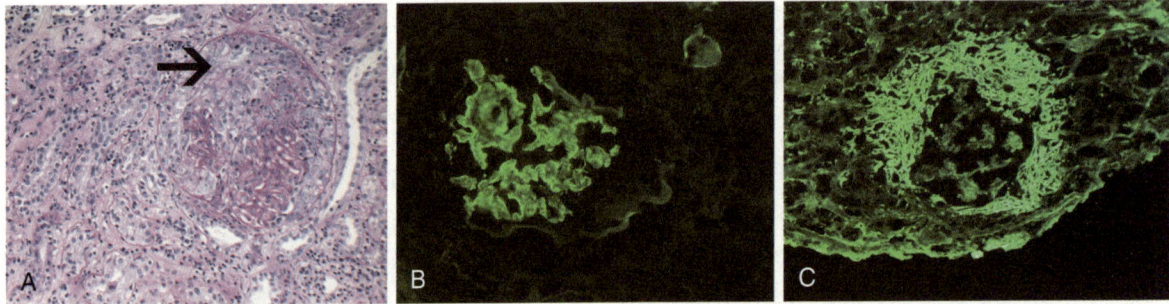

Fig. 4.12 Anti–glomerular basement membrane–mediated disease. (A) Light microscopy shows a large, circumferential crescent *(arrow)*, with collapse of the glomerular capillary tufts and many infiltrating neutrophils in the crescent (periodic acid–Schiff, ×20). Immunofluorescence microscopy shows linear staining for anti–immunoglobulin G antibody (B) along the glomerular capillary walls and bright staining for fibrinogen in the Bowman tuft (C), indicating crescent formation and fibrinoid necrosis (both, ×40).

on demonstration of amyloid deposits. After amyloid is detected, typing should be performed when possible because treatments vary according to the protein involved. The most common approach to amyloid typing involves immunofluorescence or immunohistochemistry, but genetic testing and liquid chromatography mass spectrometry are also helpful for high-resolution amyloid typing.

Treatment of amyloidosis depends on the origin of the amyloidogenic protein. In patients with amyloid light chain (AL) amyloidosis, antimyeloma therapy can be beneficial. In selected cases, bone marrow transplantation has led to resolution of the disease. Secondary amyloid A (AA) amyloidosis is most common in patients with rheumatoid arthritis, inflammatory bowel disease, chronic infection, or familial Mediterranean fever. Treatment of AA amyloidosis is directed at the underlying inflammatory process with antimicrobials or anti-inflammatory medications.

Light Chain Deposition Disease

Light chain deposition disease is a paraprotein-associated disorder. The peak incidence is in the sixth decade of life, and men are affected more commonly than women. Approximately 30% to 50% of patients with light chain deposition disease have multiple myeloma. Most have a detectable monoclonal protein (usually κ light chain) in the serum or urine, but no hematologic abnormality is identified in about 10% of cases. The clinical presentation is very heterogeneous and can vary from mild renal dysfunction, proteinuria without nephrotic syndrome, to clinically overt acute renal failure. Fanconi syndrome, characterized by normoglycemic glycosuria, aminoaciduria, and phosphaturia, is the classic presentation. Immunoglobulin deposits in other organs may result in myriad of associated clinical symptoms.

Renal biopsy specimens show acellular, eosinophilic mesangial nodules that stain strongly positive with PAS, often mimicking diabetes

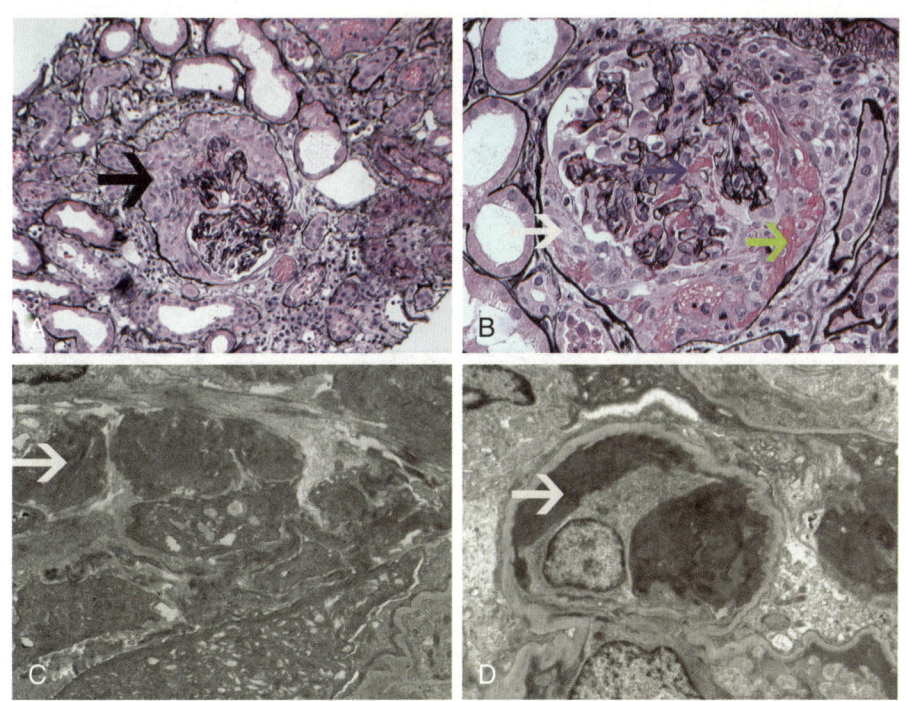

图 4.11 一例 MPO-ANCA 相关血管炎患者的新月体性肾小球肾炎。（**A** 和 **B**）光镜和六胺银染色显示一个大细胞新月体（黑色箭头）伴有纤维素样坏死（蓝色箭头），出血进入肾小囊（黄色箭头），毛细血管袢塌陷（A，×20；B，×40）。（**C** 和 **D**）电镜显示在肾小囊（白色箭头）和毛细血管袢（白色短箭头）中的纤维素样坏死（即坏死性病变）（均为 ×11100）

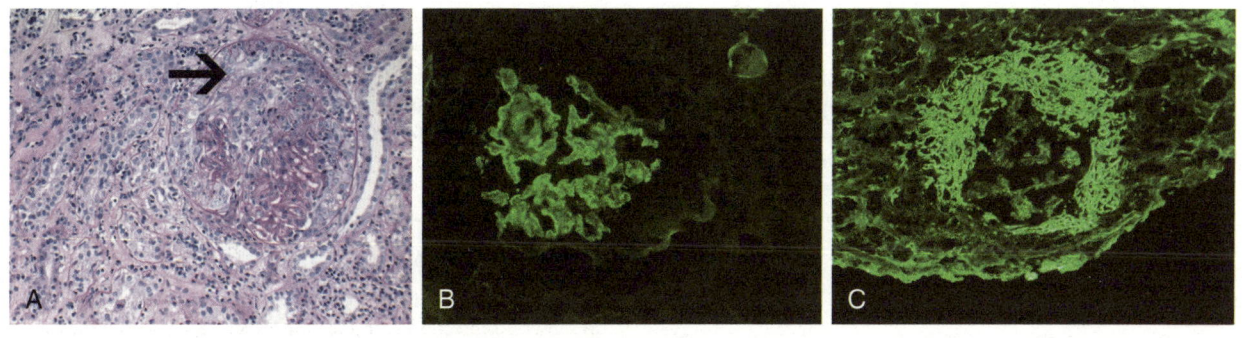

图 4.12 抗肾小球基底膜抗体介导的肾小球肾炎。（**A**）光镜下显示一个大的环状新月体（箭头），伴肾小球毛细血管袢塌陷，新月体中有大量中性粒细胞浸润（PAS，×20）。免疫荧光显微镜检查显示抗 IgG 抗体沿肾小球毛细血管壁呈线样沉积（**B**）和肾小囊中纤维蛋白原染色阳性（**C**），提示新月体形成和纤维素性坏死（均为 ×40）

脏增大，而确诊依赖淀粉样蛋白沉积的证据。检测到淀粉样蛋白后应进行分型鉴定，因为针对不同淀粉样蛋白的治疗方法不同。最常用的淀粉样蛋白分型方法是免疫荧光或免疫组化，但基因检测和液相色谱质谱法也有助于淀粉样蛋白的高分辨率分型鉴定。

淀粉样变性的治疗取决于淀粉样变性蛋白的来源。对于轻链（AL）型淀粉样变性的患者，抗骨髓瘤治疗可能获益。在某些特定的病例中，骨髓移植可治愈该病。继发性淀粉样蛋白 A（AA）型淀粉样变性最常见于类风湿关节炎、炎症性肠病、慢性感染或家族性地中海热的患者。AA 型的治疗主要是使用抗生素或抗炎药物治疗潜在的炎症反应。

轻链沉积病

轻链沉积病是一种副蛋白相关疾病。发病高峰年龄为 60~70 岁，男性患者多于女性。约 30%~50% 的轻链沉积病患者患有多发性骨髓瘤。大多数患者的血清或尿液中可检测到单克隆蛋白（通常为 κ 轻链），但约有 10% 的病例中无血液学异常发现。该病临床表现多种多样，从轻度肾功能不全、无肾病综合征的蛋白尿到临床显著的急性肾衰竭。以血糖正常的糖尿、氨基酸尿和磷酸盐尿为特征的范科尼综合征是其典型表现。免疫球蛋白沉积在其他器官也可能导致各种相关的临床症状。

肾活检组织显示系膜区无细胞性、PAS 强阳性的嗜伊红的系膜结节，类似于糖尿病表现。沉积的单克

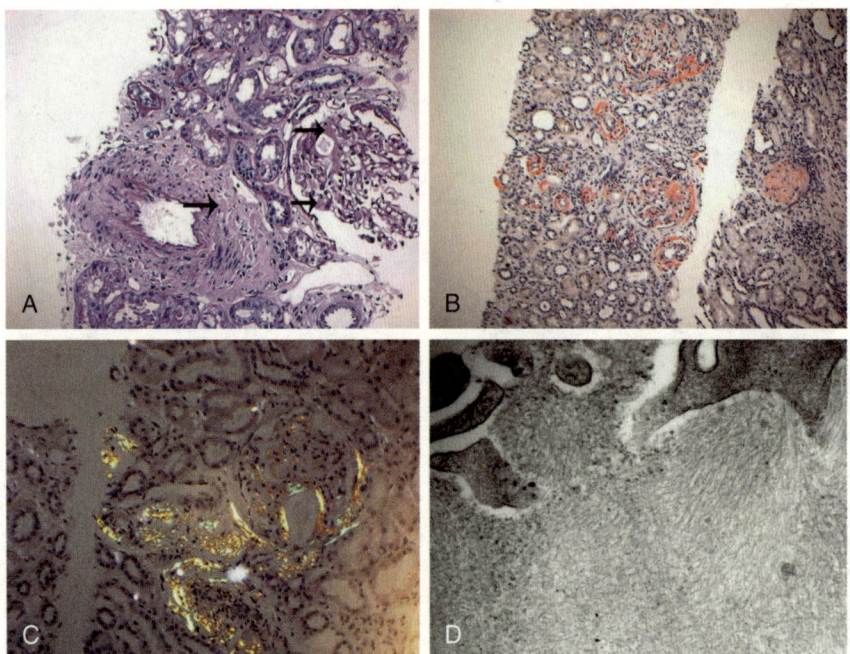

Fig. 4.13 Amyloidosis. (A) Light microscopy shows amyloid deposits characterized by mesangial expansion *(small arrows)* with material negative for staining. The material is also seen in vessel walls, where the *arrow* points to vascular deposits (periodic acid–Schiff stain, ×20). (B) Congo red staining is positive for amyloid and shows reddish-brown material in the glomeruli, interstitium, and vessel walls (×10). (C) Amyloid deposits show apple green to orange-yellow birefringence under polarized light (×20). (D) Electron microscopy shows randomly oriented amyloid fibrils. The fibrils measured 9 nm thick (×49,000).

mellitus. The deposited monoclonal proteins do not form fibrils and are Congo red negative. Immunofluorescence microscopic findings are diagnostic, with diffuse linear immunoglobulin light chain deposition (κ in 80% of cases) along the GBM and tubular basement membranes. On electron microscopy punctate powdery granular electron dense deposits are seen along the GBM and TBM (Fig. 4.14).

Encouraging results have emerged with the use of anti-plasma cells targeted therapy and autologous stem cell transplantation. Unless remission is achieved after chemotherapy, the disease will recur in the kidney allograft.

FIBRILLARY GLOMERULONEPHRITIS AND IMMUNOTACTOID GLOMERULOPATHY

See section on immune-complex glomerulonephritis.

GLOMERULONEPHRITIS ASSOCIATED WITH VIRAL INFECTIONS

Hepatitis B

HBV-mediated glomerular disease usually manifests as membranous nephropathy, especially in children. The diagnosis of HBV-mediated glomerular disease requires detection of the virus in the blood and the exclusion of other causes of glomerular diseases.

HBV-mediated glomerular disease usually has a favorable prognosis, with a high spontaneous remission rate in children, but it is often progressive in adults. Patients with HBV infection and glomerulonephritis should receive antiviral therapy (e.g., entecavir) as recommended by standard clinical practice guidelines for management of HBV infection. Those with severe vasculitis or RPGN may be candidates for immunosuppressive therapy in combination with antiviral therapy. Rituximab treatment of patients who are positive for HBV has been associated with fatal acute hepatitis. Rituximab is therefore contraindicated in patients with chronic HBV unless antiviral therapy is also given and in patients with an active hepatitis flare.

Hepatitis C

See the section on cryoglobulinemic glomerulonephritis.

HIV-Associated Nephropathy

Patients with HIV infection can have many forms of kidney injury due to sepsis, co-infection with HBV or HCV, nephrotoxic drugs, and use of antiretroviral agents. HIV-associated nephropathy (HIVAN) is a clinicopathologic entity characterized by nephrotic-range proteinuria and a collapsing form of FSGS, often with microcystic tubular dilation. On electron microscopy, tubuloreticular inclusions (i.e., interferon fingerprints) may be seen within the glomerular and vascular endothelial cells.

HIVAN occurs almost exclusively in patients of African descent when CD4 levels are low. It is thought to be caused by infection and subsequent expression of HIV viral genes in podocytes. The onset of proteinuria is typically acute. Proteinuria can be greater than 10 g/day, and renal insufficiency can progress rapidly.

THROMBOTIC MICROANGIOPATHIES

Thrombotic microangiopathy is characterized by thrombocytopenia, microangiopathic hemolytic anemia, and microvascular occlusion, resulting in various degrees of organ dysfunction. Markers of hemolysis include low haptoglobin levels, increased levels of lactate dehydrogenase and unconjugated bilirubin, and a high reticulocyte count. Schistocytes are seen in peripheral blood smears.

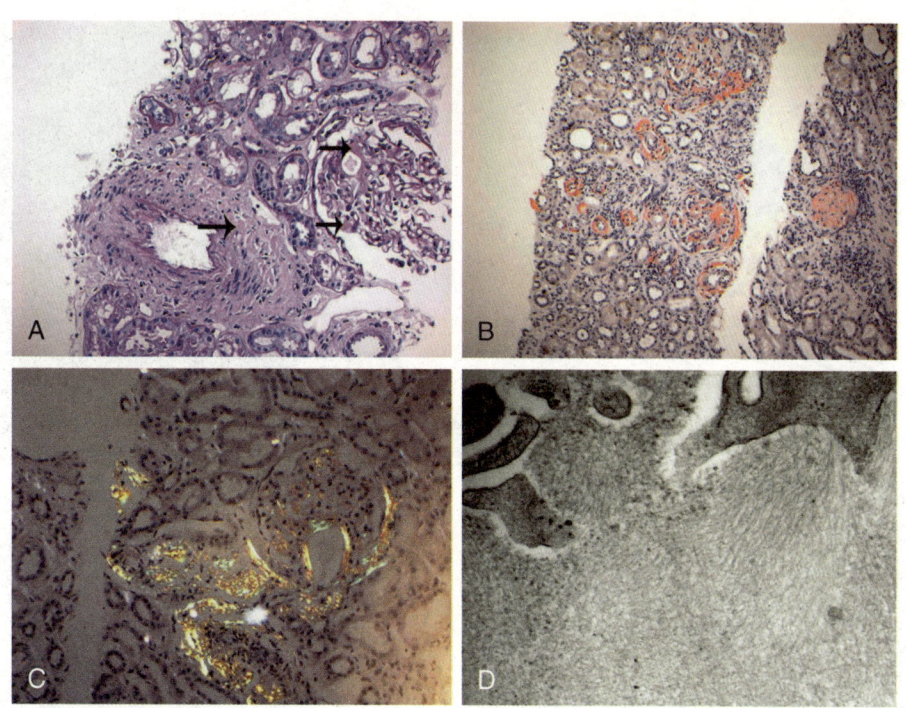

图 4.13 淀粉样变性。(**A**)光镜下显示以系膜扩张(小箭头)且染色阴性为特点的淀粉样蛋白沉积。血管壁也可见到这种物质沉积,箭头所指为血管沉积物(PAS,×20)。(**B**)淀粉样蛋白刚果红染色阳性,在肾小球、间质和血管壁可见红褐色物质(×10)。(**C**)在偏振光下,淀粉样沉积物呈现苹果绿至橙黄色双折光(×20)。(**D**)电镜显示随机排列的淀粉样蛋白纤维。纤维丝直径为 9 nm(×49 000)

隆蛋白不形成纤维,且刚果红染色阴性。免疫荧光检查具有诊断意义,可见免疫球蛋白轻链沉积(80% 的病例为 κ)沿 GBM 和肾小管基底膜的弥漫线样沉积。电镜可见沿 GBM 和 TBM 的点状颗粒样电子致密物沉积(图 4.14)。

在轻链沉积病中,抗浆细胞治疗和自体干细胞移植取得了令人鼓舞的结果。除非化疗后获得疾病缓解,否则本病将在移植肾复发。

纤维性肾小球肾炎和免疫触须样肾小球病

参见"免疫复合物介导的肾小球肾炎"部分。

病毒感染相关的肾小球肾炎

乙型肝炎

HBV 介导的肾小球疾病通常表现为膜性肾病,尤其是在儿童患者。诊断 HBV 介导的肾小球疾病需要在血液中检测到病毒并且排除其他原因引起的肾小球疾病。

HBV 介导的肾小球疾病通常预后良好,儿童患者的自发缓解率较高,但成人患者常为进展性。合并 HBV 感染和肾小球肾炎的患者应按照 HBV 感染管理的标准临床实践指南建议接受抗病毒治疗(如恩替卡韦)。具有严重血管炎或 RPGN 的患者可在联合抗病毒治疗的情况下使用免疫抑制治疗。利妥昔单抗治疗 HBV 阳性患者可出现致命的急性肝炎。因此,利妥昔单抗禁用于未接受抗病毒治疗的慢性 HBV 患者及活动期肝炎患者。

丙型肝炎

参见"冷球蛋白血症性肾小球肾炎"部分。

HIV 相关性肾病

HIV 感染者可因感染中毒症、合并 HBV 或 HCV 感染、肾毒性药物以及使用抗逆转录病毒药物而出现多种形式的肾损伤。HIV 相关性肾病(HIVAN)是一种临床病理综合征,其特征是肾病范围蛋白尿和塌陷型 FSGS,通常有微囊样肾小管扩张。电镜可见肾小球和血管内皮细胞内管网状包涵体(即干扰素印记)。

HIVAN 几乎仅发生在 CD4 细胞水平较低的非裔患者中。HIVAN 因感染 HIV 及其后 HIV 病毒基因在足细胞中表达所致。蛋白尿的发生通常较急,可超过 10 g/d,伴肾功能不全可迅速恶化。

血栓性微血管病

血栓性微血管病的特点是血小板减少、微血管病性溶血性贫血和微血管堵塞,导致不同程度的器官功能障碍。溶血的标志包括血触珠蛋白降低、乳酸脱氢酶和间接胆红素水平升高以及网织红细胞计数增高。外周血涂片中可见破碎红细胞。

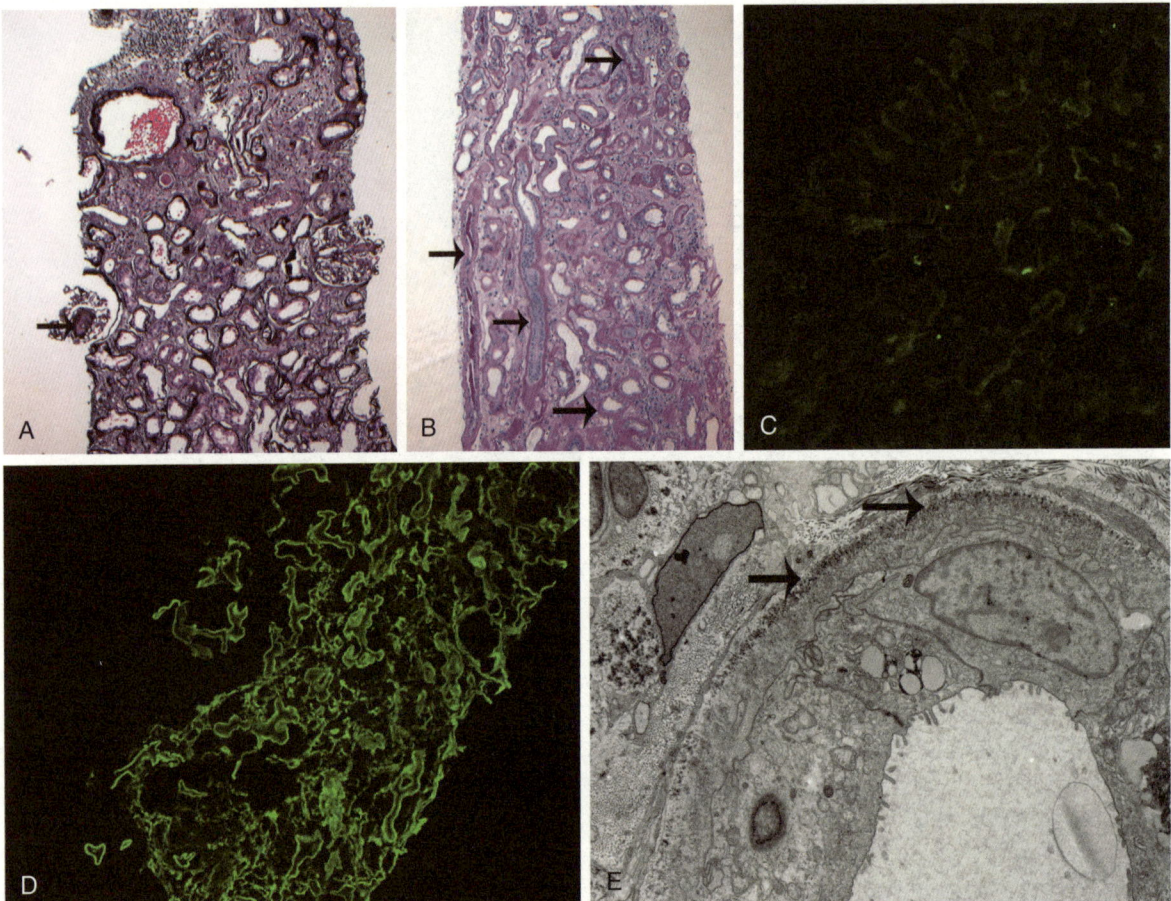

Fig. 4.14 Light chain deposition disease. (A) Light microscopy shows glomeruli with silver-positive mesangial nodules *(arrow)* and thickened tubular basement membranes (silver methenamine, ×10). (B) Periodic acid–Schiff staining shows thickened, wavy tubular basement membranes *(arrow)* (×10). Immunofluorescence studies found negative staining for λ light chains (C) and bright staining for κ light chains (D) along the tubular basement membranes (both ×10). (E) Electron microscopy shows granular, punctate, electron-dense deposits *(arrows)* along the tubular basement membranes (×5800).

The quintessential forms of thrombotic microangiopathy include hemolytic uremic syndrome (HUS) and thrombotic thrombocytopenic purpura (TTP). Although previously thought to represent different manifestations of the same disease, these disorders are distinct clinically and mechanistically. In adults, predominant neurologic involvement suggests a diagnosis of TTP, and predominant renal involvement points to HUS. In most cases, the clinical presentations are very similar, making it difficult to distinguish between HUS and TTP on clinical grounds alone. Other causes of thrombotic microangiopathy include malignant hypertension, drugs (e.g., cocaine, quinidine, ticlopidine), autoimmune diseases (e.g., SLE, scleroderma, antiphospholipid antibody syndrome), malignancy, HIV infection, and antibody-mediated rejection.

Kidney biopsy in HUS and TTP reveals microthrombi in glomerular capillaries and arterioles, and mesangial expansion with loose granular material, called *mesangiolysis*, may be seen in HUS and TTP and in malignant hypertension or autoimmune diseases (Fig. 4.15). Malignant hypertension and autoimmune diseases may also show thickening and intimal fibrosis of arteries and onion-skinning (i.e., laminated deposition of basement membrane–type material) of the vessel walls. Thrombi are common and may occlude the vascular lumen.

Hemolytic Uremic Syndrome

Two subtypes of HUS are recognized: a sporadic or diarrhea-associated form (D+ HUS) and an atypical or non–diarrhea-associated form (D– HUS). D+ HUS is the most frequently encountered form, and it is linked strongly to ingestion of meat contaminated with enterohemorrhagic *Escherichia coli* or other infectious agents. The bacterium produces a Shiga-like toxin that binds to a glycolipid receptor on renal endothelial cells and triggers activation of the alternative complement cascade, leading to endothelial damage. Therapy for D+ HUS is supportive. Children with D+ HUS have a good prognosis (90% recover renal function), but older patients have increased mortality rates and unfavorable long-term renal survival.

Atypical or D– HUS represents 10% to 15% of the cases of HUS and is more common in adults. The disease results from genetic mutations or autoantibodies against complement factors or complement factors regulating proteins (i.e., C3, factor B, factor H, factor I, MCP, CFHR1, and CFHR3) that control the activity of C3 convertase of the alternative complement pathway. The resulting defective control of C3 convertase leads to widespread activation of the complement cascade.

The complement inhibitor eculizumab has been approved for the treatment of patients with atypical HUS. Eculizumab and plasma infusion may also be considered in the treatment of children with D+ HUS and severe central nervous system involvement such as seizures, stroke, or coma.

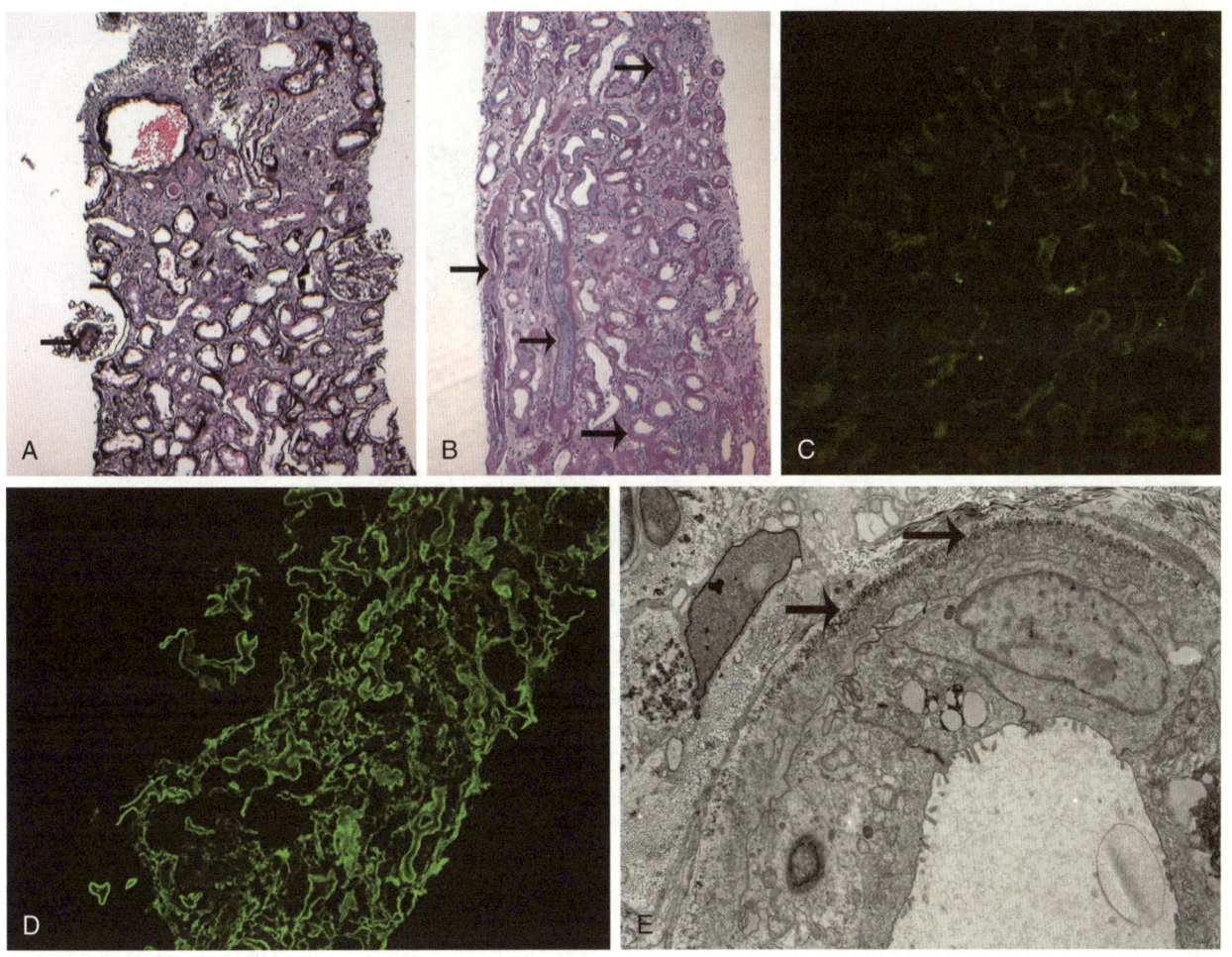

图4.14 轻链沉积病。（**A**）光镜下可见肾小球银染阳性的系膜结节（箭头）和肾小管基底膜增厚（六胺银，×10）。（**B**）PAS染色显示波浪形增厚的肾小管基底膜（箭头）（×10）。免疫荧光提示肾小管基底膜 λ 轻链染色阴性（**C**），κ 轻链染色强阳性（**D**）（均×10）。（**E**）电镜显示沿肾小管基底膜有点状、颗粒状的电子致密物沉积（箭头）（×5800）

经典的血栓性微血管病包括溶血性尿毒综合征（HUS）和血栓性血小板减少性紫癜（TTP）。尽管以往认为二者是同一种疾病的不同表现，但它们在临床和发病机制上截然不同。在成人中，以神经系统受累为主时提示 TTP，而以肾脏受累为主时则指向 HUS。在大多数情况下，二者的临床表现非常相似，因此仅凭临床表现很难区分 HUS 和 TTP。导致血栓性微血管病的其他病因包括恶性高血压、药物（如可卡因、奎尼丁、噻氯匹定）、自身免疫性疾病（如系统性红斑狼疮、硬皮病、抗磷脂综合征）、恶性肿瘤、HIV 感染和抗体介导的排斥反应。

HUS 和 TTP 的肾活检均可见到肾小球毛细血管和微动脉中的微血栓。系膜扩张伴有松散的颗粒状物质，称为系膜溶解，可以见于 HUS、TTP、恶性高血压或自身免疫性疾病中（图4.15）。恶性高血压和自身免疫性疾病还可以出现动脉管壁增厚和内膜纤维化以及血管壁的洋葱皮样改变（即基底膜样物质层状沉积）。血栓很常见并可能堵塞血管腔。

溶血性尿毒综合征

HUS 有两种亚型：散发性或腹泻相关型（D＋HUS）和非典型或非腹泻相关型（D-HUS）。D＋HUS 是最常见的形式，与进食肠出血性大肠埃希菌或其他感染性病原体污染的肉类密切相关。该细菌产生志贺毒素，志贺毒素与肾脏内皮细胞上的糖脂受体结合，继而引发补体旁路途径的激活，导致内皮损伤。D＋HUS 的治疗以支持为主。儿童 D＋HUS 预后良好（90% 患儿肾功能可恢复），但老年患者死亡率升高，长期肾脏预后不良。

非典型或 D-HUS 占 HUS 的 10%～15%，在成人中更为常见。该病是由于控制替代补体途径 C3 转化酶活性的补体因子或补体调节蛋白（即 C3、B 因子、H 因子、I 因子、MCP、CFHR1 和 CFHR3）发生基因突变或自身抗体所引起，C3 转化酶的控制缺陷导致补体系统的全面激活。

补体抑制剂依库珠单抗已获批用于治疗非典型 HUS。有严重的中枢神经系统受累（如癫痫发作、卒中或昏迷）的 D＋HUS 患儿，也可考虑使用依库珠单抗和血浆输注。

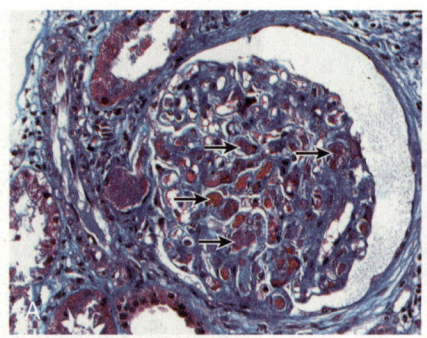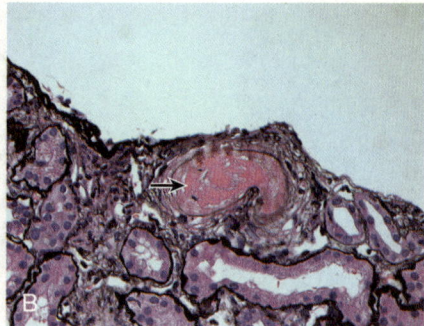

Fig. 4.15 Thrombotic microangiopathy. (A) Light microscopy shows multiple, small thrombi *(arrows)* in glomerular capillaries in the setting of hemolytic uremic syndrome (Masson trichrome, ×40). (B) Light microscopy shows a thrombus *(arrow)* in a small artery in the setting of scleroderma (silver methenamine, ×20).

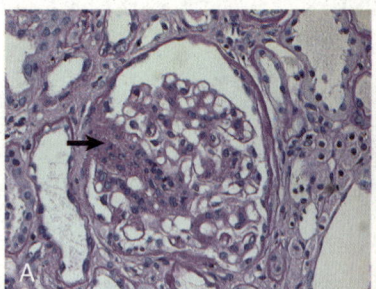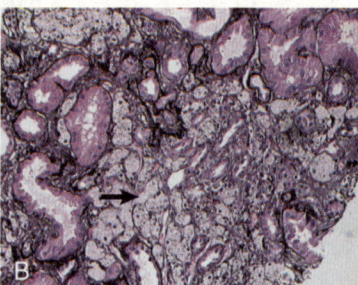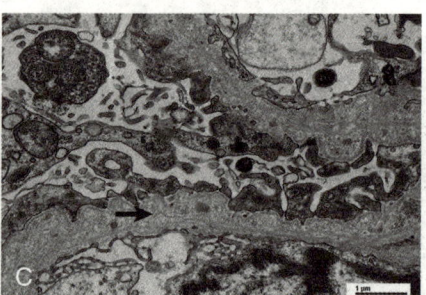

Fig. 4.16 Alport syndrome. (A) Light microscopy shows focal segmental glomerulosclerosis *(arrow)* (periodic acid–Schiff, ×40). (B) Light microscopy shows numerous foam cells *(arrow)* in the interstitium (silver methenamine, ×40). (C) Electron microscopy shows thickening of the glomerular capillary walls with multiple lamellations of basement membrane material *(arrow)* and formation of the classic basket-weave appearance (×212,000).

Thrombotic Thrombocytopenic Purpura

TTP results from mutations in the von Willebrand factor (VWF)–cleaving protease (ADAMTS13) or development of an autoantibody against ADAMTS13. ADAMTS13 cleaves large multimers of VWF, and abnormalities or deficiency of ADAMTS13 activity affects VWF function. Patients can have acute or chronic (i.e., relapsing) TTP. Microthrombi rich in large VWF multimers develop in the arterioles and capillaries of the brain and other organs.

Genetic or acquired forms of ADAMTS13 deficiency can be treated by plasma infusion or exchange to supply functional protease. Plasma exchange should be initiated promptly, based on findings of microangiopathic hemolytic anemia and thrombocytopenia without evidence of other causes of thrombotic microangiopathy (e.g., scleroderma, malignancy, antiphospholipid syndrome). Treatment should not await test results for the levels or activity of ADAMTS13.

DISEASES WITH GLOMERULAR BASEMENT MEMBRANE ABNORMALITIES

Alport Syndrome

Alport syndrome is an inherited disorder of basement membranes. In more than one half of patients, the disease results from a mutation in the *COL4A5* gene that codes for the α5 chain of type IV collagen (α5[IV]). The mutation in *COL4A5* disables a developmental switch in the GBM collagen that retains its embryonic phenotype and results in a friable GBM.

Alport syndrome is frequently associated with sensorineural hearing loss and ocular abnormalities (e.g., lenticonus of the anterior lens capsule). Patients characteristically have persistent or intermittent hematuria and usually have mild proteinuria, which progresses with age and may reach nephrotic range in up to 30%. The disease is X-linked in approximately 85% of patients, but autosomal recessive and autosomal dominant patterns of inheritance have been described.

In virtually all male patients, the syndrome progresses to ESRD, often before the age of 30 years. The disease is usually mild in heterozygous women, but some develop ESRD, usually after the age of 50 years. The rate of progression to ESRD is fairly constant among affected men within individual families, but it varies markedly from family to family. The degree of deafness correlates with the rate of progression to ESRD.

On light microscopy, the glomerular changes are nonspecific. Diagnostic features are usually seen on electron microscopy. At an early stage, thinning of the GBM may be the only visible abnormality and may suggest thin basement membrane disease. With time, the GBM thickens, and the lamina densa splits into several irregular layers that may branch and rejoin, producing a characteristic basket-weave appearance (Fig. 4.16).

Immunohistochemical studies of type IV collagen show the absence of α3(IV), α4(IV), and α5(IV) chains from the GBM and distal tubular basement membrane. This abnormality occurs only in patients with Alport syndrome and is diagnostic. In families with an unquestionable diagnosis, evaluation of patients with newly diagnosed hematuria can be limited to kidney ultrasound and urinary tract examination in most cases. If a defined mutation has been previously identified, molecular diagnosis of affected men or gene-carrying women is possible. In other cases, confirmation of the diagnosis can be obtained by examination of skin biopsy by immunofluorescence for the expression of the α5(IV)

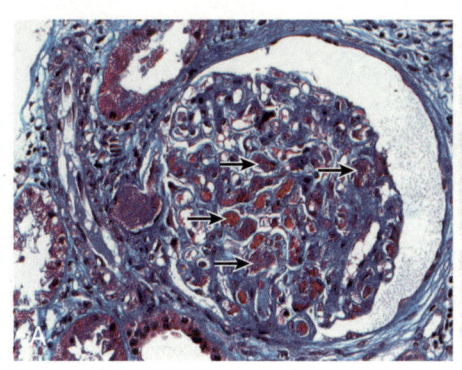
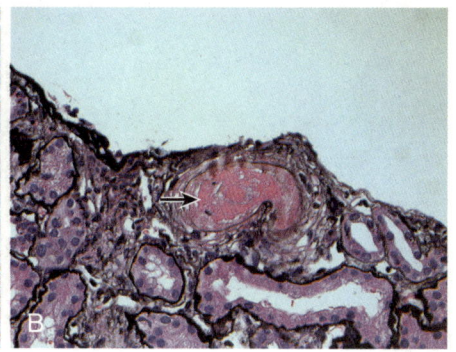

图 4.15 血栓性微血管病。(**A**) 光镜下显示溶血性尿毒综合征中的肾小球毛细血管中有多发小血栓 (箭头) (Masson 染色, ×40)。(**B**) 光镜显示硬皮病中的小动脉中血栓 (箭头) (六胺银, ×20)

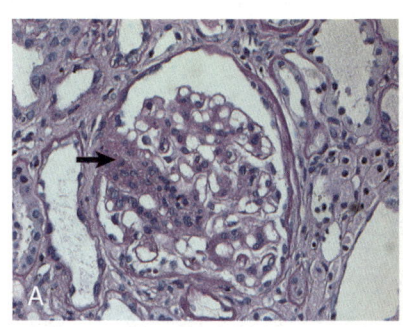
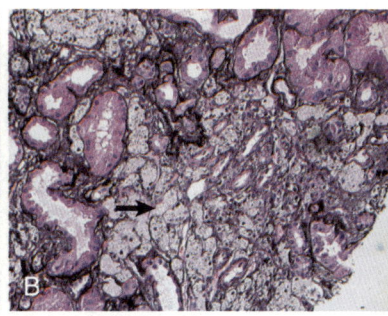
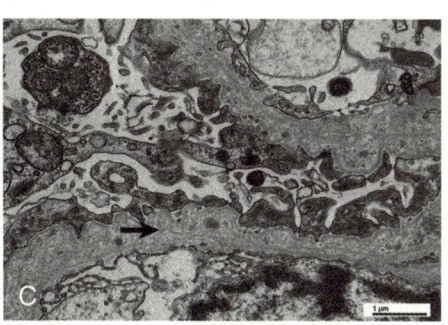

图 4.16 Alport 综合征。(**A**) 光镜下显示局灶节段性肾小球硬化 (箭头) (PAS, ×40)。(**B**) 光镜下显示间质中大量泡沫细胞 (箭头) (六胺银, ×40)。(**C**) 电镜显示肾小球毛细血管壁增厚, 伴基底膜呈多层分层状 (箭头) 并形成典型的篮网样外观 (×212 000)

血栓性血小板减少性紫癜 (TTP)

TTP 是由血管性血友病因子 (VWF) 剪切酶 (ADAMTS13) 突变或产生针对 ADAMTS13 的自身抗体引起的。ADAMTS13 可剪切 VWF 的大型多聚体, ADAMTS13 活性异常或缺乏会影响 VWF 的功能。患者可出现急性或慢性 (即复发性) TTP。在大脑和其他脏器的微动脉和毛细血管中会形成富含大型 VWF 多聚体的微血栓。

遗传性或获得性 ADAMTS13 缺乏可通过输注血浆或血浆置换来补充具有功能的 VWF 剪切酶来治疗。根据微血管病性溶血性贫血和血小板减少, 且无其他引起血栓性微血管病的病因 (如硬皮病、恶性肿瘤、抗磷脂综合征) 的证据, 即可立即开始血浆置换。无需等待 ADAMTS13 水平或活性的检测结果再开始治疗。

肾小球基底膜异常疾病

Alport 综合征

Alport 综合征是一种遗传性基底膜疾病。一半以上的患者是由于编码Ⅳ型胶原 α5 链 [α5 (Ⅳ)] 的 COL4A5 基因发生突变引起。COL4A5 基因突变使 GBM 胶原在发育中无法进行转换, 从而保留了胚胎型的脆弱的 GBM。

Alport 综合征常伴有感音神经性耳聋和眼睛异常 (如前圆锥晶状体)。患者表现为持续性或间歇性血尿, 常伴有轻度蛋白尿, 蛋白尿会随着年龄的增长而进展, 最终高达 30% 的患者会出现肾病范围蛋白尿。约 85% 的患者为 X 连锁遗传, 但也有常染色体隐性遗传和常染色体显性遗传的报道。

几乎所有男性患者会在 30 岁前进展至 ESRD。杂合子女性患者的病情通常较轻, 但有些在 50 岁以后也会进展为 ESRD。在同一个家族中的男性患者发展至 ESRD 的速度相对恒定, 但在不同家族中则有明显差异。耳聋的程度与进展至 ESRD 的速度相关。

在光镜下, 肾小球病变无特殊。电镜检查常可发现诊断性特征。在早期阶段, GBM 变薄可能是仅有的异常表现, 可提示薄基底膜肾病。随着时间的推移, GBM 增厚, 基底膜致密层分裂成几层不规则的片层, 并可形成分支并重新连接, 从而产生特征性的篮网样外观 (图 4.16)。

Ⅳ型胶原的免疫组化染色提示 GBM 和远端肾小管基底膜缺乏 α3 (Ⅳ)、α4 (Ⅳ) 和 α5 (Ⅳ) 链。这种异常仅见于 Alport 综合征患者, 具有诊断意义。在已确诊的家庭中, 多数情况下对新诊断血尿患者的评估可仅进行肾脏超声和尿路检查。如果之前已明确基因突变, 则可对受累男性或携带基因的女性进行分子诊断。在其他情况下, 可以使用皮肤活检组织的免疫荧光检测 α5 (Ⅳ) 链的表达情况来确诊。皮肤基底

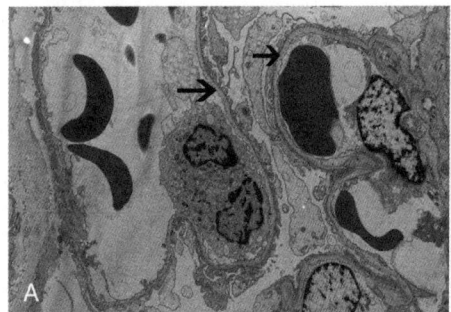
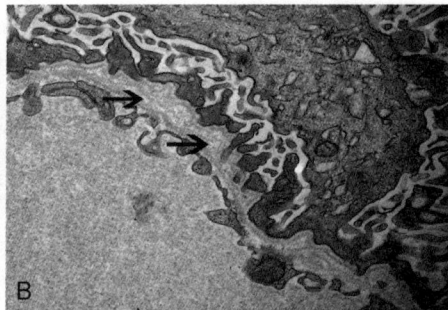

Fig. 4.17 (A) In thin glomerular basement membrane nephropathy, electron microscopy shows glomerular basement membranes *(arrows)* that are 198 nm thick (×5800). (B) Alport syndrome. Electron microscopy showing thickened glomerular capillary walls with lamellations and disorganization of the glomerular basement membranes (×30000). Arrows point to thin glomerular basement membranes in A and to the lamellations in B.

chain. Absence of the α5(IV) chain from epidermal basement membrane is diagnostic of X-linked Alport syndrome and may avoid a renal biopsy. Direct sequencing of the *COL4A5* gene can help to diagnose patients in whom a clear diagnosis cannot be made based on clinical findings and histologic methods or to identify the carrier state in asymptomatic female members of X-linked Alport syndrome families.

No specific treatment is available for Alport syndrome. Tight control of blood pressure and moderate protein restriction are recommended to retard the progression of renal disease, but the benefit is unproven. Patients with Alport syndrome are phenotypic knockouts for the α3(IV) chain. Consequently, kidney transplantation carries a 5% to 10% risk of subsequent anti-GBM GN due to the introduction of an intact α3(IV) chain with the transplanted kidney and subsequent generation of auto-antibodies to the antigen present in the intact α3(IV) chain of the transplanted kidney.

Thin Glomerular Basement Membrane Nephropathy

Thin glomerular basement membrane nephropathy, also known as benign familial hematuria, is a relatively common condition characterized by isolated glomerular hematuria and associated with the renal biopsy finding of an excessively thin GBM. It is usually transmitted as an autosomal dominant disease. Heterozygous mutations in the *COL4A3* or *COL4A4* genes have been described in numerous patients with thin glomerular basement membrane nephropathy, indicating a genetically heterogeneous condition.

The usual clinical presentation is isolated, persistent hematuria that is first detected in childhood. In some patients, hematuria is intermittent and may not manifest until adulthood. On light microscopy, glomeruli appear normal, and immunofluorescence microscopy shows no immunoglobulin or complement deposition. Electron microscopy shows diffuse thinning of the GBM (Fig. 4.17). In adults, a GBM thickness less than 250 nm strongly suggests thin GBM disease.

The condition is usually benign and requires no specific treatment. However, a few patients have progressive renal disease that leads to ESRD.

FABRY'S DISEASE

Fabry's disease is an X-linked recessive inborn error of glycosphingolipid metabolism caused by deficient activity of the lysosomal enzyme α-galactosidase A, which results in the progressive accumulation of neutral glycosphingolipids (predominately globotriaosylceramide, particularly in the vascular endothelial cells of the kidney and heart.

Early manifestations of the disease include angiokeratoma, episodic pain crises, and hypohidrosis. With time, progressive

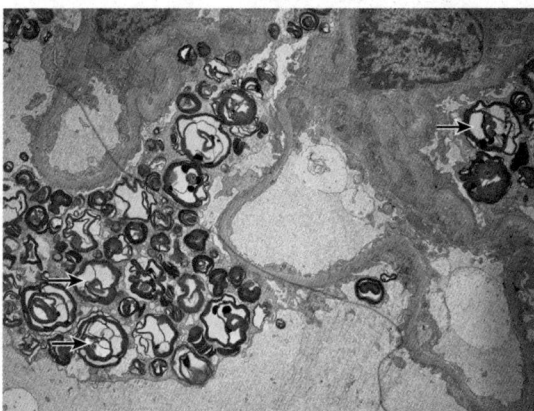

Fig. 4.18 Fabry's disease. Electron microscopy shows visceral epithelial cells (i.e., podocytes) with numerous multilamellated structures called *myelin bodies* or *zebra bodies (arrows)* that are made of glycosphingolipids (×4800).

globotriaosylceramide accumulation in the microvasculature in the kidney, heart, and brain leads to clinical manifestations such as proteinuria, renal failure, cardiac arrhythmias, and strokes, resulting in early death during the fourth and fifth decades of life of affected men.

Light microscopy reveals vacuolated glomerular cells, especially podocytes. Electron microscopy shows enlarged podocytes lysosomes filled with osmiophilic, granular to lamellated membrane structures (i.e., zebra bodies) (Fig. 4.18). Enzyme replacement therapy can lead to significant improvement of neuropathic pain, but the beneficial effects on the severity or progression of other disease manifestations are less clear.

DIABETIC NEPHROPATHY

Diabetic nephropathy accounts for more than 50% of patients on dialysis in the United States. In type 1 diabetes mellitus, nephropathy usually manifests 10 to 15 years after the initial diagnosis; and a similar natural history is likely for patients with type 2 diabetes mellitus. The main risk factors include a positive family history of diabetic nephropathy, hypertension, and poor glycemic control. The risk may be greater in some racial groups (e.g., Pima Indians, African Americans).

The pathogenesis is complex. Increased glycosylation of proteins with accumulation of advanced glycosylation end products that

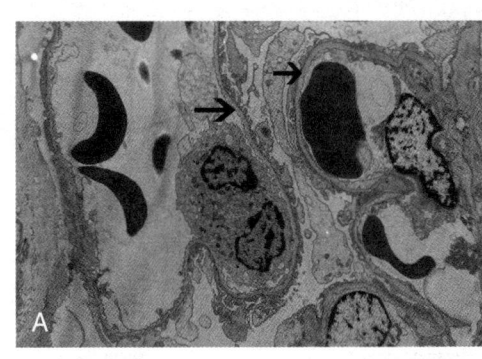 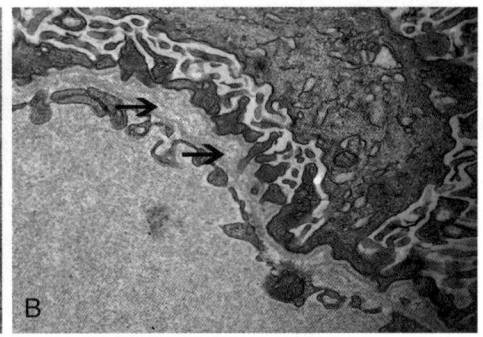

图 4.17 （A）在薄基底膜肾病中，电镜下显示肾小球基底膜（箭头）的厚度为 198 nm（×5800）。（B）Alport 综合征电镜下显示肾小球毛细血管壁增厚并伴有肾小球基底膜分层和杂乱排列（×30 000）。A 图箭头指向变薄的肾小球基底膜，B 图箭头指向分层

膜上 α5（Ⅳ）链缺失是诊断 X 连锁 Alport 综合征的标志，并且可避免肾活检。对那些根据临床表现和组织学检查无法明确诊断的患者，以及需要确定 X 连锁 Alport 综合征家族中无症状女性成员的携带状态时，进行 COL4A5 基因的直接测序将有助于诊断。

Alport 综合征目前尚无特效治疗方法。推荐严格控制血压和适度限制蛋白质摄入以延缓肾脏疾病的进展，但其益处尚未得到证实。Alport 综合征患者具有 α3（Ⅳ）链敲除的表型，肾移植后约 5%～10% 可继发抗 GBM 肾小球肾炎，这与移植肾带来了完整的 α3（Ⅳ）链，随后机体产生了针对移植肾中完整 α3（Ⅳ）链抗原的自身抗体有关。

薄基底膜肾病

薄基底膜肾病又称良性家族性血尿，是一种相对常见的疾病，其特征是孤立的肾小球性血尿，并在肾活检发现极度变薄的肾小球基底膜。该病通常为常染色体显性遗传病。在许多肾小球薄基底膜肾病患者中都发现了 COL4A3 或 COL4A4 基因的杂合突变，表明该病具有遗传异质性。

薄基底膜肾病常见的临床表现是儿童期首次发现的孤立性、持续性血尿。有些患者的血尿呈间歇性，且成年后才出现。光镜检查肾小球正常，免疫荧光镜检查无免疫球蛋白或补体沉积。电镜检查显示 GBM 弥漫性变薄（图 4.17）。在成人中，GBM 厚度小于 250 nm 高度提示薄基底膜肾病。

该病通常为良性病程，无需特殊治疗。然而，少数患者有进展性肾脏疾病，最终导致 ESRD。

法布里病

法布里病是一种由溶酶体内 α- 半乳糖苷酶 A 活性不足引起的 X 连锁隐性遗传性先天性鞘糖脂代谢异常，导致中性鞘糖脂（主要是三己糖酰基鞘脂醇）进行性积累，尤其是在肾脏和心脏的血管内皮细胞中。

该病的早期表现包括血管角化瘤、阵发性疼痛和

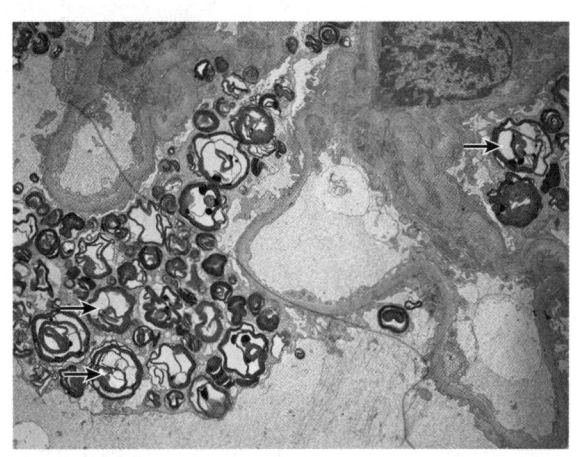

图 4.18 法布里病。电镜显示脏层上皮细胞（即足细胞）具有大量由鞘糖脂组成的多层膜结构，称为髓样小体或斑马小体（箭头），由鞘糖脂构成（×4800）

无汗症。随着时间的推移，在肾脏、心脏和大脑的微血管中逐渐积聚的三己糖酰基鞘脂醇会导致蛋白尿、肾衰竭、心律失常和卒中等临床表现，导致患病男性常在 40～50 岁早逝。

光镜下可见空泡化的肾小球细胞，尤其是足细胞。电镜显示增大的足细胞溶酶体，其内充满嗜锇性的颗粒状至层状膜结构（即斑马小体）（图 4.18）。酶替代疗法可明显改善神经性疼痛，但对其他表现的严重程度或进展的益处尚不明确。

糖尿病肾病

糖尿病肾病占美国透析患者的 50% 以上。在 1 型糖尿病患者中，通常在最初确诊糖尿病后 10～15 年出现肾脏病；2 型糖尿病患者也可能有类似的自然病史。主要风险因素包括糖尿病肾病家族史、高血压和血糖控制不佳。某些种族（如印第安人、非裔美国人）的风险可能更大。

糖尿病肾病发病机制复杂。蛋白质的糖基化增加导致晚期糖基化终产物蓄积并与胶原蛋白交联，以及

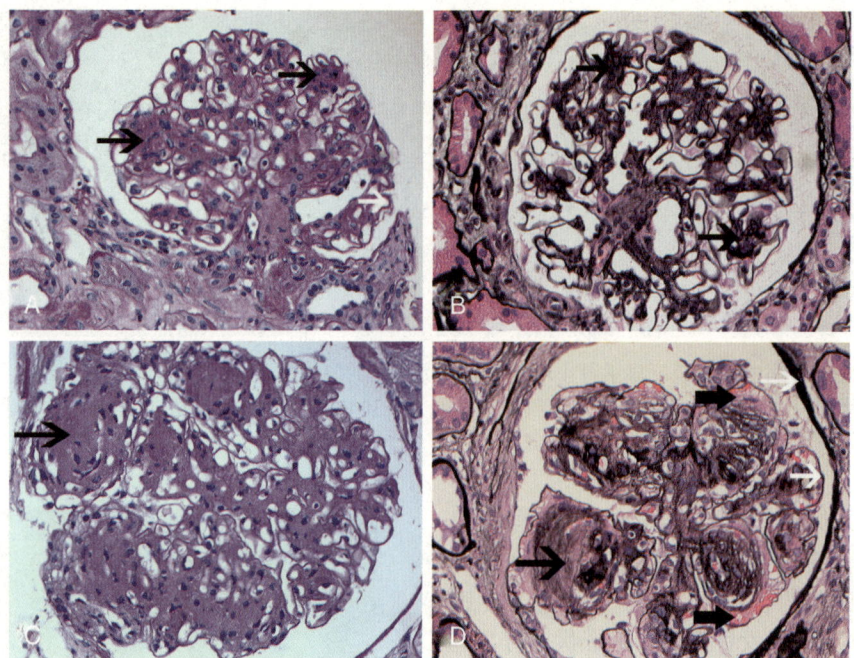

Fig. 4.19 Light microscopy shows diabetic glomerulosclerosis. (A and B) Early diabetic nodule formation *(arrows)*. (C and D) Well-formed Kimmelstiel-Wilson lesions result from mesangial expansion *(thin black arrows)*. The nodules are periodic acid–Schiff and silver methenamine positive. The glomerular capillary lumen is distended by formation of small microaneurysms *(thick black arrows)*. The glomerular basement membrane and Bowman capsule *(white arrows)* are thickened (A and C, periodic acid–Schiff; B and D, silver methenamine; all ×40).

cross-link with collagen and glomerular hyperfiltration with hypertension are important. Microalbuminuria (i.e., urinary albumin excretion >30 but <300 mg/24 h) is the initial manifestation of diabetic nephropathy. With time, microalbuminuria may evolve into overt proteinuria (>300 mg/24 h), with the degree of proteinuria correlating roughly with the renal prognosis.

After overt proteinuria develops, progression to ESRD is relentless, although rates of decline vary among patients. For patients with type 1 diabetes, there is a strong correlation (95%) between the development of nephropathy and other signs of diabetic microvascular compromise (e.g., diabetic retinopathy), but the correlation is weaker for patients with type 2 diabetes. Hypertension is almost universal among patients with proteinuria. It is difficult to control and usually requires at least three antihypertensive agents.

On renal biopsy, early signs of diabetic nephropathy include glomerular hypertrophy and thickening of the GBM. As the disease progresses, arteriolar hyalinosis, arteriosclerosis, and progressive mesangial expansion (i.e., diffuse diabetic glomerulosclerosis) and nodular formations (i.e., Kimmelstiel-Wilson nodules) develop (Fig. 4.19). For patients with a history of diabetes longer than 10 years and retinopathy, a renal biopsy may not be necessary. However, renal biopsy is indicated for patients with an atypical course of the disease (e.g., nephrotic syndrome), those with less than 10 years of type 1 diabetes, or patients with rapid loss of renal function.

Treatment with ACEIs or ARBs slows progression of diabetic nephropathy and should be used in all patients with albuminuria, even if normotensive. Tight glycemic control (i.e., glycated hemoglobin <7.0%) may also retard progression of diabetic nephropathy. Target systolic blood pressure should be less than 125 mm Hg, but this may be difficult to achieve and may require multiple medications and a strict low-salt diet.

SUGGESTED READINGS

De Vriese AS, Glassock RJ, Nath KA, et al: A proposal for a serology-based approach to membranous nephropathy, J Am Soc Nephrol 28(2):421–430, 2017.

De Vriese AS, Sethi S, Nath KA, et al: Differentiating primary, genetic, and secondary FSGS in adults: A clinicopathologic approach, J Am Soc Nephrol 29(3):759–774, 2018.

Kashtan CE: Alport syndrome: Achieving early diagnosis and treatment, Am J Kidney Dis S0272-6386(20)30734-4, 2020.

Kitching AR, Anders HJ, Basu N, et al: ANCA-associated vasculitis, Nat Rev Dis Primers 6(1):71, 2020.

McAdoo SP, Pusey CD: Anti-glomerular basement membrane disease, Clin J Am Soc Nephrol 12(7):1162–1172, 2017.

Noris M, Remuzzi G: Atypical hemolytic-uremic syndrome, N Engl J Med 361(17):1676–1687, 2009.

Ortiz A, Germain DP, Desnick RJ, et al: Fabry disease revisited: Management and treatment recommendations for adult patients, Mol Genet Metab 123(4):416–427, 2018.

Roccatello D, Saadoun D, Ramos-Casals M, et al: Cryoglobulinaemia, Nat Rev Dis Primers 4(1):11, 2018.

Sethi S, Fervenza FC: Membranoproliferative glomerulonephritis—a new look at an old entity, N Engl J Med 366(12):1119–1131, 2012.

Vivarelli M, Massella L, Ruggiero B, et al: Minimal change disease, Clin J Am Soc Nephrol 12:332–345, 2017.

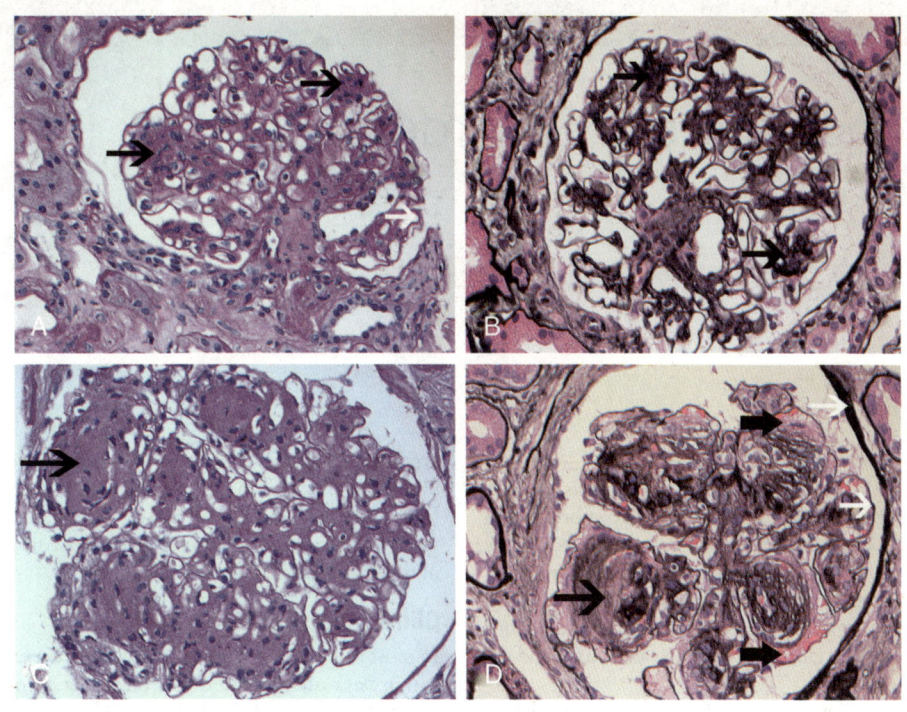

图 4.19　光镜显示糖尿病肾小球硬化。(**A 和 B**) 早期糖尿病结节形成（箭头）。(**C 和 D**) 系膜扩张形成的明显的 K-W 结节（细黑色箭头）。K-W 结节 PAS 和六胺银染色阳性。肾小球毛细血管腔因形成小的微动脉瘤而扩张（粗黑色箭头）。肾小球基底膜和肾小囊（白色箭头）增厚（A 和 C，PAS；B 和 D，六胺银；均 ×40）

高血压导致的肾小球高滤过均是重要原因。微量白蛋白尿（即尿白蛋白排泄量 30～300 mg/24 h）是糖尿病肾病的最初表现。随着时间的推移，微量白蛋白尿可能进展为显性蛋白尿（大于 300 mg/24 h），蛋白尿的程度与肾脏预后大致相关。

在出现显性蛋白尿后，尽管不同患者的肾功能下降速度不同，但进展至 ESRD 是不可避免的。对于 1 型糖尿病患者来说，肾脏病的发生与糖尿病微血管损害的其他表现（如糖尿病视网膜病变）密切相关（95%），但对于 2 型糖尿病患者来说相关性较弱。有蛋白尿的患者普遍有高血压，且难以控制，通常需要至少三种降压药。

在肾活检中，糖尿病肾病的早期表现包括肾小球肥大和肾小球基底膜增厚。随着病情进展，出现小动脉玻璃样变、小动脉硬化和进行性系膜扩张（即弥漫性糖尿病肾小球硬化）和结节形成 [即 Kimmelstiel-Wilson（K-W）结节]（图 4.19）。对于糖尿病病史超过 10 年且患有视网膜病变的患者，可能不需要进行肾活检。然而，病程不典型的患者（如肾病综合征）、1 型糖尿病病史不足 10 年或肾功能迅速下降的患者具有肾活检指征。

ACEI 或 ARB 治疗可减缓糖尿病肾病的进展，并应在所有白蛋白尿患者中使用，即使是血压正常的患者。严格控制血糖（即糖化血红蛋白 < 7.0%）也可能延缓糖尿病肾病的进展。目标收缩压应低于 125 mmHg，但可能比较难于达到该目标，常需要多种药物和严格的低盐饮食辅助。

推荐阅读

De Vriese AS, Glassock RJ, Nath KA, et al: A proposal for a serology-based approach to membranous nephropathy, J Am Soc Nephrol 28(2):421–430, 2017.

De Vriese AS, Sethi S, Nath KA, et al: Differentiating primary, genetic, and secondary FSGS in adults: A clinicopathologic approach, J Am Soc Nephrol 29(3):759–774, 2018.

Kashtan CE: Alport syndrome: Achieving early diagnosis and treatment, Am J Kidney Dis S0272-6386(20)30734-4, 2020.

Kitching AR, Anders HJ, Basu N, et al: ANCA-associated vasculitis, Nat Rev Dis Primers 6(1):71, 2020.

McAdoo SP, Pusey CD: Anti-glomerular basement membrane disease, Clin J Am Soc Nephrol 12(7):1162–1172, 2017.

Noris M, Remuzzi G: Atypical hemolytic-uremic syndrome, N Engl J Med 361(17):1676–1687, 2009.

Ortiz A, Germain DP, Desnick RJ, et al: Fabry disease revisited: Management and treatment recommendations for adult patients, Mol Genet Metab 123(4):416–427, 2018.

Roccatello D, Saadoun D, Ramos-Casals M, et al: Cryoglobulinaemia, Nat Rev Dis Primers 4(1):11, 2018.

Sethi S, Fervenza FC: Membranoproliferative glomerulonephritis—a new look at an old entity, N Engl J Med 366(12):1119–1131, 2012.

Vivarelli M, Massella L, Ruggiero B, et al: Minimal change disease, Clin J Am Soc Nephrol 12:332–345, 2017.

5

Major Nonglomerular Disorders of the Kidney

Nilum Rajora, Shani Shastri, Pooja Koolwal, Ramesh Saxena

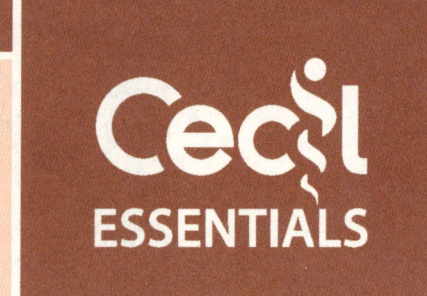

INTRODUCTION

Nonglomerular structures of the kidney include blood vessels, tubules, and interstitium. The tubulointerstitial compartment comprises 80% of kidney parenchyma, with most of the volume accounted for by tubules, interstitial cells, extracellular matrix, and interstitial fluid. Although primary glomerular and vascular diseases are associated with significant tubulointerstitial changes, the clinical presentations are dominated by injury of the glomeruli and the vasculature, and are discussed in Chapters 4 and 6.

Primary tubulointerstitial disorders are characterized by structural and functional abnormalities predominantly involving kidney tubules and the interstitium and are associated with a myriad of clinical presentations based on the principal structure involved: acute tubulointerstitial nephritis, characterized by sudden onset and a rapid decline in kidney function; chronic tubulointerstitial nephropathy, characterized by a more protracted clinical course; cystic diseases with kidney cysts and kidney failure; nephrolithiasis with pain, hematuria, and sometimes acute kidney injury (AKI). This chapter will cover primary tubulointerstitial disorders of the kidney.

ACUTE INTERSTITIAL NEPHRITIS

Definition, Epidemiology, and Pathology

Acute interstitial nephritis (AIN), also called *tubulointerstitial nephritis*, is characterized by inflammation and edema of the kidney interstitium; glomeruli and vessels are distinctly normal. AIN is associated with an acute, rapid decline in kidney function and is a common cause of AKI. AIN is seen in 1% to 3% of kidney biopsies, but if biopsy is done in the setting of AKI with clinical suspicion for AIN, 15% to 27% of biopsies show AIN.

On gross examination, the kidneys are pale and swollen. Histologically, the hallmarks of AIN include interstitial edema and infiltration of the interstitium with inflammatory cells comprising lymphocytes, monocytes, plasma cells, eosinophils, and macrophages. This inflammation can progress to fibrotic changes in 7 to 10 days. Immunofluorescence studies typically are unrevealing. Tubular basement membrane immune deposits can be seen in cases of AIN associated with some drug-induced tubulointerstitial nephritis, immunoglobulin G4 (IgG4)–associated nephritis, membranous nephropathy, membranoproliferative glomerulonephritis, lupus nephritis, Sjögren syndrome, and other autoimmune diseases.

Any drug can cause AIN but frequently used therapeutic drugs merit particular emphasis. Common causes of AIN are shown in Table 5.1. They include antibiotics, allopurinol, mesalamine, nonsteroidal anti-inflammatory drugs (NSAIDs), proton pump inhibitors, and chemotherapeutic agents. Other causes of AIN include infections, autoimmune disorders, tubulointerstitial nephritis and uveitis syndrome, snakebite, and herbal supplements. Nephrotoxicity of novel biologic agents used in cancer therapy is increasingly being recognized (see Table 5.1). Several of these drugs are associated with AIN. In many such cases, autoimmunity rather than drug sensitivity is the basis of tubulointerstitial inflammation.

Clinical Presentation

In most cases, AIN begins abruptly with a decrease in kidney function within days of exposure to the offending agent. However, AIN may ensue after several weeks of the exposure in some cases. Characteristic clinical manifestations include rash, fever, and eosinophilia. Modest proteinuria (usually <1 g/day) or hematuria may be observed, and oliguria is uncommon. A high index of suspicion is required for diagnosis because these features may be absent.

Diagnosis and Differential Diagnosis

When evaluating a patient with a recent decline in kidney function, the diagnosis of AIN is suggested by a history of exposure to the known offending agents coupled with typical clinical features. In addition to identifying elevated serum creatinine levels, a urinalysis can detect the characteristic findings of white blood cells, red blood cells, and white blood cell casts in urine. Identification of eosinophils in urine with Hansel or Wright stains is highly suggestive, but their absence does not rule out AIN. Moreover, eosinophils in urine can be observed in other diseases, including cholesterol embolism, urinary tract infections, parasitic disorders, and glomerulonephritis.

Unfortunately, there is currently no noninvasive test that reliably diagnoses drug-induced AIN. Kidney biopsy should be considered when the diagnosis is not obvious. Besides tubular injury, other histologic features may suggest the underlying disease that is associated with AIN. IgG4-related AIN has presence of tubular basement membrane immune complex deposits and an increase in IgG4-positive plasma cells in the interstitium. Sarcoidosis associated AIN may also have granulomas on biopsy, and AIN related to systemic lupus erythematosus (SLE) may also show diffused immune complex deposits on immunofluorescence. A definitive diagnosis of AIN requires a kidney biopsy, although most times it is not necessary for management when clinical features are highly suggestive.

Treatment and Prognosis

Treatment of patients with AIN consists of removal of the offending drug and management of the underlying infection or autoimmune process. The role of corticosteroids in limiting the inflammatory process is controversial, but early use (within 7 to 14 days) may decrease the duration of AIN and protect kidney function. When indicated, the usual approach includes high-dose intravenous methylprednisolone (250 mg consecutively for 3 days), followed by oral prednisone (1 mg/kg) tapering over 4 to 6 weeks. Patients who are intolerant or resistant

常见的非肾小球肾脏疾病

郑华 译　叶文玲　王玉 审校　李雪梅 通审

引言

肾脏的非肾小球结构包括血管、肾小管和肾间质。肾小管间质部分占肾脏实质的80%，其中大部分由肾小管、肾间质细胞、细胞外基质和组织间液组成。尽管原发性肾小球和血管疾病常伴有显著的肾小管间质改变，但临床主要表现为肾小球和肾血管损伤，分别于第4章和第6章中讨论。

原发性肾小管间质疾病以肾小管和间质的结构和功能异常为主要特征，因主要受累的结构不同，呈现出多种临床表现：急性肾小管间质性肾炎，以突然起病、肾功能快速下降为特征；慢性肾小管间质性肾病的临床病程更呈慢性化；囊肿性肾病则以肾囊肿和肾衰竭为特点；肾结石则表现为疼痛、血尿，有时出现急性肾损伤（AKI）。本章将介绍原发性肾小管间质疾病。

急性间质性肾炎

定义、流行病学和病理学

急性间质性肾炎（AIN），也称为肾小管间质性肾炎，以肾脏间质的炎症和水肿为特征；肾小球和血管则无明显异常。AIN表现为肾功能的急性快速下降，是AKI的常见原因。AIN占肾活检病例的1%～3%，但在临床怀疑AIN的AKI患者中，15%～27%的活检结果为AIN。

在大体检查中，肾脏呈现苍白且肿胀之态。组织学上，AIN的特征性表现为间质水肿和炎症细胞浸润，包括淋巴细胞、单核细胞、浆细胞、嗜酸性粒细胞和巨噬细胞。间质炎症可以在7～10天内进展为纤维化改变。免疫荧光检查通常没有阳性发现。在部分药物诱导的肾小管间质性肾炎、IgG4相关性肾炎、膜性肾病、膜增生性肾小球肾炎、狼疮性肾炎、干燥综合征和其他自身免疫性疾病相关的AIN病例中，肾小管基底膜可见免疫复合物沉积。

任何药物都可能引起AIN，但常用的治疗药物需要特别关注。AIN的常见原因见表5.1。常见药物包括抗生素、别嘌呤醇、美沙拉嗪、非甾体抗炎药（NSAID）、质子泵抑制剂和化疗药物。AIN的其他原因还有感染、自身免疫性疾病、肾小管间质性肾炎-葡萄膜炎综合征、蛇咬伤和草药。用于癌症治疗的新型生物制剂的肾毒性也越来越被人们所认识（见表5.1），其中一些药物的肾毒性与AIN相关。在许多这样的病例中，肾小管间质炎症的基础是自身免疫，而非药物敏感。

临床表现

在大多数案例中，AIN患者在接触致病因素几天内出现肾功能的快速下降。但在有些情况下，也可于接触致病因素几周后发生。AIN特征性的临床表现包括皮疹、发热和嗜酸性粒细胞增多。可能同时出现轻度蛋白尿（通常 < 1 g/d）或血尿，少尿则不常见。由于这些特征性表现可能不出现，因此诊断时需高度存疑。

诊断和鉴别诊断

评估近期肾功能快速下降的患者时，如果患者接触过已知的致病因素并具有典型的临床表现，需考虑AIN的诊断。除了血清肌酐水平升高外，尿常规分析可检测到白细胞、红细胞和白细胞管型等AIN特征性的表现。使用Hansel或Wright染色在尿液中发现嗜酸性粒细胞高度提示AIN，但没有嗜酸性粒细胞也并不排除AIN。此外，尿液中的嗜酸性粒细胞也见于其他疾病，包括胆固醇栓塞、泌尿道感染、寄生虫疾病和肾小球肾炎。

遗憾的是，目前没有可靠的诊断药物诱导的AIN的无创检查。当诊断不清时，应考虑进行肾活检。肾小管损伤外的其他组织学特征可能提示AIN相关的潜在疾病。IgG4相关AIN存在肾小管基底膜的免疫复合物沉积和间质中IgG4阳性浆细胞的增加。结节病相关的AIN可能在活检中发现肉芽肿，与系统性红斑狼疮（SLE）相关的AIN免疫荧光检查可能表现为弥漫的免疫复合物沉积。虽然临床表现高度符合时，多数情况下不一定需要进行肾活检，但只有肾活检才能明确诊断AIN。

治疗和预后

AIN的治疗包括停用致病药物，治疗潜在的感染或自身免疫性疾病。皮质类固醇控制炎症的作用尚有争议，但早期使用（7～14天内）可能缩短AIN的病程，并起到保护肾功能的作用。通常的方案为静脉应用大剂量甲泼尼龙（250 mg连续3天），序贯口服泼尼松（1 mg/kg），并在4～6周内逐步减量。激素不耐受

TABLE 5.1	Causes of Acute Interstitial Nephritis
Cause	Examples
Antibiotics	Penicillin
	Cephalosporin
	Sulfa drugs
	Ciprofloxacin
	Rifampin
Nonsteroidal anti-inflammatory drugs	Naproxen
	Ibuprofen
	Diclofenac
	Celecoxib
Diuretics	Thiazides
	Furosemide
	Triamterene
Other drugs	Cimetidine
	Proton pump inhibitors
	Phenytoin
	Allopurinol
Chemotherapeutic agents	Ifosfamide
	Interferon
	Sorafenib
	Sunitinib
	Adriamycin
	Ipilimumab
	Carboplatin
	Bevacizumab
Systemic infections	Legionnaires disease
	Leptospirosis
	Streptococcal infection
	Cytomegalovirus infection
Primary kidney infections	Acute bacterial pyelonephritis
Autoimmune disorders	Sarcoidosis
	Sjögren syndrome

TABLE 5.2	Clinical Findings That Suggest Chronic Interstitial Nephritis
Hyperchloremic metabolic acidosis (out of proportion to the degree of kidney injury)
Hyperkalemia (out of proportion to the degree of kidney injury)
Reduced maximal urinary concentrating ability (e.g., polyuria, nocturia)
Partial or complete Fanconi syndrome (e.g., phosphaturia, bicarbonaturia, aminoaciduria, uricosuria, glycosuria)
Modest proteinuria (<2 g/day)
Anemia
Hypertension

to steroids may benefit from mycophenolate mofetil (500 to 1000 mg twice daily).

Most cases of drug-related AIN resolve after removal of the offending drug. In tubulointerstitial nephritis and uveitis syndrome, both the ocular and kidney changes respond to a brief course of corticosteroids, but the disease can relapse. The overall prognosis depends on the duration of the AIN; a longer interval between onset of AIN and drug withdrawal can lead to irreversible kidney damage. Because of the rapid transformation of interstitial cellular infiltrates into fibrosis, up to 40% of patients may not fully recover baseline kidney function, and about 10% of the patients may become dialysis dependent.

CHRONIC INTERSTITIAL NEPHRITIS

Chronic interstitial nephritis (CIN) is a clinicopathologic diagnosis. Prolonged exposure to a causative agent initiates an indolent inflammatory process, and CIN can lead to permanent kidney damage over months to years before it manifests clinically. Patients usually have a gradual decline in kidney function. CIN is common and accounts for 15% to 30% of all cases of end-stage renal disease (ESRD).

Pathology

Histologically, CIN shows tubular atrophy, flattened epithelial cells, tubule dilation, interstitial fibrosis, and areas of mononuclear cell infiltration within the interstitial compartment. The infiltrates are typically less conspicuous compared with AIN, and there is more interstitial fibrosis. In earlier stages of CIN, glomeruli are usually spared, but with progression, glomerular abnormalities such as segmental and global sclerosis can develop.

Clinical Presentation and Laboratory Findings

Patients with CIN are usually asymptomatic until they develop overt chronic kidney disease (CKD). The features are nonspecific and include fatigue, lack of appetite, nausea, vomiting, hypertension, and sleep disturbances, and other laboratory and clinical findings may develop, as listed in Table 5.2. CIN can also cause proximal or distal tubular dysfunction, which can lead to defects in acidification of the urine, partial or complete Fanconi syndrome and decreased concentrating ability. Laboratory data for these patients may show elevated levels of creatinine, proteinuria, hematuria, glycosuria, and pyuria. Due to the destruction of erythropoietin-producing interstitial cells, anemia, associated fatigue, and decreased exercise tolerance are common as CIN progresses.

Diagnosis and Differential Diagnosis

The histologic findings of CIN are nonspecific, and the differential diagnosis can be extensive, as shown in Table 5.3. Repeated injuries from drugs, toxins, radiation nephritis, and reflux nephropathy can result in a similar histologic picture. The most common cause of CIN is chronic NSAID use. Other causes include infections, immune-mediated disorders, drug reactions, hematologic disorders, chronic urinary tract obstruction, and urinary reflux. Some metabolic disorders and exposure to heavy metals can also lead to CIN. The clinical importance, distinguishing features, causes, and management of several forms of CIN are discussed in the following sections.

Analgesic Nephropathy

Analgesic nephropathy is the prototype CIN, and it occurs commonly worldwide. This disorder is caused by long-term ingestion of aspirin in various combinations with phenacetin, caffeine, or acetaminophen. In its most severe form, analgesic nephropathy is associated with papillary necrosis.

The cumulative amount of phenacetin-acetaminophen combination required to cause CIN is estimated to be at least 2 to 3 kg. Although initially thought to be exclusively associated with phenacetin-containing combinations, all analgesics, including acetaminophen, aspirin, and NSAIDs, are capable of inducing CIN.

Analgesic nephropathy is most commonly detected in women in the sixth and seventh decades of life. Patients with analgesic nephropathy may have elevated serum creatinine, modest proteinuria, sterile pyuria, and anemia. Occasionally, patients develop flank pain and gross hematuria, suggesting papillary necrosis. Diagnosis is supported

表 5.1 急性间质性肾炎的病因	
病因	举例
抗生素	青霉素
	头孢菌素
	磺胺类药物
	环丙沙星
	利福平
非甾体抗炎药	萘普生
	布洛芬
	双氯芬酸
	塞来昔布
利尿剂	噻嗪类
	呋塞米
	氨苯蝶啶
其他药物	西咪替丁
	质子泵抑制剂
	苯妥英
	别嘌呤醇
化疗药物	异环磷酰胺
	干扰素
	索拉非尼
	舒尼替尼
	阿霉素
	伊匹木单抗
	卡铂
	贝伐珠单抗
全身感染	军团病
	钩端螺旋体病
	链球菌感染
	巨细胞病毒感染
肾脏原发感染	急性细菌性肾盂肾炎
自身免疫性疾病	结节病
	干燥综合征

表 5.2 提示慢性肾小管间质性肾炎的临床表现
与肾脏损伤程度不匹配的高氯性代谢性酸中毒
与肾脏损伤程度不匹配的高钾血症
尿液最大浓缩能力下降（如多尿、夜尿）
部分或完全的范科尼综合征（如高磷酸盐尿、高碳酸氢盐尿、氨基酸尿、高尿酸尿、糖尿）
轻度蛋白尿（< 2 g/d）
贫血
高血压

或抵抗的患者使用吗替麦考酚酯（500～1000 mg，每天两次）可能获益。

大多数药物相关的 AIN 在停用致病药物后病情缓解。在肾小管间质性肾炎-葡萄膜炎综合征中，短期皮质类固醇治疗对眼部和肾脏病变有效，但疾病可能会复发。总体预后取决于 AIN 的持续时间；AIN 发病与停药之间的时间间隔越长，越可能导致不可逆的肾脏损伤。由于间质炎症细胞浸润向纤维化的快速转变，高达 40% 的患者可能无法完全恢复至基线肾功能，大约 10% 的患者可能需要长期透析。

慢性间质性肾炎

慢性间质性肾炎（CIN）是一种临床病理诊断。长期接触致病因子会引发慢性的炎症过程，CIN 可在临床表现出现之前进展数月至数年，并导致永久性肾脏损伤。患者肾功能通常逐渐下降。CIN 很常见，占所有终末期肾病（ESRD）病例的 15%～30%。

病理学

组织学上，CIN 表现为肾小管萎缩、上皮细胞扁平、肾小管扩张、间质纤维化和单个核细胞浸润。与 AIN 相比，细胞浸润通常不太显著，间质纤维化更为明显。在 CIN 早期阶段，肾小球一般无明显异常，但随着病情进展，会逐渐出现肾小球病变，如节段性和球性硬化。

临床表现和实验室结果

CIN 患者在发展为明显的慢性肾脏病（CKD）之前通常无明显症状。临床表现缺乏特异性，包括疲劳、纳差、恶心、呕吐、高血压和睡眠紊乱，以及其他实验室和临床表现（表 5.2）。CIN 还可能导致近端或远端肾小管功能障碍，导致尿液酸化不足、部分或完全范科尼综合征以及尿浓缩能力下降。实验室检查表现为肌酐升高、蛋白尿、血尿、糖尿和脓尿。由于产生促红细胞生成素的间质细胞遭受损伤，随着 CIN 进展，贫血以及由此产生的疲劳和运动耐量降低很常见。

诊断和鉴别诊断

CIN 的病理表现缺乏特异性，因此需要与其进行鉴别诊断的疾病范围广泛，如表 5.3 所示，药物、毒素、放射性肾炎和反流性肾病的反复损伤均可产生类似的病理表现。长期使用非甾体抗炎药是 CIN 最为常见的病因，其他原因包括感染、免疫介导疾病、药物反应、血液病、慢性尿路梗阻和尿路反流。一些代谢性疾病和重金属暴露也可能导致 CIN。下文将讨论几种重要 CIN 的临床特征、病因和治疗。

镇痛剂肾病

镇痛剂肾病是 CIN 的经典类型，为全球范围的常见疾病。该病是因长期服用阿司匹林与非那西丁、咖啡因或对乙酰氨基酚的各种药物组合而引起的。最严重的表现为肾乳头坏死。

引起 CIN 所需的非那西丁-对乙酰氨基酚复合制剂的累积用量估计至少为 2～3 kg。尽管最初认为 CIN 仅与含非那西丁的药物有关，但后来发现所有的镇痛剂，包括对乙酰氨基酚、阿司匹林和非甾体抗炎药，都能引起 CIN。

镇痛剂肾病最常见于六、七十岁的女性。患有镇痛剂肾病的患者可能有血清肌酐升高、轻度蛋白尿、无菌性脓尿和贫血。偶尔，患者出现侧腹疼痛和肉眼血尿，提示肾乳头坏死。大量镇痛剂的服用史

TABLE 5.3 Conditions Associated With Chronic Interstitial Nephritis	
Associated Conditions	Examples
Hereditary diseases	Karyomegalic interstitial nephritis
Metabolic disturbances	Hypercalcemia, nephrocalcinosis
	Hyperuricemia
	Hyperoxaluria
	Hypokalemia
	Cystinosis
Drugs and toxins	Analgesics, nonsteroidal anti-inflammatory drugs
	Lead
	Nitrosoureas
	Cisplatin
	Calcineurin inhibitors
	Lithium
	Chinese herbs
	Olanzapine
Immune-mediated diseases	Granulomatosis with polyangiitis (Wegener's granulomatosis)
	Sjögren syndrome
	Systemic lupus erythematosus
	Vasculitis
	Sarcoidosis
	Crohn's disease
Hematologic disease or malignancy	Multiple myeloma
	Sickle cell disease
	Lymphoma
Infection	Chronic pyelonephritis
	Xanthogranulomatous pyelonephritis
	Hepatitis
	Epstein-Barr virus
	HIV
Obstruction	Tumors
	Stones
	Bladder outlet obstruction
	Vesicoureteral reflux
Miscellaneous disorders	Mesoamerican nephropathy
	Radiation nephritis
	Hypertensive arterionephrosclerosis
	Renal ischemic disease

by a history of heavy analgesic use, and computed tomography (CT) may reveal microcalcifications at the papillary tips.

Treatment of analgesic nephropathy is supportive and includes discontinuation of analgesic use. Long-term follow-up studies are characterized by progression to ESRD requiring renal replacement therapies. A high incidence of uroepithelial cancers is also observed in patients with long-term analgesic use.

Chinese Herb Nephropathy and Balkan Endemic Nephropathy

Chinese herb nephropathy (CHN) and Balkan endemic nephropathy (BEN), also called *aristolochic acid nephropathy* (AAN), are chronic tubulointerstitial kidney diseases associated with urothelial carcinoma. The clinical expression and pathologic lesions observed at different stages of CHN and BEN are strikingly similar except for the higher prevalence of CHN among women and familial clustering of BEN. Both have been linked to exposure to the nephrotoxin and carcinogen aristolochic acid. It has been suggested that the terms *CHN* and *BEN* should be abandoned and replaced by the term *AAN*.

Aristolochic acid is a major component of *Aristolochia*-containing herbal remedies and is commonly prescribed in China and other Asian countries. AAN was first reported in 1993 in Belgium in young women taking aristolochic acid–containing Chinese herbs for weight reduction, and the finding has been confirmed by many others. BEN was described 50 years ago in farming villages in the Balkan area, where there is dietary exposure to aristolochic acid through the contamination of flour prepared from locally grown wheat.

Unique features of AAN include clustering of the cases among adults in endemic areas and close association with upper urinary tract carcinomas. About 50% of the affected patients develop transitional cell carcinomas; aristolochic acid induces DNA damage with a distinct molecular signature. Unfortunately, no effective specific treatment for AAN is available. Management is supportive with regular monitoring for urothelial malignancy.

Heavy Metals

Heavy metals such as cadmium, lead, and chromium can cause CIN, and exposure usually represents an environmental toxin. Cadmium exposure occurs with tobacco smoke and contaminated water and food. Lead exposure occurs from contact with lead-based paint and lead-contaminated dust and soil. Chromium is used to increase the hardness and corrosion resistance of alloy steel, and chromium exposure can occur when industrial plant employees work with alloy steels, dyes, paints, inks, and plastics. Proximal tubules are the principal site of accumulation and injury, but other nephron segments also can be injured.

Heavy metal nephrotoxicity ranges from mild tubular dysfunction to advanced CKD. The extent of kidney damage depends on the nature, dose, route, and duration of exposure. With chronic exposure, changes consistent with CIN are observed on kidney biopsy. The best-characterized clinical feature of heavy metal kidney toxicity is the Fanconi syndrome, which results from proximal tubule damage. These patients have low-molecular-weight proteinuria, aminoaciduria, bicarbonaturia, glycosuria, and phosphaturia. Other clinical findings of lead toxicity include gout from decreased urate excretion in proximal tubules, hemolytic anemia, encephalopathy, and neuropathy.

Other than supportive care, no specific treatment is available for heavy metal–associated kidney disease. Chelating agents may be used in acute poisoning, but no randomized clinical trials have proved the efficacy of chelation on clinical outcomes.

Sarcoidosis

Sarcoidosis is a chronic, multisystem, inflammatory disease of unknown origin. It is characterized by noncaseating, epithelioid granulomas in affected organs, leading to organ dysfunction. The severity and diversity of the clinical manifestations related to sarcoidosis depend on the extent of the infiltrating granulomatous lesions. Granulomatous tubulointerstitial nephritis is observed in approximately 20% of patients with sarcoidosis and responds well to steroid therapy. Sarcoidosis is described in details elsewhere.

Corticosteroid therapy is effective in the acute setting and in advanced tubulointerstitial nephritis. Treatment includes prednisone (1 mg/kg/day) for 6 to 12 weeks followed by taper. Some patients with granulomatous tubulointerstitial nephritis may require long-term treatment with steroids to preserve kidney function, although the side effects of steroids limit their use in advanced kidney disease. The efficacy of corticosteroid-sparing agents such as mycophenolate mofetil or azathioprine for sarcoid-related interstitial nephritis requires further investigation.

Radiation Nephritis

Radiation exposure is a significant cause of CKD, and radiation nephritis develops in most patients if they are exposed to more than

表5.3 与慢性间质性肾炎相关的疾病

相关疾病	举例
遗传性疾病	巨核性间质性肾炎
代谢性异常	高钙血症，肾钙沉着症
	高尿酸血症
	高草酸尿症
	低钾血症
	胱氨酸病
药物和毒物	镇痛剂，非甾体抗炎药
	铅
	亚硝基脲类
	顺铂
	钙调磷酸酶抑制剂
	锂
	中草药
	奥氮平
免疫介导疾病	肉芽肿性多血管炎（韦格纳肉芽肿病）
	干燥综合征
	系统性红斑狼疮
	血管炎
	结节病
	克罗恩病
血液系统疾病或肿瘤	多发性骨髓瘤
	镰状细胞病
	淋巴瘤
感染	慢性肾盂肾炎
	黄色肉芽肿性肾盂肾炎
	肝炎
	EB病毒
	HIV
梗阻	肿瘤
	结石
	膀胱出口梗阻
	膀胱输尿管反流
其他	中美洲肾病
	放射性肾炎
	高血压肾小动脉硬化
	肾缺血性疾病

支持该诊断，计算机断层成像可能会显示肾乳头尖端微钙化灶。

镇痛剂肾病的治疗主要是支持治疗，包括停止使用镇痛剂。本病长期随访研究的特点是进展至需要肾脏替代治疗的ESRD。长期服用镇痛剂的患者尿路上皮癌发生率也升高。

中草药肾病和巴尔干地方性肾病

中草药肾病（CHN）和巴尔干地方性肾病（BEN），又称马兜铃酸肾病（AAN），是与尿路上皮癌相关的慢性肾小管间质性疾病。除了CHN在女性中的患病率更高，而BEN有家族聚集性外，这两个疾病不同阶段的临床表现和病理损伤极为相似。两者都与接触具有肾毒性和致癌作用的马兜铃酸有关。有建议称，应放弃使用CHN和BEN这两个术语，改用AAN。

马兜铃酸是含有马兜铃属植物的草药疗法的主要成分，在中国和其他亚洲国家普遍使用。1993年，比利时首次报告了AAN，为一例因减肥而服用含有马兜铃酸的中草药的年轻女性。此后有更多报道证实了此病。BEN是50年前于巴尔干农村发现报道的，人们因食用被马兜铃酸污染的小麦面粉而致病。

AAN具有在流行地区的成人聚集患病以及与上尿路癌密切相关的特点，大约50%的患者罹患移行细胞癌。马兜铃酸会诱导具有独特分子特征的DNA损伤。遗憾的是，目前没有针对AAN的有效疗法，主要是支持性治疗，并对尿路上皮癌进行定期监测。

重金属

镉、铅和铬等重金属可以引起慢性间质性肾炎，一般以环境毒素的形式接触。镉暴露发生在接触烟草烟雾和受污染的水及食物的人群。铅暴露见于接触含铅油漆和被铅污染的土壤灰尘的人群。铬用于增加合金钢的硬度和耐腐蚀性，因此，铬暴露发生于生产合金钢、染料、油漆、墨水和塑料的工厂工人中。近曲小管是毒物积累和损伤的主要部位，但肾单位的其他节段也可能受损。

重金属的肾毒性表现从轻度的肾小管功能障碍到晚期CKD均可见到，取决于毒物的性质、剂量、摄入途径和暴露时间。在慢性暴露中，肾活检可观察到和CIN一样的病变。重金属肾毒性最典型的临床表现是近曲肾小管损伤所致的范科尼综合征，包括低分子量蛋白尿、氨基酸尿、高碳酸氢盐尿、糖尿和高磷酸盐尿。铅毒性尚有因近曲肾小管尿酸排泄减少导致的痛风、溶血性贫血、脑病和神经病变等其他临床表现。

除了支持性治疗，没有针对重金属相关肾病的特殊治疗。急性中毒可使用螯合剂，但没有随机临床试验证明螯合剂对临床预后具有改善作用。

结节病

结节病是一种原因不明的慢性、多系统、炎症性疾病，特征为受累器官中非干酪性、上皮样肉芽肿，导致器官功能障碍。结节病相关临床表现的严重程度和多样性取决于肉芽肿性病变的浸润程度。大约20%的结节病患者存在肉芽肿性肾小管间质性肾炎，对糖皮质激素治疗反应良好。结节病的详细描述参见其他章节。

皮质类固醇治疗对急性期和晚期肾小管间质性肾炎均有效。治疗包括泼尼松[1 mg/（kg·d）]治疗6~12周，然后逐渐减量。一些肉芽肿性肾小管间质性肾炎患者可能需要长期应用糖皮质激素以维持肾功能，但类固醇的副作用限制其在晚期肾病中的使用。糖皮质激素的替代方案，如吗替麦考酚酯或硫唑嘌呤，对结节病相关间质性肾炎的疗效需要进一步研究。

放射性肾炎

辐射暴露是CKD的重要原因，如患者接受超过

23 Gy. Ionizing radiation directly damages all molecules, including DNA, and initiates cellular synthesis of reactive oxygen species, which cause secondary tissue damage. Hydroxyl radicals are generated within milliseconds of tissue exposure. Oxidative stress and other factors may play additional roles over time, and patients may develop severe kidney injury and impaired function 6 to 12 months (or longer) after exposure. Histopathologically, early and late changes can be seen that include cell swelling, mesangiolysis, variable tubular injury, tubular atrophy, glomerular scarring, and increased mesangial matrix.

The diagnosis is usually based on a history of radiation exposure and the clinical findings of kidney injury. Treatment is supportive.

Sickle Cell Disease

CKD is relatively common in patients with sickle cell disease, an inherited hematologic disorder characterized by hemolytic anemia and vascular occlusion by sickled red cells. Under normal conditions, the renal medullary zone is characterized by low oxygen tension, acidic pH, and high osmolality, which can predispose to increased blood viscosity and red blood cell sickling. This increases the likelihood of local ischemia and infarction of the kidney microcirculation. In the vasa recta, vascular occlusion can interfere with the countercurrent exchange system in the inner medulla, resulting in a defect in the urine-concentrating mechanism.

Patients may have nocturia or polyuria and can develop gross hematuria due to papillary necrosis resulting from medullary ischemia and infarction. The sloughed papillae can obstruct urinary tract outflow, leading to obstructive nephropathy and kidney failure. Another abnormality associated with sickle cell disease is proteinuria, a consequence of glomerular hyperfiltration that results from reduction in nephron mass.

The treatment of sickle cell nephropathy focuses on primary management of the hematologic disorder. Tubular dysfunction may require potassium and bicarbonate supplementation to treat hypokalemia and acidosis, and those with ESRD are treated with dialysis and renal transplantation.

Lithium

Lithium is a monovalent cation, which is freely filtered through the glomeruli. Up to 80% of filtered lithium is reabsorbed in the proximal tubule, and a small fraction is reabsorbed in the distal nephron through the epithelial sodium channel (E_{NaC}). Lithium causes dysregulation of the aquaporin water channel and E_{NaC} expression in the cortical collecting duct. The most common manifestation of kidney disease associated with lithium is CIN manifesting as a chronic, insidious decline in kidney function. The course of kidney disease after discontinuation of lithium is highly unpredictable, with no reliable clinical clues to identify those destined for recovery or progression.

Lithium also is associated with nephrogenic diabetes insipidus, which can occur in up to 40% of patients as early as 8 weeks after lithium initiation. Other tubular dysfunctions associated with lithium include water diuresis, natriuresis, and metabolic acidosis. Lithium-associated nephrogenic diabetes insipidus can be treated with E_{NaC} blockade by amiloride.

Mesoamerican Nephropathy

Mesoamerican nephropathy, now formally designated as CKD of nontraditional causes, is an emerging form of progressive CKD identified in the last two decades. It is primarily seen in agricultural workers (usually in sugarcane or cotton plantations) in Central America. A similar nonproteinuric CKD has been described in South Asia and Sri Lanka as well. The most significant risk factor is prolonged, strenuous physical labor in hot and humid climates. Other risk factors include male gender, low body mass, consumption of high-fructose beverages, exposure to heavy metals from soil, nephrotoxins or NSAIDs and infectious diseases such as leptospirosis and hantavirus infections. Pesticide exposure alone does not appear to increase risk. Pathogenesis is not yet clearly understood; however, current hypothesis suggests that repeat episodes of heat stress and dehydration lead to activation of renin-angiotensin-aldosterone system, vasopressin and polyol-fructokinase pathway causing increased oxidative stress and recurrent AKI, eventually leading to tubulointerstitial nephritis. Moreover, heat exposure and consequent dehydration can enhance tubular reabsorption of toxins and potentially enhance toxin-mediated kidney injury. Furthermore, heat exposure can result in heat stroke or low grade rhabdomyolysis that can exacerbate kidney injury.

Patients are usually young or middle-aged men, normotensive, have minimal edema, and may describe symptoms of dysuria or nocturia. Laboratory data are notable for elevated creatinine, hypokalemia, hypomagnesemia, hyperuricemia, and urinalysis is often unremarkable with no hematuria and minimal (if any) proteinuria. Abdominal ultrasound shows small kidneys with cortical thinning. Diagnosis requires appropriate clinical context and kidney biopsy. Histologic features show tubulointerstitial damage, glomerulosclerosis, and chronic glomerular ischemia. Treatment is supportive and further efforts should be directed to preventing disease progression.

Urinary Tract Obstruction

Urinary tract obstruction is a common cause of AKI and CKD. When kidney function is normal at baseline, unilateral or partial obstruction anywhere along the urinary tract may be asymptomatic, with no discernable change in kidney function or urine output. Bilateral urinary tract obstruction, however, can lead to acute and chronic kidney injury and ESRD. It is important to address this possibility early in the clinical course of unexplained kidney injury or uremia.

Obstruction to urine flow causes an increase in ureteral intraluminal pressure. Over time, nephron tubules are injured, and the resulting changes in thromboxane A_2 and angiotensin levels decrease renal blood flow. Tubular damage leads to urinary concentrating defects, renal tubular acidosis (RTA), and hyperkalemia. If complete obstruction is not relieved, ischemia and nephron loss decrease the glomerular filtration rate.

Common causes of obstructive nephropathy are shown in Table 5.4. Among elderly men, benign prostatic hypertrophy is of particular concern. Overall, the clinical presentation depends on the cause, site, and time course of obstruction. Patients with obstructive nephropathy may present with decreased urine output associated with suprapubic pain (i.e., bladder distention from ureteral obstruction), renal colic (i.e., nephrolithiasis), urinary tract infections, fever, AKI, hypertension, and hematuria. Pain resulting from stretching of the urinary collecting system is the most common presenting symptom. Acute ureteral obstruction usually results in severe flank pain that typically radiates to the groin and is referred to as *renal colic*. Patients with complete bladder outlet obstruction develop AKI and anuria. Patients with incomplete or intermittent bladder outlet obstruction have urinary hesitancy, dribbling, urgency, decreased urine stream, nocturia, and polyuria. These patients are usually pain free. Tubular injury from obstruction causes decreased urinary concentrating capability leading to polyuria.

The physical examination should include palpation of the kidney and bladder, as well as a rectal, pelvic, and prostate assessment. The patient may have an enlarged and palpable bladder, enlarged prostate, costovertebral tenderness, groin pain, hypertension, or gross hematuria. The mainstays of the initial evaluation include measurement of the postvoid residual volume of the bladder (>125 mL is considered

23 Gy 的辐射，大多数会出现放射性肾炎。电离辐射直接损伤包括 DNA 在内的所有分子，并促进细胞内活性氧合成，造成继发性组织损伤。羟基自由基在组织暴露于辐射后数毫秒内产生。随时间的推移，氧化应激和其他因素可能发挥额外作用，患者可能在受到辐射后的 6～12 个月（或更长时间）内出现严重的肾脏损伤和功能受损。组织病理学上可见到细胞肿胀、系膜溶解、不同程度的肾小管损伤、肾小管萎缩、肾小球瘢痕形成，以及系膜基质增加等早期和晚期改变。

诊断通常基于辐射暴露史和肾脏损伤的临床表现。治疗为对症支持。

镰状细胞病

CKD 在镰状细胞病患者中相对常见。镰状细胞病是一种以溶血性贫血和镰状红细胞引起的血管阻塞为特征的遗传性血液病。正常情况下，肾髓质区具有氧分压低、酸性 pH 值和高渗透压的特点，其对血液黏度增加和镰状红细胞更为敏感。这增加了肾脏微循环局部缺血和梗死的可能性。在肾直小血管中，血管阻塞可能干扰内髓部的逆流交换系统，导致尿液浓缩机制缺陷。

患者可能有夜尿或多尿，并且可能因髓质缺血和梗死导致的肾乳头坏死出现肉眼血尿。脱落的肾乳头会阻塞尿路，引起梗阻性肾病和肾衰竭。与镰状细胞病相关的另一种异常表现是蛋白尿，这是因肾单位减少导致肾小球高滤过的结果。

镰状细胞肾病的治疗主要是针对血液原发病的治疗。肾小管功能障碍可能需要补充钾和碳酸氢盐以纠正低钾血症和酸中毒，ESRD 患者需要透析和肾脏移植治疗。

锂

锂是一种单价阳离子，可以自由地从肾小球滤过。高达 80% 的滤过的锂在近曲肾小管中被重吸收，一小部分通过上皮钠通道（$E_{Na}C$）在远端肾单位被重吸收。锂引起皮质集合管中的水通道蛋白和 $E_{Na}C$ 表达失调。与锂相关的肾脏疾病最常见的表现是慢性间质性肾炎，表现为慢性、隐匿性肾功能下降。停用锂后的肾脏情况很难预测，没有可靠的临床线索来判定患者可能恢复或进展。

锂还与肾源性尿崩症相关，高达 40% 的患者使用锂后发生尿崩症，最早于使用后 8 周发病。其他与锂相关的肾小管功能障碍包括水钠排泄增加和代谢性酸中毒。锂相关的肾源性尿崩症可以用阿米洛利阻断 $E_{Na}C$ 来治疗。

中美洲肾病

中美洲肾病是近二十年来发现的一种新的进展性 CKD，现已被正式命名为非传统原因的 CKD。主要见于中美洲的农业工人（通常在甘蔗或棉花种植园工作）。南亚和斯里兰卡也有类似的非蛋白尿性 CKD 报道。最重要的危险因素是在炎热潮湿的气候中长时间从事繁重的体力劳动。其他危险因素包括男性、低体重、饮用高果糖饮料、接触土壤中的重金属、使用肾毒性药物或非甾体抗炎药，以及钩端螺旋体病和汉坦病毒感染等传染病。仅接触杀虫剂似乎不会增加患病风险。其发病机制尚未完全清楚。目前的学说认为，反复的热应激和脱水可能导致肾素-血管紧张素-醛固酮系统、血管加压素和多聚果糖激酶通路的激活，引起氧化应激增加和反复发作的 AKI，最终导致肾小管间质性肾炎。此外，热暴露和随之而来的脱水会增强肾小管对毒素的重吸收，可能加重毒素介导的肾脏损伤。热暴露可导致中暑或轻度横纹肌溶解，从而加剧肾脏损伤。

患者通常是年轻或中年男性，血压正常，水肿轻微，可能有排尿困难或夜尿症状。实验室检查显示血肌酐升高、低钾血症、低镁血症、高尿酸血症，而尿常规通常无异常，无血尿，蛋白尿极少（如果有的话）。腹部超声显示肾脏缩小，皮质变薄。诊断需要相符的临床背景和肾脏活检结果。病理特征包括肾小管间质损伤、肾小球硬化和慢性肾小球缺血。治疗为支持性的，重点是努力防止疾病进展。

尿路梗阻

尿路梗阻是引起 AKI 和 CKD 的常见原因。当基线肾功能正常时，泌尿道任何部位的单侧或部分梗阻可能并无症状，也无肾功能或尿量的明显变化。然而，双侧尿路梗阻可导致急/慢性肾脏损伤和 ESRD。在遇到不明原因的肾功能异常或尿毒症时尽早关注有无梗阻的可能性非常重要。

尿路梗阻导致输尿管腔内压力增加。随病程的进展，肾小管受损，引起血栓素 A2 和血管紧张素水平变化，减少肾血流量。肾小管损伤导致尿液浓缩障碍、肾小管酸中毒（RTA）和高钾血症。如果完全性梗阻不能解除，缺血和肾单位损失会降低肾小球滤过率。

梗阻性肾病的常见原因见表 5.4。在老年男性中，良性前列腺增生需要特别关注。总体而言，临床表现取决于梗阻的原因、部位和程度。梗阻性肾病患者可能出现尿量减少伴耻骨上疼痛（因尿道梗阻导致的膀胱膨胀）（译者注：原文因输尿管梗阻导致的膀胱膨胀有误）、肾绞痛（因肾结石所致）、尿路感染、发热、AKI、高血压和血尿。尿路集合系统牵拉产生的疼痛是最常见的临床表现。急性输尿管梗阻通常导致严重的腰痛，这种疼痛通常会放射至腹股沟，被称为肾绞痛。膀胱出口完全梗阻的患者会发生急性肾损伤和无尿。不完全或间歇性膀胱出口梗阻的患者可有尿等待、尿滴沥、尿急、尿流变细、夜尿和多尿。这些患者通常无明显疼痛。梗阻引起的肾小管损伤引起尿液浓缩能力下降，造成多尿。

体格检查应包括肾脏和膀胱的触诊，以及直肠、盆腔和前列腺评估。患者可能有可触及的扩张的膀胱、前列腺增大、肋脊角压痛、腹股沟疼痛、高血压或肉眼血尿。初步评估的主要内容包括测量膀胱排尿后残余尿量（一般认为 > 125 ml 有意义，可能提示梗阻），

TABLE 5.4 Causes of Urinary Obstruction

Cause	Examples
Congenital urinary tract malformation	Meatal stenosis
	Ureterocele
	Posterior urethral valves
	Urethral atresia
	Phimosis
	Megaureter–prune belly syndrome
Intraluminal obstruction (urethra and bladder outlet)	Phimosis
	Urethral strictures
	Benign prostate hyperplasia
	Pelvic tumor
	Anticholinergic drugs
	Neurogenic bladder
	Tuberculosis
	Radiation
	Trauma
	Calculi
	Blood clots
	Papillary necrosis (sickle cell disease, diabetes mellitus)
Extrinsic compression	Pelvic tumors
	Prostatic hypertrophy
	Retroperitoneal fibrosis or tumors
Acquired anomalies	Urethral strictures
	Neurogenic bladder
	Intratubular precipitates
	Bladder mass or stones

significant and may indicate obstruction) and ultrasound or CT scan of kidneys and urinary tract to evaluate the kidneys, ureters, and bladder for distention or other abnormalities.

The initial goals of therapy are to manage volume status, electrolyte abnormalities, infection, and other complications of obstructive nephropathy and to relieve the obstruction as soon as possible to prevent further damage to the kidney parenchyma. If urinary obstruction is suspected, a catheter should be placed in the bladder to address possible bladder outlet obstruction. If a large postvoid residual volume (>125 mL) is detected, the urinary catheter should remain in place while the cause is ascertained. Occasionally, relief of obstruction is associated with a large postobstructive diuresis that may be sufficient in degree to cause volume depletion and hypotension.

If the obstruction is acute, complete recovery of kidney function can be expected. If the anatomic site of the urinary tract obstruction is above the bladder, more sophisticated approaches to drainage (e.g., percutaneous nephrostomy tube placement) may be required to relieve obstruction.

CYSTIC KIDNEY DISEASES

Kidney cysts are fluid-filled tubular structures lined by a polarized epithelium. They result from defects in the structure and function of renal tubular epithelial cells. Kidney cysts can be solitary or multiple, simple or complex. Cystic kidney disease can be developmental, hereditary or acquired that develops in patients with CKD. Cystic diseases can be localized to kidneys or have systemic manifestations. Depending on the underlying cause of cysts, age of presentation can vary from prenatal to later in life. Cystic kidney diseases are also important causes of ESRD.

Several cellular and molecular mechanisms involved in cystogenesis have been uncovered in recent years.

Simple Cysts

Simple cysts are most common. Widespread use of ultrasonography and CT has resulted in frequent detection of kidney cysts. They are usually unilateral, solitary, well-defined structures, but they can be multiple and bilateral. They tend to be more common among older adults and are often benign, incidental findings on radiographic imaging. Sonography reveals a thin-walled, fluid-filled cavity with no septations or calcifications. The diameter varies between 0.5 and 1.0 cm, but a few may be as large as 3 to 4 cm in diameter.

Diagnosis: Simple cysts are usually asymptomatic but occasionally may result in a palpable abdominal mass, infection, back pain, or hematuria. Differentiation of simple cysts from cysts associated with genetic disorders is based on the cystic pattern, age at detection, and family history.

Treatment: In the absence of symptoms, no treatment is required for simple cysts. If the kidney cyst becomes infected, causes pain, or leads to renin-mediated hypertension, percutaneous drainage is often the first step in further evaluation and management.

Complex Cysts

Differentiation of simple from complex cysts is usually made radiographically. When in doubt, histologic examination is required to exclude malignancy, but imaging is sensitive and specific, and it suffices in most cases. The distinction between complex and simple cysts is important in monitoring the need for intervention because simple cysts are usually benign, whereas complex cysts have a higher risk of malignancy and other complications. In a simple cyst, complications such as hemorrhage or infection can result in the development of features of more complex cysts, including calcification, septa, irregular borders, and multilobularity.

Initial evaluation of kidney cyst includes ultrasonography and, if ultrasound is equivocal, triphasic CT is done to characterize the cyst. If the characteristics of a cyst in terms of size, nodularity, mural enhancement, or septations change over time, the likelihood of malignancy increases.

To help with diagnosis and management, the Bosniak classification of kidney cysts was introduced in 1986 and has been revised since then. This classification, which includes four categories with several important subcategories, based on triphasic CT findings, is described in Table 5.5. Category I and category II cysts are benign. Category II F cysts have a range of reported malignancy rates of 0 to 38% so requires follow-up. The risk increases to almost 50% for category III cysts. Category III and IV renal cysts are considered to be renal carcinoma unless proven otherwise, and they are usually surgically resected. While the current Bosniak classification of kidney cysts predicts likelihood of cancer, it does not assess the aggressiveness of the tumor. With the technological innovations and advancement of knowledge, new proposal for further revision of Bosniak classification was made in 2019.

Acquired Cystic Kidney Disease in CKD

Acquired cystic kidney disease (ACKD) is a disease consequent from long-term CKD. It is defined by three or more cysts per kidney in a patient with CKD or ESRD. The prevalence of ACKD increases with the duration of dialysis, reaching 87% after 10 years of dialysis. Patients of male gender, older age, with history of heart disease, larger kidneys, and kidney calcifications are more likely to develop ACKD.

表 5.4 尿路梗阻的病因	
病因	举例
先天尿路畸形	尿路狭窄
	输尿管囊肿
	后尿道瓣膜
	尿道闭锁
	包皮过长
	巨输尿管-梅干腹综合征
腔内梗阻（尿道和膀胱出口）	包皮过长
	尿道狭窄
	良性前列腺增生
	盆腔肿瘤
	抗胆碱能药物
	神经源性膀胱
	结核
	辐射
	创伤
	结石
	血凝块
	肾乳头坏死（镰状细胞病、糖尿病）
腔外压迫	盆腔肿瘤
	前列腺肥大
	腹膜后纤维化或肿瘤
获得性原因	尿道狭窄
	神经源性膀胱
	肾小管管型
	膀胱肿物或结石

以及泌尿系统的超声检查或 CT 扫描，以评估肾脏、输尿管和膀胱是否有扩张或其他异常。

治疗的初步目标是尽快解除梗阻以防止肾实质进一步受损，同时控制容量状态、电解质异常、感染以及梗阻性肾病的其他并发症。如果怀疑存在尿路梗阻，应在膀胱内放置导尿管以解决可能存在的膀胱出口梗阻。如果存在大量残余尿（> 125 ml），在明确原因的同时应继续留置导尿管。少数情况下，解除梗阻后可能出现梗阻后大量利尿，其程度可能会引起容量不足和低血压。

如果梗阻是急性的，肾功能预期可以完全恢复。如果尿路梗阻的解剖部位位于膀胱以上，则可能需要更复杂的引流方法（如经皮肾造瘘）来解除梗阻。

囊肿性肾病

肾囊肿是由极化的上皮细胞包围形成的充满液体的管状结构。它们由肾小管上皮细胞的结构和功能缺陷导致。肾囊肿可以为单发或多发，简单或复杂。囊肿性肾病可以是发育性的、遗传性的，或者是 CKD 患者后天形成的。囊肿性疾病可以仅发生于肾脏，也可以有全身表现。根据囊肿的潜在病因，发病年龄可以从出生前到晚年不等。囊肿性肾病也是 ESRD 的重要原因。

近年来，已经发现了一些参与囊肿形成的细胞和分子机制。

单纯性囊肿

单纯性囊肿最为常见。超声和 CT 的广泛应用使肾囊肿的检出更为频繁。通常是单侧、孤立、边界清楚的结构，但也可能呈多发和双侧分布。肾囊肿在老年人中更为常见，通常是影像学检查中偶然发现，为良性病变。超声上表现为一个薄壁、充满液体、没有分隔或钙化的空腔。直径一般为 0.5～1.0 cm，但有些可达 3～4 cm。

诊断：单纯性囊肿通常是无症状的，但偶尔可表现为可触及的腹部肿块、感染、背痛或血尿。单纯性囊肿与遗传相关的囊肿的鉴别点在于囊肿的分布形式、发现时的年龄和家族史。

治疗：如果没有症状，不需要对单纯性囊肿进行治疗。如果肾囊肿发生感染、疼痛或导致肾素介导的高血压，经皮引流通常是进一步评估和治疗的第一步。

复杂性囊肿

单纯性和复杂性囊肿通常通过放射影像学检查来鉴别。如有疑问，需要进行组织学检查以排除恶性肿瘤，但影像学检查敏感而特异，可满足大多数病例的需要。鉴别复杂性囊肿和单纯性囊肿对于监测是否需要干预非常重要，因为单纯性囊肿通常是良性的，而复杂性囊肿发生恶性肿瘤和其他并发症的风险较高。在单纯性囊肿中，出血或感染等并发症会导致出现包括钙化、分隔、边界不规则和多叶等更复杂的囊肿的特征。

肾囊肿的初步评估包括超声检查，如果超声检查无法确定，则进行增强 CT 检查以确定囊肿的特征。如果囊肿在大小、结节性、囊壁增强或分隔等特征上出现随时间的变化，则恶变的可能性增加。

1986 年引入并于此后进行了修订的 Bosniak 肾囊肿分类法可用于帮助诊断和治疗。该分类根据三相 CT 表现，将囊肿分为 4 个类别和几个重要亚类（表 5.5）。Ⅰ类和Ⅱ类囊肿为良性。ⅡF 类囊肿报告的恶变率从 0% 到 38% 不等，需要定期随访。Ⅲ类囊肿的恶性风险几乎增加到 50%。Ⅲ类和Ⅳ类囊肿被认为是肾癌，除非另有证明为非恶性病变，通常需手术切除。虽然当前的 Bosniak 肾囊肿分类可预测癌症的可能性，但不能评估肿瘤的侵袭性。随着技术革新和知识的进步，2019 年提出了进一步修订 Bosniak 分类的新建议。

CKD 中的获得性囊性肾病

获得性囊性肾病（ACKD）是一种由长期 CKD 引起的疾病，定义为在 CKD 或 ESRD 患者中，每个肾脏有 3 个或更多的囊肿。ACKD 的患病率随着透析时间的延长而增加，透析 10 年后达到 87%。男性、年龄较大、有心脏病史、肾脏较大和肾脏钙化的患者更有可能发生 ACKD。

TABLE 5.5 Bosniak Renal Cyst Classification Scheme

Category	Description
I. Simple cyst	A benign simple cyst with a thin wall and no septa, calcifications, or solid components.
II. Minimally complicated	A benign cystic lesion with a few thin septa. The wall or septa may contain fine calcifications or short segment of a slightly thickened calcification. (This category also includes uniformly high-attenuating lesions that are less than 3 cm in diameter, well marginated, and nonenhancing.)
IIF. Complicated	Well-marginated cysts but more complicated than category II. They have multiple thin septa or minimal smooth thickening of the septa or wall and may contain calcifications that may be thick and nodular. (This category also includes totally intrarenal, nonenhancing high-attenuating lesions that are more than 3 cm in diameter.)
III. Indeterminate	Indeterminate cystic masses that have thickened, irregular, or smooth walls or septa. These lesions are enhancing on computed tomography. Between 40% and 60% of lesions are malignant (e.g., cystic renal cell carcinoma, multiloculated cystic renal cell carcinoma). The remaining lesions are hemorrhagic, chronic, infected cysts or multiloculated cystic nephroma and are benign.
IV. Malignancy	On computed tomography, they have characteristics of category III cysts and contain enhancing soft tissue components that are adjacent to and independent of the wall or septum on the cyst. Between 85% and 100% of lesions are malignant; evaluation and surgical excision are recommended.

Neither the cause of the underlying ESRD nor the mode of dialysis influences the progression of ACKD. It has been postulated that damage to the kidney parenchyma in CKD increases local growth factors levels that promote hypertrophy and cyst generation in the remaining nephrons. In some cases, increased levels of growth factors and mutated genes (e.g., *ERBB2*) may cause the malignant transformation of cysts, the primary clinical concern in 3% to 7% of ACKD patients.

ACKD-related cyst formation is limited to the kidneys and is an incidental finding on radiographic imaging. Patients with ACKD are usually asymptomatic but may develop infectious or bleeding complications. ACKD can be differentiated from hereditary causes of cystic renal disease by presence of CKD or ESRD and the absence of any other clinical findings.

Patients with ACKD do not require specific treatment. Cysts are managed based on the Bosniak category as discussed in the section on renal cell carcinoma (RCC). Routine screening for ACKD among dialysis patients is contentious but is recommended for patients during their pretransplantation evaluation. Kidney transplant recipients with ACKD should get yearly kidney ultrasound because of higher risk of malignancy due to exposure to immunosuppression and longer life expectancy.

TABLE 5.6 Extrarenal Manifestations of ADPKD

Organ Involved	Manifestations
Liver	Polycystic liver disease
Brain	Intracranial aneurysms
Vascular	Thoracic aortic dissection
	Coronary artery aneurysm
Cardiac	Valvular heart disease
	Mitral valve prolapse and regurgitation
	Tricuspid valve prolapse and regurgitation
Other	Pancreatic cyst
	Seminal vesicle cyst
	Colonic and duodenal diverticula

Hereditary Cystic Kidney Diseases

The most common inherited cystic kidney diseases are the polycystic kidney diseases (PKDs), including autosomal dominant and autosomal recessive forms of PKD. Other hereditary cystic renal diseases include autosomal dominant tubulointerstitial kidney disease, Von Hippel–Lindau disease (VHLD), and tuberous sclerosis. In the inherited disorders, several mutations have been associated with cyst formation. In PKD, the cysts are not connected to the urinary drainage system, and cellular secretion results in cyst enlargement. Mutation of any of the tubular epithelial–related genes such as *PKD1*, *PKD2*, and mucin-1 *(MUC1)* can result in disruption of normal ciliary function, resulting in cyst formation from over-proliferation of tubular epithelium and increased fluid secretion.

Polycystic Kidney Disease

PKD consists of two main form of monogenetic cystic kidney disease: autosomal dominant polycystic kidney disease (ADPKD) and autosomal recessive polycystic kidney disease (ARPKD). Patients with PKD develop multiple fluid-filled cysts in both kidneys and sometimes in other organs as well. Cysts usually form in the distal segment of the nephron and collecting ducts from outgrowths of kidney epithelial cells, abnormal fluid secretion, and altered cell-matrix interaction. Once the cysts are formed, they detach from the tubules and progressively increase in size, compressing nearby nephrons, interstitium, and vessels. Injury to adjacent kidney structures leads to inflammation and fibrosis.

Autosomal Dominant Polycystic Kidney Disease

Definition and epidemiology. ADPKD is the most common cause of cystic renal disease and an important cause of ESRD. The monogenetic, progressive disorder is characterized by multiple cysts in kidneys and other organs, including the liver and pancreas. The incidence of ADPKD is 1 case in 400 to 1000 live births, and between 300,000 and 600,000 Americans are affected by the disease.

Pathology and pathogenesis. Mutations in the *PKD1* and *PKD2* genes are responsible for about 85% and 15% of ADPKD cases, respectively, and there is evidence for important modifier genes. *PKD1* is located on chromosome 14 and encodes the protein polycystin 1 (PC1), which functions as a membrane receptor. *PKD2* is located on chromosome 4 and encodes polycystin 2 (PC2), which functions as a calcium-permeable cation channel. PC1 and PC2 regulate intracellular calcium homeostasis and signaling pathways involved in tubular morphogenesis and cell-cell interactions. PC1 and PC2 also are integral membrane proteins of cilia, including the primary cilia of renal tubular cells. ADPKD is now classified under the new class of diseases called *ciliopathies*. In addition to renal tubules, PC1 and PC2 proteins are found in diverse cell types, including bile ducts, endothelial cells, and neurons. Consequently, ADPKD patients with mutated PC1 or PC2 proteins often have extrarenal manifestations (Table 5.6).

表 5.5	Bosniak 肾囊肿分类法
分类	描述
Ⅰ. 单纯性囊肿	良性的单纯性囊肿，壁薄，无分隔、钙化或实质性成分。
Ⅱ. 轻度复杂性囊肿	良性囊性病变，有少量薄分隔，囊壁或分隔可能有细小钙化灶或一小段轻度增厚的钙化。（这类囊肿还包括直径小于 3 cm、边界清晰且无增强的均匀高衰减病变。）
ⅡF. 复杂性囊肿	边缘清晰的囊肿，但比Ⅱ类更复杂。有多个薄的分隔，或轻度平滑增厚的分隔或囊壁，可能含有增厚和结节状的钙化。（这一类还包括完全处于肾内且直径超过 3 cm 的无增强高衰减病变。）
Ⅲ. 性质待定的囊肿	囊壁或分隔增厚、不规则或平滑的性质不确定的囊性肿块。这些病变在 CT 检查中会增强。大约 40%～60% 的病变是恶性的（如囊性肾细胞癌、多房囊性肾细胞癌）。其余病变为出血性、慢性、感染性囊肿或多房性囊性肾瘤，均为良性。
Ⅳ. 恶性囊肿	在 CT 上具有Ⅲ类囊肿的特征，并且伴有邻近且独立于囊壁或分隔的增强软组织成分。85%～100% 的病变为恶性；建议进行评估和手术切除。

ESRD 的病因或透析的方式均不影响 ACKD 的进展。推测 CKD 中肾实质的损伤增加了局部生长因子水平，这促进了剩余肾单位的肥大和囊肿生成。在某些情况下，生长因子水平的增加和基因突变（如 ERBB2）可能会导致囊肿的恶变，这是 3%～7% 的 ACKD 患者的主要临床问题。

ACKD 相关的囊肿形成局限于肾脏，在影像学检查中偶然发现。ACKD 患者通常无症状，但可能出现感染或出血并发症。ACKD 具有 CKD 或 ESRD 病史，且无其他临床表现，这是它和遗传性囊肿性肾病的鉴别点。

ACKD 不需要特殊治疗。囊肿根据 Bosniak 肾囊肿分类法进行管理，详见肾细胞癌（RCC）部分内容。对在透析患者中进行 ACKD 常规筛查存在争议，但建议在移植前进行评估。有 ACKD 的肾脏移植受者由于长期处于免疫抑制状态且预期寿命较长，恶性肿瘤风险增加，建议每年进行肾脏超声检查。

遗传性囊肿性肾病

最常见的遗传性囊肿性肾病是多囊肾病（PKD），包括常染色体显性和常染色体隐性遗传 PKD。其他遗传性囊肿性肾病包括常染色体显性肾小管间质肾病、希佩尔-林道病（VHLD）和结节性硬化症。在遗传性疾病中，已经发现几种基因突变与囊肿形成有关。在 PKD 中，囊肿不与尿路相通，细胞分泌液导致囊肿不断增大。任何与肾小管上皮相关的基因突变，如 PKD1、PKD2 和黏蛋白-1 基因（MUC1），都可能使纤毛丧失正常功能，引起肾小管上皮的过度增殖和液体分泌增加，导致囊肿形成。

多囊肾病

PKD 包含两种主要的单基因囊肿性肾病：常染色体显性遗传多囊肾病（ADPKD）和常染色体隐性遗传多囊肾病（ARPKD）。PKD 患者双肾会出现多个充满液体的囊肿，有时囊肿也出现在其他器官。囊肿通常由于肾脏上皮细胞的过度生长、液体分泌异常，以及细胞基质间相互作用改变，在肾单位远段和集合管形

表 5.6	ADPKD 的肾外表现
受累器官	表现
肝脏	多囊肝
大脑	颅内动脉瘤
血管	胸主动脉夹层 冠状动脉动脉瘤
心脏	心脏瓣膜病 二尖瓣脱垂和反流 三尖瓣脱垂和反流
其他	胰腺囊肿 精囊囊肿 结肠及十二指肠憩室

成。囊肿一旦形成，就会与肾小管分离并逐渐增大，压迫附近的肾单位、肾间质和血管。对邻近肾脏结构的损伤导致炎症和纤维化。

常染色体显性遗传多囊肾病

定义和流行病学 ADPKD 是囊肿性肾病的最常见原因，也是 ESRD 的重要原因。此病为一种单基因、进展性疾病，以肾脏和其他器官（包括肝脏和胰腺）的多发囊肿为特征。ADPKD 的发病率为每 400～1000 例活产婴儿中有 1 例。大约有 30 万到 60 万美国人罹患该病。

病理学和发病机制 PKD1 和 PKD2 基因的突变分别占 ADPKD 病例的 85% 和 15%，并且有证据提示存在重要的修饰基因。PKD1 位于 14 号染色体，编码蛋白多囊素 1（PC1），PC1 作为膜受体发挥作用。PKD2 位于 4 号染色体，编码蛋白多囊素 2（PC2），PC2 作为钙通透性阳离子通道发挥作用。PC1 和 PC2 调节细胞内钙稳态以及参与肾小管生发及细胞间相互作用的信号通路。PC1 和 PC2 也是纤毛（包括肾小管细胞初级纤毛）的完整膜蛋白。ADPKD 现在被归类为纤毛性疾病这一新的疾病类别。除肾小管外，PC1 和 PC2 蛋白还存在于包括胆管、内皮细胞和神经元等多种细胞类型中。因此，携带 PC1 或 PC2 蛋白突变的 ADPKD 患者通常有肾外表现（表 5.6）。

TABLE 5.7	Ultrasonography Criteria of ADPKD
Age	Number of Cysts
Positive family history	
<30 years	≥2 unilateral or bilateral
30-39 years	≥3 cysts unilateral or bilateral
40-59 years	≥2 cysts in each kidney
>60 years	≥4 cysts in each kidney
No family history	
16-40 years	>10 cysts in each kidney

In the kidney, increase in cyst size and number over time damages adjacent renal architecture and causes CKD and renin-mediated hypertension. Total kidney volume increases continuously and is associated with progressive decline of kidney function. Higher rates of kidney enlargement are associated with a more rapid decrease in kidney function.

Clinical presentation. ADPKD is a multisystem disease. The clinical presentation may range from no symptoms to an array of systemic manifestations, including polycystic liver disease, which is detected in about 80% of adults. Cardiac valvular abnormalities and cerebral aneurysms are key noncystic features of ADPKD, and familial clustering of cases occurs. Cerebral aneurysms are observed in about 8% of patients with ADPKD, but the incidence increases to 20% among those with a positive family history of cerebral aneurysm or subarachnoid hemorrhage. ADPKD patients, with positive family history of cerebral aneurysm or sudden death of unknown cause, should be screened for cerebral aneurysm.

Most patients with ADPKD develop cysts before the age of 30, but CKD can be delayed to beyond the fourth decade. Patients with the *PKD2* mutation have later onset and slower progression of the disease than patients with the *PKD1* mutation. Kidney survival associated with *PKD2* mutations is about 20 years longer than that associated with *PKD1* mutations. Besides the cysts, other kidney manifestations of APKD include urinary concentrating defects, hypertension, and nephrolithiasis. Twenty percent of patients with ADPKD can develop uric acid and calcium oxalate nephrolithiasis and may have renal colic, obstructive nephropathy, or urinary tract infection.

Diagnosis. ADPKD is usually diagnosed by imaging of the kidneys. The finding of three or more cysts (unilateral or bilateral) in those younger than age 30, two or more cysts in each kidney in those between 40 and 59 years of age, and four or more cysts in each kidney in patients older than 60 years is sufficient to make diagnosis of ADPKD (Table 5.7). Absence of more than two cysts in individuals older than 40 years of age makes ADPKD very unlikely. Genetic testing is usually not required for an individual with a positive family history if other diagnostic criteria for ADPKD are met, but other family members should be screened with ultrasound of kidneys.

Treatment. Total kidney volume correlates with disease manifestation of PKD. No specific treatment is available to prevent the growth of kidney or liver cysts. Tolvaptan, a vasopressin receptor 2 inhibitor, has been recently approved to slow progression of kidney disease in PKD. Given the high cost and side effect profile of the drug, it should only be given to select patients with ADPKD who will likely benefit most from it. Due to hepatotoxicity, use of tolvaptan requires close monitoring of liver enzymes. Other interventions include enhanced hydration; maintenance of healthy weight; decrease in sodium, protein, and caffeine intake; and treatment of hypertension and dyslipidemia, which may delay the progression of renal disease. Renin-mediated hypertension is a common complication of ADPKD, and it contributes to an increased incidence of cardiovascular mortality and faster progression to ESRD. The main and most effective therapy remains control of hypertension by angiotensin-converting enzyme inhibitors or angiotensin-receptor blockers to achieve a target blood pressure of less than 125/75 mm Hg. Dual blockade with angiotensin-converting enzyme inhibitors and angiotensin-receptor blockers does not provide any additional benefit and increases risk of hyperkalemia.

Renal cyst enlargement can cause pain, and cysts can be complicated by infection or bleeding that warrants specific intervention. Surgical decompression is usually reserved for patients who fail conservative management. If ESRD occurs, patients are treated with renal replacement therapy, including dialysis and kidney transplantation. Preemptive management of intracranial aneurysms is important but controversial.

Prognosis. The time of onset and rate of progression of ADPKD varies from patient to patient, even within the same family. Risk factors for progressive CKD include increases in kidney cyst volume, a *PKD1* gene mutation, and uncontrolled hypertension. Other risk factors include male gender, diagnosis of ADPKD before 30 years of age, hypertension before 35 years of age, concurrent diabetes mellitus, and hematuria. About 45% of the patients with ADPKD develop ESRD by 60 years of age, but they have a better prognosis than patients with ESRD from other causes.

Autosomal Recessive Polycystic Kidney

Definition and epidemiology. ARPKD also is classified under the ciliopathies. ARPKD is characterized by diffuse dilation of the collecting ducts and congenital hepatic fibrosis. The estimated incidence of ARPKD is 1 case in 20,000 live births.

Pathogenesis. Mutations in *HNF1B* and the polycystic kidney and hepatic disease 1 gene *(PKHD1)* are responsible for ARPKD. *PKHD1* is a large gene located on chromosome 6. More than 300 mutations have been identified at different loci of the *PKHD1* gene. Fibrocystin (i.e., polyductin) is the product of *PKHD1* and is expressed in the primary cilia of the thick ascending limb, in cortical and medullary ducts in the kidney, and in hepatic bile ducts. It has an important role in the terminal differentiation of kidney and biliary ductules.

Clinical presentation. ARPKD, phenotypically, is highly variable. Patients with ARPKD may be diagnosed at different ages, but those with a more severe phenotype present in utero or at birth because they develop enlarged kidneys, oligohydramnios, pulmonary hypoplasia, Potter facies (flattened nose, recessed chin, epicanthal folds, and low-set ears), and deformities of the spine and limb. Neonates usually have kidney enlargement and kidney failure, and older patients have liver disease, including portal hypertension, hepatosplenomegaly, variceal bleeding, and hepatic fibrosis.

Differential diagnosis. The initial diagnosis is usually suspected on the basis of kidney imaging with antenatal or infantile ultrasound. Abdominal ultrasound shows bilateral enlarged kidneys with multiple cysts. Fetal imaging shows oligohydramnios, pulmonary hypoplasia, and Potter syndrome. Although molecular diagnostic analysis is the gold standard for diagnosing ARPKD, it is difficult to perform due to the high level of heterogeneity of the *PKHD1* gene.

Treatment and prognosis. No treatment is available for ARPKD, and genetic testing is usually not performed outside of research scenarios. Most deaths occur in utero or at the time of birth, and of those with ARPKD who survive birth, 20% to 30% die within the first year of life. Neonates have more kidney manifestations, and older patients have more liver disease manifesting as portal hypertension, hepatosplenomegaly, and bleeding esophageal or gastric varices. The likelihood of patients being alive without ESRD increases with older age at presentation due to their more benign phenotypes. Due to autosomal recessive inheritance, recurrence risk of ARPKD in subsequent pregnancies of parents of an ARPKD child is 25%.

表 5.7 ADPKD 超声诊断标准	
年龄	囊肿数量
阳性家族史	
<30 岁	单侧或双侧≥3（译者注：原文≥2 有误）
30～39 岁	单侧或双侧≥3
40～59 岁	每侧≥2
>60 岁	每侧≥4
无家族史	
16～40 岁	每侧>10

译者注：原表右列内容位置有误。

在肾脏中，囊肿大小和数量随时间的推移而增加，损害邻近的肾脏结构，导致 CKD 和肾素介导的高血压。肾脏总体积持续增加，肾功能随之逐渐下降。肾脏增大的速度越快，肾功能下降的速度也越快。

临床表现 ADPKD 是一种多系统疾病。临床表现从无症状到一系列系统表现不等，包括多囊肝，可在约 80% 的成年人中检测出。心脏瓣膜异常和脑动脉瘤是 ADPKD 的主要的非囊肿性特征，病例有家族聚集性。约 8% 的 ADPKD 患者有脑动脉瘤，但在有脑动脉瘤或蛛网膜下腔出血家族史的患者中，发病率增加到 20%。有脑动脉瘤或不明原因猝死家族史的 ADPKD 患者应进行脑动脉瘤筛查。

大多数 ADPKD 患者在 30 岁之前出现囊肿，但 CKD 可延迟至 40 岁后发生。携带 PKD2 突变的患者比携带 PKD1 突变的患者发病时间晚，疾病进展慢。PKD2 突变患者的肾脏存活期比 PKD1 突变者长约 20 年。除囊肿外，ADPKD（译者注：原文 APKD 有误）的其他肾脏表现包括尿液浓缩障碍、高血压和肾结石。20% 的 ADPKD 患者可出现尿酸结石和草酸钙结石，可发生肾绞痛、梗阻性肾病或尿路感染。

诊断 ADPKD 主要依靠肾脏影像学检查诊断。40 岁以下（译者注：原文 30 岁以下有误）个体中发现 3 个或更多囊肿（单侧或双侧），40～59 岁个体每侧肾脏发现 2 个或更多囊肿，以及 60 岁以上患者每侧肾脏发现 4 个或更多囊肿，足以诊断 ADPKD（表 5.7）。40 岁以上个体少于 2 个以上的囊肿，则 ADPKD 的可能性非常小。有阳性家族史的患者如满足其他 ADPKD 的诊断标准，通常不需要进行基因检测，但其他家庭成员应该进行肾脏超声筛查。

治疗 肾脏总体积与 PKD 的疾病表现相关。目前没有防止肾脏或肝脏囊肿生长的特异性治疗方法。抗利尿激素受体 2 抑制剂托伐普坦近期被批准用于减缓 PKD 中肾脏疾病的进展。鉴于药物的高成本和副作用，应仅将其用于可能从中受益最大的 ADPKD 患者。由于有肝毒性，使用托伐普坦需要密切监测肝酶。其他干预措施包括加强水化，保持健康体重，减少钠、蛋白质和咖啡因的摄入，以及治疗高血压和血脂异常，可能延缓肾脏病的进展。肾素介导的高血压是 ADPKD 的常见并发症，可增加心血管疾病死亡率和加速 ESRD 进展。主要和最有效的治疗方法仍然是通过血管紧张素转换酶抑制剂或血管紧张素受体阻滞剂来控制高血压，以达到低于 125/75 mmHg 的目标血压。同时应用血管紧张素转换酶抑制剂和血管紧张素受体阻滞剂的双重阻断不会产生任何额外的好处，并会增加高钾血症的风险。

肾囊肿增大可引起疼痛，囊肿如发生感染或出血，需要特殊干预。外科减压通常只针对保守治疗失败的患者。如果发生 ESRD，患者需接受肾脏替代治疗，包括透析和肾脏移植。颅内动脉瘤的预防性治疗很重要，但存在争议。

预后 ADPKD 的发病时间和进展速度因人而异，即使在同一家族中也是如此。进展性 CKD 的风险因素包括肾囊肿体积、PKD1 基因突变和未控制的高血压。其他风险因素包括男性、30 岁前诊断 ADPKD、35 岁前高血压、合并糖尿病以及血尿。大约 45% 的 ADPKD 患者在 60 岁前发展为 ESRD，但他们的预后比其他病因的 ESRD 患者好。

常染色体隐性遗传多囊肾病

定义和流行病学 ARPKD 也属于纤毛病，以集合管弥漫性扩张和先天性肝脏纤维化为特征。ARPKD 的发病率估计为每 2 万例活产中有 1 例。

发病机制 HNF1B 和多囊肾病及肝脏疾病 1（PKHD1）基因的突变是 ARPKD 的原因。PKHD1 是一个位于 6 号染色体上的大基因。目前已经发现 300 多种 PKHD1 基因不同位点的突变。纤维囊蛋白（即多管蛋白）是 PKHD1 的产物，表达于肾小管升支粗段的初级纤毛、肾脏皮层和髓质集合管以及肝胆管。它在肾脏和胆管的末端分化中起着重要作用。

临床表现 ARPKD 在表型上高度可变。可能在不同年龄发病，但那些更严重的表型在胎儿或出生时就可出现，表现为肾脏增大、羊水过少、肺发育不全、波特综合征（扁平鼻、下巴后缩、内眦赘皮和低位耳朵），以及脊柱和四肢畸形。新生儿通常有肾脏增大和肾衰竭，而年长患者有肝脏疾病，包括门静脉高压、肝脾大、静脉曲张出血和肝纤维化。

鉴别诊断 初步诊断通常基于产前或婴儿期的肾脏超声。腹部超声显示双侧肾脏增大伴多个囊肿。胎儿超声显示羊水过少、肺发育不全和波特（Potter）综合征。尽管分子诊断是诊断 ARPKD 的金标准，但由于 PKHD1 基因的高度异质性，实施较为困难。

治疗和预后 目前没有治疗 ARPKD 的方法，如果不是进行研究通常也不进行基因检测。大多数个体胎死宫内或出生时夭折，20%～30% 的 ARPKD 幸存患者在出生后 1 年内死亡。新生儿有更多的肾脏表现，而年长的患者有更多肝脏疾病表现，包括门静脉高压、肝脾大，以及食管或胃静脉曲张出血。由于起病越晚的患者表型越为良性，无 ESRD 生存的可能性越高。由于此病是常染色体隐性遗传，ARPKD 患儿的父母再次妊娠时 ARPKD 再发风险是 25%。

Juvenile Nephronophthisis and Autosomal Dominant Tubulointerstitial Kidney Disease

Definition and epidemiology. Nephronophthisis (NPHP) and autosomal dominant tubulointerstitial kidney disease (ADTKD) are hereditary forms of cystic kidney disease. Both produce bilateral cysts at the corticomedullary junction of the kidney and are associated with progressive CKD and ESRD. They are clinically and pathologically indistinguishable, and they are separated only by the age of onset and mode of inheritance.

NPHP is an autosomal recessive cystic kidney disease, and the median age of onset of renal disease is 11.5 years. ADTKD has an autosomal dominant pattern of inheritance, and the median age of onset of renal disease is 28.5 years. NPHP is more common than ADTKD and is the most common cause of ESRD in the first 3 decades of life.

Pathogenesis. Several genes are associated with the NPHP and ADTKD phenotypes. Functional defects of any of the proteins associated with these genes can lead to ciliary dysfunction and development of multiple cysts. Mutations in at least three genes—*MUC1*, *REN*, and *UMOD* encoding mucin-1, renin, and uromodulin, respectively—can lead to ADTKD. *UMOD* gene mutation is the most common mutation and patients with this mutation develop gout at an early age along with CKD. NPHP is caused by mutations in at least 20 genes encoding proteins that are associated with cilia, basal bodies, and centromeres. Mutation of *NPHP1* is the most common mutation, reported in approximately 20% of the patients, whereas other mutations contribute to less than 3% each.

Clinical presentation. The three clinical forms of NPHP are based on the onset of ESRD: an infantile form with a median onset at 1 year of age, a juvenile form with a median onset at 13 years of age, and an adolescent form with a median onset at 19 years of age. Some children may present with extrarenal symptoms: retinitis pigmentosa (Senior-Løken syndrome), mental retardation, cerebellar ataxia, bone anomalies, or liver fibrosis. Situs inversus and ventricular cardiac septal defect can also be present in the infantile form of NPHP. In patients with ADTKD, symptoms usually develop in the fourth or fifth decade of life and include hematuria, infection or nephrolithiasis. ESRD develops between the ages of 50 and 70 years.

Differential diagnosis. The diagnosis of NPHP or ADTKD is based mainly on clinical features. Medullary cysts, a low urinary specific gravity, and absence of significant proteinuria may suggest either disease. Genetic testing is available for several gene mutations and can be applied based on the age at presentation. Siblings can be screened by kidney ultrasound and urine concentration test results. Kidney biopsy is usually not indicated because the findings of interstitial fibrosis and tubular atrophy are nonspecific.

Treatment and prognosis. No specific treatment is available for NPHP or ADTKD, and treatment is mainly supportive. The time of onset of ESRD varies between 30 and 60 years, depending on the type of mutation. Sodium supplementation for salt wasting, allopurinol for gout, and dialysis or renal transplantation for ESRD are part of supportive care. NPHP and ADTKD do not recur after renal transplantation.

Medullary Sponge Kidney

Medullary sponge kidney (MSK), also known as Lenarduzzi-Cacchi-Ricci disease, is a relatively uncommon cystic disorder. It usually occurs sporadically, but familial cases have been reported. MSK is characterized by ectasia and cystic dilation of medullary and papillary collecting ducts, resulting in a spongy appearance of the kidney on imaging. MSK is associated with urinary acidification and concentration defects, a high risk of nephrocalcinosis and kidney stones, and a moderate risk of urinary infections and CKD. The prevalence of MSK is 1 case in 5000 persons in the general population, and 15% to 20% of patients with nephrolithiasis have MSK.

No clear genetic basis for MSK has been established. MSK is usually detected between the ages of 30 and 50 years. Most patients with MSK are asymptomatic and may have incidental findings on imaging. The clinical course is benign and is usually not associated with ESRD.

When suspected, CT urography has replaced intravenous urography as the imaging study of choice for the diagnosis of MSK. There is retention of contrast media in renal pyramids and cystic collecting ducts, giving the appearance of blush or diffused linear striations. Nephrocalcinosis is common in patients with MSK but is not required to make the diagnosis of MSK. CT imaging may help in excluding papillary necrosis, ADPKD, obstruction, or pyelonephritis.

TUBEROUS SCLEROSIS

Definition and Epidemiology

Tuberous sclerosis complex (TSC) (i.e., Bourneville disease) is an autosomal dominant genetic disorder that affects adults and children. TSC causes benign tumors to form in multiple organ systems, including the skin, brain, and kidneys. TSC is often characterized by related neurologic disorders such as epilepsy and mental retardation.

The prevalence of TSC in the general population is approximately 1 in 10,000 and 50% to 65% of cases are sporadic. Because TSC has an autosomal dominant pattern of inheritance, there is a 50% risk of siblings being affected. Genetic counseling is important for affected families.

Pathology

TSC is caused by inactivating mutations in the *TSC1* or *TSC2* genes, located on chromosome 9, and chromosome 16, adjacent to the *PKD1* gene, respectively. They, respectively, encode the hamartin and tuberin proteins, which together form a complex that regulates specific cellular growth, motility, and migration of cells. Inactivating mutations of the *TSC1* or *TSC2* genes result in disruption of these processes and may cause unrestricted growth of cells and tumorigenesis.

TSC conveys a lifetime risk of 2% to 3% for RCC. Kidney tumors are usually bilateral and occur at an early age. More commonly, the tumors are benign angiomyolipomas, composed of abnormal, thick-walled vessels, smooth muscle cells, and adipose tissue, seen in about 80% of patients with TSC by the age of 10 years. These benign kidney tumors often require no treatment. However, they can grow, become locally invasive, and cause bleeding, pain, and hypertension.

Conclusive guidelines for surveillance are unavailable, but annual magnetic resonance imaging of kidney and brain lesions is suggested until the age of 21 years and then every 2 to 3 years to monitor their growth. Patients with progressive lesions should have yearly imaging. If the angiomyolipomas become locally invasive or cause bleeding, surgical intervention is needed.

Mutations in the *TSC1* or *TSC2* gene cause constitutive activation of mTOR. Everolimus, an inhibitor of mTOR, has been approved for the treatment of patients with TSC-associated subependymal giant cell astrocytomas, who are not surgical candidates.

VON HIPPEL–LINDAU DISEASE

VHLD is an autosomal dominant disease that affects multiple organ systems. It is caused by germline mutations in *VHL*, a tumor suppressor gene located on chromosome 3. This mutation predisposes to RCC and to tumor formation in other organs, including the eyes, cerebellum, spinal cord, adrenal glands, epididymis, and pancreas. VHLD

少年型肾消耗病和常染色体显性肾小管间质性肾病

定义和流行病学 肾消耗病（NPHP）和常染色体显性肾小管间质性肾病（ADTKD）是遗传性囊肿性肾病。两者都在双侧肾脏的皮髓交界处产生囊肿，表现为进展性CKD和ESRD（译者注：ADTKD并无突出的肾囊肿）。两者在临床和病理上无法区分，只能根据发病年龄和遗传方式来区分。

NPHP是一种常染色体隐性遗传性囊肿性肾病，肾脏疾病的中位发病年龄为11.5岁。ADTKD呈常染色体显性遗传，肾脏疾病的中位发病年龄为28.5岁。NPHP比ADTKD更常见，是30岁前最常见的ESRD原因。

发病机制 一些基因与NPHP和ADTKD表型有关。与这些基因相关的任何蛋白质的功能缺陷都可能导致纤毛功能障碍和发生多发性囊肿（译者注：ADTKD一般无突出的肾囊肿）。至少有三个基因的突变——*MUC1*、*REN*和*UMOD*，分别编码黏蛋白-1、肾素和尿调蛋白，可以导致ADTKD。*UMOD*基因突变最为常见，该基因突变的患者会在年龄较小时出现痛风以及CKD。NPHP是由至少20个基因的突变引起的，这些基因编码与纤毛、基体和中心粒有关的蛋白质。*NPHP1*突变最为常见，约占患者的20%，而其他突变各占不到3%。

临床表现 基于ESRD的发病年龄，NPHP分为三种临床类型：婴儿型，中位发病年龄为1岁；少年型，中位发病年龄为13岁；青少年型，中位发病年龄为19岁。一些儿童可能存在肾外症状：视网膜色素变性（Senior-Løken综合征）、智力发育迟缓、小脑性共济失调、骨骼异常或肝纤维化。婴儿型NPHP也可能存在内脏转位和心脏室间隔缺损。在ADTKD患者中，通常在四五十岁时出现症状，包括血尿、感染或肾结石。ESRD发生在50～70岁之间。

鉴别诊断 NPHP或ADTKD的诊断主要基于临床特征。髓质囊肿、低比重尿和无明显蛋白尿提示这两种疾病可能。基因检测可用于检测几种基因突变，并可根据发病年龄进行检测。可用肾脏超声和尿液浓缩检查对兄弟姐妹进行筛查。通常不建议进行肾活检，因为该病病理表现出的肾间质纤维化和肾小管萎缩不具有特异性。

治疗和预后 NPHP或ADTKD没有特效治疗方法，主要为支持治疗。ESRD的发生时间取决于突变类型，一般发生在30～60岁。支持治疗包括补充钠盐以治疗盐消耗、别嘌呤醇治疗痛风，对ESRD患者进行透析或肾脏移植。NPHP和ADTKD在肾脏移植后不会复发。

髓质海绵肾

髓质海绵肾（MSK），也称为Lenarduzzi-Cacchi-Ricci病，是一种相对少见的囊性疾病。通常散发，但也有家族性病例的报道。MSK的特征是髓质和乳头集合管的扩大和囊性扩张，导致肾脏在影像上呈现海绵状。MSK与尿液酸化和浓缩缺陷、肾钙质沉着症和肾结石的高风险、尿路感染及CKD的中度风险有关。MSK在普通人群中的患病率为每5000人中有1例，15%～20%的肾结石患者有MSK。

尚未确立MSK的明确遗传基础。MSK多在30～50岁之间被发现。大多数MSK患者无症状，可能在影像学检查中偶然发现。临床过程是良性的，通常与ESRD无关。

当怀疑MSK时，CT尿路造影已取代静脉尿路造影，成为MSK诊断的首选影像学检查。肾锥体和囊性集合管会出现造影剂潴留，呈现出刷状（译者注：原文blush应为brush）或弥漫性线状条纹。肾钙质沉着症在MSK患者中很常见，但不是MSK诊断的必要条件。CT成像可能有助于排除肾乳头坏死、ADPKD、梗阻或肾盂肾炎。

结节性硬化症
定义和流行病学

结节性硬化症（TSC）（即Bourneville病）是一种影响成人和儿童的常染色体显性遗传疾病。TSC导致多器官系统形成良性肿瘤，包括皮肤、大脑和肾脏。TSC常以相关的神经系统疾病为特征，如癫痫和智力下降。

TSC在普通人群中的患病率约为1/10 000，50%～65%的病例为散发。因为TSC有常染色体显性遗传模式，兄弟姐妹中患病的风险为50%。遗传咨询对受影响的家庭很重要。

病理学

TSC是由位于9号染色体的*TSC1*或16号染色体的*TSC2*基因的失活突变引起的，后者紧邻*PKD1*基因。它们分别编码错构瘤蛋白（hamartin）和结核菌素蛋白（tuberin），两者形成的复合体调节特定细胞的生长、运动和迁移。*TSC1*或*TSC2*基因的失活突变阻断了调节作用，可能导致细胞的无限制生长和肿瘤形成。

TSC患者一生中发生肾细胞癌的风险为2%～3%。肾脏肿瘤通常为双侧的，且早年发病。更为常见的肿瘤为良性血管平滑肌脂肪瘤，由异常的厚壁血管、平滑肌细胞和脂肪组织组成，约80%的TSC患者在10岁以前就可发生这种肿瘤。这些良性肾脏肿瘤通常不需要治疗。然而，肿瘤可以生长，局部浸润，并引起出血、疼痛和高血压。

尚无明确的监测指南，但建议在21岁之前每年进行肾脏和大脑病变的磁共振成像检查，之后每2～3年进行一次，以监测其生长情况。病变进展的患者应每年进行一次影像学检查。如果血管平滑肌脂肪瘤出现局部浸润或引起出血，需要手术干预。

*TSC1*或*TSC2*基因的突变导致mTOR激活。mTOR抑制剂依维莫司（Everolimus）已获批用于治疗不适合手术的TSC相关室管膜下巨细胞型星形细胞瘤的患者。

希佩尔-林道（Von Hippel-Lindau）病

希佩尔-林道病（VHLD）是一种累及多器官系统的常染色体显性遗传病。它由位于3号染色体上肿瘤抑制基因*VHL*的胚系突变引起。这种突变导致患者易

TABLE 5.8   TNM Staging System of Renal Cell Carcinoma

Primary Tumor (T)

TX	Primary tumor cannot be assessed
T0	No evidence of primary tumor
T1	**Tumor <7 cm and limited to the kidney**
T1a	Tumor <4 cm and limited to the kidney
T1b	Tumor >4 cm but <7 cm and limited to the kidney
T2	**Tumor >7 cm and limited to the kidney**
T2a	Tumor >7 cm but <10 cm and limited to the kidney
T2b	Tumor >10 cm and limited to the kidney
T3	**Tumor extends into major veins or perinephric tissues but not into the ipsilateral adrenal gland and not beyond Gerota fascia**
T3a	Tumor grossly extends into the renal vein or its segmental branches, or tumor invades perirenal and/or renal sinus fat but not beyond Gerota fascia
T3b	Tumor grossly extends into the vena cava below the diaphragm
T3c	Tumor grossly extends into the vena cava above the diaphragm or invades the wall of the vena cava
T4	**Tumor invades beyond Gerota fascia, including contiguous extension into the ipsilateral adrenal gland**

Regional Lymph Nodes (N)

NX	Regional lymph nodes cannot be assessed
N0	No regional lymph node metastasis
N1	Metastasis in regional lymph node(s)

Distant Metastasis (M)

M0	No distant metastasis
M1	Distant Metastasis

Anatomic Stage/Prognosis Groups

Stage	T	N	M
Stage I	T1	N0	M0
Stage II	T2	N0	M0
Stage III	T1 or T2	N1	M0
	T3	N0 or N1	M0
Stage IV	T4	Any N	M0
	Any T	Any N	M1

affects approximately 1 in 40,000 births, and about 7000 patients are affected in the United States. There is an important association with pheochromocytoma in some patients with VHLD that warrants consideration.

RCC occurs in up to 70% of patients with VHLD. It is usually bilateral and the clear cell type. RCC affects younger patients with a mean age at presentation of 26 years. For a high-risk patient, the diagnosis of VHLD is suggested by central nervous system or retinal hemangioblastoma, RCC, or pheochromocytoma. These patients should be referred for detailed assessment. When indicated, genetic testing can be performed to assess possible mutations of the *VHL* gene.

KIDNEY TUMORS

Each year, approximately 74,000 new cases of renal cancer are diagnosed and 15,000 deaths from RCC are reported in the United States. Most cases are sporadic, but there is an association between RCC and VHLD and tuberous sclerosis that has helped to explain the cellular mechanisms involved.

RCC originates from renal epithelial cells and accounts for 85% of renal cancers. Based on histology, the five subtypes are clear cell, papillary (chromophilic), oncocytoma, collecting duct (Bellini duct), and chromophobe RCC. Clear cell carcinoma is the most common subtype and accounts for about 75% to 85% of all cases.

The classic triad of symptoms of flank pain, hematuria, and a palpable flank mass is uncommon (10%). About 50% of cases are identified as a result of an incidental finding on radiographic imaging. Other clinical symptoms are nonspecific and include fatigue, anemia, and weight loss. Paraneoplastic syndromes associated with RCC include erythrocytosis (due to overproduction of erythropoietin), hypercalcemia (due to excess parathyroid hormone–related peptide), hepatic dysfunction (Stauffer syndrome), and cachexia.

The initial diagnosis of RCC is usually made by imaging. Unlike simple cysts, which are anechoic, round, and smooth walled, RCC is more likely to be a septate, irregular, thick-walled mass. When RCC is suspected, additional evaluation by CT urography or magnetic resonance imaging is usually required, along with complete staging and evaluation for metastases (Table 5.8). Biopsy is usually reserved, to confirm the diagnosis for medical treatment, for the patients who are not surgical candidates.

When possible, the primary treatment of localized RCC is surgical resection, which usually includes complete or partial nephrectomy. Locally advanced or metastatic RCC is treated medically with chemotherapy and immunomodulatory therapy with interleukin-2. Newer therapies include tyrosine kinase inhibitor (Sunitinib) and two immune checkpoint inhibitors, nivolumab and ipilimumab.

The prognosis for RCC depends primarily on the clinical stage at the time of presentation as assessed by the tumor-node-metastasis (TNM) criteria. TNM stages I through III have a better prognosis than TNM stage IV (metastatic) RCC. Poor prognostic factors include a lower Karnofsky performance status, elevated lactate dehydrogenase level, low hemoglobin level, and hypercalcemia. With documented

表 5.8 肾细胞癌的 TNM 系统

原发灶（T）	
TX	原发肿瘤无法评估
T0	没有原发肿瘤的迹象
T1	**肿瘤（直径）< 7 cm，局限于肾脏内**
T1a	肿瘤 < 4 cm，局限于肾脏内
T1b	4 cm < 肿瘤 < 7 cm，局限于肾脏内
T2	**肿瘤 > 7 cm，局限于肾脏内**
T2a	7 cm < 肿瘤 < 10 cm 局限于肾脏内
T2b	肿瘤 > 10 cm，局限于肾脏内
T3	**肿瘤侵犯主要的静脉或肾周围组织，但没有突破 Gerota 筋膜或侵犯肾上腺**
T3a	肿瘤侵犯肾静脉或其主要分支，或侵犯肾周和（或）肾窦脂肪，但没有突破 Gerota 筋膜
T3b	肿瘤侵犯腔静脉的膈下部分
T3c	肿瘤侵犯腔静脉的膈上部分或侵犯腔静脉壁
T4	**肿瘤已经扩散到 Gerota 筋膜之外，包括侵犯同侧肾上腺**
局部淋巴结（N）	
NX	局部淋巴结无法评估
N0	无局部淋巴结转移
N1	局部淋巴结转移
远处转移（M）	
M0	无远处转移
M1	存在远处转移

解剖/预后分期			
Ⅰ期	T1	N0	M0
Ⅱ期	T2	N0	M0
Ⅲ期	T1 或 T2	N1	M0
	T3	N0 或 N1	M0
Ⅳ期	T4	任意 N	M0
	任意 T	任意 N	M1

出现肾细胞癌和其他器官（包括眼、小脑、脊髓、肾上腺、附睾和胰腺）的肿瘤形成。VHLD 发病率大约为 1/40 000 例新生儿，美国大约有 7000 例患者。值得注意的是，部分 VHLD 患者会存在嗜铬细胞瘤。

多达 70% 的 VHLD 患者会发生肾细胞癌，通常为双侧透明细胞癌。肾细胞癌患者较年轻，平均发病年龄为 26 岁。对于高危患者，出现中枢神经系统或视网膜血管母细胞瘤、肾细胞癌或嗜铬细胞瘤提示 VHLD 可能。这些患者应接受进一步详细评估，必要时行基因检测评估 VHL 基因可能存在的突变。

肾脏肿瘤

据报道，美国每年大约新诊断 74 000 例肾癌，15 000 例死于肾细胞癌（RCC）。大多数病例是散发的，但 RCC 与 VHLD 和结节性硬化症之间存在关联，这有助于解释相关的细胞机制。

肾细胞癌起源于肾上皮细胞，占肾癌的 85%。根据组织学，可分为五种亚型：透明细胞癌、乳头状癌（嗜色）、嗜酸细胞瘤、集合管肿瘤（Bellini 管）和嫌色细胞癌。透明细胞癌是最常见的亚型，约占所有病例的 75%～85%。

典型三联征：腰痛、血尿和可触及的腰部肿块并不常见（10%）。大约 50% 的病例是在影像学检查时意外发现的。其他临床症状无特异性，包括疲劳、贫血和体重减轻。与肾细胞癌相关的副肿瘤综合征包括红细胞增多症（由于促红细胞生成素过度产生所致）、高钙血症（甲状旁腺激素相关肽产生过多）、肝功能异常（Stauffer 综合征）和恶病质。

肾细胞癌的初步诊断通常通过影像学检查进行。与单纯囊肿的无回声、圆形、壁平滑的特点不同，肾细胞癌更可能是有分隔、不规则、厚壁的肿块。当怀疑肾细胞癌时，通常需进一步行 CT 尿路造影或磁共振成像，并行完整的分期和转移评估（表 5.8）。在不适合手术的患者中，通常选择活检以确诊是否需要进行药物治疗。

局限性肾细胞癌的主要治疗方法是外科切除，通常包括全肾切除或部分肾切除。局部晚期或转移性肾细胞癌的药物治疗包括化疗和使用白细胞介素-2 的免疫调节治疗。较新的治疗方法包括酪氨酸激酶抑制剂（舒尼替尼）和两种免疫检查点抑制剂，纳武利尤单抗（nivolumab）和伊匹木单抗（ipilimumab）。

肾细胞癌的预后主要取决于就诊时基于肿瘤-淋巴结-转移（TNM）标准评估的临床分期。TNM Ⅰ 到 Ⅲ 期的肾细胞癌预后优于 Ⅳ 期（转移性）。预后不良的因素包括更低的卡氏功能状态评分（Karnofsky performance status）、乳酸脱氢酶增高、贫血和高钙血症。明确存在

metastases, the 1-year survival rate is 12% to 71%, and the 3-year survival rate is 0% to 31%, but in the past decade with availability of newer drugs, survival has improved.

NEPHROLITHIASIS

Nephrolithiasis is a major public health problem. It imposes a substantial burden on human health and considerable financial expenditure for the nation. Calcium-containing stones are the most common stones, comprising approximately 80% of all stones. Uric acid, struvite, and cysteine stones are less common, accounting for approximately 9%, 10%, and 1% of all stones, respectively, but have high recurrence rates.

Epidemiology

The prevalence of stones has been substantially increasing. National Health and Nutrition Examination Survey (NHANES) demonstrated an increase in self-reported prevalence of kidney stones in the United States from 3.2% in 1976 to 1980, to 8.8% in 2007 to 2010, to 10.1% in 2014. Moreover, the incidence of kidney stones is also increasing and is estimated to be approximately 0.5% in North America and Europe. Diet and lifestyle factors likely play significant roles in the changing epidemiology.

Nephrolithiasis increases with age. It is more common in men than in women; however, in the last 2 decades, the male to female ratio has changed from 3:1 to about 2:1. Comparison of NHANES data over time showed prevalence of kidney stones was stable in males but increased in females, with the most significant increase noted in females of childbearing age. Epidemiologic studies have noted a relationship between nephrolithiasis and metabolic syndrome, and the magnitudes of this association were greater for women compared with men. This may be one plausible explanation for the increasing incidence of kidney stones among women. The prevalence is higher in Caucasian males, intermediate in Hispanic and Asian males, and less frequent in black males. The highest risk of stone formation has been reported in men in the United Arab Emirates and Saudi Arabia and has been attributed to genetic and environmental factors. Stone recurrence is common with the relapse rate of kidney stones being 50% in 5 to 10 years and 75% in 20 years. Risk factors associated with recurrent stone formation include younger age of onset, positive family history, underlying medical conditions, and urinary infections. The Recurrence of Kidney Stone (ROKS) nomogram provides a clinical tool to estimate the risk of recurrence in first-time symptomatic stone formers. It uses participants' characteristics at baseline to estimate recurrence at varying times, thus identifying those who may benefit from dietary and medical interventions. An electronic version of the ROKS nomogram is available at https://qxmd.com/calculate/calculator_3/roks-recurrence-of-kidney-stone-2014.

Pathogenesis

Stone formation occurs as a result of supersaturation of urinary solutes, expressed as the ratio of solute concentration in urine to its known solubility. A ratio of greater than 1 indicates that urine is supersaturated with the given substance and promotes crystallization, whereas a ratio of less than 1 inhibits crystallization. Low urine volume increases supersaturation of all solutes, thereby promoting stone formation. Urine pH influences free ion activity. The main determinants for crystallization vary for different stones: low urine volume and high urinary calcium and oxalate concentration promote calcium oxalate crystals, whereas alkaline urine and high urinary calcium concentrations promote calcium phosphate crystals. Acidic urine is the main determinant for uric acid crystals, and for cystine crystals it is high urinary cystine concentration and acidic urine. Urine contains substances such as citrate, pyrophosphate, magnesium, Tamm-Horsfall glycoprotein, glycosaminoglycans, osteopontin, and calgranulin that can inhibit crystal aggregation in urine. Of these, citrate is the only inhibitor that can be measured and modified in clinical settings; thus, it is a focus of therapeutic intervention.

TABLE 5.9 Medications Associated With Stone Formation

Mechanism	Medication
Hypocitraturia	Acetazolamide
	Zonisamide
	Vitamin C
	Topiramate
Hypercalciuria	Vitamin D
	Antacids
	Theophylline
	Nifedipine
Hyperuricosuria	Probenecid
	Aspirin
Precipitation within the tubule	Indinavir
	Atazanavir
	Acyclovir
	Sulfadiazine
	Triamterene
	Guaifenesin/ephedrine

Clinical Presentation

Patients are often asymptomatic, and calculi are detected as an incidental finding on imaging studies. Flank pain with or without gross hematuria is the most common presentation. Pain can vary in intensity from mild to severe and is classically abrupt in onset, paroxysmal, waxing and waning. Other associated symptoms include dysuria, urgency, nausea, and vomiting. Location of pain is suggestive of site of obstruction and may vary as the stone migrates. Upper ureteral obstruction (as in the ureteropelvic region) can cause flank pain, while lower ureteral obstruction can cause pain to radiate to the ipsilateral testes or labium. Some patients may pass gravel, more typical with uric acid stones. Complications associated with nephrolithiasis include obstruction, hydronephrosis, infection, and AKI from obstructive uropathy in the setting of bilateral obstruction or unilateral obstruction in case of the solitary kidney. Conditions that can mimic renal colic include ectopic pregnancy in women, bleeding within the kidney leading to formation of clots, hemorrhagic cysts, loin pain hematuria syndrome, and malingering.

Diagnosis

Detailed history is crucial and should include age at the first episode, number of stones, bilateral or unilateral stones, frequency of stone formation, type of stone if known, type and number of surgical interventions, family history of stone disease, and any associated infections. Certain clues elucidated on history may point towards a systemic etiology for nephrolithiasis; for example, patients with malabsorptive states may be predisposed calcium oxalate stones. History should also include detailed dietary habits, including amount of fluid intake, dietary sodium, protein, oxalate, and calcium intake to determine the potential cause or contributors of stone formation. Certain medications can potentiate stone formation and are shown in Table 5.9. Except during an acute episode of stone passing, most patients will have a normal physical examination. However, physical examination may sometimes reveal findings of systemic condition such as presence of tophi in patients with hyperuricosuria and uric acid stones.

Laboratory testing should include complete metabolic profile and uric acid. Hypokalemia and metabolic acidosis are suggestive of RTA.

转移的患者，1年生存率为12%～71%，3年生存率为0%～31%。但随着新药的出现，过去十年的生存率有所提高。

肾结石

肾结石是重要的公共卫生问题。它是人类健康的巨大负担，也给国家带来可观的财政支出。含钙结石是最常见的结石类型，约占所有结石的80%。尿酸、磷酸铵镁和胱氨酸结石［译者注：原文有误，应为胱氨酸（cystine）而非半胱氨酸（cysteine）。下文也均为cystine stone］较少见，分别约占所有结石的9%、10%和1%，但复发率较高。

流行病学

结石的患病率一直在显著增加。国家健康和营养调查（NHANES）显示，美国自我报告的肾结石患病率从1976—1980年的3.2%增加到2007—2010年的8.8%，再到2014年的10.1%。此外，肾结石的发病率也在增加，北美和欧洲估计约为0.5%。饮食和生活方式因素可能在流行病学变化中发挥重要作用。

肾结石的患病率随年龄增长而增加。男性比女性更常见；然而，在过去20年中，男女比例已从3∶1变为大约2∶1。NHANES数据随时间变化的比较显示，男性肾结石患病率稳定，但女性患病率上升，特别是在育龄期女性中增幅最为显著。流行病学研究指出肾结石与代谢综合征之间存在关联，并且在女性中比男性更为显著。这可能是女性肾结石发病率增加的一个合理解释。白人男性患病率最高，西班牙裔和亚裔男性居中，黑人男性较少见。阿拉伯联合酋长国和沙特阿拉伯男性的结石风险最高，这与遗传和环境因素有关。结石复发很常见，5～10年肾结石复发率为50%，20年为75%。结石复发的危险因素包括发病年龄小、阳性家族史、有基础疾病和尿路感染。肾结石复发（ROKS）预测图为首次有症状的结石患者提供评估复发风险的临床工具。它使用参与者基线时的特征来估计不同时间的复发，从而识别可能从饮食和医疗干预中受益的人群。ROKS预测图的电子版本可在 https://qxmd.com/calculate/calculator_3/roks-recurrence-of-kidney-stone-2014 上获取。

发病机制

结石形成是尿溶质过饱和的结果，以尿液中溶质浓度与其已知的溶解度的比率来表示。比率大于1表示尿液中该物质过饱和，促进结晶形成，而比率小于1则抑制结晶产生。低尿量增加了所有溶质的过饱和度，从而促进结石形成。尿液pH值影响自由离子的活性。不同结石晶体形成的主要决定因素不同：低尿量、高尿钙和高尿草酸盐浓度促进草酸钙结晶形成，而碱性尿液和高尿钙浓度促进磷酸钙结晶形成。酸性尿液是尿酸结晶形成的主要决定因素，而胱氨酸结晶形成的主要决定因素

表5.9	与结石形成相关的药物
机制	药物
低枸橼酸尿症	乙酰唑胺
	唑尼沙胺
	维生素C
	托吡酯
高钙尿症	维生素D
	抑酸药
	茶碱
	硝苯地平
高尿酸尿症	丙磺舒
	阿司匹林
肾小管内沉淀	茚地那韦
	阿扎那韦
	阿昔洛韦
	磺胺嘧啶
	氨苯蝶啶
	愈创木酚甘油醚

是高尿胱氨酸浓度和酸性尿液。尿液中的枸橼酸盐、焦磷酸盐、镁、T-H（Tamm-Horsfall）糖蛋白、糖胺聚糖、骨调素和钙粒蛋白等物质，可以抑制尿液中结晶聚集。其中，枸橼酸盐是唯一可以在临床测定和干预的抑制剂，因此也是结石治疗的重点。

临床表现

患者通常无症状，在影像学检查中偶然发现结石。腰痛伴或不伴肉眼血尿是最常见的表现。疼痛程度可从轻微到严重不等，通常突然发作，呈阵发性，时强时弱。其他相关症状包括排尿困难、尿急、恶心和呕吐。疼痛的位置提示梗阻部位，并可能随结石的移动而变化。输尿管上段梗阻（如在输尿管盆腔区域）可导致腰痛，而输尿管下段梗阻疼痛可放射至同侧睾丸或阴唇。一些患者可排出碎石，这在尿酸结石中更为典型。与肾结石相关的并发症包括梗阻、肾积水、感染，以及因双侧梗阻或孤立肾单侧梗阻引起的AKI。类似肾绞痛的情况包括女性的异位妊娠、导致血凝块形成的肾内出血、出血性囊肿、腰痛-血尿综合征和诈病。

诊断

详细的病史至关重要，应包括首次发作的年龄、结石数量、双侧或单侧结石、结石形成频率、结石类型（如果知道）、手术干预的类型和次数、结石病的家族史以及任何相关的感染。病史中的某些线索可能提示肾结石的系统性病因：例如，吸收不良的患者更容易形成草酸钙结石。病史还应包括详细的饮食习惯，包括液体摄入量，饮食中的钠、蛋白质、草酸和钙摄入量，以确定结石形成的潜在原因或促成因素。某些药物可能促进结石形成，如表5.9所示。除结石急性发作期外，大多数患者的体格检查正常。然而，体格检查有时可能会揭示系统性疾病，如高尿酸尿症和尿酸结石患者中的痛风石。

实验室检测应包括完整的代谢情况和尿酸。低钾血症和代谢性酸中毒提示肾小管酸中毒。如果发现高

TABLE 5.10 Urinalysis and Radiographic Findings of Renal Calculi

Stone Type	Urine Microscopy	Radiologic Findings
Calcium oxalate monohydrate	Dumbbell shaped, appear coarse, needle-like under polarized light	Opaque, round, multiple calculi
Calcium oxalate dihydrate	Envelope-shaped	
Struvite, magnesium aluminum phosphate	Coffin lid shaped	Opaque, may be staghorn
Uric acid	Pleomorphic, often rhomboid plates or rosettes	Radiolucent
Cystine	Hexagonal	Opaque

TABLE 5.11 Treatment Modalities for Different Nephrolithiasis Risk Factors

Urinary Abnormality	Dietary Change	Medication
Hypercalciuria	Adequate dietary calcium intake Reduce animal protein intake Reduce sodium intake to <2 g/day	Thiazide diuretic
Hyperoxaluria	Adequate dietary calcium intake Avoid high oxalate foods	Consider vitamin B_6 (Pyridoxine)
Hyperuricosuria	Reduce purine intake	Allopurinol
Hypocitraturia	Increase fruit and vegetable intake Reduce animal protein intake	Potassium citrate (alkali)
Low urine volume	Increase fluid intake Goal urine output is >2-2.5 L per day.	

If hypercalcemia is noted, parathyroid hormone should be checked to assess for primary hyperparathyroidism. A careful urinalysis should be performed, and certain findings may point toward a specific diagnosis (Table 5.10). Uric acid crystals are formed in acidic urine, whereas calcium phosphate and struvite crystals are formed in alkaline urine. High urine specific gravity is suggestive of inadequate fluid intake. In patients with suspected struvite stones, urine culture should be obtained. Retrieving the stone for chemical analysis is essential to help identify the type of stone and thus guide therapy. All patients should strain their urine and retrieve any stone. A 24-hour urine collection is the cornerstone of evaluation in patients with nephrolithiasis and includes urine volume, pH, calcium, magnesium, potassium, uric acid, citrate, oxalate, sodium, urea nitrogen, ammonium, sulfate, phosphate, and creatinine (to assess the completeness of the collection). Preferably two collections should be done in outpatient settings when the patients are consuming their usual diet. Because individuals tend to change their dietary habits after an acute episode, the collection should be performed 6 weeks after an episode of renal colic. Urine collection should be repeated periodically to assess the impact of dietary changes and therapeutics.

Noncontrast helical CT has replaced intravenous urography (or intravenous pyelogram) as the diagnostic test of choice for evaluation of kidney stones. CT can detect both radiopaque and radiolucent stones with high sensitivity and specificity. Ultrasound can also detect radiolucent and radiopaque stones in kidneys but may miss ureteral stones. Ultrasound has a role in evaluating stones in pediatric and pregnant patients.

Treatment

Small (<4 mm), nonobstructive stones can be managed conservatively because they have a good chance passing spontaneously. With increase in stone size there is a progressive decrease in the spontaneous passage rate from 55% for stones smaller than 4 mm, to 35% for 4- to 6-mm stones, and 8% for stones greater than 6 mm, respectively.

During an acute colic episode, pain management is essential and can be controlled with use of NSAIDs or narcotics. Patients should be instructed to increase their fluid intake in order to increase their urine output to at least 2 liters per day to hasten stone passage. α-1 Adrenergic-receptor blockers and calcium-channel blockers can be used to facilitate stone passage. α-1 Adrenergic-receptor blockers decrease ureteral smooth muscle tone as well as frequency and force of peristalsis, whereas calcium-channel blockers suppress smooth muscle contraction and reduce ureteral spasm. Presence of any signs of urinary tract infection, inability to take oral fluids, or obstruction of a single functioning kidney requires hospitalization. In the presence of AKI, anuria, or sepsis with an obstructive stone, urgent urologic consultation should be obtained. Urology consult should also be obtained for stones larger than 10 mm, failure of conservative management, and presence of anatomic abnormalities that would prevent passage of the stone. Type of surgical intervention is determined by stone size, type, location, and presence of infection. For proximal ureteral stones, both shock-wave lithotripsy and ureteroscopy are first-line therapy. Shock-wave lithotripsy is most effective for smaller (<10 mm) calculi. For mid- or distal ureteral stones, ureteroscopy is first-line therapy. Shock-wave lithotripsy has lower morbidity and lower complication rates compared to ureteroscopy; however, the latter has a greater stone-free rate with a single procedure. Percutaneous nephrolithotomy is recommended for larger (>20 mm) or complex calculi (e.g., staghorn calculi).

Prevention of Stones

General measures to prevent recurrent stones include increasing fluid intake to greater than 2 to 2.5 L/day and limiting dietary sodium intake to less than 2 g/day and protein intake to 0.8 to 1 g/day. Dietary calcium restriction is not recommended because calcium in food binds to oxalate in the bowel and reduces urinary excretion of the highly lithogenic oxalate. On the other hand, additional calcium supplements in between meals should be avoided in patients with calcium stones.

Specific Types of Stones

Specific treatment modalities may be implemented when the metabolic risk factors for stone formation are identified (Table 5.11).

表 5.10　肾结石的尿液分析和影像学表现

结石类型	尿沉渣镜检	影像学表现
一水草酸钙	偏振光显微镜下哑铃状、粗糙、针状	不透射线、圆形、多发结石
二水草酸钙	信封状	
磷酸铵镁、磷酸镁铝	棺盖状	不透射线，可以是鹿角状
尿酸	形状多样，经常为菱形或花结样	透射线
胱氨酸	六边形	不透射线

表 5.11　不同肾结石危险因素的治疗模式

尿检异常	饮食调整	药物
高钙尿症	充足的饮食钙摄入 减少动物蛋白摄入 减少钠摄入，< 2 g/d	噻嗪类利尿剂
高草酸尿症	充足的饮食钙摄入 避免高草酸食物	考虑维生素 B6（吡哆醇）
高尿酸尿症	减少嘌呤摄入	别嘌呤醇
低枸橼酸尿症	增加水果和蔬菜摄入 减少动物蛋白摄入	枸橼酸钾（碱性）
尿量少	增加饮水量 目标尿量 > 2～2.5 L/d	

钙血症，应检查甲状旁腺激素以评估有无原发性甲状旁腺功能亢进。应仔细进行尿液分析，某些检查结果可能指向特定的诊断（表 5.10）。尿酸结晶在酸性尿液中形成，而磷酸钙和磷酸铵镁结晶在碱性尿液中形成。高尿比重提示液体摄入不足。在疑似磷酸铵镁结石的患者中，应进行尿液培养。对结石进行化学分析有助于确定结石类型，从而指导治疗。所有患者都应该过滤尿液并获取结石。收集 24 h 尿液是评估肾结石患者的基础，应包括尿量、pH 值、钙、镁、钾、尿酸、枸橼酸、草酸盐、钠、尿素氮、铵、硫酸盐、磷酸盐和肌酐（用于评估尿液收集的完整性）。最好在门诊进行两次采集，此时患者正处于正常饮食状态。因为急性发作后患者往往会改变饮食习惯，因此应在肾绞痛发作 6 周后收集尿液。应定期重复收集尿液检测，以评估饮食调整和治疗的影响。

非增强螺旋 CT 已取代静脉尿路造影（或静脉肾盂造影）成为评估肾结石的首选诊断检查。CT 对放射性透光和不透光的结石均有较高的检测敏感性和特异性。超声也能检测到肾内不透射线和透射线的结石，但可能漏诊输尿管结石。超声在儿童和孕妇的结石评估中具有一定作用。

治疗

小的（< 4 mm）非梗阻性结石可以保守治疗，因为它们很可能自发排出。随着结石大小的增加，自发排出率逐渐下降，分别从 4 mm 以下结石的 55%，到 4～6 mm 结石的 35%，以及大于 6 mm 结石的 8%。

在急性绞痛发作期间，疼痛管理至关重要，可使用非甾体抗炎药或麻醉剂类药物。应指导患者增加液体摄入，使尿量达到每天至少 2 L，以加快结石排出。可使用 α_1 受体阻滞剂和钙通道阻滞剂促进结石排出。α_1 受体阻滞剂降低输尿管平滑肌的张力以及输尿管蠕动的频率和力度，而钙通道阻滞剂抑制平滑肌收缩并减轻输尿管痉挛。有任何尿路感染的迹象、无法口服液体或孤立功能肾的梗阻需要住院治疗。如出现 AKI、无尿或梗阻性结石引起感染中毒时，应请泌尿外科紧急会诊。对于大于 10 mm 的结石、保守治疗失败以及存在阻碍结石排出的解剖异常，也应进行泌尿外科会诊。手术干预的类型由结石的大小、类型、位置和是否感染决定。对于输尿管上端结石，冲击波碎石和输尿管镜是一线治疗。冲击波碎石对较小（< 10 mm）的结石最有效。对于输尿管中段或远端结石，输尿管镜是首选治疗方法。比输尿管镜相比，冲击波碎石的并发症较少，但输尿管镜单次手术后无残石的概率更高。对于较大（> 20 mm）或复杂的结石（如鹿角状结石），建议采用经皮肾镜取石术。

结石预防

预防结石复发的一般措施包括增加液体摄入量至 2～2.5 L/d 以上，限制饮食中钠的摄入在 2 g/d 以下，蛋白质摄入限制至 0.8～1 g/d。不推荐限制饮食中的钙，因为食物中的钙与肠道中的草酸结合，减少高度致石性的草酸在尿中排泄。另一方面，对于含钙结石的患者，应避免在两餐间额外补充钙剂。

特定类型的结石

确定了结石形成的代谢危险因素后，可进行针对性的治疗（表 5.11）。

TABLE 5.12 Principle Risk Factors for Formation of Calcium Stones
Low urinary volume
High urinary oxalate
High urinary calcium
Low urinary citrate
Dietary factors
Low dietary intake of fluids, calcium, phytates, potassium
High intake of oxalates, sodium, protein, sucrose
Medical conditions: obesity, metabolic syndrome, diabetes mellitus, primary hyperparathyroidism, gout, medullary sponge kidneys

Calcium Stones

Approximately 80% of stones are calcium stones, most of which are composed primarily of calcium oxalate, mixed oxalate and phosphate, and less often, pure calcium phosphate. Calcium oxalate supersaturation is not pH-dependent in the physiologic range whereas alkaline urine promotes calcium phosphate supersaturation. The pathophysiologic mechanisms for calcium kidney stone formation are complex, diverse, and can be associated with a number of metabolic derangements (Table 5.12).

Hypercalciuria. Hypercalciuria is the most common metabolic abnormality found in recurrent calcium stones formers, detected in 30% to 60% of adults with nephrolithiasis. It is defined as calcium excretion 250 mg/day or greater in women and 300 mg/day or greater in men. It is most often familial or idiopathic. Gut calcium absorption is increased in persons with idiopathic hypercalciuria, but serum calcium values remain unchanged as the absorbed calcium is promptly excreted. There are three primary pathophysiologic mechanisms for hypercalciuria. (1) Increased intestinal calcium absorption (absorptive hypercalciuria), which is the most common abnormality. (2) Enhanced calcium mobilization from bone (resorptive hypercalciuria), which leads to urinary loss of bone calcium. This can be seen in patients with primary hyperparathyroidism, immobilization, and metastatic tumors. (3) Decreased renal calcium reabsorption (renal leak), the pathogenesis of which is unclear and is thought to be due to a primary defect in renal tubular absorption of calcium. High sodium intake results in decrease in proximal sodium reabsorption. The ensuing urinary sodium excretion results in physiologic increase in calcium excretion, thus promoting stone formation. High animal protein intake can lead to increased acid load, causing calcium release from bones and resulting in increased urinary calcium excretion. Moreover, acidosis resulting in decreased tubular calcium reabsorption and depletion of urinary citrate.

Thiazide diuretics are commonly used to decrease urine calcium excretion in recurrent calcium stone formers. They are effective in treating hypercalciuria and reducing stone recurrence regardless of the underlying pathophysiologic mechanism. They cause volume contraction-induced increased proximal tubule calcium absorption. Thiazides can cause hypokalemia-induced hypocitraturia; therefore they should be supplemented with potassium. Potassium citrate has an advantage over other agents because it because it provides both potassium and citrate.

Hyperoxaluria. Hyperoxaluria (>45 mg/day in women and 55 mg/day in men) is detected in 10% to 50% of calcium stone formers. Hyperoxaluria increases calcium oxalate supersaturation and thus promotes calcium oxalate stone formation. Hyperoxaluria can result from increased dietary intake, increased gastrointestinal absorption of oxalate, or overproduction of oxalate as a result of an inborn error in metabolism. Foods known to increase urinary oxalate excretion include rhubarb, spinach, potatoes, beetroot, most nuts, chocolate, tea, raspberries, figs, plums, and high amounts of vitamin C. Enteric hyperoxaluria occurs in patients with malabsorption of fat, which leads to binding of dietary calcium to excessive enteric fat, and subsequent increase in absorption of free oxalate in the colon. This is commonly seen in patients with chronic diarrhea, inflammatory bowel diseases, celiac disease, and intestinal resection or after bariatric surgery. In patients with enteric hyperoxaluria, cholestyramine can be used to bind bile acids and oxalate; however, it is not always well tolerated. Other concomitant stone risk factors include low urine volume, acidic urine, and hypocitraturia. Rarely, hyperoxaluria is caused by inborn errors in metabolism such as primary hyperoxaluria, a rare autosomal recessive genetic disorder of oxalate synthesis. Type 1 primary hyperoxaluria is more common and often presents in childhood with nephrolithiasis, nephrocalcinosis, and kidney failure. Type II primary hyperoxaluria has a milder course with similar clinical manifestations.

Treatment measures include a low-oxalate diet and increased calcium intake with meals to bind intestinal oxalate and prevent its absorption. Patients should be advised to avoid excessive vitamin C (>500 mg/day). In addition, for patients with enteric hyperoxaluria, measures to reduce steatorrhea such as low-fat diet, cholestyramine, and administration of medium-chain triglycerides should be instituted. Liver transplant is the definitive therapy for patients with primary hyperoxaluria. Pyridoxine, which promotes conversion of glyoxylate to glycine, may reduce oxalate production in patients with type 1 primary hyperoxaluria. *Oxalobacter formigenes*, a colonic bacteria that uses oxalate for cellular metabolism, has been shown to be associated with a decreased risk of recurrent calcium oxalate stone formation, presumably because the bacterium degrades oxalate, prevents its absorption, and thus promotes excretion. However, a randomized control trial comparing use of *Oxalobacter formigenes* to placebo in patients with primary hyperoxaluria did not show reduction in urinary oxalate levels.

Hypocitraturia. Citrate, an endogenous inhibitor of calcium stone formation, is the only inhibitor that is measured and can be modified in clinical settings. It is a tricarboxylic acid that mostly stems from endogenous oxidative metabolism, freely filtered through the glomerulus and actively reabsorbed in the proximal tubule. Citrate binds to urinary calcium to form a soluble complex and thus prevents precipitation of calcium with oxalates or phosphates. Citrate also directly inhibits crystal aggregation. Hypocitraturia, defined by citrate concentration of less than 325 mg/day, can be a consequence of metabolic acidosis, high protein intake, carbonic anhydrase inhibitors, hypokalemia, or as an idiopathic disorder. Fall in tubular fluid pH results in conversion of trivalent citrate anion into the divalent anion, which is more easily reabsorbed via the sodium-citrate cotransporter in the luminal membrane. In addition, acidosis results in increased cell citrate utilization and upregulation of proximal renal tubular reabsorption of citrate leading to hypocitraturia.

Both potassium and sodium alkali supplementation can effectively raise urinary pH and citrate. However, potassium citrate is more effective in preventing calcium stone formation compared to sodium citrate because the sodium load can worsen hypercalciuria. Required dose for potassium citrate is 15 to 25 mmol two or three times a day. One potential concern with alkali therapy is the risk of calcium phosphate stone formation. In addition, among patients with reduced kidney function, serum potassium needs to be monitored closely for hyperkalemia.

Calcium Phosphate Stones

Calcium phosphate stone formation is a result of hypercalciuria, hypocitraturia, and persistently alkaline urine. Calcium phosphate stones can be seen in conditions causing distal RTA (inherited defects,

表 5.12　钙结石形成的主要危险因素
尿量少
高草酸盐尿
高尿钙
低枸橼酸盐尿
饮食因素
饮水量不足；钙、肌醇磷酸酯、钾摄入不足
草酸、钠、蛋白、蔗糖摄入过多
共患病：肥胖、代谢综合征、糖尿病、原发性甲状旁腺功能亢进、痛风、髓质海绵肾

钙结石

大约 80% 的结石是钙结石，其中大多数主要由草酸钙、草酸/磷酸盐混合结石组成，少数为纯磷酸钙。在生理范围内，草酸钙过饱和与 pH 值无关，而碱性尿液会促进磷酸钙过饱和。肾钙结石形成的病理生理机制复杂多样，可能与多种代谢紊乱有关（表 5.12）。

高钙尿症 高钙尿症是复发性钙结石患者中最常见的代谢异常，见于 30%～60% 的成人肾结石患者。定义为女性每天钙排泄量 ≥ 250 mg，男性 ≥ 300 mg。它通常是家族性或特发性的。特发性高钙尿症患者的肠道钙吸收增加，但因为吸收的钙迅速被排泄，血清钙保持不变。高钙尿症有三个主要病理生理机制：①肠道钙吸收增加（吸收性高钙尿症），这是最常见的异常；②骨钙动员增强（再吸收性高钙尿症），导致骨钙由尿液丢失，这种情况可见于原发性甲状旁腺功能亢进、卧床不动和转移性肿瘤；③肾脏钙重吸收减少（肾性排泄增加），其发病机制尚不清楚，认为与肾小管吸收钙的原发性缺陷有关。高钠摄入导致近端钠重吸收减少。随之而来的尿钠排泄导致钙排泄的生理性增加，从而促进结石形成。高动物蛋白摄入可导致酸负荷增加，引起钙从骨骼释放，导致尿钙排泄增加。此外，酸中毒导致肾小管钙重吸收减少和尿枸橼酸盐耗竭。

噻嗪类利尿剂常用于减少复发性钙结石患者的尿钙排泄。无论潜在的病理生理机制如何，它们都有效地治疗高钙尿症，减少结石复发。它们通过减少容量使近端小管钙吸收增加。噻嗪类利尿剂可能导致低钾血症引起的低枸橼酸尿症，应用时应补充钾。枸橼酸钾比其他药物有优势，因为它同时提供钾和枸橼酸盐。

高草酸尿症 10%～50% 的钙结石患者检出高草酸尿（女性超过 45 mg/d，男性超过 55 mg/d）。高草酸尿症增加草酸钙的过饱和度，从而促进草酸钙结石的形成。高草酸尿症可由饮食摄入过多、草酸胃肠道吸收增加或先天代谢异常使生成过多而导致。已知增加尿液草酸排泄的食物包括大黄、菠菜、土豆、甜菜根、大多数坚果、巧克力、茶、树莓、无花果、李子和大量维生素 C。肠源性高草酸尿症发生在脂肪吸收不良的患者中，饮食中的钙与过多的肠内脂肪结合，进而增加结肠中游离草酸的吸收。这种情况常见于慢性腹泻、炎症性肠病、乳糜泻、肠切除或减肥手术后的患者。考来烯胺（消胆胺）可用于肠源性高草酸尿症患者以结合胆汁酸和草酸，但通常耐受不佳。其他伴随的结石危险因素包括低尿量、酸性尿液和低枸橼酸尿。极少数情况下，高草酸尿症由先天性代谢缺陷引起，如原发性高草酸尿症，这是一种罕见的引起草酸盐合成异常的常染色体隐性遗传性疾病。1 型原发性高草酸尿症较常见，通常在儿童时期出现肾结石、肾钙化和肾衰竭。2 型原发性高草酸尿症临床表现类似，但病情较轻。

治疗措施包括低草酸饮食和增加餐中钙摄入以结合肠道中的草酸，防止其被吸收。建议患者避免摄入过量维生素 C（> 500 mg/d）。此外，对于肠源性高草酸尿症患者，应采取减少脂肪泻的措施，如低脂饮食、服用消胆胺和中链甘油三酯等。肝移植是原发性高草酸尿症患者的有效治疗方法。吡哆醇促进乙醛酸转化为甘氨酸，可以减少 1 型原发性高草酸尿症患者的草酸产生。甲酸草酸杆菌（Oxalobacter formigenes）是一种利用草酸进行细胞代谢的结肠细菌，已被证明可降低草酸钙结石复发的风险。推测可能与该细菌降解草酸、防止其吸收，进而促进排泄相关。然而，一项原发性高草酸尿症患者的随机对照试验显示甲酸草酸杆菌相比安慰剂未能降低患者尿液的草酸水平。

低枸橼酸尿症 枸橼酸盐，是钙结石形成的内源性抑制剂，也是唯一能在临床测定和干预的抑制剂。它是一种主要来自内源性氧化代谢的三羧酸，通过肾小球自由过滤，并在近端小管中主动重吸收。枸橼酸盐与尿液中的钙结合形成可溶性复合物，从而防止钙与草酸盐或磷酸盐沉淀。枸橼酸盐还可直接抑制晶体聚集。低枸橼酸尿症的定义为尿液中枸橼酸盐排泄量低于每天 325 mg。它可以由代谢性酸中毒、高蛋白饮食、碳酸酐酶抑制剂、低钾血症或特发性疾病导致。肾小管内液体 pH 值下降导致三价枸橼酸阴离子转化为二价阴离子，后者更容易通过管腔膜上的钠-枸橼酸共转运蛋白被重吸收。此外，酸中毒可导致细胞枸橼酸利用增加和近端肾小管枸橼酸重吸收上调，导致低枸橼酸尿症。

补充钾和钠的碱盐均能有效提高尿液 pH 值和枸橼酸盐水平。因为钠负荷会加重高钙尿症，因此枸橼酸钾比枸橼酸钠在预防钙结石方面更为有效。枸橼酸钾的治疗剂量是每天 2～3 次，每次 15～25 mmol。补碱治疗的一个潜在问题是形成磷酸钙结石的风险。此外，在肾功能减退的患者中，需要密切监测血清钾以防止高钾血症。

磷酸钙结石

磷酸钙结石的形成是高钙尿症、低枸橼酸尿和持续碱性尿的结果。磷酸钙结石见于导致远端肾小管酸中毒的疾病（遗传缺陷、继发于自身免疫性疾病或特

secondary to autoimmune conditions or idiopathic), with use of carbonic anhydrase inhibitors such as acetazolamide (which reduces bicarbonate reabsorption in the proximal tubule), or with use of antiepileptic drugs that have carbonic anhydrase inhibitory activity such as topiramate and zonisamide. In patients with distal RTA, correction of the systemic acidosis with oral alkali (usually potassium citrate or potassium bicarbonate) is recommended with the goal of increasing serum bicarbonate level and urinary citrate excretion. Administration of alkali to maintain the serum bicarbonate level with the risk associated with a higher urine pH should be balanced. Urinary pH should be monitored closely on alkali therapy and not increased above 7 (because of increased risk for precipitating calcium phosphate crystals). A thiazide diuretic can be added to lower urinary calcium if stone formation persists, even if the urine calcium is in the "normal" range or when low bone density is present. Among patients with stone disease due to the administration of medications, discontinuation of the medication, if feasible, will prevent new stone formation.

Uric Acid Stones

The three major urinary abnormalities causing uric acid precipitation are low urinary pH (urine pH <5.5), low urine volume, and hyperuricosuria (defined as uric acid excretion >800 mg/day in men and >750 mg/day in women). Acidic urine is a more important risk factor for uric acid stones than hyperuricosuria. In low urinary pH the relatively soluble urate gets converted into insoluble uric acid, thereby facilitating lithogenesis. Excessive acid load (high animal protein diet) or chronic bicarbonate loss in patients with chronic diarrhea can result in low urinary pH, thus increasing the propensity for uric acid stone formation. Increased incidence of uric acid stones can be seen in patients with insulin resistance and type 2 diabetes mellitus and has been linked to impaired ammonia synthesis resulting in reduced urinary pH. Hyperuricosuria may be seen in certain clinical conditions such as myeloproliferative disorders, tumor lysis syndrome, and rare genetic disorders of uric acid synthetic pathway or mutations in renal uric acid transporters.

Alkaline therapy along with increasing urine volume is the most effective treatment of uric acid stones. Potassium citrate 30 to 80 mmol in divided doses is prescribed to maintain urine pH greater than 6.5 to 7. Raising the urinary pH to greater than 7 may result in calcium phosphate precipitation and should be avoided. Other measures to decrease uric acid excretion and raise urinary pH include low animal protein and low purine diet. In situations where marked hyperuricosuria persists despite dietary measures, xanthine oxidase inhibitors such as allopurinol at doses of 100 to 300 mg/day can be prescribed.

Struvite Stones

Struvite stones or triple phosphate stones are composed of magnesium ammonium phosphate and calcium carbonate-apatite. They can grow rapidly and if left untreated can fill the entire renal pelvis (i.e., staghorn calculi) and may lead to CKD and ESRD. These stones result from chronic urinary tract infections with urea-splitting organisms (Table 5.13), which increase the urine pH by generating ammonium to produce stones composed of ammonium-magnesium-phosphate.

The cornerstone of treatment for struvite stones includes early surgical removal of the bacteria-laden stones and eradicating the infection with antibiotics. Also, it is important to define and treat any metabolic abnormality. Acetohydroxamic acid, a urease inhibitor, is the only drug approved for the treatment of infectious kidney stones; however, its use is limited by its side effects such as headache, thrombophlebitis, tremor, nausea, vomiting, rash, abdominal discomfort, anemia, and reticulocytosis. This treatment should only be used if other measures are ineffective. Medical management alone for struvite stones is rarely successful and is not recommended unless patients are too ill for surgery or refuse stone removal.

TABLE 5.13 Urease-Producing Bacteria

Most species of *Proteus* and *Providencia*
Corynebacterium
Klebsiella
Pseudomonas
Serratia
Haemophilus
Staphylococcus

Cystine Stones

Cystinuria is the most common of the rare hereditary kidney stone diseases and is caused by an autosomal recessive defect in renal transport of amino acid cystine. Mutations of one of the two subunits of the amino acid transporter in the kidney leads to defective renal tubular reabsorption of dibasic amino acids such as cystine, arginine, lysine, and ornithine. Cystine stones are the main complication of this defect due to the low solubility of cystine in urine. Characteristic hexagonal cystine crystals can be seen on urine sediment (see Table 5.10). Cystinuria is diagnosed by family history of stones, stone formation at a young age, mildly radiopaque stones, and measurement of urinary cystine excretion. Patients with cystinuria excrete 250 to 1000 mg of cystine per day (normal is approximately 30 mg/day). Treatment must be aimed at decreasing the urinary cystine concentration by increasing urine volume to greater than 4 liters per day, reducing sodium intake, and alkalinizing the urine (urine pH >6.5) with potassium citrate or sodium bicarbonate and by decreasing animal protein intake. Persistence of urine cystine excretion greater than 250 mg/L, cystine crystals on urine sediment, and failure to elevate pH to greater than 7.0 despite conservative measures may require initiation of thiol-derivatives such as D-penicillamine and α-mercaptopropionylglycine (tiopronin). These drugs split cystine molecules into two cysteines and produce a highly soluble disulfide compound; however, their use may be limited by their side effect profile.

SUGGESTED READINGS

Badr M, El Koumi MA, Ali YF, et al: Renal tubular dysfunction in children with sickle cell haemoglobinopathy, Nephrology (Carlton) 18:299–303, 2013.

Bergman C, Guay-Woddford LM, et al.: Polycystic kidney disease, Nat Rev Dis Primers 50:1–24, 2018. 4.

Bosniak MA: The current radiological approach to renal cysts, Radiology 158:1–10, 2012.

Chen Z, Prosperi M, Bird VY. Prevalence of kidney stones in the USA: the National Health and Nutrition Evaluation Survey. Nov 26, 2018.

Cornec-Le Gall E, Audrezet MP, Chen JM, et al: Type of PKD1 mutation influences renal outcome in ADPKD, J Am Soc Nephrol 24:1006–1013, 2013.

Crino PB, Nathanson KL, Henske EP: The tuberous sclerosis complex, N Engl J Med 355:1345–1356, 2006.

Katabathina VS, Kota G, Dasyam AK, et al: Adult renal cystic disease: a genetic, biological, and developmental primer, Radiographics 30:1509–1523, 2010.

Khan SR, Pearle MS, Robertson WG, et al: Kidney stones, Nat Rev Dis Primers, 2016.

Moe OW: Kidney stones: pathophysiology and medical management, Lancet 367:333–344, 2006.

Moe OW, Pearle MS, Sakhaee K: Pharmacotherapy of urolithiasis: evidence from clinical trials, Kidney Int 79:385–392, 2011.

发性），使用碳酸酐酶抑制剂如乙酰唑胺（减少近端小管碳酸氢盐的重吸收），或使用具有碳酸酐酶抑制活性的抗癫痫药物如托吡酯和唑尼沙胺。在远端肾小管酸中毒患者中，建议使用口服碱剂（通常是枸橼酸钾或碳酸氢钾）纠正全身性酸中毒，以提高血清碳酸氢盐水平及尿枸橼酸盐的排泄。应平衡使用碱剂维持血清碳酸氢盐水平与尿液 pH 值升高带来的风险。补碱治疗时应密切监测尿液 pH 值，不要升至 7.0 以上（因为增加磷酸钙晶体沉淀的风险）。即使尿钙在"正常"范围内或存在低骨密度时，如果结石持续形成，可加用噻嗪类利尿剂降低尿钙。在药物相关的结石患者中，如条件许可，停药可预防新结石的形成。

尿酸结石

导致尿酸沉淀的三个主要尿液异常是尿液低 pH 值（尿液 pH < 5.5）、尿量少和高尿酸尿症（定义为男性每天尿酸排泄量 > 800 mg，女性 > 750 mg）。与高尿酸尿相比，酸性尿液是尿酸结石更为重要的危险因素。尿液 pH 值低时，相对可溶的尿酸盐转化为不溶性尿酸，从而促进结石形成。过多的酸负荷（高动物蛋白饮食）或慢性腹泻导致的长期碳酸氢盐丢失，可导致尿液 pH 值降低，增加尿酸结石形成的倾向。胰岛素抵抗和 2 型糖尿病患者的尿酸结石发病率增加，与氨合成受损导致尿液 pH 值降低有关。高尿酸尿症可见于某些临床情况，如骨髓增殖性疾病、肿瘤溶解综合征以及罕见的遗传性疾病，如尿酸合成途径或肾脏尿酸转运体的基因突变。

碱化尿液的同时增加尿量是尿酸结石最有效的治疗方法。每天分次服用 30 ~ 80 mmol 的枸橼酸钾，以维持尿液 pH 值 6.5 ~ 7。避免将尿液 pH 值提高到 7.0 以上，因为可能导致磷酸钙沉积。其他降低尿酸排泄和提高尿液 pH 值的措施包括低动物蛋白和低嘌呤饮食。在饮食干预下仍存在明显高尿酸尿症的情况下，可应用黄嘌呤氧化酶抑制剂如别嘌呤醇，每天 100 ~ 300 mg。

磷酸铵镁结石

磷酸铵镁或三磷酸盐结石由磷酸镁铵和碳酸钙-磷灰石组成。它们可以迅速增长，如不加治疗，可能会充满整个肾盂（即鹿角状结石），并可能导致 CKD 和 ESRD。这些结石是由分解尿素的微生物引起的慢性尿路感染的结果（表 5.13）。这些微生物分解尿素产生铵，导致尿液 pH 值增加，从而产生磷酸铵镁结石。

磷酸铵镁结石治疗的基石包括早期手术去除包含细菌的结石和使用抗生素根除感染。此外，确定并治疗代谢异常也很重要。脲酶抑制剂乙酰羟胺酸是唯一批准用于治疗感染性肾结石的药物。然而，头痛、血栓性静脉炎、震颤、恶心、呕吐、皮疹、腹部不适、贫血和网织红细胞增多症等副作用限制了它的应用。这一治疗只有在其他措施无效时使用。单纯药物治疗

表 5.13 产生脲酶细菌

变形杆菌属和普罗维登斯菌属的大部分菌种
棒状杆菌属
克雷伯菌
假单胞菌
沙雷氏菌属
嗜血杆菌
葡萄球菌

磷酸铵镁结石很少成功，除非患者因病情过重不能接受手术或拒绝取石，否则不建议使用。

胱氨酸结石

胱氨酸尿症是罕见遗传性肾结石疾病中最常见的一种，由肾脏胱氨酸转运蛋白的常染色体隐性缺陷引起。肾脏氨基酸转运蛋白两个亚单位之一发生的突变，可导致肾小管对胱氨酸、精氨酸、赖氨酸和鸟氨酸等二碱性氨基酸重吸收缺陷。由于胱氨酸在尿液中的溶解度低，胱氨酸结石是这一遗传缺陷的主要并发症。尿沉渣中可以看到特征性的六边形胱氨酸晶体（见表 5.10）。胱氨酸尿症可依据结石家族史、年轻时结石形成、轻度不透射线的结石，以及测定尿液胱氨酸排泄量来诊断。胱氨酸尿症患者每天排泄 250 ~ 1000 mg 的胱氨酸（正常值大约为 30 mg/d）。治疗的目标是通过以下方式降低尿胱氨酸浓度：将尿量增加至每天 4 L 以上、减少钠摄入、用枸橼酸钾或碳酸氢钠碱化尿液（尿液 pH > 6.5）和减少动物蛋白摄入。如果尿胱氨酸排泄持续超过 250 mg/L，尿沉渣中有胱氨酸晶体，并且采取上述保守措施后仍无法将尿 pH 值提高到 7.0 以上，则可能需要开始使用硫醇衍生物如 d- 青霉胺和 α- 巯基丙酰甘氨酸（硫普罗宁）。这些药物将胱氨酸分子分解为两个半胱氨酸，并产生一种高度可溶的二硫化合物，但它们的使用可能会受到副作用的限制。

推荐阅读

Badr M, El Koumi MA, Ali YF, et al: Renal tubular dysfunction in children with sickle cell haemoglobinopathy, Nephrology (Carlton) 18:299–303, 2013.

Bergman C, Guay-Woddford LM, et al.: Polycystic kidney disease, Nat Rev Dis Primers 50:1–24, 2018. 4.

Bosniak MA: The current radiological approach to renal cysts, Radiology 158:1–10, 2012.

Chen Z, Prosperi M, Bird VY. Prevalence of kidney stones in the USA: the National Health and Nutrition Evaluation Survey. Nov 26, 2018.

Cornec-Le Gall E, Audrezet MP, Chen JM, et al: Type of PKD1 mutation influences renal outcome in ADPKD, J Am Soc Nephrol 24:1006–1013, 2013.

Crino PB, Nathanson KL, Henske EP: The tuberous sclerosis complex, N Engl J Med 355:1345–1356, 2006.

Katabathina VS, Kota G, Dasyam AK, et al: Adult renal cystic disease: a genetic, biological, and developmental primer, Radiographics 30:1509–1523, 2010.

Khan SR, Pearle MS, Robertson WG, et al: Kidney stones, Nat Rev Dis Primers, 2016.

Moe OW: Kidney stones: pathophysiology and medical management, Lancet 367:333–344, 2006.

Moe OW, Pearle MS, Sakhaee K: Pharmacotherapy of urolithiasis: evidence from clinical trials, Kidney Int 79:385–392, 2011.

Perazella MA, Markowitz GS: Drug-induced acute interstitial nephritis, Nat Rev Nephrol 6:461–470, 2010.

Perazella MA, Shirali AC: Nephrotoxicity of cancer immunotherapies: past, present and future, JASN 29:2039–2052, 2018.

Pfau A, Knauf F: Update on nephrolithiasis: core curriculum, AKJD, 2016.

Rule AD, et al.: The ROKS Nomogram for predicting a second symptomatic stone episode, JASN, 2014.

Silverman SG, Pedrosa I, Ellis JH, et al: Bosniak classification of cystic renal masses, version 2019: an update proposal and needs assessment, Radiology 292:475–488, 2019.

Torres VE, Chapman AB, Devuyst O, et al: Tolvaptan in patients with autosomal dominant polycystic kidney disease, N Engl J Med 367:2407–2418, 2012.

Whelan TF: Guidelines on the management of renal cyst disease, Can Urol Assoc J 4:98–99, 2010.

Worcester EM, Coe FL: Calcium kidney stones, N Engl J Med 363:954–963, 2010.

Zeisberg M, Kalluri R: Physiology of the renal interstitium, CJASN 10(10):1831–1840, 2015.

Perazella MA, Markowitz GS: Drug-induced acute interstitial nephritis, Nat Rev Nephrol 6:461–470, 2010.

Perazella MA, Shirali AC: Nephrotoxicity of cancer immunotherapies: past, present and future, JASN 29:2039–2052, 2018.

Pfau A, Knauf F: Update on nephrolithiasis: core curriculum, AKJD, 2016.

Rule AD, et al.: The ROKS Nomogram for predicting a second symptomatic stone episode, JASN, 2014.

Silverman SG, Pedrosa I, Ellis JH, et al: Bosniak classification of cystic renal masses, version 2019: an update proposal and needs assessment, Radiology 292:475–488, 2019.

Torres VE, Chapman AB, Devuyst O, et al: Tolvaptan in patients with autosomal dominant polycystic kidney disease, N Engl J Med 367:2407–2418, 2012.

Whelan TF: Guidelines on the management of renal cyst disease, Can Urol Assoc J 4:98–99, 2010.

Worcester EM, Coe FL: Calcium kidney stones, N Engl J Med 363:954–963, 2010.

Zeisberg M, Kalluri R: Physiology of the renal interstitium, CJASN 10(10):1831–1840, 2015.

6

Vascular Disorders of the Kidney

Abdallah Geara, Jeffrey S. Berns

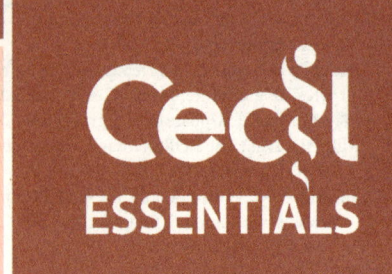

INTRODUCTION

The spectrum of vascular disorders of the kidneys is broad as a result of high renal blood flow and the intimate relationship between blood supply and fundamental glomerular and tubular functions. In this chapter, emphasis is placed on the clinical manifestations of hypertension, chronic kidney disease (CKD), end-stage kidney failure, and the many other causes of acute kidney injury (AKI).

RENAL VASCULAR ANATOMY

With a volume of around 150 mL each, the kidneys compromise less than 1% of the body mass and yet receive 20% to 25% of the cardiac output. The renal arteries arise directly from the aorta and enter the renal hilum. The right renal artery passes anterior to the inferior vena cava (IVC) and is longer than the left renal artery. In up to 30% of the population, accessory renal arteries arise from the aorta to provide blood to portions of one or both kidneys, which may become important when evaluating patients for renovascular hypertension.

The renal arteries give rise to segmental, interlobar, and arcuate arteries (Fig. 6.1). Arcuate arteries course along the corticomedullary junction and give rise to interlobular arterioles, which extend outward into the cortex before branching into afferent arterioles, from which the glomerular capillary tufts arise. The postglomerular efferent arterioles from more superficial glomeruli form a capillary network in the renal cortex, and those extending from glomeruli nearer the cortical-medullary junction (i.e., juxtamedullary glomeruli) form capillaries that extend deeper into the medulla in association with thin, descending and ascending loops of Henle as the vasa recta. The vasa recta provide the sole blood supply for the renal medulla, making this portion of the kidney particularly susceptible to ischemic injury. Venules from the ascending vasa recta and the cortical capillary network empty into the renal veins.

The left renal vein returns to the IVC anterior to the aorta and inferior to the inferior mesenteric artery, which may rarely cause compression of this vein, causing what is known as the "nutcracker syndrome," typically presenting with hematuria with or without left flank pain. The left gonadal vein also empties into the left renal vein, and a left varicocele may be evident if the renal vein is occluded by thrombosis or tumor involvement. The right renal vein is much shorter and empties directly into the IVC. The right gonadal vein empties directly into the IVC rather than into the right renal vein.

We categorize vascular diseases of the kidney based on the blood vessels typically involved (glomerulonephritis is addressed in Chapter 4):

- Main renal artery and segmental branches: Renovascular disease, fibromuscular dysplasia (FMD), aortic dissection, thromboembolic diseases and large and medium vessels vasculitis.
- Interlobular arterioles and glomerular arterioles: Hypertensive nephrosclerosis, atheroembolic disease, preeclampsia, scleroderma renal crisis, thrombotic microangiopathy (TMA) and antiphospholipid antibody syndrome (APS).
- Renal veins: Renal vein thrombosis (RVT).

RENOVASCULAR DISEASE

Any process that narrows the lumen of the main or branch renal arteries sufficiently can elicit a humoral response mediated by increased renin release from the ipsilateral kidney, which leads to increases in circulating angiotensin II and aldosterone levels. Activation of the renin-angiotensin-aldosterone system increases systemic blood pressure and renal arterial perfusion pressure and single nephron glomerular filtration rate (GFR) beyond the stenosis. This is mediated through angiotensin II-mediated preferential efferent arteriolar vasoconstriction that counterbalances the increase in resistance imposed by narrowing of the main or branch arteries.

Hemodynamically significant renal artery stenosis (RAS) requires a reduction in lumen diameter of at least 50% to 60%. In the stenotic kidney, a decrease in the glomerular capillary pressure results in activation of the renin-angiotensin-aldosterone system, systemic vasoconstriction mediated by angiotensin II, and increased renal sodium and fluid reabsorption, resulting in elevation of systemic blood pressure. If the contralateral kidney has no stenosis, the increased systemic blood pressure increases sodium excretion by that kidney (i.e., pressure natriuresis). Thus, clinically, a patient with unilateral renal artery stenosis and two functioning kidneys has hypertension secondary to angiotensin II-mediated systemic vasoconstriction without significant hypervolemia. Because hypertension in this setting is maintained by increased vasoconstriction due to angiotensin II, treatment is aimed at blocking the synthesis or effect of the elevated angiotensin II levels with an angiotensin-converting enzyme (ACE) inhibitor or angiotensin-receptor blocker (ARB).

If the arteries to both kidneys are narrowed, pressure natriuresis does not occur, and hypertension is maintained chronically by the resulting intravascular volume expansion rather than by increased total peripheral resistance. Treatment with diuretics becomes more important in this circumstance. The latter situation also occurs when there is only a single functioning kidney that has stenosis or when an initially normal contralateral kidney suffers microvascular damage from long-standing hypertension (Fig. 6.2).

The pathophysiology of hypertension with RAS is such that its treatment may also compromise kidney function and reduce the GFR. If the kidney contralateral to the one with hemodynamically significant RAS has normal function, lowering the systemic blood pressure maintains the kidney with the stenosis in a hemodynamically compromised

肾脏血管疾病

滕菲 译 郑可 张宏 审校 李雪梅 通审

引言

由于肾血流量大、肾小球及肾小管的基本功能与肾脏血供密切相关，因此肾脏血管疾病谱系宽广。本章将重点介绍（肾脏血管疾病中的）高血压、慢性肾脏病（CKD）、终末期肾病，以及许多其他原因导致的急性肾损伤（AKI）的临床表现。

肾血管解剖

尽管每侧肾脏体积约为 150 ml、双肾重量仅为体重的 1%，肾血流量却占心输出量的 20%～25%。肾动脉由主动脉直接发出，而后进入肾门。右肾动脉跨过下腔静脉（IVC）前方，长度较左肾动脉更长。人群中具有副肾动脉的比例可达 30%，副肾动脉由主动脉发出并为单肾或者双肾的部分组织供血，这对于评估肾血管性高血压患者具有重要价值。

肾动脉发出肾段动脉、叶间动脉和弓状动脉（图 6.1）。弓状动脉沿皮髓质交界走行并发出小叶间动脉，后者向外延伸进入肾皮质并发出入球小动脉、形成肾小球毛细血管丛。来自浅表部位肾小球的出球小动脉在肾皮质形成毛细血管网；而靠近皮髓质交界部位的肾小球（即，髓旁肾小球）发出的出球小动脉所形成的毛细血管则深入髓质，与 Henle 袢的细段、降支及升支相伴，即为直小血管。直小血管是肾髓质的唯一供血来源，因此肾髓质对于缺血性损伤非常敏感。从直小血管升支和皮质毛细血管网延伸出小静脉共同汇入肾静脉。

左肾静脉经过主动脉前方、肠系膜下动脉下方，后汇入 IVC，这种解剖结构关系在极少数情况下会造成左肾静脉受压，从而引起所谓的"胡桃夹综合征"，其典型临床表现为血尿、伴或不伴左侧腰部疼痛。左侧性腺静脉也汇入左肾静脉，如果左肾静脉因血栓或肿瘤侵犯而阻塞，则可能出现左侧精索静脉曲张。右肾静脉较短，直接汇入 IVC。右侧性腺静脉也直接汇入 IVC，而非右肾静脉。

基于通常受累的血管，我们将肾脏血管疾病分为如下几类（肾小球肾炎在第 4 章阐述）：

- 主肾动脉及肾段动脉：肾血管病，纤维肌发育不良（FMD），主动脉夹层，血栓栓塞性疾病以及大、中等血管血管炎。
- 小叶间动脉及肾小球小血管：高血压肾硬化，动脉粥样硬化栓塞性疾病，先兆子痫，硬皮病肾危象，血栓性微血管病（TMA）以及抗磷脂综合征（APS）。
- 肾静脉：肾静脉血栓形成（RVT）。

肾血管病

任何导致肾动脉主干或分支管腔狭窄的过程都足以引起同侧肾脏释放肾素水平增加所介导的体液反应，继而导致循环中血管紧张素Ⅱ及醛固酮水平升高。肾素-血管紧张素-醛固酮系统激活提升全身血压、肾动脉灌注压以及狭窄部位以上的单个肾单位的肾小球滤过率（GFR）。这一过程通过血管紧张素Ⅱ介导的出球小动脉优先收缩来实现，出球小动脉收缩可抵消肾动脉主干或分支狭窄造成的阻力增加。

有显著血流动力学表现的肾动脉狭窄（RAS）需要血管管腔直径减少至少大于 50%～60%。在血管狭窄侧的肾脏中，肾小球毛细血管压力的下降导致肾素-血管紧张素-醛固酮系统激活，血管紧张素Ⅱ介导全身血管收缩以及肾脏钠及液体的重吸收增加，最终造成系统性血压升高。如对侧肾脏动脉无狭窄，升高的全身血压则会增加该侧肾脏的钠排泄（即，压力利钠）。因此，在临床上，单侧肾动脉狭窄且双肾功能正常的患者会出现继发于血管紧张素Ⅱ介导的全身性血管收缩造成高血压，而并无显著的容量过多表现。由于此类高血压是由血管紧张素Ⅱ介导的血管收缩增加所维持的，因此治疗的目标就锚定于通过血管紧张素转换酶（ACE）抑制剂或血管紧张素受体阻滞剂（ARB）阻断升高的血管紧张素Ⅱ的合成或作用。

如果双侧肾动脉均存在狭窄，则不会出现压力利钠，高血压则是由血管内容量增多来长期维持，而非通过周围血管阻力增加导致。在这种情况下，应用利尿剂治疗更为重要。这种情况还可见于：仅单侧肾脏功能正常且该侧出现肾动脉狭窄，或原本功能正常的肾脏由于长期高血压出现微血管损伤的情况（图 6.2）。

鉴于 RAS 引起的高血压的病理生理机制如上，针对此类高血压的治疗同样可能引起肾功能损伤以及 GFR 下降。如果一侧肾脏具有造成血流动力学显著改变的 RAS，而对侧的肾脏功能正常，则降低全身血压可以维持患侧

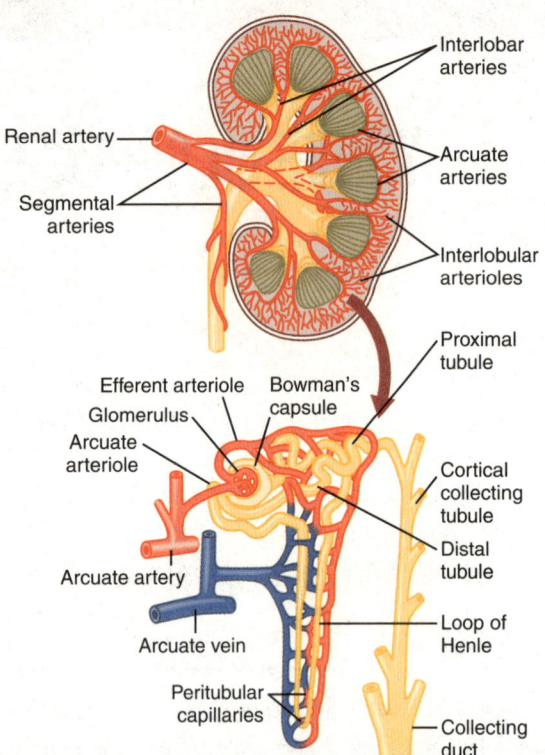

Fig. 6.1 *Top:* Cross-section of the human kidney showing renal arteries and veins. *Bottom:* Schematic of the microcirculation of each nephron. (From Guyton AC, Hall JE: Textbook of medical physiology, ed 11, 2016, Saunders, Chapter 26, 323-333.)

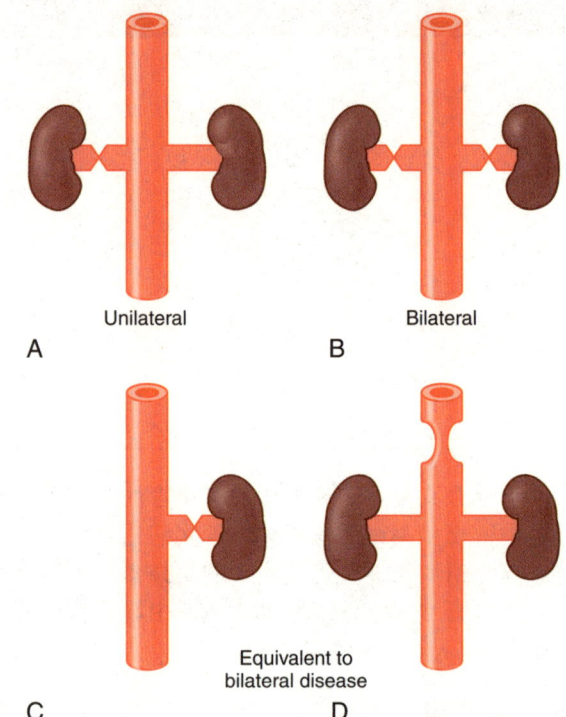

Fig. 6.2 Anatomy of renal artery stenosis. Renal artery stenosis may be unilateral (A), bilateral (B), or unilateral with a solitary kidney (C). Aortic disease may serve functionally as bilateral renal artery stenosis (D).

TABLE 6.1 Clinical Findings of Atherosclerotic Renovascular Disease
Onset of new, severe hypertension or sudden worsening of chronic hypertension at >55 years of age
Accelerated, resistant, or malignant hypertension
Unexplained atrophic kidney or size discrepancy >1.5 cm between kidneys
Sudden, unexplained ("flash") pulmonary edema
Unexplained chronic kidney disease in an individual with atherosclerotic vascular disease elsewhere
Development of acute kidney injury or worsening of chronic kidney disease after starting an ACE inhibitor or ARB

ACE, Angiotensin-converting enzyme; *ARB*, angiotensin II–receptor blocker.

state. However, this may not be detectable by measurement of the serum creatinine concentration because of the normally functioning contralateral kidney. A decline in the GFR may, however, be evident if there is underlying dysfunction of the contralateral kidney, as is often the case in long-standing hypertension, diabetes, or vascular disease. When a solitary functioning kidney or both kidneys are affected (i.e., bilateral RAS), AKI may result when ACE inhibitor or ARB treatment is initiated.

Atherosclerotic Renovascular Disease
Clinical Presentation
Atherosclerosis is the primary cause of RAS in adults, although any process that narrows one or both renal arteries may cause renal ischemia; others are discussed later in this chapter. Atherosclerotic renovascular disease is a common form of secondary hypertension, affecting up to 5% of patients with hypertension. Atherosclerotic RAS rarely occurs in patients younger than 40 years, and it is more common in men, white individuals, smokers, diabetics, and patients with atherosclerotic disease in other arterial systems. The prevalence of RAS increases to between 10% to 45% in patients with other atherosclerotic risk factors such as coronary artery disease, peripheral vascular disease, and aortic disease.

RAS should be suspected in patients with refractory hypertension or new-onset hypertension in patients older than 50 years, particularly if they have overt risk factors for atherosclerotic RAS (Table 6.1). Evaluation should always begin with a thorough history and physical examination, including attention to blood pressure and pulse amplitude in each extremity. A significant discrepancy between extremities may indicate peripheral vascular disease and increase the likelihood of RAS. An abdominal bruit is detected in about 50% of subjects but is not specific for RAS. Edema is not typically found unless significant CKD or another edematous condition also exists.

Laboratory evaluation may reveal hypokalemia (K^+ <3.5 mEq/L) or metabolic alkalosis (HCO_3^- >28 mEq/L) due to secondary hyperaldosteronism, although neither may be present. A reduced GFR with an elevated serum creatinine concentration may be found, but a normal serum creatinine concentration does not rule out hemodynamically significant RAS. Plasma renin activity and aldosterone concentrations may be elevated, but their measurement is of limited clinical utility in assessing hypertensive patients for RAS or in making therapeutic decisions. Urinalysis results are usually normal, although low-grade proteinuria (usually <1 g/day) from long-standing hypertension may be seen.

Diagnosis
Standard renal ultrasound imaging may suggest the presence of underlying RAS if it reveals a significant discrepancy in kidney size or if both

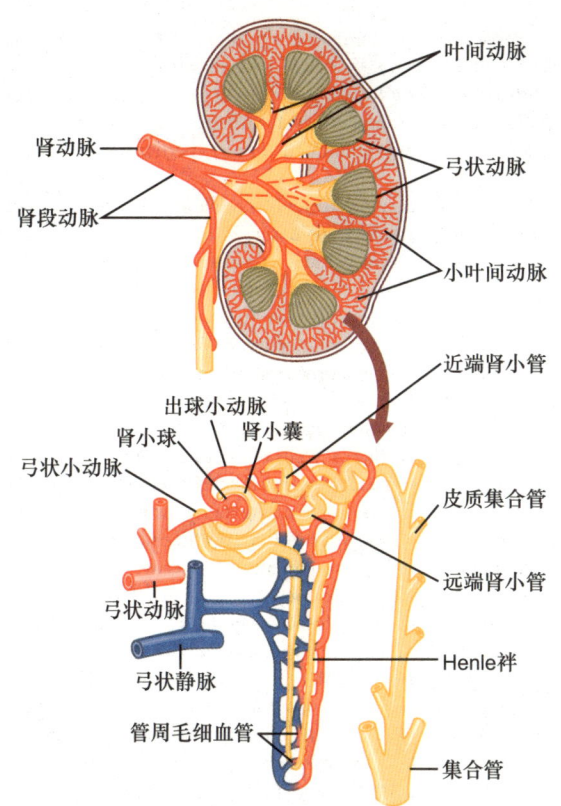
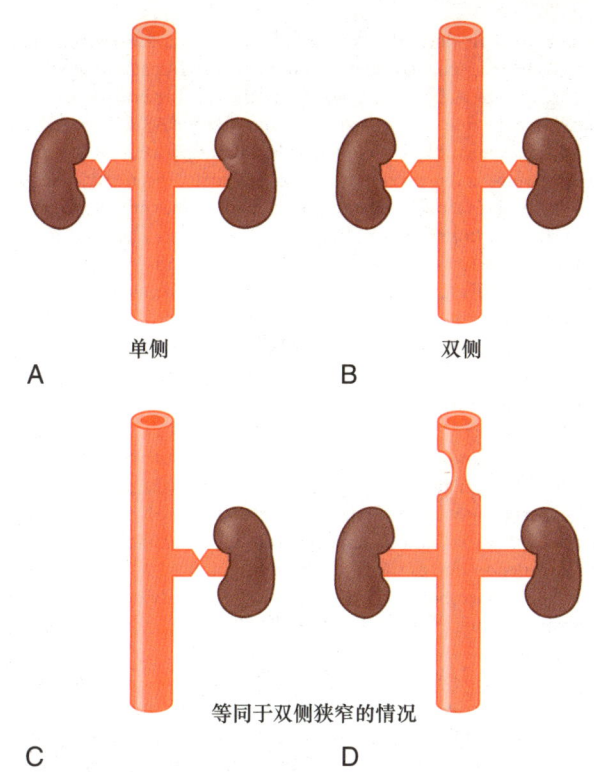

图 6.1 上图：人类肾脏横切面，显示肾动脉和肾静脉。下图：单个肾单位的微循环图解（引自 Guyton AC, Hall JE: Textbook of medical physiology, ed 11, 2016, Saunders, Chapter 26, 323-333.）译者注：原图近端肾小管指示线位置标注错误

图 6.2 肾动脉狭窄的解剖示意图。肾动脉狭窄可以是单侧（A），双侧（B），或孤立肾同侧（C）。主动脉疾病可出现类似双侧肾动脉狭窄的损伤（D）

肾脏处于血流动力学受损的状态。然而，由于对侧正常肾脏的功能足以代偿，上述变化不会反映在血清肌酐变化上。但是，如果对侧肾脏已存在损伤，如长期高血压、糖尿病或血管病变所致，则可出现 GFR 下降。当仅一个肾脏具有功能（孤立肾）或双侧肾脏均受累（即，双侧 RAS），应用 ACE 抑制剂或 ARB 治疗可能导致 AKI 发生。

动脉粥样硬化性肾血管疾病

临床表现

尽管任何引起单侧或双侧肾动脉狭窄的过程均可能导致肾缺血，动脉粥样硬化性肾血管疾病仍是成人 RAS 的主要病因；其他病因将会在下文继续讨论。动脉粥样硬化性肾血管疾病是继发性高血压的常见病因，占高血压患者的 5%。动脉粥样硬化性 RAS 很少发生于 40 岁以下的患者，在男性、白种人、吸烟、糖尿病以及存在其他动脉粥样硬化的患者中更常见。在具有其他动脉粥样硬化性疾病危险因素（如冠状动脉疾病、周围血管疾病和主动脉疾病）的患者中，RAS 的患病率会升高至 10%～45%。

对于难治性高血压或 50 岁以上的新发高血压患者需怀疑 RAS，尤其是同时合并显著的动脉粥样硬化性 RAS 危险因素的患者（表 6.1）。RAS 的评估应从详细的病史采集和全面的体格检查开始，需关注四肢的血压和脉冲幅度。四肢血压明显不对称提示可能存在周围血管病变，RAS 可能性增加。约 50% 的 RAS 患者

表 6.1　动脉粥样硬化性肾血管疾病的临床表现
新发、严重的高血压，或大于 55 岁的慢性高血压患者出现血压快速恶化
快速进展的高血压、难治性高血压，或恶性高血压
难以解释的肾萎缩，或双肾大小相差超过 1.5 cm
突发的、其他原因难以解释的（"速发"）肺水肿
存在其他动脉粥样硬化性血管病变的患者出现难以解释的慢性肾脏病
启动 ACE 抑制剂或 ARB 治疗后出现急性肾损伤或原有的慢性肾脏病恶化

ACE，血管紧张素转换酶；ARB，血管紧张素 II 受体阻滞剂。

查体可闻及腹部杂音，但其对于 RAS 诊断缺乏特异性。水肿并不常见，除非疾病已经进展至非常严重的程度。患者可合并存在 CKD 或其他原因导致的水肿。

实验室检查可出现继发于醛固酮增多症的低钾血症（$K^+ < 3.5$ mmol/L）或代谢性碱中毒（$HCO_3^- > 28$ mmol/L），但并非所有患者都会表现出上述异常。患者可出现 GFR 下降伴血清肌酐水平升高，但血清肌酐水平正常并不能除外具有血流动力学显著影响的 RAS。患者的血浆肾素和醛固酮水平可能升高，但其测量在评估高血压患者是否存在 RAS 或协助确定治疗决策中的临床价值有限。尿常规检测结果多为正常，部分长期高血压患者可出现少量蛋白尿（通常 < 1 g/d）。

诊断

标准肾脏超声影像可协助诊断潜在的 RAS，当超声发现双肾大小明显不一致，或双肾均小于正常水平（因为肾

are smaller than normal, because kidney size diminishes over time after prolonged ischemia. *Renal ultrasound with Doppler analysis* provides information about flow velocity in the renal arteries that may be helpful in detecting hemodynamically significant RAS. However, *renal duplex ultrasonography* is technically demanding, particularly in obese patients. Since at any given center, the sensitivity, specificity, and positive and negative predictive values of renal duplex ultrasonography are likely to be unknown, its clinical utility is mainly when positive for RAS; a negative test is not informative in patients with high clinical suspicion. Serial measurement of the kidney size and measurement of the renal resistive index ([peak systolic velocity − end-diastolic velocity] divided by peak systolic velocity) are helpful in assessing the potential benefit of revascularization. A high resistive index reflects an advanced degree of likely irreversible intrinsic kidney damage.

Computed tomography (CT) with intravenous iodinated contrast (i.e., CT angiography [CTA]) permits high-resolution evaluation of the arterial vasculature and can be a very useful diagnostic imaging study, particularly in patients with normal or near-normal kidney function. Its use is limited in patients with more significantly impaired kidney function due to the risk of contrast-induced AKI. Some newer CT imaging machines have a higher resolution and better tissue reconstruction allowing the visualization of RAS with lower amounts of contrast exposure.

Magnetic resonance angiography (MRA) with intravenous contrast is also useful for detecting RAS. Gadolinium administration to patients with advanced kidney disease (GFR <15 to 30 mL/min) may be contraindicated because of the risk of nephrogenic systemic fibrosis, although this appears to be much less of a concern with newer nonionic linear and macrocyclic gadolinium contrast agents. Overall, CTA and MRA appear to have similarly high sensitivity and specificity in the assessment of patients with atherosclerotic RAS. In RAS secondary to FMD, CTA and MRA are less sensitive because the disease involves the more distal part of the renal artery.

A *functional renal nuclear medicine test* might seem pathophysiologically ideal to detect RAS that is impacting kidney perfusion. Nuclear imaging has been used with various isotopes to assess isotopic uptake and excretion by each kidney before and after the administration of a short-acting ACE inhibitor (e.g., captopril). However, due to the high prevalence of baseline asymmetry of blood flow in patients with CKD and inability to accurately diagnose RAS when it is bilateral, radionuclear tests have fallen out of favor due to limited specificity and sensitivity for the diagnosis of RAS and are not commonly used any longer to assess for the presence of RAS or to determine whether RAS might be amenable to revascularization.

The most sensitive and specific test—but also the most invasive—is *renal arteriography*, which remains the gold standard for the detection of RAS. An advantage of arteriography is that angioplasty and stenting can be performed during the procedure (discussed later) if indicated. Because of the frequent occurrence of accessory renal arteries, an aortogram must be performed rather than selective renal angiography to ensure that all vessels are visualized. This also allows for detection of aortic atherosclerotic disease.

Treatment

Patients with atherosclerotic RAS typically have coexistent cerebrovascular, coronary, and peripheral vascular disease as the result of a long history of multiple risk factors such as cigarette smoking and hyperlipidemia. Clinicians should recognize this high cardiovascular risk and understand that long-term outcomes for patients with atherosclerotic RAS are often determined by coexisting atherosclerotic disease of the cerebral, cardiac, or peripheral vascular circulations. The absolute risk of developing end-stage renal disease (ESRD) is increased for patients with atherosclerotic RAS compared with those without RAS, especially in patients with bilateral RAS or RAS of a solitary kidney.

As with atherosclerotic disease in other arterial circulations, atherosclerotic RAS should prompt efforts for intensive lipid lowering, use of aspirin, smoking cessation, and control of hypertension and diabetes mellitus.

Intervention for atherosclerotic RAS remains controversial despite several randomized clinical trials designed to investigate the benefits and risks of medical management compared with angioplasty and renal artery stenting. Small clinical studies have suggested that renal artery angioplasty and stenting may improve blood pressure control in selected cases of atherosclerotic RAS, but identifying which patients may benefit has been problematic, and many have little or no improvement in blood pressure or are not able to significantly reduce the number of required antihypertensive medications. Two major randomized, controlled clinical trials of treatment of RAS with angioplasty did not demonstrate significant clinical benefit in terms of blood pressure control, kidney function, or mortality for most patients with atherosclerotic RAS, although both have been criticized for selection bias (excluding some high-risk patients with recurrent flash pulmonary edema and patients whose doctors felt they were likely to benefit from revascularization) and recruiting significant numbers of low-risk patients who were not on optimal medical therapy.

Renal artery angioplasty and stenting carry a risk of acute worsening of kidney function due to atheroembolic disease, contrast nephropathy, or in-stent thrombosis, among other technical complications, and the procedures may lead to irreversible, progressive kidney dysfunction and ESRD. Decisions to correct atherosclerotic RAS with angioplasty and stenting or surgery must be made on a case-by-case basis, considering:

- Underlying kidney function and pace of kidney function loss, if any.
- Severity and duration of hypertension: persistence of uncontrolled HTN after optimal medical therapy, intolerance to optimal medical therapy, and the short duration of blood pressure elevation prior to the diagnosis of RAS.
- Atherosclerotic disease in other vascular beds and life expectancy based on age and other comorbid conditions.
- Flash pulmonary edema.

There is no role for angioplasty alone without stenting in most patients with atherosclerotic RAS due to the high risk of recurrent stenosis.

Medical management of hypertension in patients with atherosclerotic RAS must take into consideration other comorbid conditions. Use of an ACE inhibitor or ARB and diuretics is often very effective, but patients treated with these agents must be monitored closely for further compromise of their kidney function.

Fibromuscular Dysplasia

FMD is a nonatherosclerotic, noninflammatory disease that causes RAS. FMD typically affects young women more than other groups but men and older age groups can be affected. The cause is not established, but it is thought to be a developmental defect. FMD is responsible for 35% to 50% of renovascular hypertension in children and 5% to 10% of renovascular hypertension in adults.

FMD most commonly affects the renal arteries (bilaterally in about 35% of affected patients), but carotid and vertebral arteries can also be affected.

Classification of FMD is based on the histologic layer of the artery involved (i.e., intima, media, or adventitia) (Table 6.2). Medial fibroplasia with a mural aneurysm is the most common cause of FMD in adults (70% of cases). It consists of alternating fibromuscular

脏在持续缺血后会随时间推移而缩小）则需考虑 RAS。

肾脏多普勒超声检测获得的肾动脉流速可协助检测具有血流动力学意义的 RAS。但肾脏双能超声检查的技术要求较高，特别是对于肥胖患者进行检查时。由于在任何指定机构中均尚无肾脏双能超声检查的诊断敏感性、特异性、阳性及阴性预测值的数据，因此，其临床实用性主要在于对临床高度怀疑 RAS 者呈阳性结果时支持诊断；而阴性检测结果不具参考价值。肾脏大小、肾动脉阻力指数［（收缩期峰流速－舒张末期流速）除以收缩期峰流速］的测量有助于评估血运重建的潜在获益。高阻力指数反映出肾脏损伤严重，呈不可逆性。

使用静脉注射碘造影剂的计算机断层成像（CT）［即 CT 血管造影（CTA）］提供动脉血管系统的高分辨率成像评估，是一种非常具有诊断价值的影像学检查，尤其在肾功能正常或接近正常的患者中。由于存在造影剂相关 AKI 的风险，该检查在肾功能严重受损患者中的应用受限。一些新型的 CT 成像设备可提供更高的分辨率和更好的组织重建能力，并可在更少的造影剂暴露量下显示 RAS。

使用静脉注射造影剂的磁共振血管成像（MRA）同样有助于检测 RAS。钆造影剂存在导致肾源性系统性纤维化的风险，尽管较新的非离子线性造影剂以及大环类钆造影剂已经使得该风险明显降低，晚期肾功能不全（GFR < 15～30 ml/min）仍是钆造影剂使用禁忌证。整体来说，CTA 和 MRA 对于动脉粥样硬化性 RAS 患者的评估具有相似的高敏感性以及特异性。对于继发于 FMD 的 RAS 患者，由于其病变主要累及肾动脉远端部分，因此 CTA 和 MRA 的敏感性不佳。

从病理生理角度来说，功能性肾核医学检查是检测影响肾灌注的 RAS 的理想手段。核成像使用多种同位素，在患者服用短效 ACE 抑制剂（如卡托普利）前后评估每个肾脏的同位素摄取和排泄水平。但是，由于 CKD 患者中基线双侧肾血流不对称的情况常见，且其不能准确诊断双侧 RAS，核医学检查因其诊断 RAS 的特异性和准确性均有限而不再受到青睐，也不再常用于评估 RAS 的存在或判断 RAS 是否需要血运重建治疗。

肾动脉造影是诊断 RAS 敏感性和特异性最高的检查——尽管它同时也是创伤性最大的检查，但仍是检测 RAS 的金标准。肾动脉造影的优势之一是：如有必要，可以在造影检查的同时进行血管成形术或支架植入（将在本章后续讨论）。由于人群中存在副肾动脉的比例偏高，必须先完成主动脉造影而非直接进行选择性肾动脉造影，以保证所有血管均可见。这也有助于发现主动脉粥样硬化性疾病。

治疗

动脉粥样硬化性 RAS 患者常合并脑血管、冠状动脉以及周围血管病，这是吸烟、高脂血症等多种危险因素长期存在的结果。临床医师应当认识到上述高心血管疾病风险，并理解动脉粥样硬化性 RAS 患者的预后通常取决于其共存的脑、心或周围血管的动脉粥样硬化性疾病。与无 RAS 患者相比，动脉粥样硬化性 RAS 患者，特别是双侧 RAS 或孤立肾 RAS 的患者，进展至终末期肾病（ESRD）的绝对风险升高。

与其他动脉系统的动脉粥样硬化性疾病一样，动脉粥样硬化性 RAS 的治疗应强化降脂、使用阿司匹林、戒烟、控制高血压及糖尿病。

尽管已有数个随机临床试验旨在比较药物治疗与血管成形术及肾动脉支架植入的获益与风险，动脉粥样硬化性 RAS 的介入治疗仍存在争议。一些小型临床研究表明，对于特定的动脉粥样硬化性 RAS 患者，进行血管成形术或放置支架可能有助于改善血压控制，但如何识别可能从介入治疗中获益的患者仍存在困难，许多患者血压几乎没有改善，也有患者血压改善显著、所需降压药物数量明显减少。两项大型的随机对照临床试验显示，对于大部分动脉粥样硬化性 RAS 患者而言血管成形术并未显示出血压控制、肾功能以及死亡率等方面的获益，然而上述研究均因选择偏移（排除了反复急性肺水肿的高危患者和医生认为可能从介入治疗中获益的患者）以及招募了大量未接受最佳药物治疗的低危患者而被诟病。

肾动脉血管成形术及支架植入可能引发动脉粥样硬化栓塞性疾病、造影剂肾病、支架内血栓形成等技术并发症，继而存在造成肾功能快速恶化的风险，操作过程本身可能导致不可逆性的进展性肾损害以及 ESRD。在决定动脉粥样硬化性 RAS 患者是否应进行血管成形术和支架植入或手术治疗时，必须进行个体化评估，可参考以下内容：

- 患者的肾功能以及潜在的肾功能下降速度。
- 高血压的严重程度以及持续时间：在最佳药物治疗后血压仍持续难以控制，不能耐受最佳药物治疗，在诊断 RAS 前新近出现的血压升高。
- 其他血管的粥样硬化性疾病，以及基于年龄及其他合并症情况判断的预期寿命。
- 速发性肺水肿。

由于血管再狭窄的风险高，在绝大多数动脉粥样硬化性 RAS 患者中，不考虑单独进行血管成形术而不放置支架。

动脉粥样硬化性 RAS 患者的高血压药物治疗需要充分考虑到其他合并症。ACE 抑制剂或 ARB 联合利尿剂通常可有效降压，但应用这些药物后应密切监测患者肾功能的受损情况。

纤维肌发育不良（FMD）

FMD 是一种引起 RAS 的非动脉粥样硬化性、非炎症性疾病。FMD 主要好发于年轻女性，但在男性及老年人群亦可受累。其发病机制尚不明确，但被认为是一种发育缺陷。FMD 占儿童肾血管性高血压病因的 35%～50%、成人肾血管性高血压病因的 5%～10%。

FMD 最常累及肾动脉（35% 为双侧），但颈动脉和椎动脉亦可受累。

FMD 的分类基于受累动脉的组织学分层（即，内

ridges and aneurysmal segments in the distal two thirds of the renal artery and has a classic string-of-beads appearance on angiography (Fig. 6.3). Perimedial fibroplasia of the outer one half of the media produces severe multifocal stenosis and causes about 15% of FMD in adults. Because histologic specimens are rarely obtained, FMD is classified by the angiographic appearance with multifocal disease identified as FMD involving the media and unifocal disease as FMD of the intima and/or adventitia.

Medial subtypes of FMD usually have a benign course and are responsive to angioplasty. The intimal subtype may have a higher likelihood of ischemic events and multiorgan system involvement. Symptoms are usually precipitated by stenosis, but FMD may rarely cause dissection or macroaneurysms that require intervention. Although CTA or MRA may be useful in the detection of FMD in the main renal arteries and main branch arteries, arteriography is necessary for detection of stenosis in smaller arteries.

Treatment for FMD depends on the severity of complications. Pharmacologic treatment alone may be adequate to control hypertension in many patients, with an ACE inhibitor or ARB the antihypertensives of choice. Intervention with angioplasty (with or without stenting) or surgery should be considered for patients with severe or difficult to control hypertension or declining kidney function. Angioplasty without stenting is successful in many patients, but recurrent stenosis is not uncommon, and new stenosis from FMD may develop at other sites. For this reason, regular monitoring of blood pressure and serum creatinine levels is essential, and many patients require imaging studies to detect new or recurrent lesions.

TABLE 6.2 Histologic Classification of Fibromuscular Dysplasia		
Subtype	Percentage of All Cases (%)	Radiologic Appearance
Medial fibroplasia	60-70	String of beads with aneurysms
Perimedial fibroplasia	15	String of beads without large aneurysms
Medial hyperplasia	5-15	Smooth tubular stenosis
Intimal fibroplasia	1-2	Focal or smooth stenosis
Adventitial fibroplasia	<1	Focal or smooth tubular stenosis

Aortic Dissection

Aortic dissection occurs after disruption of the intimal layer of the aorta and propagation of blood flow that dissects along the wall of the aorta, producing a false lumen and compression of the true aortic lumen. Aortic dissection is classified by the site of origin (i.e., DeBakey classification) or the segment of the aorta involved (i.e., Stanford classification). DeBakey type I and II dissections originate in the ascending aorta, and type III dissections originate in the descending aorta. Stanford type A refers to dissections involving the ascending aorta, and type B refers to all others not involving the ascending aorta.

Major branch vessels of the aorta, including the renal arteries, may become obstructed or occluded as a result of extension of the dissection. Aortic dissection frequently compromises the renal arteries (the left more commonly than the right) when it extends into the abdominal aorta and causes renal failure in approximately 20% of patients with type B dissections. When disease is extensive enough to cause AKI, vascular compromise to the intestinal and cerebral vasculature and severe aortic regurgitation often contribute to the high mortality rate.

Aortic dissection most frequently affects older patients (>50 years of age) with coexistent vascular risk factors such as hypertension, smoking, and atherosclerosis. Men are affected more commonly than women. Occasionally, a genetic connective tissue defect such as Marfan syndrome or Ehlers-Danlos syndrome type IV (about 5% of cases) causes aortic dissection, and these conditions should be considered in younger patients (<40 years of age).

AKI occurs in about 20% of patients diagnosed with acute type B aortic dissection and is an independent predictor of in-hospital mortality. Trauma or procedures (e.g., aortic catheterization) can also cause dissection of the aorta or renal artery. Isolated, spontaneous renal artery dissection may rarely occur, most commonly in the setting of polyarteritis nodosa (PAN) or FMD. Segmental arterial mediolysis is another uncommon condition of unknown origin that is characterized by vacuolar degeneration of smooth muscle cells in the arterial media, which leads to disruption of the arterial medial layer, vessel dissection, hemorrhage, and ischemia. Segmental arterial mediolysis can affect abdominal visceral arteries and virtually any other arterial system.

The most frequent symptom during aortic dissection is chest pain, which may be described as a ripping sensation. Isolated loss of pulse in one or more extremities may provide a clinical clue, and the number of

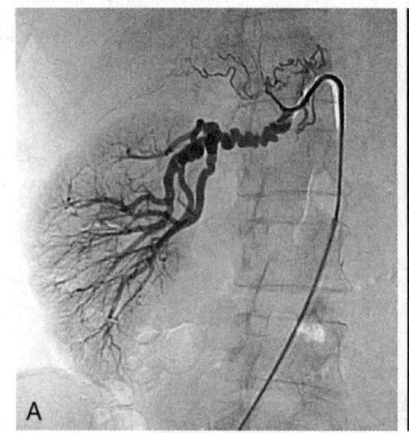 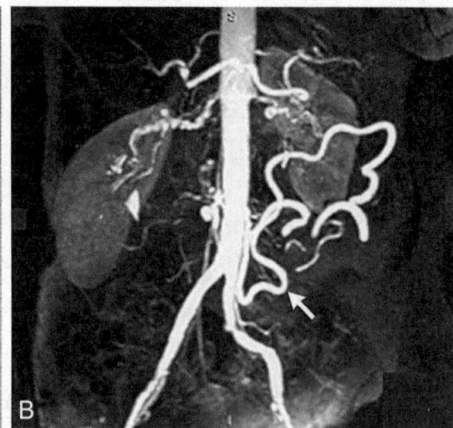

Fig. 6.3 (A) Typical medial fibroplasia (i.e., string-of-beads appearance) on an angiogram of a right renal artery. (B) Gadolinium-enhanced magnetic resonance angiography in the same patient, revealing bilateral medial fibroplasia of the renal arteries and a large marginal artery of Drummond (arrow), indicates that there is disease of the superior mesenteric artery. (From Slovut DP, Olin JW: Fibromuscular dysplasia, N Engl J Med 350:1862-1871, 2004.)

膜、中膜或外膜）（表6.2）。中膜纤维增生伴动脉瘤形成是成人FMD最主要的原因（约占70%的病例）。病变由位于肾动脉远端2/3部分的交替出现的纤维肌脊与动脉瘤节段组成，在血管造影中呈现经典的串珠样表现（图6.3）。中膜外侧一半的中膜外纤维组织增生导致严重的多灶性狭窄，约占成人FMD的15%。由于很少获得组织学标本，FMD的分类主要依据血管造影表现进行，将多灶性病变认定为累及中膜的FMD、局灶性FMD则为累及内膜和（或）外膜的FMD。

中膜型FMD通常预后良好，血管成形术疗效较好。内膜型FMD则更容易出现缺血事件以及多器官系统性受累。FMD的症状多由狭窄引起，但很少出现夹层或需要手术干预的大血管瘤。尽管CTA或MRA有助于检测主肾动脉及其主要分支的FMD，但动脉造影仍是检测更小血管的狭窄所必需的。

FMD的治疗选择主要取决于并发症的严重程度。对许多患者来说，单纯药物治疗就足以控制高血压，降压药物首选ACE抑制剂或ARB。对于严重高血压或高血压难以控制或肾功能下降的患者应考虑血管成形术介入治疗（伴或不伴支架植入）或手术治疗。多数患者单纯进行血管成形术、无需放置支架即能有效改善症状，但复发性狭窄不少见，FMD也可能在其他部位形成新狭窄。因此常规监测血压和血肌酐水平至关重要，许多患者需要影像学检查来监测新发或再狭窄病变。

表6.2 纤维肌发育不良的组织学分类		
亚型	占所有病例的百分比（%）	影像学表现
中膜纤维组织增生	60～70	串珠样动脉瘤
中膜外纤维组织增生	15	无大动脉瘤的串珠样改变
中膜增生	5～15	光滑的管状狭窄
内膜纤维组织增生	1～2	局灶或光滑的狭窄
外膜纤维组织增生	<1	局灶或光滑的管状狭窄

主动脉夹层

主动脉夹层发生于主动脉内膜破裂后，血流沿主动脉壁蔓延、撕裂动脉壁形成假腔并压迫主动脉真腔。主动脉夹层的分型可基于内膜撕裂的起始部位（即，DeBakay分型）或主动脉的受累部位（即，Stanford分型）。DeBakey Ⅰ型和Ⅱ型夹层起始于升主动脉，Ⅲ型夹层起始于降主动脉。Stanford A型夹层指累及升主动脉的夹层，B型指除升主动脉以外其他所有部位的夹层。

主动脉的主要分支血管，包括肾动脉，可能因夹层撕裂范围扩大而阻塞或闭塞。当主动脉夹层扩展至腹主动脉时，常损害肾动脉（左肾动脉比右肾动脉更常累），导致约20%的B型夹层患者发生肾衰竭。当病变范围足够广泛以致引起AKI时，肠道及脑血管的血管损害和严重的主动脉反流常是极高死亡率的重要原因。

主动脉夹层高发于年龄较大的患者（>50岁），此类患者常并合高血压、吸烟、以及动脉粥样硬化症等血管危险因素。男性较女性更易受影响。有时，遗传性结缔组织缺陷亦可导致主动脉夹层，如马方综合征或Ⅳ型埃勒斯-当洛综合征（约占病例的5%），在年轻患者（<40岁）中需考虑这些病因。

约20%的急性B型夹层患者发生AKI，AKI是院内死亡率的独立预测因素。创伤或操作（如主动脉导管检查）同样可导致主动脉或肾动脉夹层。孤立的自发性肾动脉夹层很少见，其最常见于结节性多动脉炎（PAN）或FMD。节段性动脉中膜溶解是另一种病因不明的罕见疾病，其特征性表现为动脉中膜的平滑肌细胞出现空泡变性，导致动脉中膜层破裂、血管夹层、出血以及缺血。节段性动脉中膜溶解可累及腹部内脏动脉和几乎所有其他动脉系统。

主动脉夹层最常见的症状是胸痛，可被描述为撕裂感。单个或多个肢体的脉搏消失可为主动脉夹层提供临床线索，累及血管数量的多少则与夹层的严重程度相关。

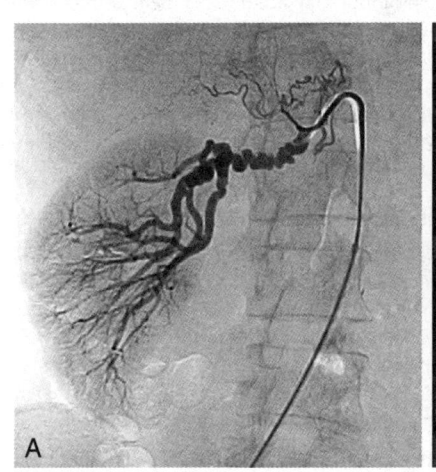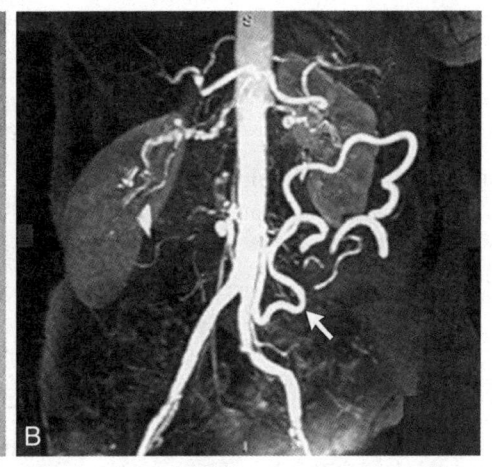

图6.3 （A）右肾动脉造影显示经典的中膜纤维组织增生表现（即，串珠样改变）。（B）同一患者的钆增强磁共振血管成像，显示双侧肾动脉中膜纤维组织增生，以及粗大的Drummond缘动脉（箭头所指），提示该患者存在肠系膜上动脉病变（引自Slovut DP, Olin JW: Fibromuscular dysplasia, N Engl J Med 350: 1862-1871, 2004.）

arteries involved correlates with the severity of dissection. A common clue to the diagnosis on a routine chest radiograph is a widened mediastinum, with or without a pleural effusion (most often on the left).

After the diagnosis of aortic dissection is established, evaluation of renal artery involvement is best undertaken noninvasively to minimize further vascular injury. Contrast-enhanced CT, magnetic resonance imaging, or MRA usually provide images capable of confirming or excluding renal involvement, although each modality carries the same limitations as outlined for the evaluation of RAS. Transesophageal echocardiography is useful for establishing the diagnosis of aortic dissection, but it does not provide information about the aorta below the diaphragm. Renal duplex ultrasonography may be useful for evaluating renal perfusion in the setting of aortic dissection, but it is not recommended for the initial investigation of aortic dissection.

Aortic dissection is a hypertensive emergency that requires aggressive reduction of blood pressure; systolic blood pressure should be maintained between 100 and 120 mm Hg. Antihypertensive medications that reduce the rate of increase in blood pressure during the cardiac cycle, such as β-adrenergic receptor blockers, have a theoretical benefit in managing aortic dissection by reducing the rate of progression.

Surgical treatment options for renal involvement due to aortic dissection depend on individual circumstances, and careful evaluation by an experienced vascular surgeon is recommended. Thoracic aortic dissection requires surgical repair due to the high mortality rate if left untreated, but isolated abdominal aortic disease may be medically managed.

Thromboembolic Disease

Systemic arterial emboli, typically originating from the left atrium or left ventricle in patients with atrial fibrillation, infectious endocarditis, cardiac valvular disease, or atrial myxoma, may cause acute obstruction of the renal arteries. Rarely, a paradoxical embolus may occur from the venous system through an atrial septal defect.

Symptoms of acute renal ischemia and infarction include flank pain, gross hematuria, and fever. Laboratory findings are nonspecific but include an elevated level of lactate dehydrogenase (LDH), hematuria, and leukocytosis. A definitive diagnosis can be based on the finding of a focal nonenhancing region on contrast-enhanced CT. Imaging studies are necessary to differentiate renal artery embolic disease from renal artery dissection.

The renal mass affected by a renal artery embolus is usually not large enough to reduce kidney function so that dialysis is necessary, although some worsening of kidney function may be observed. The diagnosis of renal infarction is rarely made early enough to initiate treatment with intra-arterial thrombolysis or thrombectomy, and it is questionable whether the risks and marginal benefit of these procedures warrant aggressive treatment except in patients where the occlusion is affecting the main renal artery and is addressed soon after occurrence. Therapy should instead address the underlying source of renal emboli with symptomatic treatment of pain as necessary. Systemic anticoagulation may be indicated to reduce the risk of further thromboembolic events.

Large and Medium-Sized Vessel Vasculitis

Systemic vasculitides such as temporal (giant cell) arteritis and Takayasu's arteritis affect primarily large and medium-sized arteries. PAN and Kawasaki disease affect primarily medium-sized and smaller arteries. These vasculitides are not associated with antineutrophil cytoplasmic antibodies (ANCAs) and do not typically cause glomerulonephritis. They are distinguished from ANCA-associated vasculitides that involve smaller blood vessels and more commonly cause glomerulonephritis.

Takayasu's arteritis and giant cell arteritis are typically associated with a granulomatous vasculitis of the aorta and its branches. Giant cell arteritis typically involves the carotid, vertebral, and temporal arteries, and renal involvement is rare. Both occur much more commonly in women than men. Takayasu's arteritis is usually diagnosed in patients younger than 50 years of age, whereas giant cell arteritis is diagnosed in those 50 years of age or older.

Involvement of the main renal arteries occurs in about 40% of patients with Takayasu's arteritis, producing areas of stenosis with renal ischemia or renal infarction. Common clinical features are constitutional symptoms, claudication, bruits, and hypertension. Pulses are often diminished or absent in one or more extremities, and a blood pressure discrepancy more than 10 mm Hg in the limbs is common. The diagnosis of Takayasu's arteritis is most often made on clinical grounds along with typical angiographic or other imaging findings. Corticosteroids are the primary treatment modality. The stenotic lesions are usually reversible when corticosteroid therapy is given during the early phase of the disease before the lesions becomes fibrotic and irreversible. About half of patients have chronic, persistent or corticosteroid-dependent disease and require therapy with additional or alternative immunosuppressants such as azathioprine, mycophenolate, methotrexate, leflunomide or cyclophosphamide. More recently targeted immunosuppression with antagonists of interleukin-6 (such as tocilizumab) and blockers of the tumor necrosis factor alpha (TNFα) pathway (such as infliximab or etanercept) may be effective in helping maintain remission.

PAN is a medium-sized or small vessel vasculitis with no gender predilection that predominantly occurs in adults between 40 and 60 years of age. It is an idiopathic systemic necrotizing vasculitis. Some cases may be secondary to hepatitis B virus infection, hepatitis C virus infection, or hairy cell leukemia. Peripheral neuropathy in the form of mononeuritis multiplex is one of the most frequent findings with PAN.

PAN affects the main renal arteries and renal interlobar arteries (less commonly, the arcuate and interlobular arteries) with a necrotizing vasculitis that typically produces microaneurysms of the intrarenal arteries. They can be seen on arteriograms in 40% to 90% of patients with renal involvement. Renal ischemia leads to loss of kidney function and renin-mediated hypertension. Low-grade proteinuria and hematuria may be seen, but the finding of acute glomerulonephritis indicates some other disorder. Renal infarction may occur, and rarely, a renal artery aneurysm may cause renal artery dissection or rupture.

The diagnosis is made on clinical grounds and by arteriography. There are no confirmatory serologic tests; PAN is not an ANCA-associated vasculitis. Arteriography appears to be superior for diagnosis compared with CTA and MRA. Progressive renal disease is not typical but may occur. Treatment with corticosteroids and immunosuppressive drugs is effective in reducing disease severity and mortality.

Kawasaki disease is an arteritis associated with the mucocutaneous lymph node syndrome that affects mostly medium-sized and small arteries, although the aorta may also be involved. It is primarily a self-limited disease of infants and young children. Renal involvement is extremely rare.

Hypertensive Nephrosclerosis

Chronic hypertension in susceptible individuals may lead to development of proteinuria, CKD, and ESRD. Hypertensive nephrosclerosis is cited as a cause of CKD and ESRD in African Americans at a much higher rate than white individuals, even with similar levels of blood pressure control and despite good control.

The renal manifestations of chronic hypertension include renal arterial and arteriolar intimal thickening and luminal narrowing with medial

主动脉夹层在常规胸部 X 线检查上的常见线索是纵隔增宽、伴或不伴胸腔积液（最常见于左侧）。

诊断主动脉夹层后，最好通过无创的手段评估肾动脉受累情况，尽量减少进一步的血管损伤。增强 CT、磁共振成像或 MRA 均可提供能够确认或除外肾动脉受累的影像，但所有检查手段均存在与前述 RAS 评估时同样的限制性。经食管超声心动图有助于诊断主动脉夹层，但不能提供膈以下主动脉的信息。肾脏双能超声有助于评估出现主动脉夹层后的肾灌注情况，但不建议应用于主动脉夹层的初始检查。

主动脉夹层是一种需要积极降压的高血压急症；收缩压应维持在 100～120 mmHg。降低心动周期血压升高率的降压药物，如 β 受体阻滞剂，理论上有益于降低主动脉夹层的进展速率。

主动脉夹层造成的肾动脉受累是否需要手术干预取决于个体情况，并且需要有经验的血管外科医师进行缜密评估。如由于不治疗的死亡率很高，因此胸主动脉夹层需要进行手术修补，但单纯腹主动脉夹层可以药物保守治疗。

血栓栓塞性疾病

系统性动脉栓子通常来源于心房颤动、感染性心内膜炎、心脏瓣膜病或心房黏液瘤患者的左心房或左心室，可导致急性肾动脉阻塞。罕见情况下，反常栓子可为通过房间隔缺损的静脉系统血栓。

急性肾缺血及梗死的症状包括腰痛、肉眼血尿和发热。实验室检查缺乏特异性，可出现乳酸脱氢酶（LDH）水平升高、血尿和白细胞增多。增强 CT 出现肾脏局灶性非增强区域即可确诊。有必要通过影像学检查来进一步鉴别肾动脉栓塞性疾病和肾动脉夹层。

尽管肾动脉栓塞可导致一定程度的肾功能恶化，其累及肾实质部分通常不足以造成需透析支持的肾功能下降。肾梗死很难能够早期诊断、从而及时启动动脉内溶栓或动脉内取栓治疗；同时，除非血栓累及肾动脉主干且迅速被识别，鉴于这些上述操作的风险及边界效益，是否值得进行这些侵入性操作仍值得商榷。治疗上应着重解决肾栓子的来源，并进行必要的止痛治疗。应启动系统性抗凝以减少更多的动脉粥样硬化性栓子事件风险。

大血管和中血管血管炎

系统性血管炎如颞动脉炎（巨细胞动脉炎）和大动脉炎主要累及大血管和中等大小的血管。PAN 和川崎病主要累及中等大小以及更小的血管。这些血管炎与抗中性粒细胞胞质抗体（ANCA）无关，且通常不引起肾小球肾炎。ANCA 相关性血管炎与之有所区别，ANCA 相关性血管炎累及更小的血管且更常引起肾小球肾炎。

大动脉炎和巨细胞动脉炎通常会伴有主动脉及其分支的肉芽肿性血管炎。巨细胞动脉炎主要累及颈动脉、椎动脉及颞动脉，较少出现肾动脉受累。两种疾病都在女性中更常见。大动脉炎常在小于 50 岁的患者中被诊断，而巨细胞动脉炎则多在大于 50 岁或年龄更大的患者中被诊断。

约 40% 的大动脉炎患者出现肾动脉受累，造成狭窄区域出现肾缺血及肾梗死。常见的临床表现包括全身症状、跛行、血管杂音和高血压。患者存在单个或多个肢体的脉搏减弱或消失，肢体血压往往相差 10 mmHg 以上。大动脉炎的诊断主要依据临床表现以及典型的血管造影或其他影像学表现。皮质类固醇是主要的治疗手段。在疾病早期、尚未形成不可逆的纤维化病变的阶段给予皮质类固醇治疗后，狭窄病变通常是可逆的。约一半的患者病变为慢性、持续性或皮质类固醇依赖性，需要联合或改用免疫抑制剂治疗，如硫唑嘌呤、霉酚酸酯、甲氨蝶呤、来氟米特或环磷酰胺。近年来，白介素-6 拮抗剂（如托珠单抗）及肿瘤坏死因子 α（TNFα）通路阻滞剂（如英夫利昔单抗或依那西普）等靶向免疫抑制治疗的应用可有效帮助维持缓解期。

PAN 是一类累及中型血管或小血管的血管炎，好发于 40～60 岁的成年人且无性别差异。它是一类特发性系统性坏死性小血管炎。部分病例继发于乙型肝炎病毒感染、丙型肝炎病毒感染或毛细胞白血病。PAN 最常见的周围神经病表现形式为多发性单神经炎。

PAN 累及主肾动脉以及肾脏叶间动脉（较少见情况为累及弓状动脉以及小叶间动脉），导致坏死性血管炎并常形成肾内动脉微动脉瘤。40%～90% 的肾脏受累患者可在动脉造影中观察到上述表现。肾脏缺血造成肾功能下降以及肾素介导的高血压。患者可出现少量蛋白尿和血尿，但若出现急性肾小球肾炎表现则提示其他疾病。患者可发生肾梗死，同时，在罕见情况下肾动脉动脉瘤可导致肾动脉夹层或破裂。

PAN 诊断依据临床表现及动脉造影。PAN 并非 ANCA 相关性血管炎，缺乏确诊性的血清学指标。相较于 CTA 和 MRA，动脉造影在诊断上更佳。急进性肾脏疾病偶可发生、但其并非 PAN 的典型表现。皮质类固醇联合免疫抑制剂治疗可有效减低疾病严重程度和死亡率。

川崎病是一类与黏膜皮肤淋巴结综合征相关的血管炎，尽管主动脉亦可受累，但主要累及的是中等及小动脉，该病为婴幼儿的一类自限性疾病。肾脏受累极为罕见。

高血压性肾硬化症

在易感个体中慢性高血压可能导致蛋白尿、CKD 以及 ESRD。高血压性肾硬化症被认为是非裔美国人 CKD 和 ESRD 的病因之一，其发生率远高于白人个体，即使二者的血压控制水平相似且控制良好。

慢性高血压的肾脏表现包括肾动脉和小动脉内膜增厚及中膜肥厚伴管腔狭窄、动脉内膜成纤维细胞性增厚、

hypertrophy and fibroblastic intimal thickening of arteries and deposition of hyaline-like material (plasma proteins) in the walls of arterioles. Glomeruli show global and focal glomerulosclerosis; the former likely results from glomerular ischemia and the latter from increased intracapillary pressure and compensatory hypertrophy and injury in response to nephron loss. Wrinkled glomerular basement membranes due to glomerular ischemia are seen on electron microscopy. Chronic interstitial nephritis with tubular atrophy and interstitial fibrosis is another manifestation of chronic ischemic tubular injury seen with hypertensive nephrosclerosis, particularly in patients with other disorders such as diabetes mellitus, atheroembolic disease, and atherosclerotic RAS.

The overall risk of hypertensive nephrosclerosis with progressive CKD is low in the general hypertensive population, and most patients with hypertensive nephrosclerosis have mild hypertension. The risk is greater for those who have had poorly controlled hypertension and for those of African descent, who are at particularly high risk for hypertensive nephrosclerosis. Polymorphisms in the gene that encodes for apolipoprotein L1 (*APOL1*) is found more commonly in African Americans compared with European Americans and strongly associated with the risk of hypertensive nephrosclerosis. A diagnosis of hypertensive nephrosclerosis as the cause of otherwise unexplained CKD is much less likely to be made in white patients compared with black patients, particularly in the absence of long-standing, severe hypertension or a history of malignant hypertension.

The diagnosis of hypertensive nephrosclerosis is typically made clinically based on a history of long-standing hypertension that precedes development of proteinuria and CKD in the absence of other causes. Kidney biopsy is rarely performed except when other disorders are suggested clinically or by laboratory evaluation. The urinary sediment is typically bland, with only low-grade proteinuria (<1 g/day). Symmetrical loss of renal cortical thickness is commonly found on renal ultrasound.

Pharmacologic treatment of severe hypertension reduces the risk for progression of CKD to ESRD in many patient populations, providing further evidence for the causative role of hypertension. The optimal blood pressure for patients with hypertensive nephrosclerosis has not been determined. For black patients, this was best addressed by the African American Study of Kidney Disease (AASK) trial, which examined more than 1000 African Americans with long-standing hypertension, slowly progressive CKD, and low-grade proteinuria. Subjects were allocated to treatment with ramipril, metoprolol, or amlodipine to a blood pressure goal of 125/75 mm Hg or 140/90 mm Hg. The mean rate of change in GFR and the rate of other secondary outcomes were similar in the two groups, suggesting that lowering blood pressure to less than 140/90 mm Hg does not provide further benefit in slowing CKD progression in black patients with hypertensive nephrosclerosis. However, there was a trend favoring the lower blood pressure goal for patients with higher baseline proteinuria.

Lower blood pressure goals may also be appropriate for patients with other comorbid conditions such as diabetes mellitus. Besides affecting CKD progression, blood pressure control reduces the risk of heart failure and stroke. Most patients with hypertensive nephrosclerosis and CKD require multiple antihypertensive medications to control blood pressure, typically including a thiazide or thiazide-like diuretic (when GFR is well preserved) and a loop diuretic (as the GFR declines to less than 25 to 30 mL/min), along with an ACE inhibitor or ARB, calcium-channel blocker, and β-blocker.

Atheroembolic Disease

Atheroembolic disease is the result of cholesterol embolization from atherosclerotic plaques, most commonly from the aorta and typically dislodged during an invasive arterial procedure such as cardiac catheterization, aortic angiography, cardiac surgery, or surgery on the aorta. Cholesterol emboli may occur spontaneously or may be precipitated by systemic anticoagulation, such as with heparin, or during systemic administration of thrombolytic agents. Because patients must have underlying atherosclerosis, the incidence increases with age, and atheroembolic disease rarely occurs before 40 years of age.

As the result of systemic embolization from atheromatous plaques, cholesterol crystals lodge in small arterial vessels, including the arcuate or interlobular arteries of the kidneys. Cholesterol emboli frequently involve other organs, and the pattern of organ involvement depends in part on whether disrupted plaque is in the ascending or descending aorta. The extremities are commonly affected with digital ischemia and gangrene, the skin with livedo reticularis, and the gastrointestinal tract with intestinal ischemia, but any organ can be affected. Embolization from the ascending aorta can cause cardiac ischemia, and emboli arising from the ascending aorta or carotid arteries (e.g., after carotid endarterectomy) can cause stroke.

Cholesterol embolization to the eye may be recognized by finding Hollenhorst plaques on funduscopic examination, which are whitish yellow flecks at retinal arteriole bifurcations. They are often asymptomatic but may cause retinal ischemia with usually transient visual field defects.

Patients with atheroembolic disease may have fever, eosinophilia, eosinophiluria, and hypocomplementemia, particularly acutely. Laboratory findings include an elevated erythrocyte sedimentation rate and elevated levels of amylase or liver enzymes. The widespread systemic clinical and laboratory manifestations of atheroemboli can lead to a clinical picture suggesting systemic vasculitis.

The typical pattern of renal atheroembolic disease is a decline in kidney function that first becomes apparent 3 or more days after an inciting procedure or other event. The degree of acute and chronic kidney injury that follows is determined by the magnitude of the embolic burden, whether atheroembolism is a one-time or ongoing process, and the degree of inflammation induced by the plaque material. Many patients have stabilization of the process after the initial insult, whereas others progress with various patterns and tempos to advanced CKD and ESRD. Cholesterol embolization also may cause severe hypertension due to acute renal ischemia leading to renin release.

Diagnosis of renal atheroembolic disease is usually made clinically in the appropriate setting, but for some patients, a kidney biopsy is needed to confirm the diagnosis and exclude others. Because the fixation process washes out the cholesterol crystals from the renal biopsy sample, the pathologic examination reveals a typical needle-shaped disruption in the arterial lumen surrounded by reactive inflammatory and fibrous intimal proliferation leading to a luminal occlusion and distal ischemic injury.

There is no specific treatment for cholesterol emboli. Because an inflammatory reaction typically results from the emboli, some physicians advocate corticosteroids, but their use is unproved for preventing further atheroembolism or progression of kidney failure. Avoidance of anticoagulation has been recommended to prevent dissolution and embolization of thrombus that may overlie an atheromatous plaque. Statin therapy is recommended for most patients for treatment of their underlying atherosclerotic disease, but it has not been shown to influence the renal manifestation of atheroemboli. Treatment with ACE inhibitors or ARBs may be effective for hypertension control in the acute setting, but worsening kidney function may limit their use. Dialysis may be necessary if AKI and ESRD develop.

Preeclampsia

Preeclampsia is characterized by the new onset of sustained hypertension (blood pressure ≥140/90 mm Hg) and proteinuria (>300 mg/day)

小动脉管壁玻璃样物质（血浆蛋白）沉积。肾小球可出现球性及局灶性肾小球硬化；前者为肾小球缺血所致，后者则是毛细血管内压升高、肾单位丢失导致肾小球代偿性肥大及损伤所致。电镜下可观察到缺血导致肾小球基底膜皱缩。慢性间质性肾炎伴肾小管萎缩和间质纤维化是高血压性肾硬化症慢性缺血性小管损伤的另一个征象，这些肾小管间质改变在伴糖尿病、动脉粥样硬化栓塞性疾病、动脉粥样硬化性 RAS 等疾病患者中更加常见。

在整体高血压人群中，高血压性肾硬化症的 CKD 总体进展风险不高，绝大部分高血压性肾硬化症的患者为轻度高血压。血压控制不佳的患者和非裔患者的 CKD 进展风险更高，此类患者同样为发生高血压性肾硬化症的高危人群。编码载脂蛋白 L1（APOL1）的基因多态性在非裔美国人较欧裔美国人更为常见、且与高血压性肾硬化症的风险密切相关。相较于黑人患者，在白人患者中将其他原因难以解释的 CKD 归因于高血压性肾硬化症的可能性要小得多，尤其是没有长期、严重的高血压或恶性高血压病史的情况下。

高血压性肾硬化症的诊断通常是基于长期高血压病史，而后在没有其他病因的基础上出现尿蛋白和 CKD。除非存在临床或实验室检查提示的其他病因，该病较少需要进行肾活检。尿液检查中常仅有少量的蛋白尿（< 1 g/d），而尿沉渣没有明显异常。肾脏超声常见双肾对称性的皮质厚度减低。

在多个患者人群中，针对严重高血压进行药物治疗可降低 CKD 进展至 ESRD 的风险，进一步证明了高血压的致病作用。高血压性肾硬化症患者的最佳血压尚不明确。对于黑人患者，非裔美国人肾脏病研究（AASK）对此做出了最好的回答，该研究纳入了超过 1000 名长期高血压、伴有缓慢进展的 CKD 及少量蛋白尿的非裔美国患者。受试者被分配使用雷米普利、美托洛尔或氨氯地平治疗，目标血压分组为 125/75 mmHg 或 140/90 mmHg。不同血压分组的患者中，平均 GFR 变化率以及其他次要终点均无显著差异，这表明将血压控制到 140/90 mmHg 以下对于减缓黑人高血压性肾硬化症 CKD 进展并不能带来额外获益。然而，对于基线尿蛋白高的患者更倾向于较低的目标血压（125/75 mmHg）。

更低的目标血压可能更适合于伴发糖尿病等合并症的患者。除了延缓 CKD 进展外，控制血压可降低心力衰竭和卒中的风险。多数高血压性肾硬化症和 CKD 患者需要多种降压药物来控制血压，经典用药包括噻嗪或类噻嗪利尿剂（当 GFR 正常时）以及袢利尿剂（当 GFR 降至 25～30 ml/min 以下时），联合一种 ACE 抑制剂或 ARB、钙通道阻滞剂和 β 受体阻滞剂。

动脉粥样硬化栓塞性疾病

动脉粥样硬化栓塞性疾病是由动脉粥样硬化斑块脱落的胆固醇栓子栓塞所造成的，栓子最常见来源于主动脉，通常在有创动脉操作过程中脱落，如心导管检查、主动脉造影、心脏手术或主动脉手术。胆固醇栓塞可自发发生，或在全身抗凝治疗（如应用肝素）或全身应用溶栓药物时发生。由于患者必须有潜在动脉粥样硬化性疾病、而动脉粥样硬化的发生率随着年龄增长而升高，因此 40 岁以下人群很少发生动脉粥样硬化栓塞性疾病。

粥样硬化斑块导致全身性栓塞，胆固醇结晶堵塞于小动脉血管内，包括肾脏的弓状动脉或小叶间动脉。胆固醇栓子常累及其他器官，受累器官的形式部分取决于破裂的斑块位于升主动脉还是降主动脉。四肢受累常表现为指端缺血和坏疽，皮肤则表现为网状青斑，胃肠道受累可出现肠缺血，实际上任何器官均可受累。升主动脉来源的栓塞可能导致心肌缺血，升主动脉或颈动脉脱落的栓子（如，颈动脉内膜切除术后）可导致卒中。

眼部胆固醇栓塞可通过眼底检查中发现 Hollenhorst 斑而识别，其特征为视网膜小动脉分叉处的淡黄色斑点。眼部胆固醇栓塞通常无临床症状，但可能导致视网膜缺血，常伴随短暂性的视野缺损。

动脉栓塞性疾病患者可出现发热、嗜酸性粒细胞增多、嗜酸性粒细胞尿以及低补体血症，尤其是在急性期。实验室检查结果包括红细胞沉降率增快、淀粉酶或肝酶升高。广泛的多系统受累的动脉粥样硬化栓塞在临床和实验室检查表现上类似于系统性血管炎的临床特征。

肾脏动脉粥样硬化栓塞性疾病的典型临床表现为肾功能减退，通常在诱发栓子脱落的操作或其他事件后 3 天或更长时间才逐渐显露。随后发生的急性或慢性肾损伤的严重程度取决于栓子负荷的大小、动脉粥样硬化栓塞是一次性事件还是持续性过程，以及斑块物质诱发的炎症反应程度。许多患者在最初栓塞损伤后病情可维持稳定，但另一部分患者则以不同模式及速度进展至 CKD 或 ESRD。胆固醇栓塞还可因其引起急性肾缺血导致肾素释放，从而引发严重的高血压。

肾脏动脉粥样硬化栓塞性疾病的诊断通常基于相应临床情景，但对于某些患者则需肾穿刺活检以明确诊断，并除外其他疾病。由于肾活检组织的标本固定过程会将肾组织中的胆固醇结晶冲刷掉，所以在病理检查中仅可见到典型的动脉管腔内的针形裂隙、周围伴随反应性炎症性以及纤维性内膜增生，进而导致管腔闭塞、远端缺血性损伤。

胆固醇栓塞缺乏特异性治疗手段。由于栓塞的物质可引起炎症反应，部分临床医师推荐应用皮质类固醇，但其对于随后的动脉粥样硬化栓塞和肾功能进展的预防作用未被证实。推荐避免使用抗凝药物，以防覆盖在动脉粥样硬化斑块上的血栓溶解、脱落导致新的栓塞事件。对于绝大多数患者，推荐加用他汀类药物治疗潜在的动脉粥样硬化性疾病，但其并未显示出对于动脉粥样硬化栓塞的肾脏改变有影响。加用 ACE 抑制剂或 ARB 可有效治疗急性高血压，但对肾功能的恶化限制了其应用。如进展至 AKI 或 ESRD，则可能需要透析支持。

先兆子痫

先兆子痫的特点为：孕前血压正常的女性，在妊娠 20 周后新发的持续性高血压（血压 ≥ 140/90 mmHg）和

that develops after 20 weeks' gestation in a previously normotensive woman. Although hypertension and proteinuria are the principal features of preeclampsia, it is a systemic vascular disease that may also cause central nervous system symptoms (e.g., visual disturbances, headache, altered mental status), abdominal pain, nausea and vomiting, liver dysfunction, thrombocytopenia, pulmonary dysfunction, impaired fetal growth, nephrotic-range proteinuria, and AKI. If grand mal seizures develop without other explanation, a diagnosis of eclampsia is made. The HELLP syndrome, characterized by *h*emolysis, *el*evated *l*iver enzymes, and a *l*ow *p*latelet count, may be a manifestation of severe preeclampsia, although some consider it to be a separate disorder. It is also associated with increased maternal and fetal mortality. History of hypertension and CKD are risk factors for preeclampsia. Other major risk factors are nulliparity, preeclampsia in previous pregnancy, multifetal gestation, autoimmune disease, and family history of preeclampsia.

Preeclampsia should be distinguished from other hypertensive conditions that can occur during pregnancy, including preexisting hypertension that occurs before 20 weeks' gestation and persists after delivery, preeclampsia superimposed on preexisting chronic hypertension, and gestational hypertension (i.e., new-onset hypertension after 20 weeks' gestation without proteinuria or other related manifestations).

Progress has been made in understanding the pathogenesis of preeclampsia, and maternal and placental or fetal factors have been implicated. Abnormal development of placental vasculature in early pregnancy is thought to lead to some degree of placental hypoperfusion that releases antiangiogenic factors into the maternal circulation, disturbing the delicate balance of angiogenic and antiangiogenic factors. This causes systemic endothelial dysfunction in the mother that leads to hypertension, proteinuria, and other manifestations of the disease.

Soluble FMS-related tyrosine kinase 1 (sFLT1) is a placenta-derived circulating antiangiogenic factor that appears to play a central role in the pathogenesis of preeclampsia. It antagonizes the proangiogenic effects of vascular endothelial growth factor (VEGF) and placental growth factor (PGF) by binding to them and preventing interaction with their receptors. Soluble endoglin (sENG), another antiangiogenic factor that is widely expressed on vascular endothelium, is thought to be an important mediator of preeclampsia. Endothelial dysfunction in preeclampsia is associated with increased sensitivity to vasopressor agents, including angiotensin II, systemic vasoconstriction, and reduced fibrinolytic function.

Kidney biopsy findings include glomerular endothelial cell swelling (i.e., endotheliosis) and occlusion of the capillary lumen with ischemia. These findings are also seen with other microangiopathic disorders, although fibrin thrombi in glomerular capillaries are less commonly seen than with other causes. Foot process effacement is not usually seen.

The only effective treatment for preeclampsia is delivery of the fetus and placenta. The timing of delivery must take into account gestational age, severity of preeclampsia, presence or absence of systemic features, and status of the fetus and mother. Proper obstetric care is essential to balance the risk to the mother against the risk for prematurity of the fetus. In high-risk pregnancies, low-dose aspirin is started in the second and third trimester to reduce the risk of developing preeclampsia.

Treatment of mild hypertension in women with preeclampsia should be avoided because it does not treat the underlying disease process, alter the course of disease, or reduce clinical sequelae. In the absence of clinical manifestations other than proteinuria, it is usually unnecessary to start antihypertensive medications unless the systolic blood pressure is greater than 150 mm Hg or the diastolic blood pressure is higher than 100 mm Hg. Labetalol and hydralazine, both of which can be given intravenously or orally, are often recommended as first-line therapy for acute management. For chronic treatment, methyldopa or labetalol are often recommended initially, with extended-release nifedipine added if necessary. Diuretics and dietary sodium restriction usually are avoided unless the patient has pulmonary edema.

The risk profile of these medications is poorly defined in pregnancy. ACE inhibitors, ARBs, and direct renin inhibitors are contraindicated during pregnancy because of the risk of fetal abnormalities. Magnesium sulfate is used in severe cases of preeclampsia to reduce the risk of seizures, but it does not treat other manifestations of the disease or reduce maternal or fetal mortality rates.

Most manifestations of preeclampsia begin to improve shortly after delivery, but in some women, hypertension, proteinuria, and other manifestations may persist for several weeks or months before resolving completely. Because preeclampsia is a risk factor for future hypertension, kidney disease, and cardiovascular events, continued medical follow-up is essential.

Scleroderma Renal Crisis

Systemic sclerosis (i.e., scleroderma) is an idiopathic connective tissue disorder associated with deposition of collagen and other extracellular matrix proteins that produces inflammation and fibrosis of the skin and internal organs. Proliferative endovascular lesions may lead to obliteration of the vascular internal lumina and renal ischemia, with hypertension, increased renin activity, and elevated levels of angiotensin II and aldosterone.

AKI and rapidly worsening hypertension in patients with scleroderma is called *scleroderma renal crisis*. It occurs in approximately 5% to 10% of patients with scleroderma, typically within the first few years after onset and primarily in those with systemic rather than localized cutaneous scleroderma who also have progressive skin and cardiac involvement. Subclinical renal involvement with mild proteinuria, hypertension, and elevated serum creatinine concentration occurs much more frequently. Scleroderma renal crisis occasionally develops before the clinical diagnosis of scleroderma has been made.

Scleroderma renal crisis is often associated with rapid and severe loss of kidney function, oliguria, hypertensive encephalopathy, and heart failure. Microangiopathic hemolytic anemia (MAHA) may also occur. Low-grade proteinuria is often present but the urinalysis is not usually otherwise "active" (red blood cells, casts, etc.). About 10% of patients with scleroderma renal crisis do not have hypertension. This occurs more commonly among patients being treated with ACE inhibitors or high-dose corticosteroids.

Anti–RNA polymerase III antibodies are strongly associated with the risk of scleroderma renal crisis and have been suggested as markers for scleroderma renal crisis. Other risk factors include diffuse and rapidly progressive skin involvement and high-dose glucocorticoid use.

Renal biopsy may reveal interlobular artery involvement with intimal thickening, endothelial cell proliferation, and edema with obliteration of the vessel lumen with concentric onion-skinning of the wall of arterioles. Fibrinoid necrosis occurs in afferent arterioles with intravascular fibrin accumulation extending into the glomeruli, often with ischemic collapse, but without features of glomerulonephritis.

Activation of the renin-angiotensin-aldosterone system appears to play an important role in the progression of the disease. Before the advent of ACE inhibitors and hemodialysis, scleroderma renal crisis was fatal in about 75% of patients at 1 year. ACE inhibitor therapy has reduced this 1-year mortality rate to less than 15%. Captopril is often recommended as the ACE inhibitor of choice due to its short half-life and ease of dose titration. If the diagnosis of scleroderma renal crisis is made before advanced renal failure is established, ACE inhibition may halt or reverse the decline in renal function. Some experts recommend

蛋白尿（> 300 mg/d）。尽管高血压和蛋白尿是先兆子痫的主要特征，而它是一类系统性血管疾病，还可引起中枢神经系统症状（如，视力视野障碍、头痛、精神状态改变）、腹痛、恶心呕吐、肝功能障碍、血小板减少症、肺功能障碍、胎儿生长受限、肾病水平的蛋白尿，及 AKI。如果出现其他原因难以解释的癫痫大发作，则可以诊断子痫。HELLP 综合征以溶血、肝酶升高、血小板减低为典型表现，可能是重度先兆子痫的一种表现，尽管有学者认为它是一种独立的疾病。HELLP 综合征还与母婴死亡增加密切相关。高血压和 CKD 病史是先兆子痫的危险因素。其他主要危险因素为未经产、既往妊娠发生过先兆子痫、多胎妊娠，以及先兆子痫家族史。

先兆子痫应与其他妊娠期间可能出现的高血压疾病进行鉴别，包括孕 20 周前已出现且在生产后持续的高血压、长期慢性高血压合并先兆子痫、妊娠期高血压（即，孕 20 周后出现的新发高血压、但无蛋白尿和其他相关表现）。

目前对于先兆子痫致病机制的认识逐渐已深入，母体以及胎盘或胎儿互相牵连。孕早期胎盘血管的异常发育被认为会造成一定程度的胎盘低灌注，从而释放抗血管生成因子至母体循环中，扰乱血管生成和抗血管生成因子间的微妙平衡。这导致母体系统性内皮功能紊乱，造成高血压、蛋白尿以及疾病的其他表现。

可溶性 FMS 相关酪氨酸激酶 1（sFLT1）是一种胎盘来源的循环抗血管生成因子，其在先兆子痫的致病机制中起核心作用。sFLT1 通过结合血管内皮生长因子（VEGF）以及胎盘生长因子（PGF）以阻止其与受体的相互作用，从而拮抗这些生长因子的促血管生成作用。可溶性内皮糖蛋白（sENG）是另一种在血管内皮广泛表达的抗血管生成因子，被认为是先兆子痫发病的重要介质。先兆子痫的内皮功能障碍与对血管收缩物质（包括血管紧张素Ⅱ）的敏感性增加、系统性血管收缩，以及纤溶功能减退有关。

肾活检结果包括肾小球内皮细胞肿胀（即，内皮增生）以及毛细血管管腔闭塞伴缺血。上述表现也可见于其他微血管病性病变，但与其他病因相比肾小球毛细血管内纤维蛋白血栓更少见。足突融合也不常见。

先兆子痫唯一的有效治疗措施是娩出胎儿及胎盘。分娩的时机必须考虑孕龄、先兆子痫的严重程度、是否出现系统性症状，以及胎儿和母体状态。恰当的围产期管理对于平衡母体风险与胎儿早产的风险至关重要。为了减少高风险孕妇出现先兆子痫的风险，应在孕中期及孕晚期加用低剂量阿司匹林。

对于仅表现为轻度血压升高的先兆子痫孕妇，无需特殊干预，因为它并不能控制潜在的疾病过程、不能改变病程，或减少临床后遗症。对于除蛋白尿以外没有其他临床表现的患者通常不需要降压治疗，除非收缩压高于 150 mmHg 或舒张压高于 100 mmHg。拉贝洛尔和肼屈嗪是推荐的急性血压管理的一线降压药物，二者均可静脉或口服给药。甲基多巴和拉贝洛尔则常被推荐为慢性降压的初始药物，必要时可联合硝苯地平缓释片。除非患者出现肺水肿，否则通常应避利尿剂或限制膳食钠摄入的方式降压。

上述药物在妊娠期间使用的风险情况尚不明确。ACE 抑制剂、ARB 以及直接肾素抑制剂因存在致畸风险而在妊娠期禁用。硫酸镁可用来降低严重的先兆子痫患者癫痫发作的风险，但并不能治疗疾病的其他临床表现，也不能降低母体或胎儿的死亡率。

先兆子痫的绝大多数症状在胎儿娩出后不久即开始改善，但在部分女性中，高血压、蛋白尿以及其他症状可能会持续数周甚至数月才能完全缓解。由于先兆子痫是患者未来出现高血压、肾脏疾病及心血管疾病的危险因素之一，因此对其进行持续的医疗随访至关重要。

硬皮病肾危象

系统性硬化症（即，硬皮病）是一类特发性结缔组织病，与胶原和其他细胞外基质蛋白沉积有关，导致皮肤以及内脏的炎症和纤维化。血管内增生性病变可能导致血管内腔闭塞以及肾缺血，伴高血压、肾素活性增加、血管紧张素Ⅱ和醛固酮水平升高。

在硬皮病患者中的 AKI 和快速恶化的高血压被称为硬皮病肾危象。约 5% ～ 10% 的硬皮病患者会出现硬皮病肾危象，常发生于疾病初期几年内，主要见于常伴有进行性加重的皮肤损害及心脏受累的弥漫型硬皮病患者，而不是局限性皮肤硬皮病患者。亚临床的肾脏受累表现更加常见，包括少量蛋白尿、高血压、血肌酐水平升高。硬皮病肾危象偶可先于临床诊断硬皮病发生。

硬皮病肾危象常出现肾功能快速且严重地下降、少尿、高血压脑病，以及心力衰竭。微血管病性溶血性贫血（MAHA）也可能发生。低水平的尿蛋白常见，但尿常规中通常没有活动性尿沉渣（红细胞、管型等）。约 10% 的硬皮病肾危象患者并无高血压。这种情况在已加用 ACE 抑制剂或皮质类固醇治疗的患者中更加常见。

抗 RNA 聚合酶Ⅲ抗体与硬皮病肾危象的风险呈强相关性，已被建议作为硬皮病肾危象的标志物。其他危险因素包括弥漫性且快速进展的皮肤受累以及应用大剂量皮质类固醇。

肾活检可发现小叶间动脉受累，其表现为血管内膜增厚、内皮细胞增生和肿胀，小动脉管壁呈同心圆状的洋葱皮样改变导致管腔闭塞。入球小动脉可出现纤维蛋白样坏死、伴血管内纤维蛋白积聚并沿伸入肾小球内，常导致肾小球缺血性塌陷，但并无肾小球肾炎表现。

肾素-血管紧张素-醛固酮系统激活在疾病的进展中起到重要作用。在 ACE 抑制剂及血液透析问世前，75% 的硬皮病肾危象患者在 1 年内死亡。ACE 抑制剂治疗将患者的 1 年死亡率降至 15% 以下。由于半衰期短且容易进行剂量滴定，卡托普利被推荐为首选的 ACE 抑制剂。如果在出现晚期肾功能衰竭前诊断硬皮病肾危象，ACE 抑制剂可能中止或逆转肾功能减退。一些专家建议即使

continuing ACE inhibitors even if kidney function declines and temporary dialysis is necessary, citing an increased chance of renal recovery, which has been described in scleroderma renal crisis patients even after 18 to 24 months of dialysis dependence. ACE inhibitors are not useful for prevention of scleroderma renal crisis, and their use in this setting has been associated with a poorer outcome, including greater risk of requiring permanent dialysis if renal crisis occurs. Use of ACE inhibitors rather than ARBs is recommended because of the long track record of success with ACE inhibitors in this disease. Patients with ESRD secondary to scleroderma renal crisis have a high mortality on dialysis, poor dialysis access maturation, and reduced allograft survival following renal transplantation.

THROMBOTIC MICROANGIOPATHY OF THE KIDNEY

TMA is a pathologic lesion secondary to various distinct pathogenic mechanisms leading to endothelial injury, microvascular thrombosis, and MAHA. These syndromes each lead to organ dysfunction due to microvascular thrombosis, but each syndrome has distinct clinical, pathophysiologic, and epidemiologic features. AKI is commonly seen in TMA due to the propensity of the glomerular endothelium to damage.

The traditional classification of TMA into thrombotic thrombocytopenic purpura (TTP) and hemolytic uremic syndrome (HUS) has undergone evolution and currently TMAs are subclassified based on the underlying pathogenic process (Fig. 6.4 and Table 6.3). Although many processes cause microvascular endothelial injury, renal involvement from these disorders affects the vasculature at different levels. Renal involvement by HUS and TTP primarily affects the glomeruli, whereas scleroderma often extends to the interlobular arteries, and malignant hypertension more often affects the afferent arterioles. However, there is significant overlap and similar histologic features among these diseases, making careful clinical evaluation essential for accurate determination of the cause.

Thrombotic Thrombocytopenic Purpura

TTP is characterized by MAHA and thrombocytopenia. Patients may also have fever, AKI, and neurologic impairment. Purpura is only rarely observed, and it is not necessary to make the diagnosis. TTP occurs with a female-to-male ratio of 4:3 and a peak incidence in the third and fourth decades of life. MAHA and thrombocytopenia manifesting similar to TTP may occur in response to some drugs (e.g., ticlopidine, cyclosporine, tacrolimus), after stem cell transplantation, in association with human immunodeficiency virus (HIV) infection, and in patients with malignant hypertension, sepsis, disseminated intravascular coagulation, or advanced cancers.

TTP is caused by a deficiency or reduced activity of ADAMTS13 (a disintegrin-like and metalloproteinase with thrombospondin-1–like domains). ADAMTS13 is a plasma protease that normally cleaves von Willebrand factor (VWF) and limits the extent of intravascular thrombosis (Fig. 6.5). Microthrombi composed primarily of platelets and VWF accumulate in the vascular bed of multiple organs, leading to a MAHA. Deficiency in ADAMTS13 may be acquired, caused by anti-ADAMTS13 autoantibodies (mostly immunoglobulin G [IgG]), or, much less commonly, genetic.

Other laboratory abnormalities are manifestations of the MAHA and include thrombocytopenia; an elevated LDH concentration, indirect bilirubin concentration, and reticulocyte count; and a low haptoglobin concentration. Coagulation laboratory test results (e.g., prothrombin time, activated partial thromboplastin time, fibrinogen level) are typically normal, although levels of fibrin split products may be elevated. AKI, microscopic hematuria, and low-grade proteinuria are frequently detected.

Without treatment, TTP has a mortality rate of about 90%, with most deaths occurring within 3 months of the onset of symptoms. Treatment with plasma infusion can normalize ADAMTS13 levels, reducing intravascular hemolysis and mortality rates. Plasmapheresis and replacement with fresh-frozen plasma has the advantage of removing inhibitory autoantibodies in addition to normalizing ADAMTS13 levels because of the large volume of plasma that can be infused.

ADAMTS13 activity must be assayed before therapy is initiated to obtain accurate results, but treatment should not be delayed for the results to return. The severity of ADAMTS13 deficiency (<5%) predicts future relapse, although those with severe deficiency are just as likely to respond initially to plasmapheresis as those with a mild deficiency. Patients with MAHA due to other causes not associated with ADAMTS13 deficiency usually have a minimal response to plasmapheresis or plasma infusion. Patients with HUS do not have abnormalities in ADAMTS13 levels or function.

Hemolytic-Uremic Syndrome
Shiga Toxin-Producing *Escherichia coli*

Gastrointestinal tract infection with the Shiga-toxigenic *Escherichia coli* (STEC) strain O157:H7 produces a diarrheal illness that is complicated in about 15% of cases by a MAHA with intraglomerular thrombosis and AKI. STEC-HUS most commonly affects infants and children, although adults may also be affected. Cases are often clustered because of outbreaks of *E. coli* O157:H7, with peaks occurring in summer and autumn. *E. coli* is endemic in the gastrointestinal tract of cattle, and cases are often tracked to undercooked meat, exposure to bovine fecal matter, animal exposure, or other contaminated food products. In May 2011, an outbreak of STEC-HUS in Germany was tracked back to fenugreek sprouts grown from contaminated seeds. The pathogenic agent, *E. coli* O104:H4, was particularly virulent with 30% of infected patients, mostly adults, developing HUS.

Shiga-toxigenic bacterial strains commonly produce a prodrome of painful, bloody diarrhea, which precedes the development of HUS by 2 to 12 days (median, 3 days). Shiga toxin is directly thrombogenic in the renal vasculature. Although intravascular coagulation in STEC-HUS is usually limited to the kidney, the heart, gastrointestinal tract, and central nervous system may also be affected.

Laboratory abnormalities in HUS include elevated creatinine levels, anemia, schistocytes on the peripheral smear, elevated reticulocyte count, and thrombocytopenia. In contrast to disseminated intravascular coagulation, fibrinogen levels are normal or high, and the prothrombin time is normal or only slightly prolonged. Fresh stool should be sent for culture of *E. coli* O157:H7, which can aid in tracing the source of an outbreak. Stool studies should also be performed for patients without diarrhea because *E. coli* O157:H7 may rarely cause HUS in the absence of intestinal symptoms. If *E. coli* O157:H7 is not detected, culture for other Shiga-toxigenic organisms should be pursued.

The pathologic renal lesions of HUS include vessel wall thickening with endothelial cell swelling and intraglomerular thrombosis with platelet- and fibrin-rich thrombi. Fragmentation of red blood cells may be seen in the renal vasculature and within the vessel wall.

Treatment of STEC-HUS is supportive, including adequate volume repletion with isotonic intravenous fluids, transfusion for severe anemia, and avoidance of other nephrotoxic agents (e.g., nonsteroidal anti-inflammatory drugs, aminoglycoside antibiotics, iodinated contrast). Platelet transfusion is not recommended because it may worsen the ongoing microvascular thrombosis. Antibiotic treatment of patients with bloody diarrhea is controversial. Corticosteroids, anticoagulation (e.g., aspirin, heparin), thrombolytic agents, and plasma administration have proved ineffective for the treatment of STEC-HUS. In very severe cases, especially with central nervous system involvement, eculizumab (a complement pathway inhibitor) can be used.

肾功能已经下降或需要临时透析，仍应继续使用ACE抑制剂，因为有文献报道即使在透析依赖达到18～24个月的硬皮病肾危象患者中，ACE抑制剂也可增加肾功能恢复的概率。ACE抑制剂并不适用于硬皮病肾危象的预防，预防性用药可能导致更差的结局，包括如果后续发生硬皮病肾危象则永久透析风险更高。由于ACE抑制剂有悠久的成功治疗记录，因此相较于ARB，更推荐应用ACE抑制剂。因硬皮病肾危象进入ESRD的患者，透析死亡率高、透析通路成熟差、肾移植后异体移植肾存活率低。

肾脏的血栓性微血管病（TMA）

TMA是一种继发于不同致病机制的病理损害，导致内皮损伤、微血管内血栓形成，以及MAHA。这些综合征都可通过微血管血栓形成造成脏器功能异常，但每种综合征都有独特的临床、病理生理以及流行病学特征。由于肾小球内皮细胞的易损性，AKI在TMA中常见。

TMA的传统分类包括血栓性血小板减少性紫癜（TTP）和溶血性尿毒综合征（HUS），历经演变，目前TMA的分类基于潜在的致病过程进行了细化分类（图6.4及表6.3）。尽管许多过程均可能导致微血管内皮损伤，不同疾病的肾脏受累的血管层级不同。HUS和TTP的肾脏受累主要影响肾小球，而硬皮病则常扩展到小叶间动脉，恶性高血压则更多影响入球小动脉。然而，这些疾病之间存在高度重叠和组织学相似特征，因此需要谨慎的临床评估以做出精准的病因判断。

血栓性血小板减少性紫癜

TTP的特征是MAHA和血栓性血小板减少。患者可出现发热、AKI、神经功能损害。紫癜较少出现，也并非诊断的必备条件。TTP的女/男比例为4:3，发病高峰为30～40岁。类似TTP的MAHA和血栓性血小板减少可能发生于应用某些药物（如噻氯匹啶、环孢素、他克莫司）的患者；在干细胞移植后发生，与人类免疫缺陷病毒感染（HIV）相关；以及出现在恶性高血压、感染中毒症、弥散性血管内凝血、晚期肿瘤的患者中。

TTP是由ADAMTS13（一种具有血小板反应蛋白-1-样结构域的类解整合素和金属蛋白酶）的缺陷或活性减低导致的。ADAMTS13是一种血浆蛋白酶，通常作用是切割血管性血友病因子（VWF）、限制血管内血栓的形成（图6.5）。主要由血小板和VWF组成的微血栓聚集在多个组织的血管床中，导致MAHA。ADAMTS13缺陷可以是获得性的，由抗ADAMTS13抗体［主要是免疫球蛋白G（IgG）型］造成，或者在更为罕见的情况下由遗传因素导致。

其他实验室异常为MAHA的相关表现，包括：血小板减少；LDH浓度、间接胆红素浓度和网织红细胞水平升高；结合珠蛋白水平降低。凝血相关实验室检查结果（如，凝血酶原时间、活化部分凝血酶原时间、纤维蛋白原水平）通常正常，而纤维蛋白裂解产物水平可能升高。经常可发现AKI、镜下血尿、低水平的尿蛋白。

如不进行治疗，TTP的死亡率约90%，绝大多数死亡发生在症状发作的3个月内。血浆输注治疗可以将ADAMTS13水平纠正至正常，从而减少血管内溶血、降低死亡率。血浆置换联合新鲜冰冻血浆补充，除了通过在治疗过程中输注大量血浆以使ADAMTS13水平正常化以外，还具有去除抑制性抗体的优势。

在治疗开始前必须测定ADAMTS13的活性，以获得准确的结果，但不应因等待结果回报而延误启动治疗。ADAMTS13缺乏的严重程度（<5%）可预测未来的复发，尽管严重缺乏的患者最初对于血浆置换治疗的反应与ADAMTS13轻度缺乏患者一样良好。无ADAMTS13缺乏的其他原因导致的MAHA患者则对于血浆置换或血浆输注的反应甚微。HUS患者的ADAMTS13水平以及功能均无异常。

溶血性尿毒综合征
产志贺毒素大肠埃希菌

胃肠道感染产志贺毒素大肠埃希菌（STEC）O157:H7菌株会导致腹泻，其中15%的患者会并发MAHA、伴肾小球内血栓形成以及AKI。尽管成年人也会发病，STEC-HUS最常见于婴儿以及儿童。由于大肠埃希菌O157:H7的暴发，病例多呈现聚集性，发病高峰在夏季和秋季。大肠埃希菌主要定植在牛的胃肠道中，感染者通常能追溯出进食生肉，接触牛的粪便、动物或其他被污染食物的情况。2011年5月，在德国暴发的STEC-HUS追溯到由被污染的种子种植的葫芦巴芽。致病性毒株大肠埃希菌O104:H4毒力尤其强大，约30%的感染患者出现HUS，其中主要是成人患者。

产志贺毒素的细菌菌株会引起疼痛性、血性腹泻的前驱症状，并在2～12天（中位时间3天）后发生HUS。志贺毒素在肾脏血管中具有直接致血栓形成的作用。尽管STEC-HUS的血管内凝血通常仅局限在肾脏，但心脏、胃肠道、中枢神经系统均有可能受累。

HUS的实验室检查异常包括肌酐水平升高、贫血、外周血涂片见到破碎红细胞、网织红细胞计数升高，以及血小板减少。与弥散性血管内凝血不同，纤维蛋白原水平正常或升高，凝血酶原时间正常或仅轻度延长。应通过新鲜粪便培养大肠埃希菌O157:H7，以帮助追踪暴发的疫情来源。在没有腹泻症状的患者中也应进行粪便检查，在罕见情况下，大肠埃希菌O157:H7可在没有肠道症状的情况下造成HUS。如果没有检测到大肠埃希菌O157:H7，应进行其他产志贺毒素微生物的培养。

HUS的肾脏病理损害为血管壁增厚、内皮细胞肿胀、肾小球内富含血小板及纤维蛋白的血栓形成。肾脏血管内及血管壁中可观察到红细胞碎片。

STEC-HUS的治疗为支持性治疗，包括静脉输注等渗液体进行适当的补充容量、对于严重贫血患者输血支持、避免应用其他肾毒性药物（如非甾体抗炎药、氨基糖苷类抗生素、碘造影剂）。不推荐输注血小板，

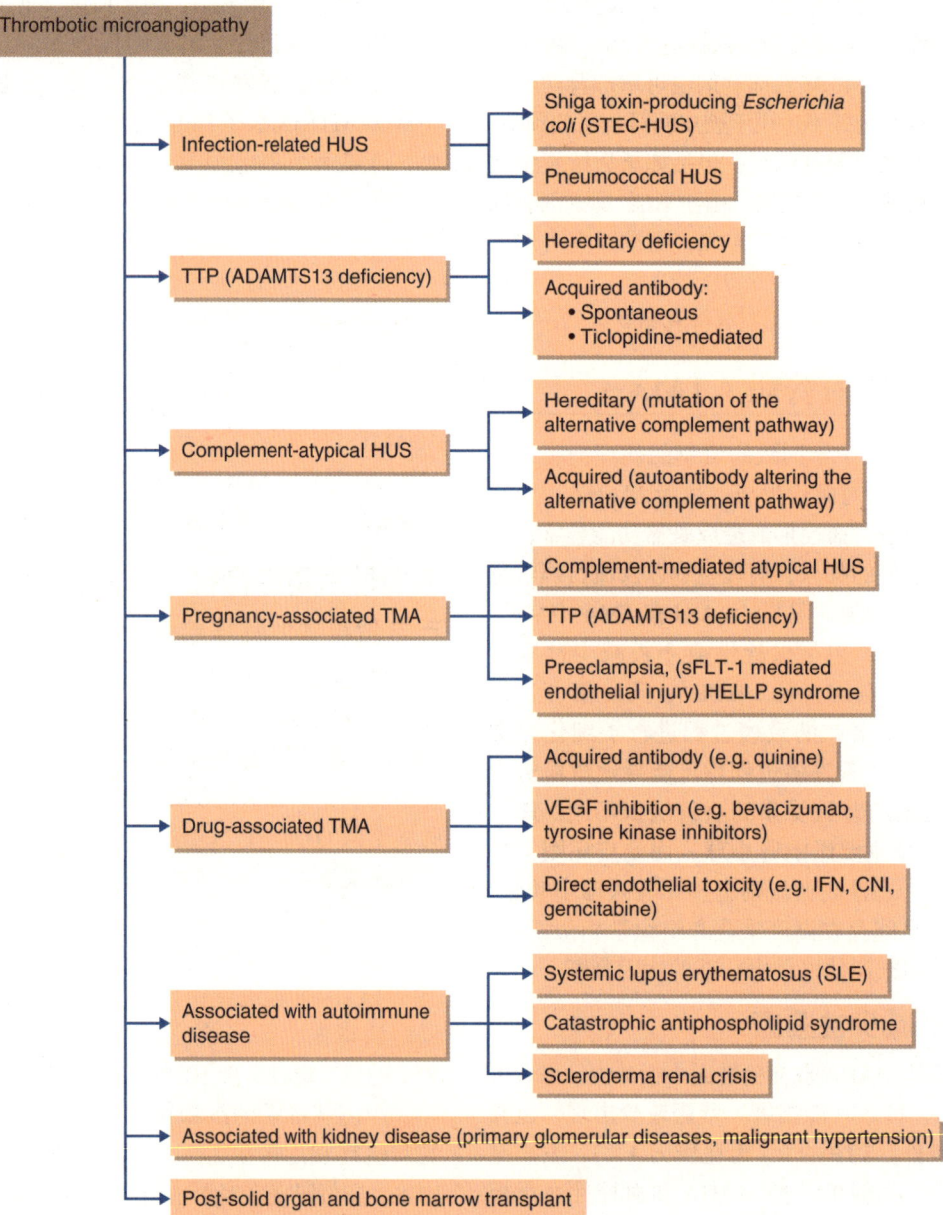

Fig. 6.4 Thrombotic microangiopathy (TMA). *CNI*, Calcineurin inhibitor; *HELLP*, hemolysis, elevated liver enzymes, and a low platelet count; *HUS*, hemolytic uremic syndrome; *IFN*, interferon; *sFLT-1*, soluble fms-like tyrosine kinase-1; *TTP*, thrombotic thrombocytopenic purpura; *VEGF*, vascular endothelial growth factor.

With supportive care alone, most patients with STEC-HUS recover with normalization of renal function or only mild residual CKD, although about 25% may develop advanced CKD or ESRD over the next 1 to 2 decades of life. Risk for CKD is increased with cortical necrosis and involvement of more than 50% of glomeruli identified on renal biopsy. The risk for complications and death increases with age, with the mortality rate increasing from about 5% to 10% for children to about 30% for adults.

Complement-Mediated Atypical HUS

The alternative complement pathway is the amplification loop of the complement system. Dysregulation of this pathway due to either hereditary or acquired causes may lead to complement-mediated endothelial damage and atypical HUS (aHUS). Mutations of genes for components of the alternative complement pathway, including C3, factor B, regulators of factor H (CFH/CFHR fusions), factor I, and CD46, have been implicated. These mutations have an incomplete penetrance and frequently a triggering factor such as infection or pregnancy precedes the onset of clinical manifestations. In some childhood forms of complement-mediated aHUS, an acquired autoantibody against factor H can be detected and gastrointestinal prodrome is often reported. Failure to detect a genetic maturation or autoantibody does not rule out this disease because it is likely that not all responsible causes have been identified.

Complement-mediated aHUS historically has had a very poor prognosis with high likelihood of ESRD and death. The disease frequently recurs in a renal allograft with the recurrence rate depending on the underlying mutation, with the highest risk for CFH, CFB,

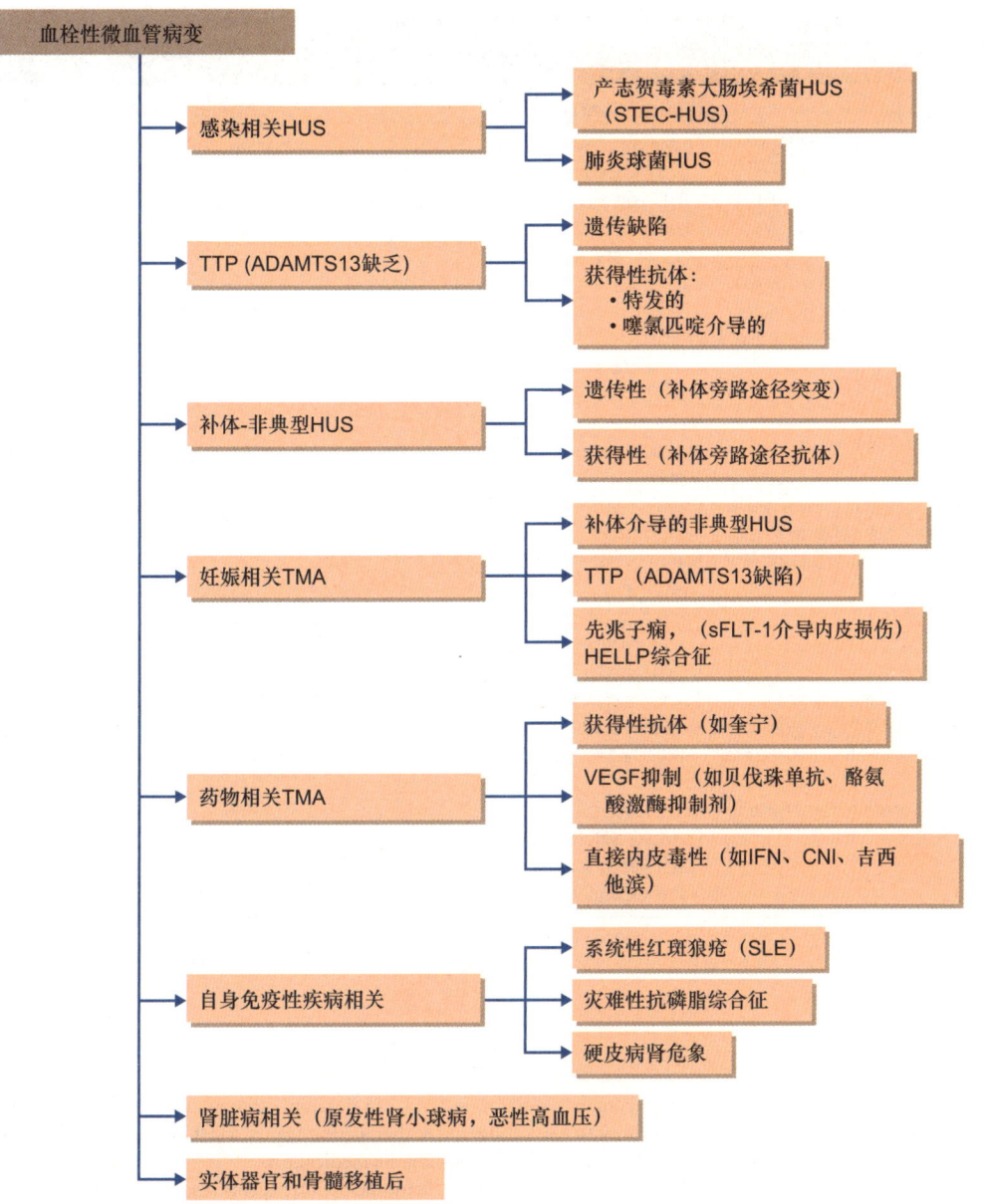

图 6.4 血栓性微血管病（TMA）。CNI，钙调磷酸酶抑制剂；HELLP，溶血、肝酶升高、血小板减少；HUS，溶血性尿毒综合征；IFN，干扰素；sFLT1，可溶性 FMS 相关酪氨酸激酶 1；TTP，血栓性血小板减少性紫癜；VEGF，血管内皮生长因子

因其可能加重进行中的微血管血栓形成。对于血性腹泻患者是否需应用抗生素仍存在争议。在 STEC-HUS 治疗中皮质类固醇、抗凝药物（如阿司匹林、肝素）、溶栓药物，以及血浆输注被证实无效。在非常危重的病例中，尤其是中枢神经系统受累者，可使用依库珠单抗（一种补体通路抑制剂）治疗。

仅通过单纯支持治疗，大部分 STEC-HUS 患者的肾功能可恢复正常，或仅残留轻度 CKD，然而约 25% 患者在未来 10～20 年可能发展至晚期 CKD 或 ESRD。当皮质坏死以及肾脏病理显示 50% 以上肾小球受累时，患者的 CKD 风险增加。并发症和死亡的风险随年龄增长而增加，死亡率从儿童的 5%～10% 增长至成年人的 30%。

补体介导的非典型 HUS

补体旁路途径是补体系统的放大环路。遗传性或获得性因素导致该途径失调，可引起补体介导的内皮损伤以及非典型 HUS（aHUS）。补体旁路途径成分，包括 C3、B 因子、H 因子的调控因子（CFH/CFHR 融合）、Ⅰ 因子以及 CD46，均可能出现基因突变。这些突变多具有不完全外显率，常常在发生感染或妊娠等诱发因素后出现临床表现。在一些补体介导的儿童期 aHUS 中，可检测到针对 H 因子的获得性自身抗体，且经常报告有胃肠道前驱症状。由于并非所有的致病原因均已被确认，因此未检测到基因突变或自身抗体并不能除外本病。

补体介导的 HUS 的预后历来都极差，伴有很高的 ESRD 和死亡可能性。本病常在异体肾移植术后复发，其复发率取决于潜在的基因突变，CFH、CFB 和 C3 突变的复发率最高，而 CD46 突变的复发率最低。依库珠单抗是一种人源化单克隆抗体，与补体蛋白 C5 具有高

TABLE 6.3 Pathogenesis, Clinical/Diagnostic Characteristics, and Management of Main Thrombotic Microangiopathic Syndromes

	Pathogenesis	Clinical Characteristics	Diagnostic Characteristics	Management
Shiga toxin–producing *Escherichia coli* (STEC-HUS)	Enteric infection with Shiga toxin–producing pathogen (*E. coli* O157; *E. coli* O104)	All age groups with peak incidence in children for the *E. coli* O157 pathogen. Enteric prodrome is common (5% do not have diarrhea)	Fibrin predominates intravascular thrombi. Swollen endothelial cells. STEC isolated in the stool	Supportive. No role for plasma exchange. Possible role for eculizumab in severe CNS involvement. Antibiotics (controversial)
TTP	ADAMTS 13 deficiency (hereditary or acquired autoantibody). Ticlopidine-induced autoantibody	Other affected family members if hereditary. In women with predisposition presents clinically in the 2nd and 3rd trimester of pregnancy. No diarrheal prodrome. Neurologic symptoms predominate	Low ADAMTS 13 activity (<10%). VWF predominates Intravascular thrombi. Absence of swollen endothelial cells	Plasma exchange. Immunosuppression (e.g. rituximab for acquired autoantibody). Stop ticlopidine
Complement-mediated aHUS	Dysregulation of the alternative complement pathway: Hereditary or acquired (anti-FH Ab)	Diarrhea can be present (30% at presentation). Hereditary disease has incomplete penetrance. Trigger (e.g., infection, pregnancy) often identified. High recurrence in kidney allograft	C3 can be low (normal levels do not exclude the disease). ADAMTS13 activity >10%. Negative genetic and autoantibody testing does not exclude the diagnosis	Eculizumab. Partial response to plasma exchange. Liver transplant may be considered
Pneumococcal HUS	Neuraminidase-mediated exposure of the endothelium antigens leading to endothelial injury	Mainly children <2 years. Frequently associated with pneumonia and empyema	Positive Coombs test	Supportive care. Treatment of the infection
Quinine-induced TMA	Autoantibodies against GP Ib/IX or IIb/IIIa	Not dose related. Can occur early (after single exposure) or late (up to 10 years after exposure)	ADAMTS13 activity ≥10%	Supportive. Plasma exchange not effective

ADAMTS3, A disintegrin and metalloproteinase with thrombospondin-1–like domains; *anti-FH Ab*, anti-factor H antibody; *CNS*, central nervous system; *GP*, glycoprotein platelets; *HUS*, hemolytic uremic syndrome; *TMA*, thrombotic microangiopathy; *TTP*, thrombotic thrombocytopenic purpura; *VWF*, von Willebrand factor.

and C3 mutations and the lowest with CD46 mutations. Eculizumab is a humanized monoclonal antibody that binds with high affinity to complement protein C5 and prevents the generation of C5a, C5b, and the terminal complement complex C5b-9. In patients with complement-mediated HUS, eculizumab inhibits complement-mediated TMA. It is used both to treat the disease and to prevent recurrence after kidney transplantation. Because complement components are mainly produced by the liver, a combined liver kidney transplant can be curative.

Malignancy-Associated TMA

In patients with a cancer diagnosis, TMA can be due to the cancer or its therapy. Disseminated malignancy can produce embolic tumor cells leading to endothelial damage and erythrocytes shearing. It has a very poor prognosis. TMA has also been described with cancer therapeutic agents that interfere with the VEGF pathway such as bevacizumab and tyrosine-kinase inhibitors (e.g., sunitinib). The VEGF pathway is upregulated in the majority of human tumors and it is thought to be important for expanding neovascularization of the tumor. In the kidney glomeruli, VEGF is produced locally by podocytes and endothelial cells express tyrosine kinase VEGF receptors. A disruption of this balance will lead to endothelial injury and TMA. Clinically, most patients present with hypertension and proteinuria. In rare cases, a severe systemic TMA can develop, often associated with use of higher doses of the cancer therapeutic agents. Most of these disorders are reversible after stopping the medication.

Other chemotherapeutic agents associated with TMA include gemcitabine, mitomycin C, vincristine, and proteasome inhibitors (e.g., bortezomib, carfilzomib, and ixazomib). Gemcitabine-related TMA is directly related to the cumulative dose. Usually treated conservatively, in severe cases with persistent TMA eculizumab therapy may be considered.

In patients receiving an allogenic bone marrow transplant, TMA occurs in 10% to 40% of patients and is considered a manifestation of graft versus host disease (GVHD) or radiation therapy. Therapy for this form of TMA is controversial and mainly directed toward treating GVHD, although eculizumab may be tried.

Pregnancy-Related TMA

Pregnancy acts as a trigger for both TTP and complement-mediated aHUS. TTP occurs mainly during the second and third trimester of pregnancy. Normal pregnancy is associated with an augmentation of VWF antigen release leading to TTP in patients who are already predisposed by a congenital or acquired ADAMTS13 deficiency.

Pregnancy-related aHUS occurs in the postpartum period. Delivery acts as a triggering factor for aHUS in patients with certain genetic

表 6.3　主要血栓性微血管病综合征的发病机制、临床/诊断特征和处理

	发病机制	临床特征	诊断特征	处理
产志贺毒素大肠埃希菌 HUS（STEC-HUS）	产志贺毒素的病原体（大肠埃希菌 O157；大肠埃希菌 O104）导致的肠道感染	大肠埃希菌 O157 在各年龄段均可发病，儿童为发病高峰 常见肠道前驱症状（5% 无腹泻）	纤维蛋白为主要成分的血管内血栓 内皮细胞肿胀 粪便中分离出 STEC	支持治疗 不推荐血浆置换 在严重 CNS 受累的患者中依库珠单抗可能有用 抗生素（存在争议）
TTP	ADAMTS13 缺乏（遗传性或获得性自身抗体） 噻氯匹啶诱发的自身抗体	若为遗传性，其他家属同样受累 存在易感倾向的女性在孕中期和孕晚期出现临床症状 无前驱腹泻症状 神经系统症状为主	ADAMTS13 活性降低（<10%） VWF 为主要成分的血管内血栓 无血管内皮肿胀	血浆置换 免疫抑制（如利妥昔单抗治疗获得性自身抗体） 停用噻氯匹啶
补体介导的 aHUS	补体旁路途径调节异常 遗传性或获得性（抗 FH 抗体）	可以出现腹泻（30% 出现） 遗传性疾病具有不完全外显率 通常可找到触发因素（如感染、妊娠） 肾移植后高复发率	C3 水平可下降（水平正常不能除外诊断） ADAMTS13 活性 >10% 基因和自身抗体检测阴性不能除外诊断	依库珠单抗 血浆置换部分有效 肝移植或可考虑
肺炎球菌 HUS	神经氨酸酶介导的内皮抗原暴露，导致内皮损伤	主要见于 <2 岁的儿童 常伴肺炎和脓胸	Coombs 试验阳性	支持治疗 抗感染
奎宁诱发的 TMA	抗 GP Ⅰb/Ⅸ 或 Ⅱb/Ⅲa 的自身抗体	与剂量无关 可早发（单次暴露后）或晚发（用药达 10 年）	ADAMTS13 活性 ≥10%	支持治疗 血浆置换无效

ADAMTS13：一种具有血小板反应蛋白 -1- 样结构域的类解整合素和金属蛋白酶；抗 -FH 抗体：抗 H 因子抗体；CNS：中枢神经系统；GP：糖蛋白血小板；HUS：溶血性尿毒综合征；TMA：血栓性微血管病；TTP：血栓性血小板减少性紫癜；VWF：血管性血友病因子

亲和力，阻止 C5a、C5b、末端补体复合物 C5b-9 的产生。在补体介导的 HUS 患者中，依库珠单抗可抑制补体介导的 TMA。它不仅用于治疗疾病，还用于预防肾移植后复发。因为补体成分主要由肝产生，联合进行肝肾移植可达到治愈疗效。

恶性肿瘤相关 TMA

在诊断为肿瘤的患者中，TMA 可能直接由肿瘤本身或其治疗导致。播散性恶性肿瘤可产生肿瘤细胞栓子、导致内皮损伤以及破碎红细胞。这类疾病预后极差。TMA 还与干扰 VEGF 通路的肿瘤治疗药物相关，如贝伐单抗和酪氨酸激酶抑制剂（如舒尼替尼）。由于 VEGF 通路对于肿瘤新生血管形成、扩张具有重要作用，在大部分人类肿瘤中该通路均有上调。在肾小球中，VEGF 主要在足细胞局部产生，而内皮细胞则表达酪氨酸激酶 VEGF 受体。这种平衡的破坏则会导致内皮损伤和 TMA。临床上，大部分患者表现为高血压和蛋白尿。罕见情况下可进展为严重的系统性 TMA，通常与应用较高剂量的肿瘤治疗药物相关。上述大部分病症在停止用药后可以逆转。

其他与 TMA 相关的化疗药物包括吉西他滨、丝裂霉素 C、长春新碱和蛋白酶抑制剂（如硼替佐米、卡非佐米、伊沙佐米）。吉西他滨相关的 TMA 与其累积剂量直接相关。通常采用保守治疗，在严重的持续性 TMA 病例中，可考虑应用依库珠单抗治疗。

在接受异基因骨髓移植的患者中，10%～40% 的患者会发生 TMA，这被认为是移植物抗宿主病（GVHD）或放射治疗的一种表现。对于这种形式的 TMA 的治疗存在争议，尽管也可以尝试依库珠单抗，但主要为针对 GVHD 的治疗。

妊娠相关 TMA

妊娠是 TTP 和补体介导的 aHUS 的触发因素。TTP 主要在孕中期和孕晚期发生。正常妊娠时存在 VWF 抗原释放增加，而这将导致已存在先天性或获得性 ADAMTS13 缺乏的易患患者发生 TTP。

妊娠相关 aHUS 在产后发病。在存在补体旁路途径某些特定基因突变的患者中，分娩是 aHUS 的触发因

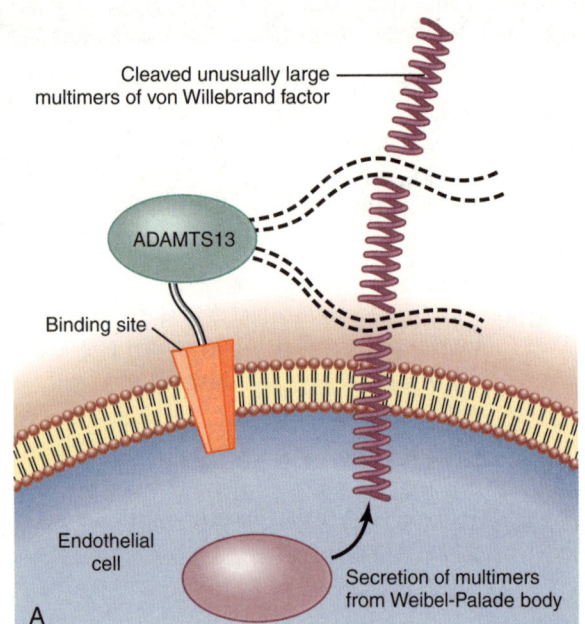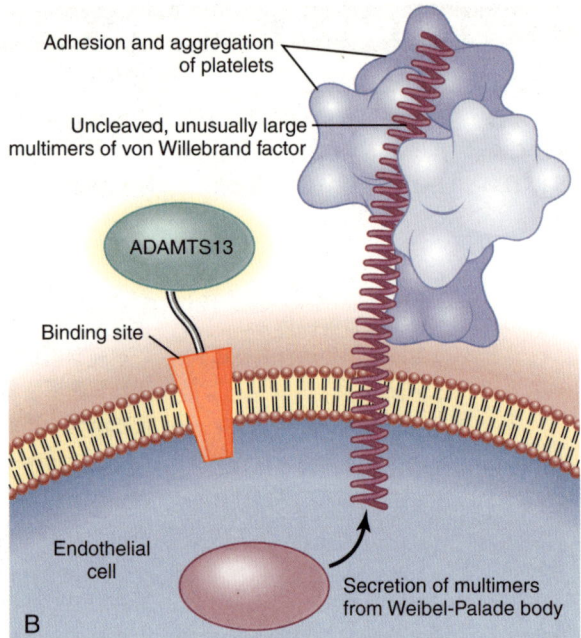

Fig. 6.5 Relation between ADAMTS13 activity, excessive adhesion and activation of platelets, and thrombotic thrombocytopenic purpura. (A) In normal subjects, ADAMTS13 (i.e., von Willebrand factor–cleaving metalloprotease) molecules attach to binding sites on endothelial cell surfaces and cleave unusually large multimers of von Willebrand factor as they are secreted by stimulated endothelial cells. The smaller von Willebrand factor forms that circulate after cleavage do not induce the adhesion and aggregation of platelets during normal blood flow. (B) Absent or severely reduced activity of ADAMTS13 in patients with thrombotic thrombocytopenic purpura prevents timely cleavage of unusually large multimers of von Willebrand factor as they are secreted by endothelial cells. The uncleaved multimers induce the adhesion and aggregation of platelets in flowing blood. (From Moake JL: Thrombotic microangiopathies, N Engl J Med 347:589-600, 2002.)

mutations of the alternative complement pathway. Historically the outcomes were very poor, with more than 75% of patients developing ESRD. Eculizumab is an effective therapy and can be used during pregnancy.

The HELLP syndrome is a TMA of the liver sinusoids that can have a presentation similar to TTP or aHUS. Although rare, AKI can occur due to an acute tubular necrosis type of injury that is rapidly reversible with recovery from the HELLP syndrome.

ANTIPHOSPHOLIPID ANTIBODY SYNDROME

Antiphospholipid antibodies (APAs) refer to autoantibodies such as lupus anticoagulants or IgG or immunoglobulin M (IgM) anticardiolipin antibodies or anti-$β_2$-glycoprotein that interfere with phospholipid-binding proteins and in vitro phospholipid-dependent clotting assays such as the partial thromboplastin time. Because not all lupus anticoagulants cause prolongation of the partial thromboplastin time, other tests of the coagulation system, such as the dilute Russell viper venom time, may need to be obtained. The diagnosis of APS is based on the occurrence of arterial or venous clotting events or fetal loss during pregnancy after 10 or more weeks' gestation or multiembryonic losses before 10 weeks' gestation in the setting of laboratory detection of an APA. Lupus anticoagulant and anticardiolipin antibodies are detectable in up to 10% of healthy populations, and their presence alone is insufficient for a diagnosis of APS. Apolipoprotein H (apo H, formerly $β_2$-glycoprotein 1) is the main antigenic target of anticardiolipin antibodies.

In the absence of an underlying autoimmune disease, the syndrome is referred to as primary APS. Secondary APS occurs when associated with other diseases such as systemic lupus erythematosus (SLE). APAs are detectable in 30% to 50% of patients with SLE, and renal involvement is often observed in this setting.

The procoagulant effect of APAs may result from interference with the anticoagulant apo H, inhibition of fibrinolysis, direct endothelial injury, accelerated atherosclerosis, and activation of platelet, monocyte, and endothelial cells. Renal involvement occurs in about 25% of patients with primary APS and can occur in patients with SLE or other causes of APS. Thrombosis may occur throughout the renal vasculature, including main or branch renal arteries, arterioles, glomeruli, and veins. These findings resemble those found in other diseases associated with a TMA. Focal atrophy of the cortex in association with interstitial fibrosis may be observed due to resulting ischemia.

The renal manifestations of APS vary. Some patients have mild proteinuria with preserved kidney function, and others develop severe hypertension, nephrotic-range proteinuria, and AKI or CKD. Renal arterial thrombosis can cause infarction, acute onset of flank pain, hematuria, and decreased kidney function. RVT may be silent or, if acute and complete, may manifest with sudden flank pain and reduced kidney function. Pathologic changes seen on renal biopsy of patients with primary APS are small vessel vaso-occlusive disease with fibrous intimal hyperplasia of interlobular arteries, recanalizing thrombi in arteries and arterioles, focal cortical atrophy, and TMA. Other manifestations of APS include thrombocytopenia, hemolytic anemia, and

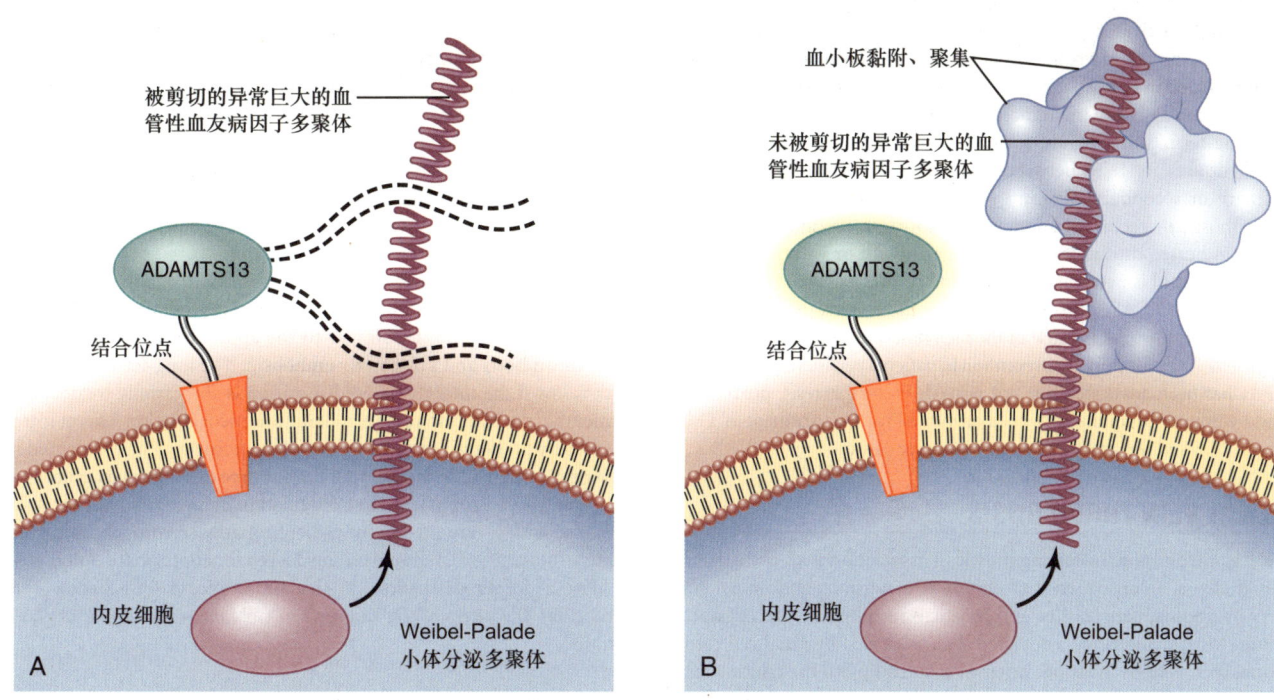

图 6.5 ADAMTS13 活性、血小板过度黏附与激活与血栓性血小板减少性紫癜之间的关联。(A) 在正常个体中,ADAMTS13(即,血管性血友病因子-剪切金属蛋白酶)分子连接到内皮细胞表面的结合位点上,当内皮细胞受到刺激后分泌异常巨大的血管性血友病因子多聚体时,ADAMTS1 将其剪切。剪切后形成的较小形式的血管性血友病因子进入循环,不会诱导血小板在正常血流中黏附和聚集。(B) 血栓性血小板减少性紫癜患者中存在 ADAMTS13 缺乏或活性严重减低,不能及时剪切内皮细胞分泌的异常巨大的血管性血友病因子多聚体。这些未被剪切的多聚体诱导血流中血小板黏附和聚集(引自 Moake JL: Thrombotic microangiopathies, N Engl J Med 347: 589-600, 2002.)

素。妊娠相关 aHUS 历来预后极差,超过 75% 的患者进展至 ESRD。依库珠单抗是一种有效治疗,且可在妊娠期间应用。

HELLP 综合征是肝血窦的 TMA,可出现类似 TTP 或 aHUS 的表现。虽然罕见,但可因急性肾小管坏死型的损伤导致 AKI,并在 HELLP 综合征缓解后可快速逆转。

抗磷脂综合征

抗磷脂抗体(APA)指的是一类自身抗体,如狼疮抗凝物,或 IgG 型或免疫球蛋白 M(IgM)型抗心磷脂抗体或抗 β2 糖蛋白抗体,这类抗体干扰磷脂结合蛋白和体外的磷脂依赖性凝血试验(如部分凝血活酶时间)。由于并非所有狼疮抗凝物均导致部分凝血活酶时间延长,因此可能需要进行其他的凝血系统检测,如稀释蝰蛇毒时间。APS 的诊断基于在实验室检测到 APA 的前提下,出现动脉或静脉血栓事件,或妊娠 10 周后发生妊娠丢失,或妊娠 10 周内发生的多胎妊娠丢失。在 10% 的健康人群中可检测到狼疮抗凝物和抗心磷脂抗体,仅有上述抗体阳性不足以诊断 APS。载脂蛋白 H(apo H,以前被称为 β2 糖蛋白 1)是抗心磷脂抗体的主要抗原靶点。

如果没有潜在的自身免疫性疾病,这类综合征被称为原发性 APS。当其与其他疾病相关时,如系统性红斑狼疮(SLE),则为继发性 APS。在 30%~50% 的 SLE 患者中可检测到 APA,这种情况下肾脏受累常见。

APA 的促凝作用可能源自干扰抗凝物 apo H、抑制纤维蛋白溶解、直接内皮损伤、加速动脉粥样硬化,以及激活血小板、单核细胞和内皮细胞。约 25% 的原发 APS 患者出现肾脏受累,SLE 或其他原因继发的 APS 中也可出现肾脏受累。整个肾脏血管系统均可出现血栓形成,包括主肾动脉及其分支、小动脉、肾小球,以及静脉。这些表现与其他 TMA 相关疾病的发现类似。可观察到缺血导致的局灶性皮质萎缩伴间质纤维化。

APS 的肾脏表现多样。一些患者仅有少量蛋白尿、肾功能正常,而其他患者可出现严重的高血压、肾病水平的蛋白尿,以及 AKI 或 CKD。肾动脉血栓可能导致梗死、急性腰痛、血尿以及肾功能减退。肾静脉血栓形成(RVT)可无症状,如果为急性且完全性的栓塞,则可表现为突发腰痛及肾功能减退。原发性 APS 的肾活检病理表现为小血管的血管闭塞性疾病,伴有小叶间动脉的纤维性内膜增生、动脉和小动脉中血栓再通、局灶性皮质萎缩,以及 TMA。APS 的其他表现包括血小板减少、溶血性贫血、未经肝素治疗情况下

a prolonged activated partial thromboplastin time in the absence of heparin therapy. It is worth noting that a high prevalence of APAs has been reported in ESRD patients undergoing hemodialysis, with dialysis access thrombosis as a main manifestation.

Long-term warfarin anticoagulation with a target international normalized ratio (INR) between 2 and 3 is indicated for patients with primary or secondary APS and prior deep vein thrombosis, arterial thrombosis, or recurrent spontaneous abortion. Because warfarin is contraindicated during pregnancy, heparin with or without low-dose aspirin (81 mg) is necessary until the end of pregnancy.

Treatment of APA-positive patients in the absence of prior clinical events is controversial because of the high false-positive rate for the tests. Aspirin therapy for primary prevention in patients persistently positive for APAs has been advocated but not proved. Plasmapheresis, prednisone, and hydroxychloroquine have been advocated for the treatment of TMA due to APS and should be considered in severe cases.

RENAL VEIN THROMBOSIS

RVT is uncommon, occurring mostly in association with malignancy, but it also is a consequence of nephrotic syndrome, abdominal surgery or trauma, pancreatitis, and genetic or acquired hypercoagulable states. Most malignancy-associated RVT is caused by renal cell carcinoma with venous invasion, often with spreading to the contralateral kidney, which may cause bilateral renal vein occlusion.

The nephrotic syndrome is associated with a risk for venous thrombosis throughout the circulation, including RVT. The RVT risk in patients with nephrotic syndrome correlates with severity of proteinuria and hypoalbuminemia; patients with a serum albumin concentration of less than 2 g/dL and/or proteinuria more than 10 g/day are at particular risk. Some studies have documented an incidence of RVT as high as 30% among patients with nephrotic syndrome, but most cases are not clinically apparent. Patients with membranous nephropathy seem to be at greatest risk for RVT for reasons that are not known, but RVT can also occur with nephrotic syndromes due to focal segmental glomerular sclerosis, membranoproliferative glomerulonephritis, minimal change disease, and diabetic kidney disease. Hypercoagulability is thought to result from loss of the antithrombotic protein antithrombin III in urine, although other factors such as increased procoagulant factors and platelet activation may also be involved.

RVT may manifest with symptoms attributable to renal cell carcinoma, such as flank pain, gross hematuria, nausea, anorexia, or lower extremity swelling. In male patents, left renal vein occlusion may cause a left varicocele, a result of the venous drainage of the left gonadal vein. In patients without a malignancy, symptoms of RVT depend on the acuity of the thrombosis. Acute, complete thrombosis may manifest with hematuria, flank pain, abdominal distention, and acute renal failure. RVT in adults usually occurs gradually because of collateral venous drainage return; in this setting, symptoms of AKI are uncommon, although proteinuria and creatinine levels may be mildly elevated. In these cases of chronic RVT, patients will typically come to clinical attention for pulmonary embolus.

Because patients often do not have symptoms, RVT is likely more common than reported in the literature. Some have suggested CT screening of asymptomatic, high-risk patients, particularly those with membranous nephropathy and severe proteinuria and hypoalbuminemia.

The standard method for diagnosis is renal venography, but because it has the risks of clot dislodgment, bleeding, and use of iodinated contrast, less invasive methods are commonly used. Contrast-enhanced CT venography appears to have a relatively high sensitivity and specificity, although it carries some risk for contrast nephropathy. Magnetic resonance imaging using gadolinium-based contrast or time-of-flight sequencing without contrast may also be useful. Renal Doppler ultrasound is useful, but it is operator dependent and has lower sensitivity than CT venography.

Treatment with systemic anticoagulation is recommended in the absence of contraindications. Most clinicians maintain anticoagulation for 6 to 9 months, similar to the approach for nonrenal deep vein thrombosis and pulmonary embolism. The long-term recurrence risk is low if the underlying predisposition is successfully treated, and patients are unlikely to require indefinite anticoagulation. Direct intravenous thrombolysis or operative thrombectomy may be considered in severe cases, particularly if the RVT is a source of pulmonary emboli or is causing AKI. Prophylactic anticoagulation in high-risk patients, such as those with severe membranous nephropathy (serum albumin concentration <2.8 g/dL) should be considered for appropriate candidates.

For a deeper discussion on this topic, please see Chapter 116, ❖ "Vascular Disorders of the Kidney," in *Goldman-Cecil Medicine*, 26th Edition.

SUGGESTED READINGS

ASTRAL Investigators, Wheatley K, Ives N, Gray R, et al.: Revascularization versus medical therapy for renal-artery stenosis, *N Engl J Med* 361(20):1953, 2009.

Barbour T, Johnson S, Cohney S, et al: Thrombotic microangiopathy and associated renal disorders, *Nephrol Dial Transplant* 27:2673–2685, 2012.

Brocklebank V, Wood KM, Kavanagh D: Thrombotic microangiopathy and the kidney, *Clin J Am Soc Nephrol* 13(2):300–317, 2018 Feb 7.

Cooper CJ, Murphy TP, Cutlip DE, Jamerson K, et al.: CORAL Investigators. Stenting and medical therapy for atherosclerotic renal-artery stenosis, *N Engl J Med* 370(1):13, 2014.

Fattori R, Cao P, De Rango P: et al: Interdisciplinary expert consensus document, on management of type B aortic dissection, *J Am Coll Cardiol* 61:1661–1678, 2013.

Friedman DJ, Pollak MR: Genetics of kidney failure and the evolving story of APOL1, *J Clin Invest* 121:3367–3374, 2011.

Jennette JC, Nachman PH: ANCA glomerulonephritis and vasculitis, *Clin J Am Soc Nephrol* 12(10):1680–1691, 2017 Oct 6.

Krüger T, Conzelmann LO, Bonser RS: et al: Acute aortic dissection type A, *Br J Surg* 99:1331–1344, 2012.

Maynard SE, Thadhani R: Pregnancy and the kidney, *J Am Soc Nephrol* 20:14–22, 2009.

Noris M, Mescia F, Remuzzi G: STEC-HUS, atypical HUS and TTP are all diseases of complement activation, *Nat Rev Nephrol* 8:622–633, 2012.

Ruiz-Irastorza G, Crowther M, Branch W, et al: Antiphospholipid syndrome, *Lancet* 376:1498–1509, 2010.

Sadler JE: Von Willebrand factor, ADAMTS13, and thrombotic thrombocytopenic purpura, *Blood* 112:11–18, 2008.

Scolari F, Ravani P: Atheroembolic renal disease, *Lancet* 375:1650–1660, 2010.

Shanmugam VK, Steen VD: Renal disease in scleroderma: an update on evaluation, risk stratification, pathogenesis and management, *Curr Opin Rheumatol* 24:669–676, 2012.

Specks U, Merkel PA, Seo P, et al: Efficacy of remission-induction regimens for ANCA-associated vasculitis, *N Engl J Med* 369:417–427, 2013.

Textor SC, Misra S, Oderich GS: Percutaneous revascularization for ischemic nephropathy: the past, present, and future, *Kidney Int* 83:28–40, 2013.

出现活化部分凝血活酶时间延长。值得注意的是，有报道称在血液透析的 ESRD 患者中 APA 的阳性率较高，其主要表现为透析通路血栓形成。

在原发性或继发性 APS 以及合并有既往深静脉血栓形成、动脉血栓形成，或复发性自然流产的患者中，有指征使用华法林长期抗凝，且将国际标准化比值（INR）目标定位为 2～3。由于华法林在妊娠期禁用，因此需要使用肝素联合或不联合低剂量阿司匹林（81 mg）直到孕期结束。

鉴于 APA 的检测假阳性率高，因此对于没有既往临床事件而仅有 APA 阳性患者的治疗存在争议。有学者建议在持续 APA 阳性的患者中使用阿司匹林作为一级预防，但该观点尚未被证实。有人提倡血浆置换、泼尼松，以及羟氯喹治疗 APS 继发的 TMA，上述治疗应在重症病例中考虑使用。

肾静脉血栓形成（RVT）

RVT 不常见，主要与恶性肿瘤相关，但也可以是肾病综合征、腹部手术或创伤、胰腺炎，以及遗传性或获得性高凝状态导致的后果。绝大部分恶性肿瘤相关的 RVT 是由肾细胞癌侵犯静脉所导致的，常扩散至肾脏，可引起双侧肾静脉闭塞。

肾病综合征与整个循环系统中静脉血栓形成的风险相关，包括 RVT。肾病综合征患者中 RVT 的风险与蛋白尿和低白蛋白血症的严重程度相关；血清白蛋白浓度低于 20 g/L 和（或）尿蛋白大于 10 g/d 的患者尤其高危。一些研究报道肾病综合征患者发生 RVT 的比例高达 30%，但大部分病例无明显临床症状。尽管原因尚不明确，膜性肾病患者的 RVT 风险似乎最高，但 RVT 同样可在由局灶节段性肾小球硬化、膜增生性肾小球肾炎、微小病变，以及糖尿病肾病导致的肾病综合征患者中出现。高凝倾向被认为与尿液中抗血栓蛋白抗凝血酶Ⅲ丢失相关，然而促凝因子升高以及血小板激活等其他因素也可能参与其中。

RVT 可出现肾透明细胞癌相关的症状，如腰痛、肉眼血尿、恶心、食欲减退，或下肢水肿。在男性患者中，左肾静脉阻塞可引起左侧精索静脉曲张，这是左侧性腺静脉回流的结果。在没有恶性肿瘤的患者中，RVT 的症状取决于血栓形成的急性程度。急性的、完全血栓形成可表现为血尿、腰痛、腹胀，以及急性肾衰竭。成人 RVT 常由于存在侧支静脉回流而缓慢进展；在这种情况下，尽管尿蛋白和肌酐水平可能轻度升高，却不常出现 AKI 症状。在这些慢性 RVT 病例中，患者常因肺栓塞才引起临床注意。

由于患者通常没有症状，RVT 实际上可能比文献报道的更为常见。一些学者建议在无症状、高风险的患者中进行 CT 筛查，特别是膜性肾病以及严重蛋白尿和低蛋白血症患者。

肾静脉造影是标准诊断方法，但由于其具有血凝块脱落、出血的风险，也需要应用碘造影剂，因此通常使用其他更加无创的方式。尽管仍存在一些造影剂肾病的风险，增强 CT 静脉成像似乎有更高的敏感性和特异性。应用钆造影剂或无造影剂的飞行时间序列的磁共振成像也可能有用。肾脏多普勒超声对诊断有价值，但其依赖操作者技术，并且敏感性低于 CT 静脉造影。

如无禁忌，推荐系统性抗凝治疗。与非肾脏深静脉血栓和肺栓塞的治疗方法类似，大部分临床医师会维持 6～9 个月的抗凝治疗。如果潜在的血栓易感因素已成功治愈，则长期复发风险低，患者不太可能需要接受无限期抗凝治疗。严重的病例，特别是当 RVT 为肺栓塞的栓子来源或造成 AKI 时，可考虑直接静脉溶栓或手术取栓。对于高风险患者应考虑进行预防性抗凝，如严重膜性肾病（血清白蛋白浓度小于 28 g/L）患者［译者注：膜性肾病（血清白蛋白浓度小于 28 g/L）认定为预防性抗凝的标准有不同结论：KDIGO2021 肾小球病指南中为高血栓且低出血风险者血清白蛋白低于 25 g/L 使用华法林，低血栓或高出血风险者血清白蛋白低于 32 g/L 使用阿司匹林］。

有关此专题的深入讨论，请参阅 *Goldman-Cecil Medicine* 第 26 版第 116 章"肾脏血管疾病"。

推荐阅读

ASTRAL Investigators, Wheatley K, Ives N, Gray R, et al.: Revascularization versus medical therapy for renal-artery stenosis, *N Engl J Med* 361(20):1953, 2009.

Barbour T, Johnson S, Cohney S, et al: Thrombotic microangiopathy and associated renal disorders, *Nephrol Dial Transplant* 27:2673–2685, 2012.

Brocklebank V, Wood KM, Kavanagh D: Thrombotic microangiopathy and the kidney, *Clin J Am Soc Nephrol* 13(2):300–317, 2018 Feb 7.

Cooper CJ, Murphy TP, Cutlip DE, Jamerson K, et al.: CORAL Investigators. Stenting and medical therapy for atherosclerotic renal-artery stenosis, *N Engl J Med* 370(1):13, 2014.

Fattori R, Cao P, De Rango P: et al: Interdisciplinary expert consensus document, on management of type B aortic dissection, *J Am Coll Cardiol* 61:1661–1678, 2013.

Friedman DJ, Pollak MR: Genetics of kidney failure and the evolving story of APOL1, *J Clin Invest* 121:3367–3374, 2011.

Jennette JC, Nachman PH: ANCA glomerulonephritis and vasculitis, *Clin J Am Soc Nephrol* 12(10):1680–1691, 2017 Oct 6.

Krüger T, Conzelmann LO, Bonser RS: et al: Acute aortic dissection type A, *Br J Surg* 99:1331–1344, 2012.

Maynard SE, Thadhani R: Pregnancy and the kidney, *J Am Soc Nephrol* 20:14–22, 2009.

Noris M, Mescia F, Remuzzi G: STEC-HUS, atypical HUS and TTP are all diseases of complement activation, *Nat Rev Nephrol* 8:622–633, 2012.

Ruiz-Irastorza G, Crowther M, Branch W, et al: Antiphospholipid syndrome, *Lancet* 376:1498–1509, 2010.

Sadler JE: Von Willebrand factor, ADAMTS13, and thrombotic thrombocytopenic purpura, *Blood* 112:11–18, 2008.

Scolari F, Ravani P: Atheroembolic renal disease, *Lancet* 375:1650–1660, 2010.

Shanmugam VK, Steen VD: Renal disease in scleroderma: an update on evaluation, risk stratification, pathogenesis and management, *Curr Opin Rheumatol* 24:669–676, 2012.

Specks U, Merkel PA, Seo P, et al: Efficacy of remission-induction regimens for ANCA-associated vasculitis, *N Engl J Med* 369:417–427, 2013.

Textor SC, Misra S, Oderich GS: Percutaneous revascularization for ischemic nephropathy: the past, present, and future, *Kidney Int* 83:28–40, 2013.

Acute Kidney Injury

Mark A. Perazella, Jeffrey M. Turner

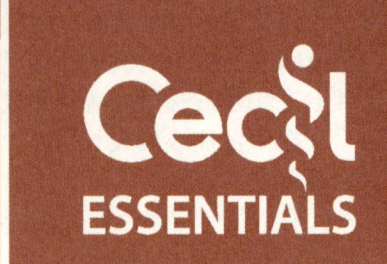

DEFINITION

Acute kidney injury (AKI) is a syndrome defined as an abrupt decrease in glomerular filtration rate (GFR) sufficient to promote the retention of nitrogenous waste products (blood urea nitrogen [BUN] and creatinine); disturb the regulation of extracellular fluid volume, electrolyte balance, and acid-base homeostasis; and impair drug excretion. Importantly, even mild abnormalities in kidney structure and function are associated with other end-organ complications and increased mortality.

AKI includes a spectrum of clinical conditions. The numerous causes of AKI vary based on individual comorbidities (and risk for AKI) and whether kidney injury develops in the outpatient setting or in hospital. The incidence of AKI is rising, and its complications include progression to more severe kidney failure, need for renal replacement therapy (RRT), chronic kidney disease (CKD), and death. Several consensus groups have produced definitions and diagnostic criteria for AKI. Table 7.1 describes the diagnostic criteria for the Risk, Injury, Failure, Loss, and End-stage renal disease (ESRD) (RIFLE); Acute Kidney Injury Network (AKIN); and Kidney Disease: Improving Global Outcomes (KDIGO) classifications.

In 2004, the RIFLE classification was put forth to standardize the definition of AKI. Changes in serum creatinine concentration (over 7 days), reductions in estimated glomerular filtration rate (eGFR), and urine output parameters were used in this diagnostic system. The Risk (R), Injury (I), and Failure (F) categories were applicable to AKI, whereas the Loss (L) and ESRD (E) categories were CKD stages. In 2007, the AKIN group modified the RIFLE criteria definition of AKI by adding an absolute increase in serum creatinine of only 0.3 mg/dL, eliminating the eGFR criteria, and changing the time frame for AKI to develop (to 48 hours, compared with the 7 days for RIFLE diagnosis). Focusing on AKI, the AKIN criteria replaced the R, I, and F categories from the RIFLE criteria with stages 1, 2, and 3 and eliminated the L and E categories. In 2012, the KDIGO group combined parts of the RIFLE and AKIN criteria to capture AKI with increased sensitivity.

Understanding of the pathophysiology underlying development of AKI has advanced, and better diagnostic tools have moved the field forward. However, specific directed therapies remain limited for the most common forms of AKI. Although technical advances in RRT and supportive care have improved, patients commonly develop other end-organ disease in the setting of AKI. More concerning is the relatively high mortality rate associated with AKI, particularly when it develops in the hospital setting and requires RRT.

ETIOLOGY

In most cases, more than one process contributes to AKI, but for ease of classification, three broad categories (Fig. 7.1) are used: (1) *prerenal AKI*, the result of a decrease in renal blood flow and perfusion of the kidney; (2) *intrinsic AKI*, the result of disease affecting one of the renal parenchymal compartments; and (3) *postrenal AKI*, the result of obstruction to urinary flow anywhere along the urinary tract starting from the renal calyces/pelves and involving the ureters, bladder, or urethra.

The most common form of AKI is due to prerenal physiology, particularly in the outpatient setting, but also in the hospital. Postrenal AKI is more common in elderly men with prostatic hyperplasia, patients with bladder dysfunction, and patients with certain malignancies. Intrinsic AKI may be due to a vascular process, glomerular disease, interstitial disease, or tubular injury. The most common intrinsic AKI is an entity known as *acute tubular necrosis* (ATN), or more recently *acute tubular injury* (ATI), which is histologically more accurate. This is a clinical syndrome characterized by an abrupt and sustained decline in GFR due to an acute ischemic injury, nephrotoxic insult, or a combination of both. The clinical recognition of ATN is based primarily on exclusion of prerenal and postrenal causes of AKI, as well as other causes of intrinsic AKI (glomerulonephritis [GN], acute interstitial nephritis [AIN], and vasculitis). Once other intrinsic causes of AKI are excluded, it is reasonable to conclude ATN is the cause or major contributor to AKI. Although the name *acute tubular necrosis* is not an entirely valid histologic description of the lesion, the term will be utilized as it is part of the language of clinical medicine.

EPIDEMIOLOGY

AKI occurs more commonly in hospitalized patients as compared to the community setting. Community-acquired AKI defined by various step-wise increases in serum creatinine has an incidence of approximately 1%. Nearly half of the patients involve AKI superimposed on CKD. Prerenal AKI accounts for approximately 70% of cases, obstructive uropathy approximately 17%, and intrinsic AKI from various etiologies approximately 11% of the AKI cases. In contrast, hospital-acquired AKI has an incidence ranging from 4.9% to 7.2%. The incidence of AKI is higher in intensive care unit (ICU) admissions, approximating 30%. CKD, older age, and other comorbidities are important risk factors for AKI. Prerenal AKI remains the most common cause, followed by intrinsic AKI from nephrotoxic medications and ischemic ATN.

急性肾损伤

马杰 译　李明喜　赵明辉 审校　李雪梅 通审

定义

急性肾损伤（AKI）是一种综合征，定义为肾小球滤过率（GFR）的急剧下降，足以导致氮质废物［血尿素氮（BUN）和肌酐］的滞留；引起细胞外液容量、电解质及酸碱平衡调节的紊乱，并损害药物的排泄。重要的是，即使是轻微的肾脏结构和功能异常也与其他终末器官并发症和死亡率的增加相关。

AKI 包括一系列临床状况。AKI 的众多病因因个体的合并症（和 AKI 风险）以及肾损伤发生在院内或院外而有所不同。AKI 的发病率正在上升，其并发症包括进展为更严重的肾衰竭、需要肾替代治疗（RRT）、慢性肾脏病（CKD）和死亡。几个共识小组已经制定了 AKI 的定义和诊断标准。表 7.1 描述了风险、损伤、衰竭、丧失和终末期肾脏病（ESRD）（RIFLE），急性肾损伤协作网（AKIN），以及改善全球肾脏预后联盟（KDIGO）的分类诊断标准。

2004 年提出了 RIFLE 分类法，旨在标准化 AKI 的定义。该诊断系统基于血清肌酐浓度变化（7 天内）、估算肾小球滤过率（eGFR）的降低以及尿量参数来判定。在 RIFLE 分类法中，风险（R）、损伤（I）和衰竭（F）类别适用于 AKI，而丧失（L）和终末期肾病（E）类别则为慢性肾脏病（CKD）阶段。2007 年，AKIN 工作组修改了 RIFLE 标准中关于 AKI 的定义，增加了血清肌酐绝对增加 0.3 mg/dl 的标准，去除了 eGFR 标准，并将 AKI 发展的时间范围更改为 48 h（相比于 RIFLE 诊断的 7 天）。针对 AKI，AKIN 标准用 1、2、3 阶段取代了 RIFLE 标准中的 R、I 和 F 类别，并取消了 L 和 E 类别。2012 年，KDIGO 工作组综合了 RIFLE 和 AKIN 标准的部分内容，以提高 AKI 判定的敏感性。

人们对 AKI 发病机制的了解不断深入，而更好的诊断工具也推动了该领域的发展。然而，对于最常见形式的 AKI，特定的治疗方法仍然有限。尽管 RRT 和支持治疗技术有所进步，但患者在 AKI 背景下通常会发展为其他终末器官疾病。更令人担忧的是与 AKI 相关的相对较高的死亡率，特别是住院时发生并需要 RRT 时。

病因

在大多数情况下，AKI 的发生是多种因素共同作用的结果，但为了便于分类，将其分为三大类（图 7.1）：①肾前性 AKI，由肾血流减少和肾灌注不足引起；②肾实质性 AKI，由影响肾实质任一部分的疾病引起；③肾后性 AKI，从肾盏/肾盂开始，涉及输尿管、膀胱或尿道的尿流阻塞引起。

最常见的 AKI 是由肾前性生理因素引起的，尤其是院外患者，但在医院内也有发生。肾后性 AKI 主要见于老年男性前列腺增生、膀胱功能障碍及某些恶性肿瘤患者。肾实质性 AKI 可能由血管病变、肾小球疾病、间质性疾病或肾小管损伤引起。最常见的肾实质性 AKI 是急性肾小管坏死（ATN），最近更精确地称为急性肾小管损伤（ATI）。这是一种临床综合征，其特征是由于急性缺血性损伤、肾毒性损伤或两者结合导致 GFR 突然且持续下降。ATN 的临床识别主要基于排除肾前性和肾后性 AKI 原因，及其他肾实质性 AKI 原因［如肾小球肾炎（GN）、急性间质性肾炎（AIN）和血管炎］。一旦排除了 AKI 的其他内在原因，就可以合理地推断 ATN 是 AKI 的原因或主要促成因素。虽然急性肾小管坏死这个名称并不是病变的完整有效的组织学描述，但由于它是临床医学常用语，因此仍沿用这个术语。

流行病学

与社区环境相比，AKI 在住院患者中更为常见。社区获得性 AKI 一般为血清肌酐逐步升高，其发病率约为 1%。近一半患者为 CKD 基础上的 AKI。肾前性 AKI 约占病例的 70%，尿路梗阻性 AKI 约占 17%，各种病因引起的肾实质性 AKI 约占 11%。与社区获得性 AKI 相比，住院患者 AKI 的发病率在 4.9% 至 7.2% 之间。在重症监护病房（ICU）患者中，AKI 的发病率更高，约为 30%。CKD、高龄及其他共病是 AKI 的重要风险因素。肾前性 AKI 仍然是最常见的原因，其次是由肾毒性药物和缺血性 ATN 引起的肾实质性 AKI。

TABLE 7.1	Classification of Acute Kidney Injury	
Stage	Serum Creatinine Increase Within 7 Days	Urine Output
Kidney Disease: Improving Global Outcomes (KDIGO) Classification (2012)		
1	1.5-1.9 times baseline *or* ≥0.3 mg/dL within 48 hr	<0.5 mL/kg/hr × 6-12 hr
2	2-2.9 times baseline	<0.5 mL/kg/hr ≥12 hr
3	3 times baseline *or* an increase in the serum creatinine to ≥4 mg/dL with an absolute increase ≥0.3 mg/dL within 48 hr or 1.5 times baseline within 7 days *or* initiation of RRT *or* in patients aged <18 yr, eGFR decreased to <35 mL/min/1.73 m²	<0.3 mL/kg/hr × ≥24 hr
Acute Kidney Injury Network (AKIN) Classification (2007)		
1	1.5-1.9 times baseline *or* ≥0.3 mg/dL within 48 hr	<0.5 mL/kg/hr × 6-12 hr
2	2-2.9 times baseline	<0.5 mL/kg/hr ≥12 hr
3	3 times baseline *or* increase in serum creatinine ≥4 mg/dL with an increase ≥0.5 mg/dL *or* initiation of RRT	<0.3 mL/kg/hr × ≥24 hr *or* anuria ≥12 hr
RIFLE Classification (2004)		
Risk	1.5-1.9 times baseline *or* GFR decrease >25%	<0.5 mL/kg/hr × 6 hr
Injury	2-2.9 times baseline *or* GFR decrease >50%	<0.5 mL/kg/hr × 12 hr
Failure	3 times baseline *or* GFR decrease >75% *or* serum creatinine ≥4 mg/dL with an increase ≥0.5 mg/dL	<0.3 mL/kg/hr × 24 hr *or* anuria × 12 hr
Loss	Complete loss of renal function for >4 wk	
ESRD	End-stage renal disease >3 mo	

eGFR, Estimated glomerular filtration rate; *GFR*, glomerular filtration rate; *RRT*, renal replacement therapy.

DIAGNOSTIC EVALUATION

History and Physical Examination

Evaluation of the patient with AKI should be methodical and systematic to ensure that potentially reversible causes are diagnosed and treated expeditiously to preserve kidney function and limit development of permanent kidney injury, as depicted in Table 7.2. Part of the difficulty in arriving at a correct diagnosis is that several potential causes of AKI often coexist. Emphasis is placed on thorough analysis of available data and examination of the sequence of deterioration in kidney function and urine volume in relation to the chronologies of the potential causes of AKI.

Knowledge of the natural history of the various causes of AKI also is critical. The evaluation should include a thorough patient history and chart review to identify risk factors for prerenal AKI (e.g., vomiting, diuretics, diarrhea, heart failure, cirrhosis); potential nephrotoxic drugs (prescribed or over-the-counter, including alternative/complementary medications); risk factors for prostate disease, cervical cancer, or bladder cancer; and symptoms of urinary tract obstruction (e.g., prostatism, overflow incontinence, anuria). The urine volume is less than 400 mL/day with oliguric AKI, less than 100 mL/day with oligo-anuric AKI, and less than 50 mL/day with anuric AKI. Normal urine output does not exclude the diagnosis of AKI: Nonoliguric AKI (>400 mL/day) can be associated with nephrotoxic AKI and partial urinary obstruction. Wide variation in daily urine output also suggests AKI due to partial urinary tract obstruction. Anuria has a limited differential diagnosis, suggesting complete urinary obstruction, a vascular catastrophe, or severe cortical necrosis.

A thorough physical exam is critical in patients with AKI, and particular attention should be given to determining the patient's volume status. Reduced body weight, hypotension, an orthostatic fall in blood pressure (BP), or flat neck veins may be present in patients with prerenal AKI or ischemic ATN caused by true volume depletion. On the other hand, the presence of edema, pulmonary rales, or an S_3 gallop signals venous congestion from cardiac dysfunction that can be the cause of cardiorenal syndrome. Alternatively, edema, ascites, and asterixis suggest acute liver dysfunction or cirrhosis, which can be the cause of AKI due to hepatorenal syndrome. It is important to differentiate these disorders, because their appropriate therapies differ. Some individuals can have signs of increased total body water in the form of edema, while simultaneously having signs of reductions in their intravascular volume in the form of hypotension and weak pulses. In these individuals, invasive intravascular monitoring may be helpful. This includes measurement of cardiac filling pressures or central venous pressures with an indwelling catheter. In addition, recent research has shown that noninvasive techniques including respiratory variations in systolic blood pressure, pulse pressure, calculated stroke volume, or the collapsibility of the inferior vena cava measured on bedside ultrasound are also useful methods for volume assessment that do not require the placement of a vascular catheter.

Evidence of systemic disease also should be sought. Findings may include signs of pulmonary hemorrhage indicative of a vasculitis or Goodpasture's syndrome, skin rash as a manifestation of systemic lupus erythematosus, atheroemboli, vasculitis, cryoglobulins, or AIN, as well as joint disease making lupus or rheumatoid arthritis a consideration.

Basic Laboratory Tests

Laboratory tests are directed by the differential diagnosis that is postulated after a complete history, chart review, and physical examination have been performed. Basic tests include a complete blood count to assess for anemia (microangiopathic or immune-mediated) and thrombocytopenia (thrombotic thrombocytic purpura [TTP], hemolytic-uremic syndrome [HUS], and disseminated intravascular coagulation [DIC]). Other tests to evaluate the cause of AKI include various serologic measurements (antinuclear antibody [ANA], antineutrophil cytoplasmic antibodies [ANCA], anti–glomerular basement membrane antibody [anti-GBM], anti–double-stranded DNA antibodies [anti-dsDNA], and hepatitis B and C viral serologies), complement levels, cryoglobulin levels, blood cultures, serum lactate dehydrogenase (LDH) and haptoglobin measurements, serum and urine immunoelectrophoresis, and serum free light chain assay.

表 7.1 急性肾损伤的分类		
阶段	血清肌酐在 7 天内升高	尿量
肾脏疾病：改善全球肾脏预后（KDIGO）分类（2012）		
1	1.5～1.9 倍基线或 48 h 内升高≥ 0.3 mg/dl	< 0.5 ml/（kg·h）×（6～12）h
2	2～2.9 倍基线水平	< 0.5 ml/（kg·h）×≥ 12 h
3	3 倍基线或血清肌酐升高至≥ 4 mg/dl 伴 48 h 内绝对值升高≥ 0.3 mg/dl 或 7 天内升高至 1.5 倍基线或开始接受 RRT 或年龄< 18 岁、eGFR 降低至< 35 ml/（min·1.73 m^2）的患者	< 0.3 ml/（kg·h）×≥ 24 h
急性肾损伤协作网（AKIN）分类（2007）		
1	1.5～1.9 倍基线或 48 h 内升高≥ 0.3 mg/dl	< 0.5 ml/（kg·h）×（6～12）h
2	2～2.9 倍基线水平	< 0.5 ml/（kg·h）×≥ 12 h
3	3 倍基线或血清肌酐升高至≥ 4 mg/dl 伴绝对值升高≥ 0.5 mg/dl 或开始接受 RRT	< 0.3 ml/（kg·h）×≥ 24 h 或无尿≥ 12 h
RIFLE 分类（2004）		
风险（R）	1.5～1.9 倍基线或 GFR 下降> 25%	< 0.5 ml/（kg·h）×6 h
损伤（I）	2～2.9 倍基线或 GFR 下降> 50%	< 0.5 ml/（kg·h）×12 h
衰竭（F）	3 倍基线或 GFR 下降> 75% 或血清肌酐≥ 4 mg/dl 伴绝对值升高≥ 0.5 mg/dl	< 0.3 ml/（kg·h）×24 h 或无尿×12 h
丧失（L）	肾功能完全丧失超过 4 周	
终末期肾病（E）	终末期肾病> 3 个月	

eGFR：估测肾小球滤过率；GFR：肾小球滤过率；RRT，肾脏替代治疗。

诊断性评估

病史和体格检查

应针对 AKI 患者进行有序和全面评估，及时诊断并治疗潜在的可逆性病因，以保护肾功能并延缓进展至永久性肾损伤（表 7.2）。正确诊断的困难在于多种潜在 AKI 病因通常共存。因此，重点是对现有数据进行详细分析，并判断肾功能恶化、尿量变少与 AKI 潜在病因的时间顺序。

了解 AKI 各种病因的自然病程也很重要。评估应包括详细的病史和病历回顾，以识别肾前性 AKI 的风险因素（如呕吐、利尿剂、腹泻、心力衰竭、肝硬化）、潜在的肾毒性药物（处方或非处方药，包括替代/补充药物）、前列腺疾病、宫颈癌或膀胱癌的风险因素，以及尿路梗阻的症状（如前列腺肥大、溢出性尿失禁、无尿）。少尿性 AKI 的尿量少于 400 ml/d，少尿-无尿性 AKI 的尿量少于 100 ml/d，无尿性 AKI 的尿量少于 50 ml/d。但尿量正常不能排除 AKI 的诊断：非少尿性 AKI（> 400 ml/d）可能与肾毒性 AKI 和部分性尿路梗阻有关。每日尿量变化过大也提示部分尿路梗阻导致的 AKI。无尿的鉴别诊断不多，其提示完全性尿路梗阻、灾难性血管病变或重度肾皮质坏死。

对 AKI 患者进行全面体检至关重要，尤其要注意确定患者的血容量状态。体重减轻、低血压、直立性低血压或颈静脉不充盈可见于真性血容量减少导致的肾前性 AKI 或缺血性 ATN 患者。另一方面，水肿、肺部啰音或 S3 奔马律的出现可能提示心功能障碍导致的静脉淤血，这可能是心肾综合征的原因。此外，水肿、腹水和扑翼样震颤则提示急性肝功能不全或肝硬化，这可能是由于肝肾综合征导致的 AKI。区分这些疾病非常重要，因为它们的治疗方法各不相同。有些患者可能表现为水肿等全身水分增加的症状，但也同时出现低血压和脉搏微弱等血管内血容量减少的症状。对这些患者，侵入性血管内监测可能有帮助，包括用留置导管测量心脏充盈压或中心静脉压。此外，最近的研究表明，非侵入性技术，包括收缩压、脉压、计算的每搏输出量的呼吸变化或床旁超声测量的下腔静脉塌陷度，也是评估血容量的有用方法，这些检查无须放置血管导管。

同时，也应寻找系统性疾病的证据。包括提示血管炎或 Goodpasture 综合征的肺出血体征，提示系统性红斑狼疮的皮疹，动脉栓塞，血管炎，冷球蛋白或急性间质性肾炎（AIN），以及提示狼疮或类风湿关节炎的关节病变。

基本实验室检查

实验室检查应以鉴别诊断为导向，鉴别诊断应在全面的病史采集、病历回顾和体格检查后提出。基础检查包括全血细胞计数，以评估是否存在贫血（微血管病性或免疫相关）和血小板减少症［血栓性血小板减少性紫癜（TTP）、溶血性尿毒综合征（HUS）和弥散性血管内凝血（DIC）］。其他评估 AKI 病因的检查包括各种血清学检测［抗核抗体（ANA）、抗中性粒细胞胞质抗体（ANCA）、抗肾小球基底膜抗体（anti-GBM）、抗双链 DNA 抗体（anti-dsDNA）及乙型和丙型肝炎病毒血清学检测］、补体水平、冷球蛋白水平、血培养、血清乳酸脱氢酶（LDH）和结合珠蛋白测量、血清和尿液免疫电泳以及血清游离轻链测定。

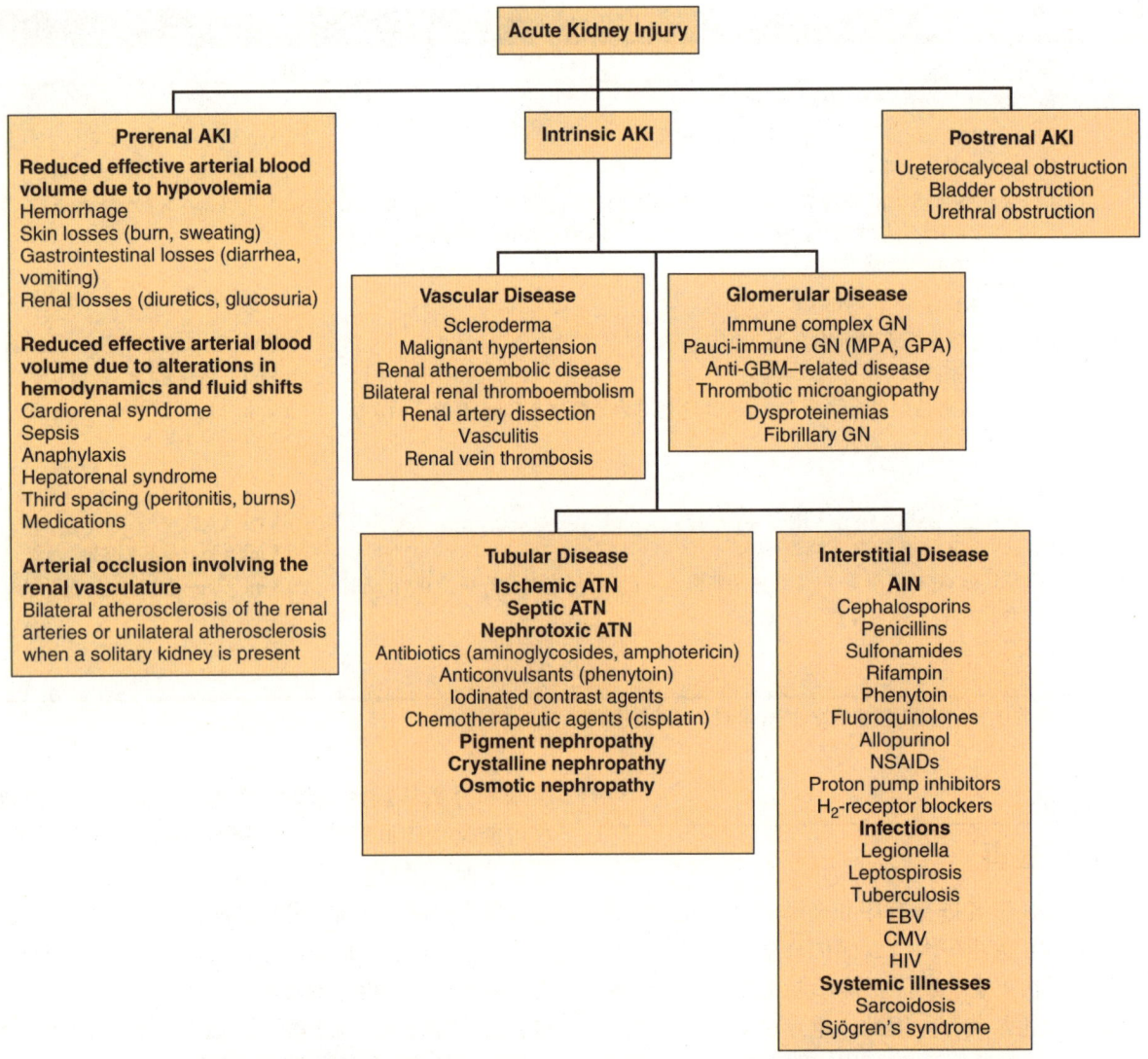

Fig. 7.1 Common causes of acute kidney injury (AKI). *AIN*, Acute interstitial nephritis; *ATN*, acute tubular necrosis; *CMV*, cytomegalovirus; *EBV*, Epstein-Barr virus; *GBM*, glomerular basement membrane; *GN*, glomerulonephritis; *GPA*, granulomatosis with polyangiitis; H_2, histamine 2; *HIV*, human immunodeficiency virus; *HUS*, hemolytic uremic syndrome; *MPA*, microscopic polyangiitis; *NSAIDs*, nonsteroidal anti-inflammatory drugs; *TTP*, thrombotic thrombocytopenic purpura.

TABLE 7.2 Diagnostic Approach to the Patient With Acute Kidney Injury

1. Record review; special attention to evidence of recent reduction in glomerular filtration rate and sequence of events leading to deterioration of kidney function to determine possible causative factors
2. Physical examination, including evaluation of hemodynamic status
3. Urinalysis and urine microscopy with thorough sediment examination
4. Determination of urinary indices, including fractional excretion of sodium and urea
5. Catheterization and measurement of postvoid residual urine volume if outlet obstruction is suspected
6. Fluid challenge in cases of suspected prerenal AKI
7. Radiologic studies, particular as dictated by the clinical setting (e.g., ultrasonography to look for obstruction)
8. Kidney biopsy

AKI, Acute kidney injury.

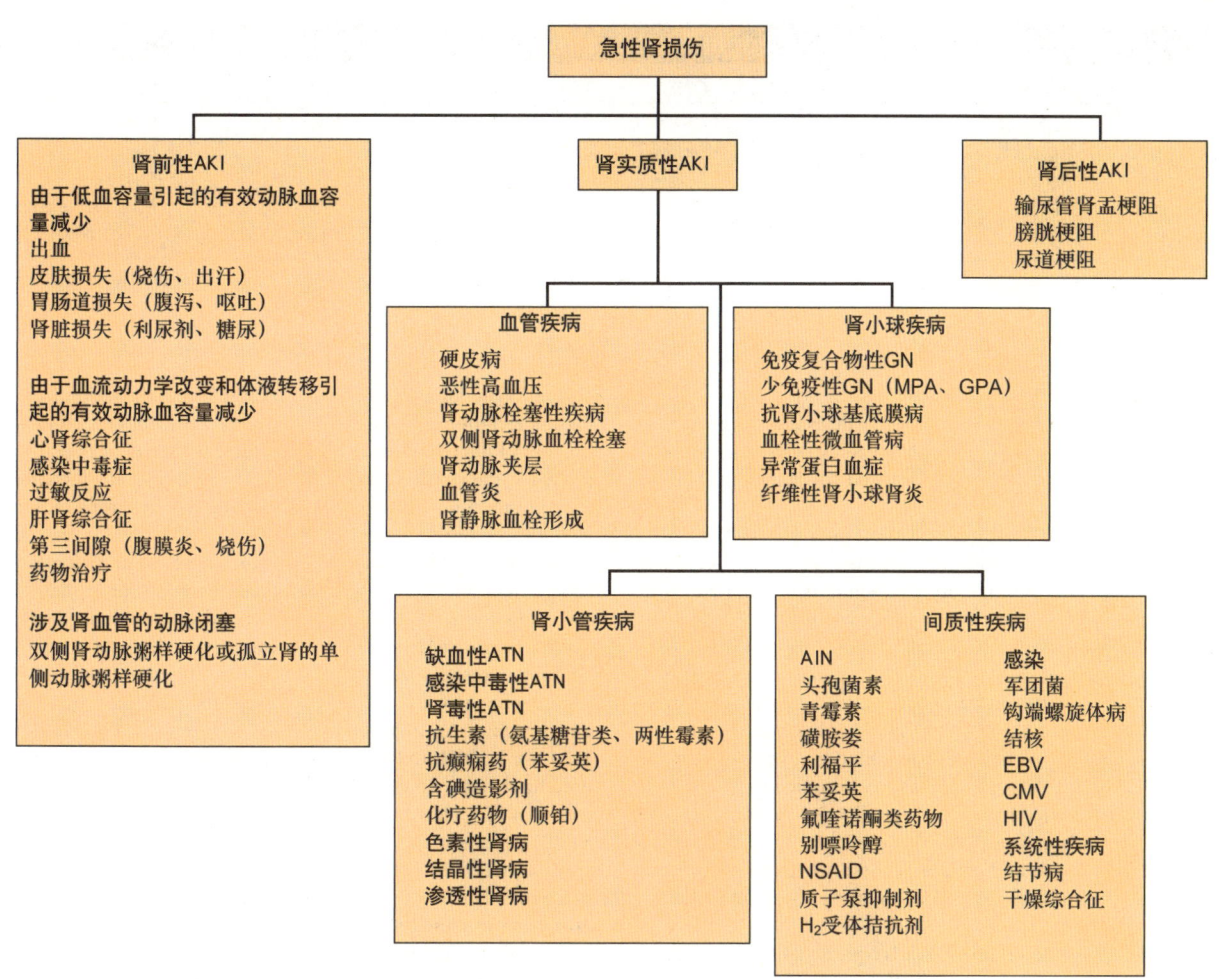

图 7.1 急性肾损伤（AKI）的常见病因。AIN，急性间质性肾炎；ATN，急性肾小管坏死；CMV，巨细胞病毒；EBV，Epstein-Barr 病毒；GN，肾小球肾炎；GPA，肉芽肿性多血管炎；H_2，组胺 2；HIV，人类免疫缺陷病毒；MPA，显微镜下多血管炎；NSAID，非甾体抗炎药

表 7.2　急性肾损伤患者的诊断流程
1. 回顾病历记录，特别注意近期肾小球滤过率降低的证据以及导致肾功能恶化的事件顺序，以确定可能的致病因素。
2. 体格检查，包括血流动力学状态的评估。
3. 尿液分析和尿液显微镜检查，包括对尿沉渣的全面检查。
4. 确定尿液指标，包括钠和尿素的排泄分数。
5. 如果怀疑尿路出口梗阻，则进行导尿并测量排尿后残余尿量。
6. 对于疑似肾前性 AKI 的病例，进行补液试验。
7. 根据临床情况进行影像学检查（如超声检查以查找梗阻部位）。
8. 肾活检。

AKI：急性肾损伤。

TABLE 7.3	Urinalysis and Microscopic Examination of the Urine Sediment					
Test	Prerenal	Vasculitis	GN	ATN	AIN	Postrenal
Specific gravity	High	Normal/high	Normal/high	Isosmotic	Isosmotic	Isosmotic
Dipstick blood	Negative	Positive	Positive	±	±	Negative
Dipstick protein	Negative	Positive	Positive	Negative	±	Negative
Urine sediment examination	Negative, hyaline casts	RBC casts, dysmorphic RBCs	RBC casts, dysmorphic RBCs	Granular casts, RTECs	WBC casts, eosinophils	Negative, sometimes WBCs/RBCs

AIN, Acute interstitial nephritis; *ATN*, acute tubular necrosis; *GN*, glomerulonephritis; *RBCs*, red blood cells; *RTECs*, renal tubular epithelial cells; *WBCs*, white blood cells.

Urinalysis and Urine Microscopy

Urinalysis is a key component of the diagnostic evaluation of AKI, as summarized in Table 7.3. It is important to evaluate urine specific gravity (SG), as well as the presence of blood (or heme), protein, or leukocyte esterase.

A very high urine SG typically suggests prerenal AKI, whereas isosthenuria (SG = 1.010) indicates intrinsic AKI (e.g., ATN). A thorough microscopic examination of the spun urine sediment, with quantification of the urinary elements, adds essential information to the case. Bland urine with no blood or protein and few to no cells or casts favors a diagnosis of prerenal AKI. Vascular causes of AKI have a variable urine tonicity and sometimes hematuria (isomorphic or dysmorphic red blood cells [RBCs]) and granular casts. GN exhibits variable urine tonicity, positive blood and protein on the dipstick, RBCs, and RBC casts. ATN shows isotonic urine with variable protein and variable heme on urine dipstick (heme is positive with rhabdomyolysis and hemolysis). Renal tubular epithelial cells (RTECs), RTEC casts, and fine or coarse pigmented granular casts (sometime muddy brown) may be present on the sediment examination.

Urine in patients with postrenal AKI is typically isotonic and bland unless there is associated infection (pyuria), nephrolithiasis (hematuria), or concomitant ATN (RTECs, RTEC casts, granular casts).

With certain processes, crystals may be indicative of the underlying cause of AKI. For example, calcium oxalate crystals may suggest enteric hyperoxaluria or ethylene glycol intoxication, uric acid crystals may point to acute urate nephropathy, and various other crystals may indicate a drug-induced form of AKI (see Figs. 2.2, 2.3, and 2.4).

Urinary Indices

Spot urine chemistry testing (sodium, creatinine, and urea), along with plasma samples (sodium, creatinine, and BUN), has been used to evaluate renal tubular function in the setting of AKI, primarily to distinguish prerenal AKI from ATN. These measures allow the clinician to calculate fractional excretion of sodium (FE_{Na}) and fractional excretion of urea (FE_{Urea}); they are thought to be more accurate indicators than urine sodium concentration, which is less than 10 to 20 mEq/L with prerenal AKI and greater than 20 mEq/L with ATN.

The ratio of the clearance of sodium (Na) to that of creatinine (Cr) is calculated as a percentage:

$$FE_{Na} = (U_{Na}/P_{Na}) \times (P_{Cr}/U_{Cr}) \times 100$$

where U and P are the concentrations in urine and plasma, respectively. Likewise, the ratio of urea clearance to creatinine clearance is

$$FE_{Urea} = (U_{Urea}/P_{Urea}) \times (P_{Cr}/U_{Cr}) \times 100$$

The rationale for the use of these indices is that the ratio of urine to plasma creatinine concentrations (U_{Cr}/P_{Cr}) provides an index of the fraction of filtered water excreted. Assuming that all of the creatinine filtered at the glomerulus is excreted into the urine, any increment in the concentration of creatinine in urine over that in plasma must result from the removal of water.

In prerenal AKI, because of the increased stimulus for salt and water retention, U_{Cr}/P_{Cr} typically is considerably greater than it is in ATN; moreover, FE_{Na} is less than 1%, and urine sodium concentrations are characteristically low. In contrast, in AKI due to ATN, the nephrons excrete a large fraction of their filtered sodium and water, resulting in a lower U_{Cr}/P_{Cr}, higher urine sodium concentrations, and a higher FE_{Na}. An important clinical exception to this finding is that FE_{Na} can be high (>1% to 2%) with prerenal AKI in the setting of diuretic therapy. To counter this effect, calculation of FE_{Urea} has been used: An FE_{Urea} less than 35% favors a diagnosis of prerenal AKI and an FE_{Urea} greater than 50% favors ATN.

Interpretations of these tests, therefore, must be made in conjunction with other assessments of the patient, because clinically important exceptions to these generalizations exist. As an example, prerenal AKI can manifest with an elevated FE_{Na} or FE_{Urea} in the setting of glycosuria, metabolic alkalosis, bicarbonaturia, salt-wasting disorders, or CKD. Similarly, ATN with low FE_{Na} and FE_{Urea} occurs with pigmenturia, sepsis, radiocontrast injury, severe heart or liver failure, and nonoliguric ATN.

Renal Imaging

If either prerenal AKI or ATN is the likely cause of AKI, and if the clinical setting does not require the exclusion of another cause, then no further diagnostic evaluation is required. Further assessment may be necessary if the diagnosis is uncertain, especially if the clinical setting suggests other possibilities (e.g., obstruction, vascular accident); if clinical findings make the diagnosis of prerenal AKI or ATN unlikely; or if oliguria persists without a good reason. When indicated, diagnostic renal imaging is important in the evaluation of AKI. Retroperitoneal ultrasonography of the kidneys, ureters, and bladder is the first test used because it is readily available, noninvasive, free of radiation exposure, and fairly accurate.

Ultrasonography provides information about kidney size (large, normal, or small) and the parenchyma (normal or increased echogenicity), the status of the pelvis and urinary collecting system (normal or hydronephrotic), and the presence of structural abnormalities (e.g., stones, masses, enlarged lymph nodes). In the setting of AKI, this test can rapidly confirm or exclude the presence of hydronephrosis and a diagnosis of obstructive uropathy. Interrogation of the renal arteries by Doppler ultrasonography provides important information about renal blood flow and renal artery stenosis; however, this test is highly operator dependent.

表 7.3　尿液分析及尿沉渣显微镜检查

检查	肾前性	血管性	GN	ATN	AIN	肾后性
尿比重	高	正常/高	正常/高	等渗	等渗	等渗
试纸法检测血尿	阴性	阳性	阳性	±	±	阴性
试纸法检测尿蛋白	阴性	阳性	阳性	阴性	±	阴性
尿沉渣检查	阴性/透明管型	RBC管型/异形红细胞	RBC管型/异形红细胞	颗粒管型/RTEC	WBC管型/嗜酸性粒细胞	阴性/有时有WBC或RBC

AIN，急性间质性肾炎；ATN，急性肾小管坏死；GN，肾小球肾炎；RBC，红细胞；RTEC，肾小管上皮细胞；WBC，白细胞。

尿液分析和尿液显微镜检查

尿液分析是 AKI 诊断评估的关键内容，如表 7.3 所示。评估尿比重（SG）以及是否存在血液（或血红素）、蛋白或白细胞酯酶非常重要。

尿 SG 非常高常提示肾前性 AKI，而等渗尿（SG = 1.010）提示肾实质性 AKI（例如 ATN）。对离心后的尿沉渣进行全面的显微镜检查，并对尿液成分进行定量分析，能为疾病提供重要信息。无血尿或蛋白尿、细胞或管型数量也很少的清淡尿液有助于肾前性 AKI 的诊断。血管性 AKI 的尿液张力变化不定，有时伴血尿（正常形态或异形红细胞）和颗粒管型。肾小球肾炎表现为尿渗透压变化不定、尿试纸检测呈血液和蛋白阳性、存在红细胞和红细胞管型。而 ATN 则表现为等渗尿、尿试纸显示不同程度的蛋白和血红素（横纹肌溶解和溶血时血红素阳性）；尿沉渣检查可能显示肾小管上皮细胞（RTEC）、RTEC 管型和细或粗的色素颗粒管型（有时呈浑浊棕色）。

肾后性 AKI 患者的尿液通常是等渗且清亮的，除非伴随感染（脓尿）、肾结石（血尿）或并发 ATN（RTEC、RTEC 管型、颗粒管型）。

在某些情况下，结晶可能提示 AKI 的潜在原因。例如，草酸钙结晶可能提示肠源性高草酸尿或乙二醇中毒，尿酸结晶可能指向急性尿酸肾病，而其他各种结晶可能表明药物引起的 AKI（见图 2.2 至图 2.4）。

尿液指标

即刻尿液化学检测（钠、肌酐和尿素）结合血浆样本检测（血钠、肌酐和血尿素氮）可用于评估 AKI 的肾小管功能，主要是用于区分肾前性 AKI 和 ATN。这些测量值使临床医生能够计算钠排泄分数（FE_{Na}）和尿素排泄分数（FE_{Urea}），它们是比尿钠浓度（肾前性 AKI 时尿钠浓度小于 10～20 mmol/L，而在 ATN 时大于 20 mmol/L）更准确的指标。

钠（Na）清除率与肌酐（Cr）清除率的比值以百分比计算：

$$FE_{Na} = (U_{Na}/P_{Na}) \times (P_{Cr}/U_{Cr}) \times 100$$

U 和 P 分别表示尿液和血浆中的浓度。同样，尿素清除率与肌酐清除率的比值为：

$$FE_{Urea} = (U_{Urea}/P_{Urea}) \times (P_{Cr}/U_{Cr}) \times 100$$

使用这些指标的依据是尿液与血浆肌酐浓度比值（U_{Cr}/P_{Cr}）提供了一个滤过水排泄分数的指数。假设肾小球滤过的所有肌酐都被排泄到尿液中，则尿液中肌酐浓度相对于血浆中的任何增加都必定是由于去除水分所致。

在肾前性 AKI 中，由于对盐和水潴留的刺激增加，U_{Cr}/P_{Cr} 通常比 ATN 时大得多；此外，FE_{Na} 小于 1%，尿钠浓度通常较低。相反，在 ATN 引起的 AKI 中，肾单位排出了大量滤过的钠和水，导致 U_{Cr}/P_{Cr} 较低，尿钠浓度升高和 FE_{Na} 升高。一个重要的临床例外：在使用利尿剂的情况下，肾前性 AKI 的 FE_{Na} 可能会升高（>1%～2%）。为了抵消这种影响，常计算 FE_{Urea}，FE_{Urea} 小于 35% 倾向于肾前性 AKI，FE_{Urea} 大于 50% 则倾向于 ATN。

因此，这些检测结果的解读必须与患者其他评估的结果相结合，因为临床上存在重要的例外情况。例如，在糖尿、代谢性碱中毒、碳酸氢盐尿、盐消耗性疾病或 CKD 的情况下，肾前性 AKI 可能表现为升高的 FE_{Na} 或 FE_{Urea}。同样，ATN 在色素尿、感染中毒症、造影剂损伤、严重的心脏或肝衰竭以及非少尿型 ATN 情况下，可能出现低 FE_{Na} 和 FE_{Urea}。

肾脏影像学

如果肾前性 AKI 或 ATN 是 AKI 的可能原因，且临床不需要排除其他原因，那么不需要进一步的诊断评估。如果诊断不确定，尤其是临床上提示其他可能性（如梗阻、血管意外）；或者临床表现提示肾前性 AKI 或 ATN 的诊断不太可能；或者少尿持续存在且没有明确原因，则可能需要进一步的评估。在这些情况下，诊断性肾脏影像学检查在 AKI 的评估中非常重要。肾、输尿管和膀胱超声通常是首选的检查方法，因为它易于操作、无创、无辐射暴露且相当准确。

超声检查能够提供关于肾脏大小（增大、正常或缩小）和肾实质（正常或回声增强）、肾盂和集合系统的状况（正常或肾盂积水），以及结构异常（如结石、肿块、淋巴结肿大）的信息。在 AKI 的情况下，该检查可以迅速确认或排除肾积水的可能，并有助于梗阻性尿路疾病的诊断。通过多普勒超声检查肾动脉，可提供有关肾血流和肾动脉狭窄的重要信息；然而，这种检查高度依赖操作者的技术水平。

Computed tomography (CT) of the retroperitoneum provides important information about the cause of postrenal AKI (e.g., tumor, stones, retroperitoneal fibrosis) when ultrasound findings are negative or inconclusive. CT angiography can also accurately diagnose renal artery disease and renal infarction, but there is a risk of nephrotoxicity in those patients with underlying acute or chronic kidney disease. *Magnetic resonance (MR) imaging* does not add much to CT scanning except in the diagnosis of retroperitoneal fibrosis. Gadolinium MR angiography can safely provide important information about renal artery stenosis or thrombosis, but it should be used cautiously in patients with AKI or stage 4 or greater CKD. Nephrogenic systemic fibrosis can develop in these patients, especially with nonionic or linear gadolinium contrast agents and in the setting of inflammation.

Radionuclide tests are used to assess the presence or absence of renal blood flow, differences in flow to the two kidneys, and excretory (secretory) function. However, these studies have limited utility in AKI and have reduced accuracy in quantitating absolute rates of flow.

Kidney Biopsy

When prerenal AKI, ATN, and obstructive uropathy are unlikely, percutaneous kidney biopsy is sometimes required to determine the cause of AKI and to direct appropriate therapy. Reasonable criteria to support use of kidney biopsy include absence of an obvious cause of AKI such as hypotension or nephrotoxin exposure and prolonged oliguria, usually for more than 2 to 3 weeks. Other potential indications include evaluation for myeloma-related kidney disease in an elderly patient with unexplained AKI; extrarenal manifestations of systemic diseases such as systemic lupus erythematosus, rheumatoid arthritis, or vasculitis; and determination of whether AIN is present in patients receiving a potential culprit drug.

Kidney tissue should be thoroughly examined with the use of light microscopy, immunofluorescence staining, and electron microscopy to facilitate an accurate diagnosis. This ensures a diagnosis of the cause of AKI in most patients. However, kidney biopsy should be employed judiciously to avoid complications such as traumatic renal arteriovenous malformation, severe bleeding requiring transfusion or embolization, other organ injury (liver, spleen, bowel), and nephrectomy for intractable bleeding.

Future Tests for AKI

The limitations of currently available tests to estimate GFR and kidney injury have led to proteomics-based studies to identify novel biomarkers of AKI. The hope is that novel biomarkers will improve the diagnosis and prognosis of AKI. For example, early AKI diagnosis would permit implementation of appropriate preventive strategies and treatment regimens to abrogate permanent loss of kidney function. In patients who develop AKI, biomarker concentrations demonstrate changes earlier than serum creatinine concentrations and appear to distinguish between prerenal AKI, ATN, and other glomerular disorders, which may allow directed interventions and avoidance of potentially harmful therapies. One such example is aggressive intravenous fluid therapy in patients with ATN, which risks volume overload and other end-organ consequences. Finally, biomarkers may allow clinicians to better predict outcomes such as worsening kidney function, RRT requirement, and mortality in patients with hospital-acquired AKI.

CLINICAL PRESENTATION, DIFFERENTIAL DIAGNOSIS, AND MANAGEMENT OF AKI

Prerenal AKI

Prerenal AKI is primarily the result of inadequate blood flow to the kidneys. Renal blood flow approximates more than 1 L/minute, which is necessary to maintain GFR, preserve oxygen delivery, and sustain ion transport and other energy-requiring processes. Therefore, normal kidney function depends on adequate perfusion; a significant reduction in renal perfusion diminishes filtration pressure and lowers GFR.

Volume Depletion

Both "true" and "effective" hypovolemia activate several neurohormonal vasoconstrictor systems as mechanisms to protect circulatory stability. The substances released include catecholamines from the sympathetic nervous system, endothelin from the vasculature, angiotensin II from the renin-angiotensin system (RAS), and vasopressin. They raise BP through arterial and venous constriction but also can constrict afferent arterioles and reduce GFR, especially when systemic BP is inadequate to maintain renal perfusion pressure.

Structural lesions in the renal arterial and arteriolar tree can also reduce perfusion and promote prerenal AKI. Kidney adaptive responses are stimulated to counterbalance diminished renal perfusion in these circumstances. These adaptive processes include the myogenic reflex, which is activated by low distending pressures sensed in the renal baroreceptors and causes afferent arteriolar vasodilatation. Prostaglandins (e.g., PGE_2, PGI_2), nitric oxide, and products from the kallikrein-kinin system modify the effects of these vasoconstrictors on the afferent arteriole. Importantly, disturbance of the balance between afferent vasodilatation and efferent vasoconstriction can disrupt intrarenal hemodynamics and precipitate AKI.

Medications

The balance of vasoconstricting and vasodilating processes may be altered by medications such as nonsteroidal anti-inflammatory drugs (NSAIDs) and selective cyclooxygenase 2 (COX2) inhibitors. These drugs act to cause prerenal AKI through inhibition of vasodilatory prostaglandins in patients who require prostaglandin effects to maintain renal perfusion. Despite its vasoconstrictor properties, angiotensin II acutely preserves glomerular filtration pressure and GFR in states of reduced renal perfusion by constricting the efferent arteriole more than the afferent arteriole. This salutary effect in part explains the GFR reduction that occurs when a patient who is dependent on angiotensin II to constrict the efferent arteriole is treated with an ACE inhibitor or an angiotensin II receptor blocker (ARB).

Cardiorenal Syndrome

The cardiorenal syndrome (CRS) is an umbrella term that encompasses a number of coexistent cardiac or kidney derangements. Although there are five subtypes of CRS, hospital-acquired AKI due to CRS is most often of the type 1 variety. Reduced cardiac output, arterial underfilling, elevated atrial pressures, and venous congestion, independently or in combination, can impair the renal circulation and reduce GFR, thereby causing a form of prerenal AKI. These processes stimulate neurohumoral adaptations such as activation of the sympathetic nervous system and RAS and increases in vasopressin and endothelin-1, in an attempt to preserve perfusion to vital organs. However, these adaptations enhance salt and water retention and systemic vasoconstriction, which ultimately promote or exacerbate prerenal AKI by two mechanisms: (1) They increase cardiac afterload and further reduce cardiac output and renal perfusion, and (2) they increase central venous pressure, renal venous pressure, and/or intra-abdominal pressure, ultimately lowering GFR.

AKI in patients with heart failure is often caused by CRS type 1, but certainly these patients can also suffer true prerenal AKI from overzealous diuresis or from ischemic or nephrotoxic ATN. Prerenal AKI from true volume depletion is responsive to judicious administration of intravenous fluids and diuretic withdrawal, making it easy

当超声检查结果阴性或不确定时，经腹计算机断层成像（CT）可提供有关肾后性 AKI 原因（如肿瘤、结石、腹膜后纤维化）的重要信息。CT 血管造影也能准确诊断肾动脉疾病和肾梗死，但对于急性或慢性肾病患者，存在肾毒性风险。除了腹膜后纤维化的诊断之外，磁共振成像（MR）并未比 CT 扫描提供更多的信息。钆造影剂 MR 血管造影可以安全地提供关于肾动脉狭窄或血栓形成的重要信息，但在 AKI 或 4 期及以上的 CKD 患者中应谨慎使用。这些患者尤其在使用非离子或线性钆造影剂和存在炎症的情况下，可能会发生肾源性系统性纤维化。

放射性核素检查用于评估肾血流的存在或缺乏、两肾血流差异以及排泄（分泌）功能。然而，这些检查在 AKI 中的实用性有限，并且在量化绝对血流速率方面的准确性较低。

肾活检

如不考虑肾前性 AKI、ATN 和梗阻性肾病时，有时需要经皮肾活检以确定 AKI 的原因并指导适当的治疗。肾活检的适应证包括：AKI 无明显原因（如低血压或肾毒性药物暴露），以及长时间少尿（通常超过 2～3 周）。其他潜在的适应证包括：评估不明原因 AKI 的老年患者中与骨髓瘤相关的肾病；有系统性疾病（如系统性红斑狼疮、类风湿关节炎或血管炎）的肾外表现；以及确定接受潜在致病药物治疗的患者是否存在 AIN。

肾组织应通过光学显微镜、免疫荧光染色和电子显微镜进行全面检查，以便明确诊断。这确保了大多数 AKI 患者的病因得到确诊。然而，肾活检应谨慎应用，以避免并发症，如创伤性肾动静脉畸形、需输血或介入性栓塞治疗的严重出血、其他器官损伤（肝、脾、肠）以及因无法控制的出血导致肾切除。

未来可用于 AKI 的检查

目前用于评估 GFR 和肾损伤的检测方法存在诸多局限性，这推动了基于蛋白质组学的研究，以寻找识别 AKI 的新型生物标志物。人们期待这些新型生物标志物能够改进 AKI 的诊断和预后。例如，早期 AKI 的诊断将允许实施适当的预防策略和治疗方案，从而避免肾功能的永久性丧失。在发生 AKI 的患者中，生物标志物浓度的变化通常早于血清肌酐浓度的变化，并且似乎能够区分肾前性 AKI、ATN 和其他肾小球疾病。这可能允许针对性的干预并避免潜在有害的治疗，其中一个例子是对 ATN 患者进行激进的静脉补液治疗而带来容量过多和其他终末器官损伤的风险。最后，生物标志物可能帮助临床医生更好地预测医院获得性 AKI 患者的各种结局，包括肾功能恶化、需要肾替代治疗以及死亡等。

AKI 的临床表现、鉴别诊断及处理

肾前性 AKI

肾前性 AKI 主要是由于肾血流不足导致的。肾脏血流量大约每分钟 1 L 以上，这对于维持 GFR、保证氧供应、维持离子转运和其他需要能量的过程是必要的。因此，正常的肾功能依赖于充足的灌注；肾灌注显著减少会降低滤过压并导致 GFR 降低。

容量不足

"真正"和"有效"的低血容量都会激活多种神经激素缩血管系统，以维持循环稳定。释放的物质包括交感神经系统的儿茶酚胺、血管的内皮素、肾素-血管紧张素系统（RAS）的血管紧张素 II 以及血管加压素。它们通过收缩动脉和静脉来提高血压，但也会收缩入球小动脉并降低 GFR，尤其当全身血压不足以维持肾灌注压时。

肾动脉和小动脉树的结构性病变也会减少灌注并促进肾前性 AKI。在这些情况下，肾脏的适应性反应被激活，以抵消减少的肾灌注。这些适应性过程包括肾压力感受器感知低张压力而激活肌源性反射，引起入球小动脉扩张。前列腺素（如 PGE2、PGI2）、一氧化氮以及激肽释放酶-激肽系统的产物会调节这些缩血管物质对入球小动脉的影响。重要的是入球小动脉扩张和出球小动脉收缩之间平衡的紊乱会破坏肾内血流动力学而诱发 AKI。

药物

非甾体抗炎药（NSAID）和选择性环氧化酶 2（COX-2）抑制剂等药物可能会改变血管收缩和血管舒张的平衡。对于依赖前列腺素的扩血管作用而维持肾灌注的患者，这些药物可抑制前列腺素作用而导致肾前性 AKI。尽管血管紧张素 II 具有血管收缩特性，但在肾灌注减少的状态下，它通过收缩出球小动脉多于入球小动脉来迅速维持肾小球滤过压和 GFR。这种有益的作用部分解释了当依赖血管紧张素 II 收缩出球小动脉的患者接受了 ACE 抑制剂或 ARB 治疗时发生的 GFR 降低。

心肾综合征

心肾综合征（CRS）是一个涵盖多种共存的心脏或肾脏疾病的总称。尽管 CRS 有五种亚型，但 CRS 引起的医院获得性 AKI 通常属于 1 型。心脏输出减少、动脉充盈不足、心房压力升高和静脉淤血，这些因素单独或共同作用，可损害肾循环并降低 GFR，从而导致肾前性 AKI。这些过程刺激神经激素的适应性，如交感神经系统和肾素-血管紧张素系统（RAS）的激活，以及血管升压素和内皮素-1 的增加以试图保持对重要器官的灌注。然而，这些适应性反应也会增加体内水钠潴留以及全身血管收缩，并最终通过两种机制促进或加剧肾前性 AKI：①增加心脏后负荷，进一步减少心输出量和肾灌注；②增加中心静脉压、肾静脉压和（或）腹内压，最终降低 GFR。

心力衰竭患者的 AKI 通常由 1 型心肾综合征（CRS）引起，但这些患者也可能因过度利尿、缺血或因肾毒性药物引起 ATN。由于真正的容量减少引起的肾前性 AKI 对合理的静脉补液和利尿剂撤药有反应，因此易

to recognize. It is sometimes more difficult to distinguish CRS type 1 from ATN because the processes often coexist.

Identification of AKI in the setting of heart failure is clinically relevant because reduced GFR is generally associated with a worse prognosis. Therapy is directed at improving cardiac function, especially in patients with low cardiac output, and relieving pulmonary and renal congestion. Small to moderate increases in serum creatinine (0.5 mg/dL) that occur in the setting of effective therapy for venous congestion in acute heart failure are acceptable and typically lead to improved long-term outcomes at 30 days and beyond. Loop diuretics are part of the central treatment strategy for relieving venous congestion; however, these agents can directly stimulate maladaptive neurohormonal responses, transiently worsening kidney function after their introduction. Patients with congestive heart failure often have some degree of diuretic resistance. Strategies to overcome this resistance include combination therapy with thiazide diuretics and rarely device-driven ultrafiltration. With advanced AKI, RRT is required to treat uremia, metabolic complications, and volume overload. Therapies for end-stage cardiac failure include cardiac transplantation and placement of a left ventricular assist device for long-term destination therapy or as a bridge to transplantation.

Hepatorenal Syndrome

A strong physiologic interplay also occurs between liver disease and kidney impairment. Patients with advanced, decompensated cirrhosis or fulminant acute hepatic failure develop a unique form of prerenal AKI called hepatorenal syndrome (HRS). The International Ascites Club diagnostic criteria for HRS include (1) the presence of cirrhosis and ascites, (2) serum creatinine levels higher than 1.5 mg/dL, (3) no improvement in kidney function after at least 48 hours of diuretic withdrawal and volume expansion with albumin, (4) absence of shock, (5) no nephrotoxic drug exposure, and (6) absence of parenchymal kidney disease. There are two subtypes of HRS based on rapidity and severity of kidney impairment. Type 1 HRS is characterized by rapidly progressive renal failure, defined by doubling of the initial serum creatinine concentration (to >2.5 mg/dL in <2 weeks). Type 2 HRS is characterized by moderate kidney failure (serum creatinine increase from 1.5 to 2.5 mg/dL). The hallmark of HRS is profound renal vasoconstriction in the setting of systemic and splanchnic arterial vasodilatation.

There is no test that is specific for the diagnosis of HRS, and diagnosis requires exclusion of other causes of AKI. The main differential diagnoses of type 1 HRS are prerenal AKI and ATN, which have an acute onset with progressive deterioration of kidney function. Recognition of prerenal AKI is typically easier, because it responds to intravenous fluids (albumin and saline), whereas HRS type 1 and ATN are more difficult to differentiate. Distinguishing ATN from HRS is crucial, because therapies for these two forms of AKI are very different, as are their prognoses and outcomes. For HRS, midodrine and octreotide, vasopressin (or its analogue terlipressin outside of the United States), or norepinephrine is used, whereas ATN requires primarily supportive therapy with initiation of RRT if necessary. Liver (or combined liver-kidney) transplantation is the definitive therapy for HRS.

Intrinsic AKI

Intrinsic AKI reflects kidney injury that arises from a process that damages one of the compartments of the renal parenchyma. To simplify the approach, kidney disease is organized into anatomic sites of injury in the vasculature, glomerulus, tubules, and interstitium.

Vascular Disease

Intrinsic AKI may result from vascular disease in large or medium-sized arteries, small arteries, and arterioles within the renal parenchyma and veins draining the kidneys. Bilateral renal artery thrombosis superimposed on underlying high-grade stenoses, significant cardiac or aortic thromboembolism occluding the renal arteries, or dissection of the renal arteries may cause AKI. With acute presentations, the clinical features often include flank or abdominal pain, fever, hematuria, and oligo-anuria or anuria. Therapy with thrombolytics may reverse acute thrombosis and thromboembolism and restore renal blood flow with early diagnosis. Percutaneous angioplasty with stent placement can non-invasively correct significant underlying renal artery stenosis. Renal artery dissection often requires surgical repair, but at times stent placement may suffice. Vasculitis of large renal vessels (e.g., Takayasu's arteritis, giant cell arteritis) is an extremely rare cause of AKI.

Induction of AKI by renal atheroemboli occurs less commonly than before due to changes in techniques that now include more commonly inserting the catheter into the radial artery for cardiac procedures as opposed to the more traditional method of inserting the catheter into the femoral artery to approach the heart, and perhaps due to the use of softer wires during vascular procedures. Cholesterol crystal embolization is caused most often by invasive vascular procedures in patients with atherosclerotic disease that disrupt the fibrous cap on the ulcerated plaque. However, thrombolytic therapy and therapeutic anticoagulation can also precipitate embolization in patients who have a significant burden of renal artery or aortic plaque. When it occurs, atheromatous material may lodge in interlobar, arcuate, or interlobular arteries in the kidneys. In addition to AKI, clinical manifestations include abrupt onset of severe hypertension, livedo reticularis, digital or limb ischemia, abdominal pain from pancreatitis or bowel ischemia, gastrointestinal bleeding, muscle pain, central nervous system symptoms such as focal neurologic deficits, confusion, amaurosis fugax, and retinal ischemic symptoms. Peripheral eosinophilia, hypocomplementemia, elevated sedimentation rate, and eosinophiluria variably accompany the syndrome. Treatment is primarily preventive by avoiding the factors known to precipitate atheroembolization. BP control, treatment with statins, amputation of necrotic limbs, aggressive nutrition, avoidance of anticoagulation (to reduce the risk for further embolization), and RRT for severe AKI may improve the dismal prognosis associated with this syndrome. Steroids and iloprost are sometimes used, but their therapeutic role is uncertain.

AKI from vasculitis involving the medium and small vessels has been described with classical polyarteritis nodosa. It is either idiopathic or secondary to hepatitis B antigenemia and manifests with severe hypertension and AKI. Renal arteriography demonstrating beading in the arterial tree of the kidney (and other organs) is diagnostic. Scleroderma is a disorder characterized by arterial and arteriolar narrowing due to deposition of mucinous material. Scleroderma renal crisis manifests as AKI and severe hypertension, often malignant, in a patient with a disease flare. Urinalysis and urine microscopy may be bland or may show cellular activity. Fibrinoid necrosis with ischemic injury occurs in the kidney. ACE inhibitors effectively control BP and improve AKI.

Rarely, AKI may develop in the setting of renal vein thrombosis, a well-known complication of nephrotic syndrome. Imbalance of anticoagulant substances lost in the urine and procoagulant substances produced by the liver leads to a hypercoagulable state and renal vein thrombosis. AKI is thought to develop from raised intrarenal pressures and reduced kidney perfusion. Therapy includes acute thrombolysis and chronic anticoagulation as well as treatment of the underlying glomerular lesion (often membranous nephropathy) and reduction in proteinuria.

于识别。然而，有时更难区分 1 型 CRS 和 ATN，因为这两种过程常常共存。

在心力衰竭背景下识别 AKI 具有重要的临床意义，因为降低的 GFR 通常与较差的预后相关。治疗的重点是改善心功能，尤其是对于心输出量较低的患者，同时缓解肺部和肾脏充血。在急性心力衰竭治疗中，通过有效治疗静脉充血，出现小到中度血清肌酐升高（0.5 mg/dl）是可以接受的，通常会在 30 天及以后改善长期预后。袢利尿剂是缓解静脉充血的核心治疗策略之一，然而，这些药物可以直接刺激不良的神经激素反应，可能导致肾功能暂时恶化。充血性心力衰竭患者常常具有某种程度的利尿剂抵抗。克服这种抵抗的策略包括与噻嗪类利尿剂联合应用，极少数情况下使用设备驱动的超滤。对于进展期 AKI，需要肾脏替代来治疗尿毒症、代谢并发症和容量超负荷。终末期心脏衰竭的治疗包括心脏移植和放置左心室辅助装置（LVAD）用于长期治疗或作为移植的过渡。

肝肾综合征

肝病与肾损伤之间也存在强烈的生理相互作用。患有晚期失代偿性肝硬化或暴发性急性肝衰竭的患者会出现一种独特形式的肾前性 AKI，称为肝肾综合征（HRS）。国际腹水组织对 HRS 的诊断标准包括：①存在肝硬化和腹水，②血清肌酐水平高于 1.5 mg/dl，③停用利尿剂和白蛋白扩容治疗至少 48 h 后，肾功能无改善，④无休克，⑤无肾毒性药物暴露，⑥无实质性肾病。根据肾损伤的进展速度和严重程度，HRS 有两种亚型。1 型 HRS 的特点是快速进展的肾衰竭，定义为初始血清肌酐浓度升高 2 倍（2 周内＞ 2.5 mg/dl）。HRS 的特点是在全身及内脏动脉血管舒张情况下肾血管严重收缩。

目前没有针对 HRS 诊断的特异性检查，诊断需要排除 AKI 的其他病因。1 型 HRS 的主要鉴别诊断是肾前性 AKI 和 ATN，这两者都具有急性起病和肾功能进行性恶化的特点。识别肾前性 AKI 通常较为容易，因为它对静脉输液（白蛋白和生理盐水）有反应，而 1 型 HRS 和 ATN 则较难区分。区分 ATN 和 HRS 至关重要，因为这两种形式的 AKI 治疗方法截然不同、预后和结局也不同。对于 HRS，通常使用米多君和奥曲肽、血管加压素（或在美国以外的地区使用其类似物特利加压素）或去甲肾上腺素；而 ATN 主要需支持治疗，必要时开始肾替代治疗。肝移植（或肝肾联合移植）是 HRS 的根治性疗法。

肾实质性急性肾损伤

肾实质性 AKI 反映了肾实质内某个部位病变引起的肾损伤。为了简化分类，肾脏疾病按损伤的解剖部位分为血管、肾小球、肾小管和肾间质疾病。

血管疾病

肾实质性 AKI 可以由血管疾病引起，包括大或中型动脉，小动脉、肾实质内的细小动脉以及引流肾脏的静脉血管病变。双侧肾动脉重度狭窄基础上的动脉血栓形成，严重的心脏或主动脉的血栓栓塞阻塞了肾动脉，或肾动脉夹层均可导致 AKI。急性发作时，临床表现通常包括侧腹或全腹痛、发热、血尿以及少尿或无尿。早期诊断后，使用溶栓药物可能逆转急性血栓形成和血栓栓塞，恢复肾血流。经皮血管成形术结合支架植入可以无创地纠正严重的肾动脉狭窄。肾动脉夹层通常需要外科修复，但有时放置支架就足够了。肾脏大血管炎（如大动脉炎、巨细胞动脉炎）是极为罕见的 AKI 原因。

肾动脉粥样硬化栓塞引起的 AKI 发生率较以往减少，这主要归功于技术的改进。现在心脏手术中更常见的是将导管插入桡动脉，而不是传统的经股动脉插入导管进入心脏；此外，还可能因为血管操作中使用了更柔软的导丝。胆固醇结晶栓塞通常见于动脉粥样硬化患者接受侵入性血管手术后，这些手术会破坏溃疡斑块上的纤维帽。然而，溶栓治疗和抗凝治疗也可能在有大量肾动脉或主动脉斑块负荷的患者中促发栓塞。当这种情况发生时，粥样斑块内物质可能会滞留在肾脏的叶间动脉、弓形动脉或小叶动脉中。除了 AKI 外，临床表现还包括突发严重高血压、网状青斑、指端或肢体缺血、胰腺炎或肠缺血引起的腹痛、胃肠道出血、肌肉疼痛、中枢神经系统症状如局灶性神经功能缺损、意识混乱、一过性黑矇和视网膜缺血症状。此外，外周嗜酸性粒细胞增多、低补体血症、红细胞沉降率（血沉）加快和嗜酸性粒细胞尿可能伴随这种综合征。治疗主要是通过避免已知可诱发动脉栓塞的因素来进行预防。控制血压、他汀类药物治疗、坏死肢体的截肢、积极营养支持、避免抗凝（以降低进一步栓塞的风险）和对严重 AKI 的肾替代治疗，可能会改善与这种综合征相关的不良预后。类固醇和伊洛前列素有时被使用，但其治疗作用尚不确定。

涉及中小血管的血管炎引起的 AKI 可见于经典的结节性多动脉炎。它可能是特发性的，也可能继发于乙型肝炎抗原血症，表现为严重高血压和 AKI。肾动脉造影显示肾脏（及其他器官）动脉树的串珠样改变具有诊断意义。硬皮病是一种由于黏液物质沉积导致的动脉和小动脉狭窄的疾病。硬皮病肾危象见于急性发作的患者，表现为 AKI 和严重高血压，通常为恶性高血压。尿检分析和尿液显微镜检查可能无明显异常，也可能显示活动性尿沉渣。肾脏发生纤维素样坏死伴缺血性损伤。ACE 抑制剂能有效控制血压并改善 AKI。

极少数情况下，AKI 也可见于肾静脉血栓形成（肾病综合征的一种常见并发症）。尿液丢失的抗凝物质与肝脏产生的促凝物质的不平衡导致高凝状态和肾静脉血栓形成。AKI 是由于肾内压力升高和肾灌注减少引起的。治疗包括急性溶栓和长期抗凝治疗，以及治疗基础肾小球病变（通常是膜性肾病）和减少蛋白尿。

Glomerular Disease

A number of glomerular diseases can cause AKI, and the more common entities are reviewed here. Acute proliferative GN may be broadly classified as (1) immune complex disease, (2) pauci-immune disease, or (3) anti-GBM–related disease. They are all characterized by glomerular cell proliferation and necrosis, polymorphonuclear cell infiltration, and, with severe injury, epithelial crescent formation. Acute proliferative GN manifests with hypertension and edema formation and with laboratory results pertinent for hematuria and proteinuria, described as *nephritic sediment*. Examination of the urine sediment classically reveals dysmorphic RBCs and RBC casts (see Figs. 2.2 and 2.3). Therapy is directed at the underlying cause, with supportive measures and RRT as necessary.

TTP and HUS are two of the more common causes of thrombotic microangiopathy, which is marked by platelet deposition and endothelial injury with thrombosis of arterioles and glomerular capillaries. AKI results from severe glomerular damage with profound ischemia and necrosis. The thrombotic microangiopathies may manifest with nephritic sediment. Patients with HUS may have severe AKI, or it may be mild, as in patients with TTP. Microangiopathic hemolytic anemia and thrombocytopenia are key features. Therapy often includes modulation of the immune system with plasma exchange or eculizumab, in addition to supportive measures.

The dysproteinemias, which deposit monoclonal immunoglobulin light or heavy chains (or both) in the kidney, may also promote glomerular lesions. The type, metabolism, and packaging of the immunoglobulin determine which type of glomerular lesion develops: light or heavy chain deposition disease, amyloidosis, or one of the fibrillary GNs. The immunoglobulin deposition diseases often manifest with nephrotic proteinuria and AKI, rarely with hematuria.

Light chain deposition disease, heavy chain deposition disease, and light/heavy chain deposition disease cause nodular glomerular lesions. Amyloidosis is also associated with the formation of acellular glomerular nodules. The fibrillary GNs (fibrillary and immunotactoid) may be associated with mesangial expansion or glomerular nodules. More commonly, they appear as a mesangial proliferative, mesangiocapillary, or membranous lesion, sometimes with formation of epithelial crescents. These diseases can be distinguished by electron microscopy. Light and heavy chain diseases produce granular deposits, whereas amyloidosis appears as haphazard fibrils in the 8- to 12-nm size range. Fibrillary GN has fibrils in the 20- to 30-nm range, and immunotactoid GN shows fibrils in the 30- to 50-nm range with organized microtubular fibrils. In addition, positive immunohistochemistry staining for DNAJB9 is highly specific for fibrillary GN.

Tubular Disease

Acute tubular necrosis. ATN is the most common form of hospital-acquired intrinsic AKI, accounting for more than 80% of AKI episodes. It is classically divided into ischemic ATN, which makes up almost 50% of the cases, nephrotoxic ATN, and combinations of both. In many instances, ATN results from multiple insults acting together to injure the kidney. The end result of either ischemic or toxic insult is tubular cell injury and death.

Ischemic ATN. Ischemic ATN is, for the most part, an extension of severe and uncorrected prerenal AKI. Prolonged renal hypoperfusion causes tubular cell injury, which persists even after the underlying hemodynamic insult resolves and may be associated with ischemia-reperfusion injury. Intraoperative and postoperative hypotension impairs renal perfusion and occurs relatively frequently after cardiac and vascular surgical procedures. Ischemic, nephrotoxic, and multifactorial ATN are common on the medical wards and in the ICU. Risk for ischemic ATN is increased by the comorbidities these patients possess. Sepsis and septic shock, severe intravascular volume depletion, cirrhotic physiology, and cardiogenic shock are examples of situations that confer high risk for development of ischemic ATN. Employment of vasopressors to restore BP may further reduce renal perfusion and exacerbate ischemia. In some cases, ischemic ATN is so profound that cortical necrosis (ischemic atrophy of the renal cortex) develops.

Nephrotoxic ATN. Nephrotoxic ATN occurs when exogenous substances injure the tubules, primarily through direct toxic effects but also through perturbations in intrarenal hemodynamics or a combination of these factors. In the past, organic solvents and heavy metals (e.g., mercury, cadmium, lead) were a frequent cause of ATN. Since then, many potentially toxic medications have been synthesized and observed to cause tubular injury by multiple mechanisms.

Aminoglycosides cause proximal tubular injury. AKI rarely develops within the first week of therapy, and injury initially manifests with subtle changes in urine concentrating ability and increased RTECs and granular casts in the urine sediment. The antifungal agent amphotericin B induces AKI through two distinct mechanisms: destruction of cellular membranes through sterol interactions and vasoconstriction-induced tubular ischemia. ATN develops in a dose-dependent fashion and manifests with increasing serum creatinine levels and RTECs and granular casts in the urine. Liposomal and lipid complex formulations are less nephrotoxic but can precipitate AKI in high-risk patients.

Radiocontrast material is a common cause of AKI because it is so widely used with imaging procedures. AKI develops in patients with underlying risk factors such as CKD (estimated GFR <30 mL/min), especially diabetic nephropathy, "true" or "effective" intravascular volume depletion, advanced age, and exposure to other nephrotoxins. The incidence of AKI may be 25% and approaches 50% in patients with underlying risk factors. ATN occurs from both ischemic tubular injury (prolonged decrease in renal blood flow) and direct toxicity (osmotic cellular injury, oxidative stress, inflammation). Large radiocontrast volumes increase risk, whereas low-osmolar and iso-osmolar radiocontrast agents are less nephrotoxic than high-osmolar material.

The antiviral agents cidofovir and tenofovir, once they have entered the cell from the peritubular blood via the human organic anion transporter 1 on the basolateral membrane, cause AKI through disruption of mitochondrial and other cellular functions. Several chemotherapeutic agents, including the platinum-based drugs, ifosfamide, mithramycin, imatinib, pentostatin, and pemetrexed, cause ATN through direct toxic effects. As with other nephrotoxins, part of their ability to induce ATN resides in the renal handling by the kidneys (transport through tubular cells) as they are being excreted. In addition, zoledronate, the polymixins, high-dose vancomycin, foscarnet, and deferasirox also cause nephrotoxic ATN. Vancomycin may cause a unique form of AKI known as cast nephropathy. Also, the combination of vancomycin plus piperacillin-tazobactam increases risk for AKI. AKI prevention is best achieved by judicious prescription of these drugs to high-risk patients, appropriate dose adjustments, avoidance of superimposed volume depletion, and close monitoring with early markers of injury such as urine microscopy.

Pigment nephropathy. Pigment nephropathy represents the nephrotoxic renal tubular effects of endogenously produced substances. The most common examples are overproduction of heme moieties in serum that are eventually filtered at the glomerulus and excreted in urine. With severe rhabdomyolysis, the heme pigment released from muscle is myoglobin. AKI develops in the setting of myoglobinuria from the combination of direct myoglobin tubular toxicity (in an

肾小球疾病

多种肾小球疾病可导致 AKI，在此回顾常见的几种类型。急性增殖性肾小球肾炎可大致分为：①免疫复合物疾病，②少免疫疾病，和③抗肾小球基底膜（GBM）相关疾病。它们的共同特点是肾小球细胞增殖和坏死、多形核细胞浸润，以及在严重损伤时，形成上皮性新月体。急性增殖性肾小球肾炎表现为高血压和水肿，并伴有血尿和蛋白尿，被描述为肾炎性尿沉渣。尿沉渣检查通常显示变形红细胞和红细胞管型（见图 2.2 和 2.3）。治疗主要针对病因，同时采取支持性措施，必要时进行肾替代治疗。

TTP（血栓性血小板减少性紫癜）和 HUS（溶血性尿毒综合征）是血栓性微血管病（TMA）的两种常见原因。TMA 的特征是血小板沉积、内皮细胞损伤伴小动脉和肾小球毛细血管的血栓形成。严重的肾小球损伤导致明显的缺血和坏死引发 AKI。TMA 可能表现为肾炎性尿沉渣。HUS 患者可能会出现严重的 AKI，而 TTP 患者的 AKI 可能较轻。微血管病性溶血性贫血和血小板减少是 TTP 的主要特征。治疗通常包括使用血浆置换或依库珠单抗调节免疫系统，此外还需要支持性措施。

异常蛋白血症通过在肾脏中沉积单克隆免疫球蛋白轻链或重链（或两者兼有），也可能导致肾小球病变。免疫球蛋白的类型、代谢和组装决定了发生哪种类型的肾小球损伤：轻链或重链沉积病、淀粉样变性或某种纤维性肾小球病。免疫球蛋白沉积病通常表现为肾病性蛋白尿和 AKI，很少伴有血尿。

轻链沉积病、重链沉积病以及轻/重链沉积病均会导致结节性肾小球病变。淀粉样变性也与寡细胞性肾小球结节的形成有关。纤维性肾小球病（纤维性和免疫触须样肾小球病）可能与系膜扩张或肾小球结节有关。更常见的是，它们表现为系膜增生性、系膜毛细血管性或膜性病变，有时伴有上皮新月体的形成。这些疾病可以通过电子显微镜进行区分。轻链和重链病产生颗粒状沉积物，而淀粉样变性表现为 8～12 nm 范围内的无序纤维。纤维性肾小球病的纤维直径为 20～30 nm，而免疫触须样肾小球病的纤维直径为 30～50 nm，为有序的微管状纤维。此外，DNAJB9 的免疫组化染色阳性对纤维性肾小球病具有高度特异性。

肾小管疾病

急性肾小管坏死（ATN） 是医院获得性 AKI 最常见的类型，占 AKI 病例的 80% 以上。ATN 传统上分为缺血性 ATN（约占 50% 的病例）、肾毒性 ATN 和两者的组合。在多种情况下，ATN 是由多种损伤共同作用导致的。无论是缺血还是毒性损伤，最终结果都是肾小管细胞损伤和死亡。

缺血性 ATN 缺血性 ATN 大多是严重且未经纠正的肾前性 AKI 的延续。长时间的肾脏低灌注导致肾小管细胞损伤，即使在基础血流动力学损害解决后仍可能持续，并可能与缺血-再灌注损伤有关。术中和术后低血压会影响肾灌注，这在心脏和血管手术后相对常见。缺血性、肾毒性和多因素 ATN 在内科病房和重症监护病房中常见。这些患者的并发症增加了缺血性 ATN 的风险。例如，感染中毒症和感染中毒性休克、严重的血管内容量不足、肝硬化及心源性休克都是高风险因素。使用血管加压药物来恢复血压可能进一步减少肾脏灌注并加剧缺血。在某些情况下，缺血性 ATN 可能非常严重，以至于发生皮质坏死（肾皮质的缺血性萎缩）。

肾毒性 ATN 肾毒性 ATN 发生在外源性物质损伤肾小管时，主要通过直接毒性作用，但也可能源于扰乱肾内血流动力学或这些因素的组合。在过去，有机溶剂和重金属（如汞、镉、铅）是 ATN 的常见原因。从那之后，许多潜在的有毒药物被合成出来，并通过多种机制导致肾小管损伤。

氨基糖苷类药物会导致近端肾小管损伤。在治疗的第 1 周内很少发生 AKI，损伤最初表现为尿液浓缩能力的轻微变化，以及尿沉渣中肾小管上皮细胞（RTEC）和颗粒管型的增加。抗真菌药物两性霉素 B 通过两种不同机制引起 AKI：通过与固醇的相互作用破坏细胞膜，以及由血管收缩引起的肾小管缺血。ATN 以剂量依赖性方式发展，表现为血清肌酐水平升高以及尿液中 RTEC 和颗粒管型的增加。脂质体和脂质复合物制剂的肾毒性较低，但在高风险患者中仍可引发 AKI。

造影剂因其在影像学检查中广泛使用而成为 AKI 的常见原因。具有潜在风险因素的患者更容易发展成 AKI，如 CKD（eGFR < 30 ml/min），特别是糖尿病肾病、"真性"或"有效"血管内容量不足、高龄以及暴露于其他肾毒性物质时。AKI 的发生率可能达 25%，在具有这些风险因素的患者中接近 50%。ATN 由缺血性肾小管损伤（肾血流持续减少）和直接毒性（渗透性细胞损伤、氧化应激、炎症）共同引起。大量使用造影剂增加了风险，而低渗和等渗造影剂比高渗造影剂的肾毒性小。

抗病毒药物西多福韦和替诺福韦通过基底外侧膜上的人类有机阴离子转运体 1 从管周血液进入细胞，通过破坏线粒体和其他细胞功能引起 AKI。多种化疗药物，包括铂类药物、异环磷酰胺、光辉霉素、伊马替尼、喷司他丁和培美曲塞，通过直接毒性作用引起 ATN。与其他肾毒性物质一样，它们诱发 ATN 的部分能力在于肾脏排泄过程中的处理方式（通过肾小管细胞转运）。此外，唑来膦酸、多黏菌素、高剂量万古霉素、磷甲酸钠和地拉罗司及去铁胺也会导致肾毒性 ATN。万古霉素可能引起一种独特形式的 AKI，称为管型肾病。此外，万古霉素与哌拉西林-他唑巴坦联合使用会增加 AKI 的风险。预防 AKI 的最佳方法是对高风险患者谨慎使用这些药物，适当调整剂量，避免容量不足，并通过早期损伤标志物（如通过尿液显微镜检）进行密切监测。

色素肾病 色素肾病是由内源性产生的物质对肾小管的肾毒性作用所致。最常见的例子是血清中含血红素物质的过量产生，最终在肾小球过滤并随尿液排出。严重横纹肌溶解症时，肌肉释放的含血红素色素

acid urine), volume depletion, and obstructing myoglobin casts. Therapy includes intravenous fluids (the addition of bicarbonate is questionable), supportive care, and sometimes RRT. Most patients recover kidney function to near-baseline.

Massive intravascular hemolysis from various causes (e.g., immune-mediated, microangiopathic) is associated with hemoglobinuria, which induces tubular injury by promoting the formation of reactive oxygen species and by reducing renal perfusion through inhibition of nitric oxide synthesis. Therapy is directed at the primary cause, with intravenous fluids and supportive care. Most patients ultimately recover kidney function.

Crystalline nephropathy. AKI may result from crystal deposition in distal tubular lumens after massive rises in uric acid or therapy with certain medications. Risk factors for AKI due to crystal deposition are underlying kidney disease and intravascular volume depletion. Acute uric acid nephropathy from urate crystal deposition and tubular obstruction develops in patients with massive tumor lysis syndrome.

Drugs such as sulfadiazine promote intratubular deposition of sulfa crystals in acid urine, whereas acyclovir crystal deposition occurs after large, rapid intravenous doses of the drug, and atazanavir and indinavir crystal deposition occurs in the setting of volume contraction and urine pH higher than 5.5. Ciprofloxacin can cause AKI due to intratubular crystal deposition when administered in excessive doses, primarily in patients with unrecognized kidney disease and those with alkaline urine. In addition, methotrexate or large doses of intravenous vitamin C (producing oxalate) can cause AKI due to intratubular crystal deposition.

Weight loss therapies such as bariatric surgery with small bowel bypass and orlistat, through induction of malabsorption, cause enteric hyperoxaluria and calcium oxalate crystal deposition, an entity known as acute oxalate nephropathy. Sodium phosphate–containing bowel purgatives have also been associated with AKI due to acute phosphate nephropathy, an entity characterized by calcium phosphate intratubular crystal deposition.

Diagnosis of crystalline nephropathy is based on a history of exposure to a culprit agent or an underlying disease state associated with excessive crystal production (see Fig. 2.4).

Osmotic nephropathy. Osmotic nephropathy is a little known entity that can promote AKI through the induction of proximal tubular swelling, cell injury, and occlusion of intratubular lumens. The hyperosmolar and unmetabolizable nature of substances such as sucrose, dextran, mannitol, the sucrose excipient of intravenous immune globulin, and hydroxyethylstarch underlies the pathophysiology of this kidney lesion. Cells develop severe swelling with cytoplasmic vacuoles that form due to accumulation of the offending substance within intracellular lysosomes, disturbing cellular integrity and occluding tubular lumens. AKI results from this abnormal tubular process when patients with underlying kidney disease or other risk factors for kidney injury (e.g., intravascular volume depletion, older age) receive these hyperosmolar substances. AKI is dose related and may require RRT. Although most patients recover from AKI, CKD can result. Therapy is primarily supportive, along with avoidance of further exposure to these agents.

Interstitial Disease

Interstitial disease develops in the setting of infection with certain agents, systemic diseases, infiltrative malignancies, and exposure to some medications. Of these, drug-induced disease is by far the most common entity, especially in the hospitalized patient. The syndrome of AIN is characterized by AKI and a variety of clinical findings. The clinical presentation varies based on the offending agent and the host response. As an example, β-lactam antibiotics frequently cause the classic triad of fever, maculopapular skin rash, and eosinophilia. Arthralgias, myalgias, and flank pain may also occur. Aside from causing AKI, NSAIDs can rarely lead to allergic or extrarenal manifestations such as fever, rash, or eosinophilia.

Urinalysis may reveal dipstick-positive (trace to 1+) protein, blood, and leukocyte esterase. Urine microscopy may be bland (≈20%), but more often, the urine sediment demonstrates white blood cells (WBCs), RBCs, WBC casts, and granular casts. Wright or Hansel stain may reveal eosinophils in the urine, but neither of these tests is sensitive or specific for AIN. The urine cytokine TNF-alpha and IL9 appear to possess excellent sensitivity and specificity for diagnosing AIN.

The diagnosis is best confirmed by kidney biopsy. A cellular infiltrate consisting of lymphocytes, monocytes, eosinophils, and plasma cells is typically present; interstitial edema and fibrosis vary based on the time of drug exposure. Tubulitis, or invasion of lymphocytes into the tubular cells, is frequently part of AIN. Granuloma formation and interstitial inflammation occur with certain drugs such as anticonvulsants and sulfonamides, systemic diseases such as sarcoidosis, tubulointerstitial nephritis with uveitis, and idiopathic granulomatous interstitial nephritis. The glomeruli and vasculature are spared until very late in the disease. If kidney biopsy is not possible, gallium scanning or positron emission tomography of the kidneys may help with diagnosis, especially when the differential diagnosis is primarily between AIN and ATN.

Early diagnosis of AIN, coupled with rapid drug withdrawal before advanced tubulointerstitial fibrosis develops, maximizes successful renal recovery. Corticosteroid therapy is controversial but may reduce the duration of AKI and perhaps improve recovery of kidney function in patients with severe AKI if it is used early (within 2 weeks of diagnosis).

Before development of antibiotics and other drugs that have been associated with AIN, interstitial infection was the major cause of tubulointerstitial nephritis. Microbial agents such as staphylococci, streptococci, mycoplasma, diphtheroids, and legionella are well-described causes of AIN. Several viral agents including cytomegalovirus, Epstein-Barr virus, human immunodeficiency virus (HIV), Hantaan virus, parvovirus, and rubeola also are associated with AIN. In addition, infectious agents that cause rickettsial diseases, leptospirosis, and tuberculosis also invade the renal interstitium.

The renal interstitium is the target of a number of systemic illnesses. Sarcoidosis causes a lymphocyte-dominant AIN, which can be associated with noncaseating granulomas. AKI and urine sediment containing WBCs and WBC casts point to this disease, along with other systemic findings. Steroids reduce the severity of AIN, but CKD is a potential long-term complication. Systemic lupus erythematosus is more commonly associated with various forms of proliferative GN; AIN may coexist with glomerular disease, or, in rare instances, it may be present in isolation. The interstitial inflammatory lesion is caused by immune complex deposition in the tubulointerstitium. AIN usually responds to the cytotoxic therapy given for lupus nephritis. Sjögren's syndrome also causes a lymphocyte-dominant AIN; it appears to be another immune complex–mediated disease of the renal interstitium.

Patients with HIV infection may develop interstitial disease that appears immune related. Diffuse infiltrative lymphocytosis syndrome (DILS) is a Sjögren-like syndrome associated with multivisceral infiltration of CD8-positive T lymphocytes. DILS appears to be a host-determined response to HIV. Immune reconstitution inflammatory syndrome (IRIS) is another multivisceral disease characterized by an interstitial infiltrate. This disease occurs when combination antiretroviral therapy reconstitutes the immune system in the setting of a previous or occult opportunistic infection. An exuberant immune reaction results in T cell infiltration of several organs, including the kidneys, which develop AIN. Therapy involves treatment of the opportunistic

是肌红蛋白。AKI 由肌红蛋白直接肾小管毒性（在酸性尿液中）、容量不足和阻塞性肌红蛋白管型共同作用所致。治疗包括静脉输液（加入碳酸氢盐的效果尚有争议）、支持治疗，有时还需要肾替代治疗。大多数患者的肾功能可恢复至接近基线水平。

由各种原因（如免疫介导和微血管病变）引起的大量血管内溶血与血红蛋白尿有关，血红蛋白尿会促进活性氧的形成，并通过抑制一氧化氮的合成减少肾灌注，从而诱导肾小管损伤。治疗主要针对原发病因，同时辅以静脉输液和支持性治疗。大多数患者最终可以恢复肾功能。

晶体肾病 AKI 可能是由于尿酸急剧升高或某些药物治疗后，晶体在远端肾小管腔内沉积而导致。晶体沉积引起的 AKI 风险因素包括基础肾病和血管内容量减少。严重肿瘤溶解综合征时，由于尿酸晶体沉积和肾小管阻塞可引起急性尿酸性肾病。

药物如磺胺嘧啶在酸性尿液中促进磺胺晶体的肾小管内沉积，而阿昔洛韦晶体沉积发生在药物大剂量快速静脉注射后。阿扎那韦和茚地那韦晶体沉积则在容量减少和尿液 pH 值高于 5.5 的情况下发生。环丙沙星过量使用时，主要在无明确肾病患者和碱性尿液患者中，通过肾小管内晶体沉积引起 AKI。此外，甲氨蝶呤或大量静脉注射维生素 C（产生草酸盐）也可通过肾小管内晶体沉积导致 AKI。

减重疗法如小肠旁路的减肥手术和奥利司他通过诱导吸收不良，引起肠源性高草酸尿症和草酸钙晶体沉积，这种情况被称为急性草酸盐肾病。含磷酸钠的肠道泻药也与 AKI 有关，这是由于急性磷酸盐肾病引起的，其特征是肾小管内钙磷酸盐晶体沉积。

晶体性肾病的诊断基于病史，即暴露于致病药物，或与过量晶体生成相关的潜在疾病状态（见图 2.4）。

渗透性肾病 渗透性肾病是一类少见疾病，通过诱导近端小管上皮肿胀、细胞损伤和肾小管腔阻塞而促进 AKI。蔗糖、右旋糖酐、甘露醇、静脉注射免疫球蛋白的蔗糖赋形剂以及羟乙基淀粉等物质的高渗和不可代谢的特性，是这种肾损伤的病理生理基础。这些致病物质在细胞溶酶体内累积而形成细胞质空泡，导致细胞严重肿胀，破坏细胞完整性并阻塞肾小管腔。当具有潜在肾病或其他肾损伤风险因素（如血管内容量减少、年龄较大）的患者接受这些高渗物质时会导致 AKI。AKI 与药物剂量相关，可能需要肾替代治疗。虽然大多数患者可从 AKI 中恢复，但也可能导致 CKD。治疗主要是支持性治疗，并避免进一步接触这些物质。

间质性肾病

间质性肾病发生在某些病原体感染、全身性疾病、浸润性恶性肿瘤和暴露于某些药物的情况下。其中，药物导致的间质性肾炎最为常见，尤其在住院患者中。急性间质性肾炎（AIN）综合征的特征是 AKI 和各种临床表现。临床表现因致病因素和宿主反应而异。例如，β-内酰胺类抗生素经常引起经典的三联征：发热、斑丘疹和嗜酸性粒细胞增多，还可能出现关节痛、肌痛和腰痛。除了引起急性肾损伤外，非甾体抗炎药较少会导致过敏或肾外表现，如发热、皮疹或嗜酸性粒细胞增多。

尿液分析可能显示试纸上蛋白（微量至 1+）、血液和白细胞酯酶阳性。尿液显微镜检查可能无阳性发现（约 20%），但更常见的是尿沉渣中显示白细胞（WBC）、红细胞（RBC）、白细胞管型和颗粒管型。Wright 或 Hansel 染色可能显示尿液中的嗜酸性粒细胞，但这两项检测对 AIN 既不敏感也不特异。尿液细胞因子 TNF-α 和 IL-9 对诊断 AIN 的敏感性和特异性较好。

肾活检是确诊的最佳方法。通常可见淋巴细胞、单核细胞、嗜酸性粒细胞和浆细胞组成的细胞浸润，间质水肿和纤维化程度因药物暴露时间的不同而有所差异。肾小管炎，即淋巴细胞侵入肾小管细胞常见于 AIN。某些药物（如抗癫痫药和磺胺类药物）、系统性疾病如结节病、伴葡萄膜炎的肾小管间质性肾炎和特发性肉芽肿性间质性肾炎会引起肉芽肿形成和间质性炎症。直到疾病晚期，肾小球和血管才会受累。如无法进行肾活检，肾脏镓扫描或正电子发射断层成像有助于诊断，尤其当需要鉴别 AIN 和 ATN 时。

早期诊断 AIN，并在肾小管间质发生严重纤维化前及时停药，可最大限度地提高肾功能恢复的成功率。类固醇激素疗法尚存争议，但在严重 AKI 患者中，如果早期（诊断后 2 周内）使用，可能会缩短 AKI 的持续时间，并可能有利于肾功能恢复。

在抗生素和其他与 AIN 相关药物问世之前，间质感染是肾小管间质性肾炎的主要原因。葡萄球菌、链球菌、支原体、类白喉杆菌和军团菌等微生物是已知的 AIN 病因。多种病毒，包括巨细胞病毒、Epstein-Barr 病毒、人类免疫缺陷病毒（HIV）、汉坦病毒、细小病毒和风疹病毒也与 AIN 有关。此外，引起立克次体病、钩端螺旋体病和结核病的感染性病原体也会侵入肾间质。

肾间质是多种系统性疾病的靶标。结节病导致以淋巴细胞为主的 AIN，这可能与非干酪样肉芽肿有关。AKI 和含有白细胞和白细胞管型的尿沉渣提示这种疾病，同时还伴有其他系统性发现。类固醇可减轻 AIN 的严重程度，但 CKD 是一个潜在的长期并发症。系统性红斑狼疮更常与各种形式的增殖性肾小球肾炎相关；AIN 可能与肾小球疾病并存，或在罕见情况下单独存在；间质炎性病变是由免疫复合物在肾小管间质中沉积引起的。AIN 通常对用于治疗狼疮性肾炎的细胞毒性治疗有反应。干燥综合征也导致以淋巴细胞为主的 AIN，它似乎是另一种免疫复合物介导的肾间质疾病。

HIV 感染患者可能会出现与免疫相关的间质性疾病。弥漫性浸润性淋巴细胞增多综合征（DILS）是一种类似于干燥综合征的疾病，与 CD8 阳性 T 淋巴细胞多脏器浸润有关。DILS 似乎是宿主对 HIV 的反应。免疫重建炎症综合征（IRIS）是另一种以间质浸润为特征的多脏器疾病，在预先或隐匿性机会性感染的情况

infection. Occasionally, corticosteroids are required to suppress the inflammatory response.

Infiltration of the kidney by cancer is an uncommon cause of AKI. Autopsy studies confirm a high rate of asymptomatic renal infiltration. The malignancies most often associated with interstitial infiltration are the lymphomas and leukemias. Lymphomatous infiltration of the kidney parenchyma can occur in the form of discrete nodules or diffuse interstitial infiltration. Lymphoma may cause massive kidney enlargement (nephromegaly) and AKI. Leukemic infiltration also causes nephromegaly, AKI, and, rarely, renal potassium wasting from either tubulointerstitial damage or lysozyme production. Successful treatment of the underlying malignancy typically improves the infiltrative lesion; however, irradiation of the kidneys may provide additional benefit. Exclusion of obstructive uropathy from bulky retroperitoneal lymph node disease is also required.

Postrenal AKI

AKI can develop when obstruction to urine flow occurs along the genitourinary system. The process causing postrenal AKI is called *obstructive uropathy*, whereas the dilated urinary collecting system identified on imaging is termed *hydronephrosis*. Tubular defect with AKI that results from urinary obstruction is called *obstructive nephropathy*. AKI can develop only when obstruction is bilateral, involving both ureters or the bladder, or unilateral in a person with a single functioning kidney. Importantly, either complete or partial obstruction can cause AKI. In general, complete obstruction is associated with more severe AKI and hypertension, intravascular volume overload, hyperkalemia, metabolic acidosis, and hyponatremia.

A wide variety of disorders, originating anywhere from the renal calyces to the urethra, can cause AKI due to urinary obstruction. The most common causes of obstructive uropathy in the upper urinary tract are stones and retroperitoneal disease; in the lower tract, at the level of the bladder and below, prostatic hyperplasia and bladder dysfunction most often obstruct urinary flow. Obstructive uropathy should be considered in many patients with AKI, especially those with a history suggesting risk. A history of nephrolithiasis or certain cancers, along with flank pain, suggests upper tract disease; a history of prostate or bladder disease, together with symptoms of prostatism and urinary retention, points to lower tract obstruction. A directed physical examination of the flanks, suprapubic area, and prostate for flank tenderness, a palpable bladder, or prostatic enlargement is required. Large residual urine demonstrated on straight catheterization of the bladder bespeaks lower tract obstruction.

Ultrasonography of the kidneys and retroperitoneum is the most appropriate initial test to evaluate the patient with AKI and possible urinary tract obstruction. The sensitivity and specificity of renal ultrasonography for the detection of urinary obstruction are approximately 90%. Several processes blunt dilatation of the collecting system and the formation of hydronephrosis, including acute obstruction of less than 48 to 72 hours' duration, severe intravascular volume depletion superimposed on obstruction, and retroperitoneal disease involving the kidneys and ureters that encases the collecting system. If ultrasonographic findings are equivocal or negative but high suspicion for urinary obstruction persists, a CT scan may provide more information. One of the major benefits of CT imaging is the ability to detect stones, tumor, enlarged lymph nodes, and other processes causing obstruction despite the absence of hydronephrosis. As last resort, if obstruction as the cause of AKI is still considered likely, retrograde pyelography may provide a diagnosis of upper tract obstruction.

Therapy for AKI due to obstructive uropathy requires rapid diagnosis and intervention to relieve the obstructive process. Delayed interventions, especially in patients with complete obstruction, compromise recovery of kidney function. Upper urinary tract obstruction requires either retrograde ureteral stent placement or nephrostomy tube insertion when it is caused by severe retroperitoneal disease such as ureteral or bladder cancer. Relief of lower tract obstruction with a bladder catheter, a suprapubic tube (rarely), or a nephrostomy tube is the first step in treatment. Electrolyte and fluid management also are required to ensure patient safety in developing postobstructive diuresis. It is a phenomenon that occurs primarily in patients with bilateral, complete obstruction and is characterized by large urine volumes after relief of obstruction. Postobstructive diuresis is physiologic in that excess sodium and water are being excreted from the hypervolemic patient, but impaired tubular function (sodium and water) may lead to excessive diuresis and volume depletion. In this setting, judicious fluid repletion is required to avoid iatrogenic postobstructive diuresis as well as underresuscitation and hypotension.

COMPLICATIONS OF AKI

Considering the normal functions of the kidneys, it is not surprising that a number of metabolic complications develop in the setting of AKI. Hyperkalemia is a potentially life-threatening complication that often requires urgent intervention. Hyperkalemia disturbs the magnitude of the action potential in response to a depolarizing stimulus. The electrocardiogram (ECG) is a better guide to therapy than a single measurement of potassium concentration. The sequential ECG changes observed in hyperkalemia are peaked T waves, PR prolongation, QRS widening, and a sine wave pattern. The presence of any of these ECG changes mandates prompt therapy.

Metabolic acidosis is common in AKI. However, it is usually well tolerated and does not require therapy unless arterial pH declines to less than 7.1. Hyperkalemia and severe metabolic acidosis not responsive to medical therapy are indications for initiation of RRT. Hypocalcemia is a common but asymptomatic finding and usually does not require therapy. Significant hyperphosphatemia may occur but often can be managed with oral phosphate binders. Anemia typically does not require treatment unless it is severe, is symptomatic, or contributes to cardiac dysfunction. Uremic manifestations of AKI may be subtle findings, or they may be obvious and life-threatening, requiring urgent RRT.

Importantly, infectious complications are the main cause of death because of the immune compromise, edema with end-organ dysfunction and skin breakdown, and numerous indwelling catheters in these patients.

GENERAL MANAGEMENT OF AKI

Management of AKI begins with identification of the cause and pathogenesis of the inciting process. In addition, the complications associated with AKI need to be recognized and rapidly treated to avoid serious adverse events. Prerenal AKI requires optimization of renal perfusion by repletion of intravascular volume in those who are volume depleted and correction of heart failure, liver failure, and other "effective" causes of reduced intravascular volume. Intrinsic AKI requires directed therapy of the disturbed kidney compartment. Management of postrenal AKI mandates early intervention to relieve obstruction and preserve kidney function.

Most consequences of AKI are managed initially with conservative measures. These include interventions to correct hypovolemia or hypervolemia, improvement of hemodynamics, and correction of hyponatremia, hyperkalemia, metabolic acidosis, and hyperphosphatemia. Conversion of patients from oliguric to nonoliguric AKI makes management easier but does not improve outcomes in terms

下联合抗逆转录病毒治疗重建免疫系统时，就会发生这种疾病。强烈的免疫反应导致 T 细胞浸润多个器官，包括肾脏，进而发展成 AIN。治疗包括处理机会性感染，有时需要使用类固醇来抑制炎症反应。

癌症浸润肾脏是急性肾损伤的罕见原因。尸检研究证实了无症状肾浸润的高发生率。与间质浸润最常相关的恶性肿瘤是淋巴瘤和白血病。肾实质淋巴瘤浸润可以离散结节或弥漫性间质浸润的形式发生。淋巴瘤可能导致肾明显增大（肾肿大）和 AKI。白血病浸润也会导致肾肿大、AKI，并且少见情况下，由于肾小管间质损伤或溶菌酶产生引起肾性失钾。成功治疗潜在的恶性肿瘤通常会改善浸润性病变，肾脏放疗可能会提供额外的益处。有时还需要排除由巨大腹膜后淋巴结病引起的尿路梗阻。

肾后性 AKI

当泌尿生殖系统尿流受阻时，可能会发生 AKI。引起肾后性 AKI 的过程称为梗阻性尿路病，而影像学上发现的尿路集合系统扩张称为肾积水。由尿路梗阻引起的肾小管缺陷伴 AKI 称为梗阻性肾病。AKI 只有在双侧梗阻（涉及两侧输尿管或膀胱），或孤立肾患者发生单侧梗阻时才会出现。重要的是，无论是完全梗阻还是部分梗阻都可能引起 AKI。通常，完全梗阻与更严重的 AKI、高血压、血管内容量过多、高钾血症、代谢性酸中毒和低钠血症有关。

各种起源于肾盏到尿道的疾病都可能因尿路梗阻导致 AKI。上尿路梗阻性尿路病最常见的原因是结石和腹膜后疾病；在下尿路（膀胱及以下部位），前列腺增生和膀胱功能障碍是最常见的尿路梗阻原因。在许多 AKI 患者，尤其是有风险的患者，应考虑梗阻性尿路病。既往有肾结石或某些癌症病史，以及腰痛提示上尿路疾病；有前列腺或膀胱疾病病史，伴前列腺增生症状和尿潴留，提示下尿路梗阻。需要对腰部、耻骨上区和前列腺进行针对性体检，检查腰部压痛、可触及的膀胱或前列腺增大。膀胱插管导尿显示的大量残余尿提示下尿路梗阻。

肾脏和腹膜后超声检查是评估 AKI 及可能的尿路梗阻患者的最合适的初步检查。肾脏超声检查检测尿路梗阻的灵敏度和特异度约为 90%。有几种情况会减弱集合系统扩张和肾积水的形成，包括急性梗阻持续时间少于 48～72 h、梗阻基础上的严重血管内容量不足，以及涉及肾脏和输尿管的腹膜后疾病，这些情况会包裹住集合系统。如果超声结果不明确或呈阴性，但高度怀疑尿路梗阻，可进行 CT 扫描以提供更多信息。CT 的主要优势之一是即使没有肾积水，也能检测到结石、肿瘤、肿大的淋巴结和其他导致梗阻的病变。最后，如果仍认为梗阻是 AKI 的可能原因，逆行肾盂造影可能有助于上尿路梗阻的诊断。

治疗因梗阻性尿路病变引起的 AKI 需要快速诊断和干预，以缓解梗阻过程。延迟干预，尤其是在完全梗阻的患者中，会影响肾功能的恢复。上尿路梗阻需要通过逆行输尿管支架植入或经皮肾造瘘术来缓解，尤其是在梗阻由严重的腹膜后疾病（如输尿管或膀胱癌）引起时。下尿路梗阻的缓解首先需使用膀胱导尿管、耻骨上区置管（很少使用）或经皮肾造瘘。电解质和液体管理也很重要，以确保在解除梗阻后出现利尿现象时患者安全。解除梗阻后利尿现象主要发生在双侧完全梗阻的患者中，表现为解除梗阻后大量排尿。解除梗阻后利尿是生理性的，使高容量的患者排出过多的钠和水，但肾小管（钠和水的重吸收）功能受损可能导致过度利尿和容量不足。在这种情况下，需要谨慎补液以避免医源性解除梗阻后利尿现象，同时避免液体补充不足和低血压。

AKI 并发症

考虑到肾脏的正常功能，在 AKI 的情况下出现多种代谢并发症并不令人意外。高钾血症是一种潜在的危及生命的并发症，通常需要紧急干预。高钾血症会干扰去极化过程中的动作电位幅度。心电图（ECG）比单次钾浓度测量更能指导治疗。高钾血症的 ECG 变化依次为 T 波高尖、PR 间期延长、QRS 波增宽以及正弦波图形。任何这些心电图变化的存在都需要立即治疗。

代谢性酸中毒在 AKI 中很常见。然而，通常情况下它是可以耐受的，除非动脉血 pH 值降至 7.1 以下，否则不需要治疗（译者注：单纯肾功能损伤造成的酸中毒，通常 pH 值未降低至 7.1 时即需要接受碳酸氢钠治疗，当 pH 值小于 7.1 时需考虑 RRT）。高钾血症和对药物治疗无反应的严重代谢性酸中毒是启动 RRT 的指征。低钙血症常见但无症状，通常不需要治疗。显著的高磷血症可能会发生，但通常可以通过口服磷结合剂来管理。贫血通常不需要治疗，除非它很严重、有症状或导致心脏功能障碍。AKI 的尿毒症表现可能是轻度异常，也可能是明显且危及生命的，需要紧急肾替代治疗。

重要的是，感染性并发症是导致死亡的主要原因，源于这些患者免疫功能受损、水肿伴终末器官功能障碍和皮肤破损，以及体内留置的众多导管。

AKI 的一般管理

AKI 的管理首先要确定病因和发病机制。此外，还需识别和迅速治疗与 AKI 相关的并发症，以避免严重的不良事件。肾前性 AKI 需要通过补充血容量来改善肾灌注，对于血容量不足的患者，需纠正心力衰竭、肝衰竭和其他导致血管内血容量减少的"有效"原因。肾实质性 AKI 需要针对受损的肾脏部位进行定向治疗。肾后性 AKI 的管理需要早期干预以解除梗阻并保护肾功能。

继发于 AKI 的多数合并症最初可通过保守措施进行管理。这些措施包括纠正低血容量或高血容量、改善血流动力学以及纠正低钠血症、高钾血症、代谢性酸中毒

of morbidity or mortality. Manifestations of severe uremia and the other consequences of AKI, may necessitate RRT if conservative measures are unsuccessful or incompletely reverse the complication. Despite significant research efforts in recent years to determine if earlier versus later initiation of RRT improves outcomes in those with AKI, mixed results amongst the various studies has left clinicians with no clear consensus on this topic. Therefore, the timing of RRT initiation is often individualized to each clinical scenario based on a number of factors including the severity of metabolic disturbances, the likelihood of rapid renal recovery in subsequent hours and days, and the preferences of both the treating clinician and the patient and his or her surrogates.

Hospital-based RRT, which includes primarily acute hemodialysis and continuous renal replacement therapies (CRRTs), is required in certain patients with AKI. Continuous therapies, which can be employed only in the ICU, include continuous venovenous hemofiltration, hemodialysis, hemodiafiltration, slow low-efficiency dialysis, and extended daily dialysis. Emergent indications include severe hyperkalemia, uremic end-organ damage (e.g., pericarditis, seizure), refractory metabolic acidosis, and severe volume overload including pulmonary edema. Although the data do not support a cutoff BUN value to initiate RRT, it is sensible to initiate therapy before severe uremic complications develop. Intractable volume overload with anasarca complicated by skin breakdown is another potential indication. Acute hemodialysis is the modality most commonly employed to treat the consequences of AKI. However, critically ill patients who are hemodynamically unstable benefit most from continuous therapies. CRRT allows more precise control of volume, uremia, acid-base disturbances, and electrolyte disorders with less hemodynamic instability. CRRT also allows aggressive nutritional support. Peritoneal dialysis is rarely used for AKI but is a reasonable modality.

OUTCOME AND PROGNOSIS OF AKI

Despite the significant advances in supportive care and RRT technology, acute and long-term complications, including mortality, remain common. The mortality associated with AKI in the hospital setting depends on the patient's severity of illness and burden of organ dysfunction. As the number of failed organs increases from 0 to 4, the mortality rate associated with AKI increases from less than 40% to more than 90%. Also, in-hospital mortality increases with AKI that develops in the medical or surgical ICU. Long-term outcomes for patients with AKI include increased risk for death (compared with hospitalized patients without AKI). Furthermore, patients with CKD who have a prehospitalization eGFR lower than 45 mL/min/1.73 m^2 who develop RRT-requiring AKI have a much higher mortality rate than patients with CKD not complicated by AKI. On the whole, all forms of AKI, including the RRT-requiring forms, appear to be associated with an increased risk for development of new CKD, progression of CKD, ESRD, and death.

For a deeper discussion on this topic, please see Chapter 112, "Acute Kidney Injury," in *Goldman-Cecil Medicine*, 26th Edition .

SUGGESTED READINGS

Bellomo R, Ronco C, Kellum JA: Acute kidney injury, *Lancet* 380:756–766, 2012.

Coca SG, Yusuf B, Shlipak MG, et al.: Long-term risk of mortality and other adverse outcomes after acute kidney injury: a systematic review and meta-analysis, *Am J Kidney Dis* 53:961–973, 2009.

Cruz DN, Ricci Z, Ronco C: Clinical review: RIFLE and AKIN—time for reappraisal, *Crit Care* 13:211, 2009.

Haase M, Bellomo R, Devarajan P, et al.: Accuracy of neutrophil gelatinase-associated lipocalin (NGAL) in diagnosis and prognosis in acute kidney injury: a systematic review and meta-analysis, *Am J Kidney Dis* 54:1012, 2009.

Hertzberg D, Ryden L, Pickering JW, et al.: Acute kidney injury-an overview of diagnostic methods and clinical management, *Clin Kidney J* 10(3):323–331, 2017.

Hsu RK, Hsu CY: The role of acute kidney injury in chronic kidney disease, *Semin Nephrol* 36(4):283–292, 2016.

Hsu RK, McCulloch CE, Dudley RA, et al.: Temporal changes in incidence of dialysis-requiring AKI, *J Am Soc Nephrol* 24:37–42, 2013.

KDIGO: 2012 clinical practice guideline for acute kidney injury. Chapter 2.5: Diagnostic approach to alterations in kidney function and structure, *Kid Intl Suppl* 2:33–36, 2012.

Mehta RL, Kellum JA, Shah SV, et al.: Acute Kidney Injury Network: report of an initiative to improve outcomes in acute kidney injury, *Crit Care* 11:R31, 2007.

Moreau R, Lebrec D: Acute kidney injury: new concepts, *Nephron Physiol* 109:73–79, 2008.

Perazella MA: The urine sediment and a biomarker of kidney disease, *Am J Kidney Dis* 66(5):748–755, 2015.

Rosner NH, Perazella MA: Acute kidney injury in the cancer patient, *N Engl J Med* 376(18):1770–1781, 2017.

Uchino S, Kellum J, Bellomo R, et al.: Acute renal failure in critically ill patients, *JAMA* 294:813–818, 2005.

和高磷血症。将患者从少尿性 AKI 转变为非少尿性 AKI 可使管理更容易，但在发病率或死亡率方面并没有改善预后。对于严重尿毒症的表现和 AKI 的其他后果，如果保守治疗无效或未能完全逆转并发症，可能需要 RRT。尽管近年来在确定早期与晚期启动 RRT 是否能改善 AKI 患者的预后方面进行了大量研究，但各研究结果不一，使临床医生在此问题上没有明确的共识。因此，RRT 启动的时机通常根据每个临床场景的多个因素进行个性化处理，包括代谢紊乱的严重程度、未来数小时和数天内肾功能快速恢复的可能性，以及治疗医生和患者及其监护人的偏好。

某些 AKI 患者需要住院进行 RRT，主要包括急性血液透析和连续性肾替代治疗（CRRT）。连续性治疗只能在 ICU 进行，包括连续性静脉-静脉血液滤过、血液透析、血液透析滤过、慢速低效透析和日间长程透析。紧急指征包括严重高钾血症、尿毒症终末期器官损伤（如心包炎、癫痫发作）、难治性代谢性酸中毒，以及包括肺水肿在内的严重体液过多。尽管数据不支持以特定的尿素氮（BUN）值作为启动 RRT 的标准，但在严重尿毒症并发症出现之前开始 RRT 治疗是明智的。伴有皮肤破损的难治性全身水肿是另一种潜在的指征。急诊血液透析是治疗 AKI 一系列不良后果最常用的方法。然而，血流动力学不稳定的危重患者最获益于连续性治疗。CRRT 能够更精确地控制体液、改善尿毒症症状、酸碱失衡和电解质紊乱，同时减少血流动力学不稳定。CRRT 还允许进行积极的营养支持。腹膜透析很少用于 AKI 患者，但也是一种合理的治疗方法。

AKI 的结局和预后

尽管支持性治疗和 RRT 技术有了显著进步，但 AKI 的短期和长期并发症（包括死亡）仍然很常见。医院中与 AKI 相关的死亡率取决于患者的疾病严重程度和器官功能障碍的负担。随着器官衰竭数量从 0 增加到 4，AKI 相关的死亡率从低于 40% 增加到超过 90%。此外，在内科或外科重症监护病房中发生的 AKI 住院死亡率更高。AKI 患者的长期结局包括死亡风险增加（与未患 AKI 的住院患者相比）。此外，患有 CKD 且在住院前 eGFR 低于 45 ml/（min·1.73 m^2）的患者，如果发展为需要肾替代治疗的 AKI，其死亡率远高于无 AKI 的 CKD 患者。总体而言，所有形式的 AKI，包括需要 RRT 者，似乎都与新发 CKD、CKD 进展、终末期肾病（ESRD）和死亡风险增加有关。

有关此专题的深入讨论，请参阅 *Goldman-Cecil Medicine* 第 26 版第 112 章"急性肾损伤"。

推荐阅读

Bellomo R, Ronco C, Kellum JA: Acute kidney injury, *Lancet* 380:756–766, 2012.

Coca SG, Yusuf B, Shlipak MG, et al.: Long-term risk of mortality and other adverse outcomes after acute kidney injury: a systematic review and meta-analysis, *Am J Kidney Dis* 53:961–973, 2009.

Cruz DN, Ricci Z, Ronco C: Clinical review: RIFLE and AKIN—time for reappraisal, *Crit Care* 13:211, 2009.

Haase M, Bellomo R, Devarajan P, et al.: Accuracy of neutrophil gelatinase-associated lipocalin (NGAL) in diagnosis and prognosis in acute kidney injury: a systematic review and meta-analysis, *Am J Kidney Dis* 54:1012, 2009.

Hertzberg D, Ryden L, Pickering JW, et al.: Acute kidney injury-an overview of diagnostic methods and clinical management, *Clin Kidney J* 10(3):323–331, 2017.

Hsu RK, Hsu CY: The role of acute kidney injury in chronic kidney disease, *Semin Nephrol* 36(4):283–292, 2016.

Hsu RK, McCulloch CE, Dudley RA, et al.: Temporal changes in incidence of dialysis-requiring AKI, *J Am Soc Nephrol* 24:37–42, 2013.

KDIGO: 2012 clinical practice guideline for acute kidney injury. Chapter 2.5: Diagnostic approach to alterations in kidney function and structure, *Kid Intl Suppl* 2:33–36, 2012.

Mehta RL, Kellum JA, Shah SV, et al.: Acute Kidney Injury Network: report of an initiative to improve outcomes in acute kidney injury, *Crit Care* 11:R31, 2007.

Moreau R, Lebrec D: Acute kidney injury: new concepts, *Nephron Physiol* 109:73–79, 2008.

Perazella MA: The urine sediment and a biomarker of kidney disease, *Am J Kidney Dis* 66(5):748–755, 2015.

Rosner NH, Perazella MA: Acute kidney injury in the cancer patient, *N Engl J Med* 376(18):1770–1781, 2017.

Uchino S, Kellum J, Bellomo R, et al.: Acute renal failure in critically ill patients, *JAMA* 294:813–818, 2005.

8
Chronic Kidney Disease

T. Alp Ikizler, Anna Marie Burgner, Beatrice P. Concepcion

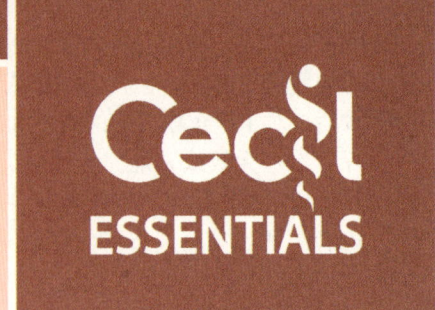

DEFINITION AND EPIDEMIOLOGY

Chronic kidney disease (CKD) is defined as persistent abnormalities of kidney structure or function. Markers of kidney damage *or* glomerular filtration rate (GFR) less than 60 mL/1.73 m² per minute must be present to meet the diagnostic criteria of CKD. The CKD spectrum includes patients with a normal GFR and kidney damage characterized by proteinuria or electrolyte abnormalities, to elevated serum creatinine, representing a decrease in GFR, to kidney failure or end-stage renal disease (ESRD). Additionally, these must be present and persistent for at least 3 months to differentiate CKD from acute kidney injury (AKI). According to the Kidney Disease Improving Global Outcomes (KDIGO) 2012 guidelines, CKD is classified based upon the underlying cause of kidney disease, GFR category, and albuminuria category. There are six GFR category levels ranging from normal or high (G1 ≥90 mL/min/1.73 m²) to kidney failure (G5 <15 mL/min/1.73 m²), and three albuminuria category levels based upon severity (Table 8.1). The rationale for these classification domains is because of differences in observed risk of health consequences and prognosis depending upon each domain's severity.

CKD is a worldwide public health problem. In the United States, the prevalence of CKD is estimated to affect 14.8% of the population, and most have mildly decreased GFR with mild to moderate increased albuminuria (Fig. 8.1). Yet, many people with CKD will progress to ESRD and require maintenance dialysis or kidney transplantation. The crude rate of new ESRD patients in the United States was relatively stable from 2000 to 2010 but started rising again in 2011; however, the United States Renal Data System (USRDS) reported in 2016 that the standardized incidence rate has appeared to plateau (348.2 per million population). Trends in overall prevalence of ESRD suggest a continuing increase in the numbers of patients requiring care, although in 2016 the increase was only 3%—the lowest rate recorded since the inception of the USRDS. Care of the ESRD patient is costly, accounting for $35.4 billion (7.2%) of the U.S. Medicare budget in 2016. In addition to concern about progression to ESRD, decreased GFR and proteinuria have each been increasingly recognized as independent risk factors for cardiovascular disease and death. Thus, diagnosis of CKD will identify those at risk not only for kidney function loss but also for decreased survival.

The most common causes of ESRD include diabetes mellitus (40%), hypertension (28%), glomerulonephritis (6% to 7%), and cystic or congenital conditions (2% to 3%). During the evaluation of CKD, every attempt should be made to arrive at the specific cause of kidney disease. Kidney biopsy is the most specific tool to reach a definitive diagnosis and guides treatment, informs prognosis, and determines suitability for kidney transplantation. However, the procedure itself has potential complications, and clinical information, including present, past, and family histories, serology, examination of the urine sediment, and kidney imaging may be sufficient to provide a conclusive diagnosis.

PATHOLOGY

To ensure adequate solute, water, and acid-base balance, the surviving nephrons must adjust by increasing their filtration and excretion rates. Patients with CKD, especially more advanced stages, are vulnerable to edema formation and severe volume overload, hyperkalemia, hyponatremia, and azotemia. During progressive kidney disease, sodium balance is maintained by increasing fractional excretion of sodium by the nephrons. Acid excretion is maintained until late stages of CKD, when the GFR falls to less than 30 mL per minute. Initially, increased tubular ammonia synthesis provides an adequate buffer for hydrogen in the distal nephron. Later, a significant decrease in distal bicarbonate regeneration results in hyperchloremic metabolic acidosis. Further nephron loss leads to retention of organic ions such as sulfates, which results in an anion gap metabolic acidosis. Metabolic acidosis appears to contribute to progression of CKD, and correction by base supplementation may be a potential treatment, although large multicenter randomized clinical trials are lacking.

Once GFR has decreased to below a critical level, CKD tends to progress to ESRD, regardless of the initial insult. Fig. 8.2 shows how risk factors may interact with pathophysiologic mechanisms to accelerate CKD progression. Detailed studies have elucidated interrelated mechanisms, including glomerular hemodynamic responses to nephron loss, proteinuria, and proinflammatory responses. Activation of the renin-angiotensin-aldosterone system (RAAS) pathway and increased transforming growth factor-β (TGF-β) also contribute to kidney fibrosis. Interventions that reduce intraglomerular pressure, such as protein restriction and the use of angiotensin-converting enzyme (ACE) inhibitors or angiotensin-receptor blockers (ARBs), help attenuate progression of kidney disease and further support the importance of glomerular hemodynamics and RAAS in progressive kidney disease.

CLINICAL PRESENTATION

General Features of Uremic Syndrome

Evidence of kidney disease commonly presents not with overt signs or symptoms, but first as abnormalities on laboratory or other diagnostic tests. Patients with CKD may not have symptoms until advanced stages where the GFR is less than 15 mL per minute. *Uremia* is a syndrome that affects every organ system. Uremic syndrome is likely the consequence of many factors, including retained molecules, deficiencies of important hormones, and metabolic abnormalities, rather than the effect of a single uremic toxin. Among these toxins, urea can cause symptoms of fatigue, nausea, vomiting, and headaches. Its breakdown product (cyanate) can result in carbamylation of lipoproteins and peptides, leading to multiple organ dysfunctions. Guanidines, byproducts of protein metabolism, are increased and can inhibit $α_1$-hydroxylase activity within the kidney leading to secondary hyperparathyroidism.

慢性肾脏病

樊晓红 译　秦岩　崔昭 审校　李雪梅 通审

定义和流行病学

慢性肾脏病（CKD）定义为肾脏结构或功能持续异常。CKD 的诊断标准需满足存在肾损伤标志物或肾小球滤过率（GFR）低于 60 ml/（min·1.73 m²）。CKD 囊括了从 GFR 正常但以蛋白尿或电解质异常为特征的肾损伤患者、血肌酐升高（GFR 下降）患者，以及肾衰竭或终末期肾病（ESRD）患者。而且，这些临床表现必须持续存在至少 3 个月，以区分 CKD 与急性肾损伤（AKI）。根据改善全球肾脏预后联盟（KDIGO）2012 指南，CKD 可根据肾脏病潜在病因、GFR 水平和白蛋白尿程度进行分类分级。按 GFR 水平分为 6 级，包括了从正常或 GFR 升高 [G1 ≥ 90 ml/（min·1.73 m²）] 到肾功能衰竭 [G5 < 15 ml/（min·1.73 m²）]。根据白蛋白尿严重程度分为 3 级（表 8.1）。之所以划分类别分级，源于 CKD 患者的健康结局和预后的风险差异依赖于每个分类的严重程度分级。

CKD 是一个全球性的公共卫生问题。美国 CKD 患病率约占总人口的 14.8%，大多数患者表现为 GFR 轻度下降，伴轻到中度的白蛋白尿（图 8.1）。但仍有许多 CKD 患者发展至 ESRD，需要维持性透析或肾移植治疗。美国新发 ESRD 的粗发病率在 2000 年至 2010 年间相对稳定，但自 2011 年再次开始上升；2016 年美国肾脏病数据系统（USRDS）报告显示，其标准化发病率已趋于稳定（每百万人口 348.2 例）。从 ESRD 总体患病率趋势看，需要照护的 ESRD 患者数量持续增加，尽管 2016 年增幅仅为 3%——USRDS 成立以来的最低增幅。ESRD 患者的医疗照护费用较高，2016 年占用美国医疗保险预算 35.4 亿美元（7.2%）。除了对进展至 ESRD 的关注外，GFR 下降和蛋白尿也分别被公认为心血管疾病和死亡的独立风险因素。因此，CKD 的诊断不仅识别出有肾功能丧失风险的人群，也识别出生存率降低的高危人群。

ESRD 最常见的病因包括糖尿病（40%）、高血压（28%）、肾小球肾炎（6%~7%）、囊性或先天性疾病（2%~3%）等。评估 CKD 过程中，应尽一切努力确定肾脏疾病的具体病因。肾活检是最具特异性的工具，能够协助明确诊断、指导治疗、提供预后信息，以及确定是否适合肾移植。但因肾活检本身存在潜在的并发症，需先评估临床信息，包括现病史、既往史和家族史、血清学检查、尿沉渣检查和肾脏影像学检查，可能足以提供明确的诊断。

病理学

为了确保足够的溶质、水分和酸碱平衡，存活的肾单位必须通过增加滤过和排泄率来进行调整。CKD 患者，尤其是晚期患者，很容易发生水肿和严重的容量超负荷、高钾血症、低钠血症和氮质血症。在肾脏疾病进展期，钠平衡是通过增加肾单位的钠的排泄分数来维持的。酸的排泄一直维持到 CKD 晚期，直到 GFR 下降至 30 ml/min 以下。最初，肾小管氨合成的增加为远端肾小管中的氢提供了充足的缓冲。后来，远端碳酸氢盐再生显著减少导致高氯性代谢性酸中毒。肾单位的进一步丧失导致硫酸盐等有机离子的潴留，从而导致阴离子间隙正常的代谢性酸中毒。代谢性酸中毒可能促进 CKD 的进展，通过补充碱剂纠正代谢性酸中毒可能是一种潜在的治疗方法，尽管目前还缺乏大型多中心随机临床试验的支持。

一旦 GFR 下降到临界水平以下，无论最初的损害原因为何，CKD 往往会进展为 ESRD。图 8.2 显示了危险因素如何与病理生理机制相互作用，加速 CKD 的进展。详细的研究阐明了相互关联的机制，包括肾单位丧失引起的肾小球血流动力学反应、蛋白尿和促炎症反应。肾素-血管紧张素-醛固酮系统（RAAS）通路的激活和转化生长因子-β（TGF-β）的增加也促进了肾脏纤维化。降低肾小球内压的干预措施，如限制蛋白质摄入和使用 ACE 抑制剂或 ARB，有助于减缓肾脏疾病的进展，并进一步支持了肾小球血流动力学和 RAAS 在进展性肾脏疾病中的重要性。

临床表现

尿毒症综合征的一般特征

肾脏疾病通常不表现为明显的体征或症状，而首先表现为实验室或其他诊断检查的异常。CKD 患者可能进展到 GFR 低于 15 ml/min 的晚期时才会出现症状。尿毒症是一种影响每个器官系统的综合征。尿毒症综合征可能是多种因素共同作用的结果，包括潴留的分子、重要激素的缺乏和代谢异常，而不是单一尿毒症毒素的影响。在这些毒素中，尿素可引起疲劳、恶心、呕吐和头痛等症状。其分解产物（氰酸盐）可导致脂蛋白和肽的氨甲酰化，从而导致多器官功能障碍。胍类是蛋白质代谢的副产物，其增加会抑制肾脏内 α_1-羟化酶活性，导致继发性甲状旁腺功能亢进。

TABLE 8.1 Categories of Glomerular Filtration Rate and Albuminuria in CKD

Category	GFR (mL/1.73 m²/min)	Terms
G1[a]	≥90	Normal or high
G2[a]	60-89	Mildly decreased
G3a	45-59	Mildly to moderately decreased
G3b	30-44	Moderately to severely decreased
G4	15-29	Severely decreased
G5	<15	Kidney failure

Category	AER (mg/24 hours)	ACR (mg/g)	(mg/mmol)	Terms
A1	<30	<30	<3	Normal to mildly increased
A2	30-300	30-300	3-30	Moderately increased
A3	>300	>300	>30	Severely increased

ACR, Albumin-to-creatine ratio; *AER*, albumin excretion rate; *GFR*, glomerular filtration rate.
[a]G1 and G2 alone, without other evidence of kidney damage, do not meet the criteria for CKD.

				Albuminuria categories			
				A1 Normal to mildly increased	A2 Moderately increased	A3 Severely increased	
				<30 mg/g <3 mg/mmol	30-300 mg/g 3-30 mg/mmol	>300 mg/g >30 mg/mmol	Total
GFR categories (ml/min/1.73 m²)	G1	Normal to high	≥90	54.9	4.2	0.5	59.6
	G2	Mildly decreased	60–89	30.2	2.9	0.3	33.5
	G3a	Mildly to moderately decreased	45–59	3.6	0.8	0.3	4.7
	G3b	Moderately to severely decreased	30–44	1.0	0.4	0.2	1.7
	G4	Severely decreased	15–29	0.13	0.10	0.15	0.37
	G5	Kidney failure	<15	0.01	0.04	0.09	0.13
			Total	89.9	8.5	1.6	100

Fig. 8.1 Distribution of CKD in the United States by GFR and albuminuria categories.

β_2-microglobulin accumulation in patients with ESRD has been associated with neuropathy, carpal tunnel syndrome, and amyloid infiltration of the joints. Finally, certain protein-bound solutes such as indoxyl sulfate and the conjugates of p-cresol, may confer cardiovascular toxicity by affecting leukocyte, endothelial, and vascular smooth muscle cell function. Major manifestations of uremia are summarized in Fig. 8.3.

Cardiovascular
In addition to hypertension, cardiovascular disorders are common in patients with CKD. More than 60% of patients with ESRD who start dialysis have echocardiographic manifestations of left ventricular hypertrophy, dilation, and systolic or diastolic dysfunction. Metabolic consequences of CKD, including accelerated atherogenesis, contribute to metastatic calcification in the myocardium, cardiac valves, and arteries. Arrhythmias, including those resulting in sudden death, may be caused by electrolyte abnormalities, cardiac structural changes or ischemic cardiovascular disease. Pericarditis can occur in patients with uremia before they start dialysis, as well as in ESRD patients receiving inadequate dialysis.

Gastrointestinal
Gastrointestinal disturbances are among the earliest and most common signs of the uremic syndrome. Patients describe a metallic taste and loss of appetite. Later, they experience nausea, vomiting, and weight loss, and those with severe uremia may also experience stomatitis and enteritis. There may be gastrointestinal bleeding caused by gastritis, peptic ulceration, and arterial venous malformations in the setting of platelet dysfunction.

Neurologic
Central nervous system (CNS) manifestations are frequent in advanced CKD and characterized predominantly by changes in cognitive function and sleep disturbances. Lethargy, irritability, asterixis, seizures, and frank encephalopathy with coma are late manifestations of uremia and are usually avoided by timely initiation of kidney replacement therapy. Peripheral neurologic manifestations appear as a progressive symmetrical sensory neuropathy in a glove-and-stocking distribution. Patients have decreased distal tendon reflexes and loss of vibratory perception. Peripheral motor impairment can result in restless legs, footdrop, or wristdrop. The majority of these neurologic manifestations reverse with maintenance dialysis or kidney transplantation.

Musculoskeletal
Alterations in calcium and phosphate homeostasis, with hyperparathyroidism and disturbance of vitamin D metabolism, are also common. Hypocalcemia and secondary hyperparathyroidism are the result of phosphate retention and the lack of α_1-hydroxylase activity in the failing

表 8.1 慢性肾脏病中肾小球滤过率和白蛋白尿的分类

分类	GFR [ml/(1.73 m² · min)]		定义
G1[a]	≥ 90		正常或增高
G2[a]	60~89		轻度下降
G3a	45~59		轻至中度下降
G3b	30~44		中至重度下降
G4	15~29		重度下降
G5	< 15		肾衰竭

分类	AER (mg/24 h)	ACR (mg/g)	(mg/mmol)	定义
A1	< 30	< 30	< 3	正常至轻度增加
A2	30~300	30~300	3~30	中度增加
A3	> 300	> 300	> 30	显著增加

ACR，白蛋白肌酐比值；AER，白蛋白排泄率；GFR，肾小球滤过率。
[a] 仅 G1 和 G2，无其他肾损害证据，不满足 CKD 标准。

			白蛋白尿分类			
			A1 正常至轻度增加 <30 mg/g, <3 mg/mmol	A2 中度增加 30~300 mg/g, 3~30 mg/mmol	A3 显著增加 >300 mg/g, >30 mg/mmol	总计
GFR分类 [ml/(min·1.73 m²)]	G1	正常至增高 ≥90	54.9	4.2	0.5	59.6
	G2	轻度下降 60~89	30.2	2.9	0.3	33.5
	G3a	轻至中度下降 45~59	3.6	0.8	0.3	4.7
	G3b	中至重度下降 30~44	1.0	0.4	0.2	1.7
	G4	重度下降 15~29	0.13	0.10	0.15	0.37
	G5	肾衰竭 <15	0.01	0.04	0.09	0.13
		总计	89.9	8.5	1.6	100

图 8.1 在美国根据 GFR 和白蛋白尿分类的 CKD 分布情况

ESRD 患者体内 β_2-微球蛋白的沉积与神经病变、腕管综合征和关节淀粉样蛋白浸润有关。最终，这些与蛋白质结合的溶质，如硫酸吲哚酚和对甲酚（p-cresol）的偶联物，可能通过影响白细胞、内皮细胞和血管平滑肌细胞的功能，从而引起心血管毒性。尿毒症的主要表现总结详见图 8.3。

心血管

除高血压外，心血管疾病在 CKD 患者中很常见。超过 60% 的 ESRD 患者开始透析时，超声心动图显示有左心室肥厚、扩张以及收缩或舒张功能障碍。包括加速动脉粥样硬化在内的 CKD 的代谢后果，参与心肌、心脏瓣膜和动脉的转移性钙化。电解质异常、心脏结构改变或缺血性心血管疾病可能导致心律失常，可致猝死。尿毒症患者在开始透析前以及透析不充分时，可发生心包炎。

胃肠道

胃肠功能紊乱是尿毒症综合征最早也是最常见的症状之一。患者会主诉口腔有金属味和食欲减退。随后，他们可能出现恶心、呕吐和体重减轻，严重尿毒症患者还可能出现口腔炎和肠炎。尿毒症患者存在血小板功能障碍，可能出现胃炎、消化性溃疡和动静脉畸形引起的胃肠出血。

神经系统

中枢神经系统（CNS）表现在晚期 CKD 患者中很常见，主要表现为认知功能的改变和睡眠障碍。倦怠、易激惹、扑翼样震颤、癫痫发作和伴有昏迷的脑病是尿毒症晚期表现，及时开始肾替代治疗通常可以避免。周围神经表现为进行性对称性感觉神经病变，呈手套和袜套状分布。患者的远端腱反射减弱，振动觉丧失。外周运动障碍可导致不安腿、足下垂或腕下垂。这些神经系统表现大多会随着维持性透析或肾移植而逆转。

肌肉骨骼

钙磷稳态的改变、甲状旁腺功能亢进和维生素 D 代谢紊乱也很常见。磷潴留和衰竭肾中 α1-羟化酶活性缺乏导致低钙血症和继发性甲状旁腺功能亢进症，从而引起活性维生素 D 缺乏。随着时间的推移，甲状

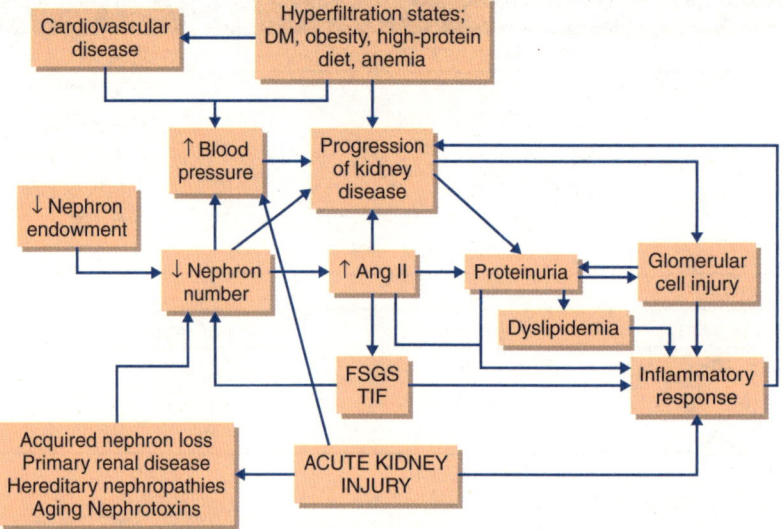

Fig. 8.2 A simplified depiction of risk factors interacting with pathophysiologic mechanisms to accelerate chronic kidney disease progression. *DM*, Diabetes mellitus; *FSGS*, focal segmental glomerulosclerosis; *TIF*, tubulointerstitial fibrosis. (Adapted from Taal MW, Brenner BM: Predicting initiation and progression of chronic kidney disease: Developing renal risk scores. Kidney Int 70:1694-1705, 2006.)

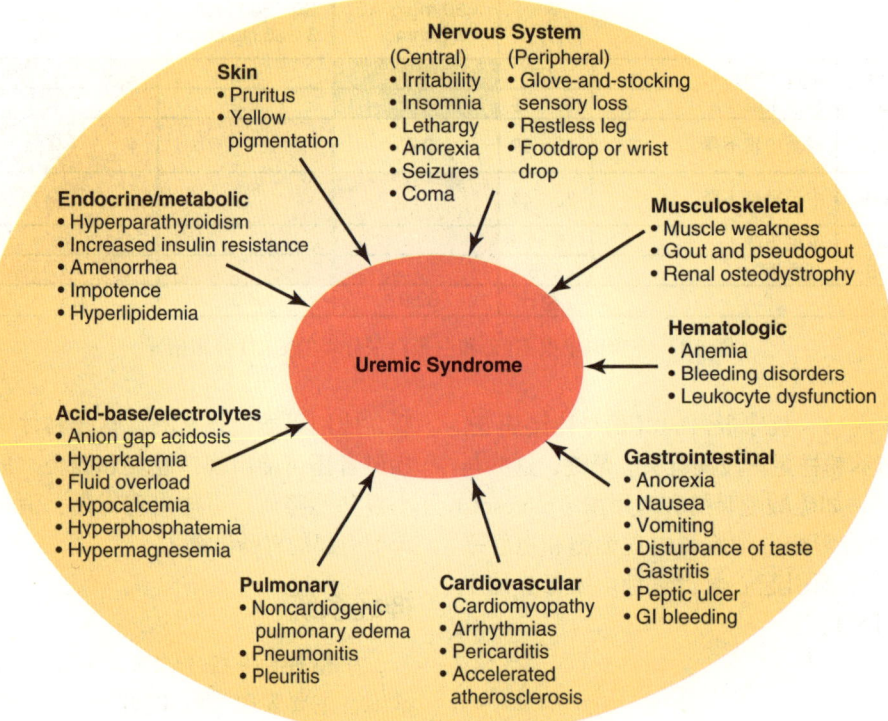

Fig. 8.3 Diagrammatic summary of the major manifestations of the uremic syndrome. *GI*, Gastrointestinal.

kidney, with consequent deficiency of the most active form of vitamin D. Over time, maladaptive parathyroid hypertrophy (i.e., tertiary hyperparathyroidism) leads to bone disease and tissue calcification.

Hematologic and Immunologic

Erythropoietin (EPO), a hormone produced by the kidney that regulates erythrocyte production, becomes progressively deficient as CKD progresses. EPO and iron deficiency are common causes of anemia in CKD. Administration of synthetic EPO results in correction of anemia, improved quality of life and anemia-related symptoms, and decreased dependence on blood transfusions. Caution must be exercised because higher doses of EPO resulting in elevations of the serum hemoglobin to more than 13 g/dL may be associated with a higher risk for adverse cardiovascular events. Bleeding disorders, primarily from defects in

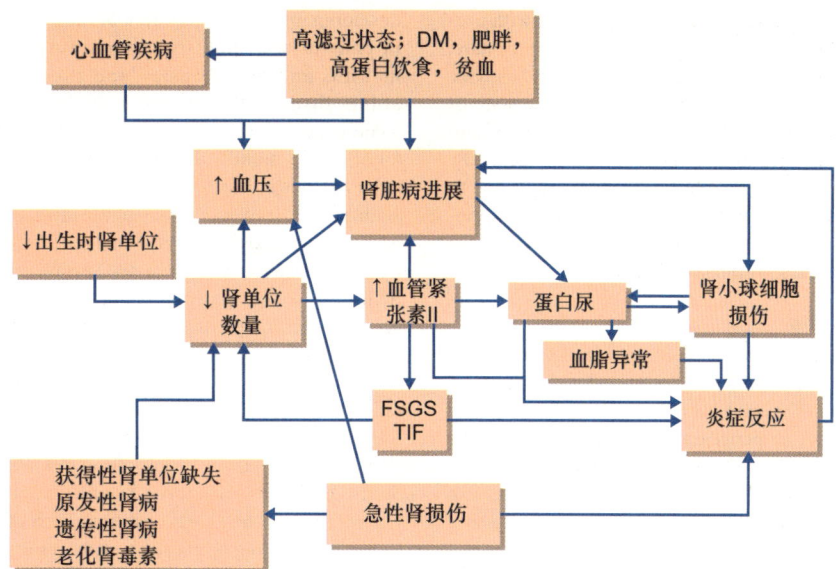

图8.2 简述危险因素与病理生理机制相互作用加速慢性肾脏病进展。DM，糖尿病；FSGS，局灶节段性肾小球硬化；TIF，肾小管间质纤维化（引自 Taal MW, Brenner BM: Predicting initiation and progression of chronic kidney disease: Developing renal risk scores. Kidney Int 70: 1694-1705, 2006.）

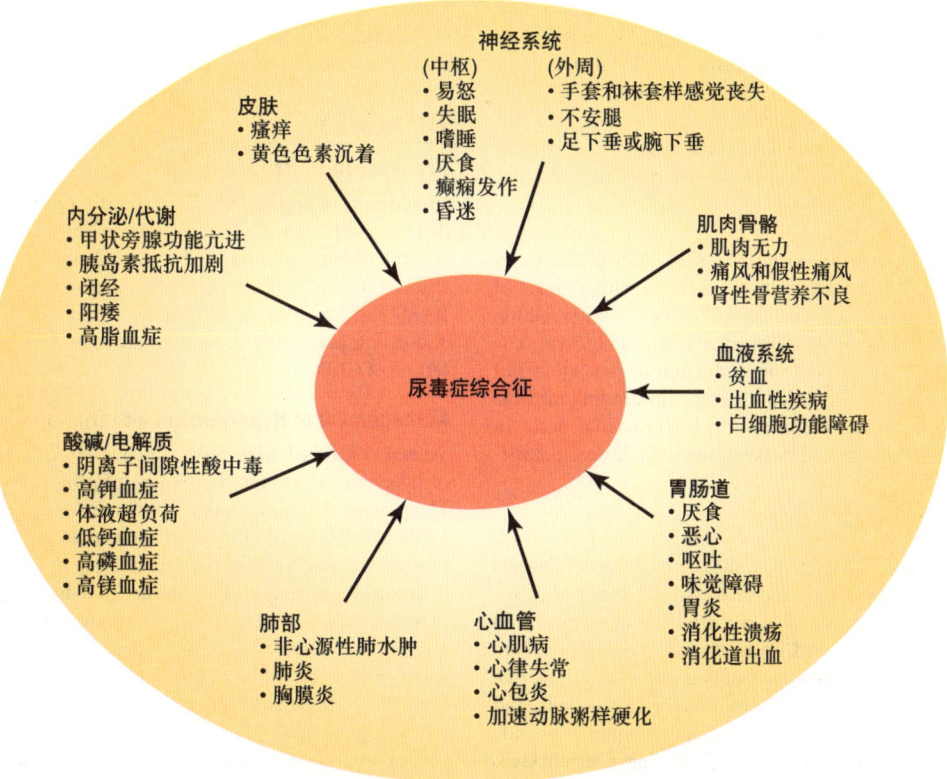

图8.3 尿毒症综合征主要表现图示

旁腺持续增生（如三发性甲状旁腺功能亢进）会导致骨病和组织钙化。

血液和免疫系统

促红细胞生成素（EPO）是一种由肾脏产生的激素，可调节红细胞的生成。随着 CKD 的进展，EPO 生成逐渐减少。EPO 减少和缺铁是导致 CKD 患者贫血的常见原因。使用合成的 EPO 可以纠正贫血，改善生活质量和贫血相关症状，减少对输血的依赖。但应注意的是，较高剂量的 EPO 导致血红蛋白升高超过 13 g/dl，可能会增加心血管不良事件的风险。尿毒症患者中常见出血性疾病，主要是由于血小板黏附和聚集功能缺陷

platelet adherence and aggregation, are common in patients with uremia. Uremic bleeding can be generally controlled with cryoprecipitate, desmopressin, conjugated estrogens, treatment of anemia, and dialysis.

Defects occur in both the humoral and cellular immune systems in patients with CKD. Although the leukocyte count is normal and appropriately responsive in advanced CKD, patients are generally immunosuppressed and susceptible to infections. This may be due to functional abnormalities of polymorphonuclear leukocytes, lymphocytes, and other cellular host defenses. Additionally, patients with CKD may have a variable immune response to vaccination.

Endocrine and Metabolic

Thyroid function testing may be less reliable in uremia. Common laboratory findings include an increased triiodothyronine resin uptake, a low triiodothyronine level resulting from the impaired conversion of thyroxine to triiodothyronine peripherally, and normal thyroxine levels. Thyroid-stimulating hormone levels are usually normal.

A deranged pituitary-gonadal axis can result in sexual dysfunction exhibited by impotence, decreased libido, amenorrhea, sterility, and uterine bleeding. Patients have decreased plasma levels of testosterone, estrogen, and progesterone, with normal or increased levels of follicle-stimulating hormone, luteinizing hormones, and prolactin. Pregnancy is uncommon in female patients who have a GFR of less than 30 mL per minute.

Lipid abnormalities are also common in CKD. They are most consistent with type IV hyperlipoproteinemia, with a marked increase in plasma triglycerides and less of an increase in total cholesterol. The activity of lipoprotein lipase is decreased in uremia, with a reduction in the conversion of very-low-density lipoprotein to low-density lipoprotein and thus hypertriglyceridemia. The treatment of choice is the hydroxymethylglutaryl–coenzyme A reductase (HMG-CoA) inhibitor class of drugs, especially in CKD patients not yet on maintenance dialysis, because of their pluripotent effects on inflammation and atherosclerosis.

Electrolytes

Hyperkalemia occurs in patients with CKD as a result of decreased renal clearance of potassium, intracellular to extracellular shifts of potassium in the setting of metabolic acidosis related to kidney failure, and the concomitant use of medications such as RAAS blockers. The primary method of treatment is dietary reduction of potassium but may also include use of loop diuretics or potassium-binding medications. Hypokalemia is much less common in CKD but may occur in the setting of very poor nutritional intake or use of high-dose potassium-wasting diuretic medications.

Skin

Uremic hue, a yellowish skin color, is likely the result of retained liposoluble pigments, such as lipochromes and carotenoids. Uremic hue usually responds to dialysis, control of hyperparathyroidism, improved calcium and phosphate balance, and, occasionally, ultraviolet rays. Nail findings of uremia include the half-and-half nail, characterized by red, pink, or brownish discoloration of the distal nail bed, pale nails, and splinter hemorrhages. Other common signs and symptoms include pruritus, and ecchymoses due to disorders of bleeding. Calciphylaxis, or calcific uremic arteriolopathy, results in painful skin calcification and is often seen in patients with uncontrolled hyperparathyroidism. Use of warfarin is suggested to be a risk factor for this condition.

DIAGNOSIS

Comprehensive care of kidney disease includes screening, diagnosing, and treating CKD and complications of CKD to prevent CKD development and progression. Screening for CKD is recommended in patients with high-risk comorbid disease, including diabetes mellitus and hypertension and those with a family history of kidney disease. The diagnosis of chronic kidney disease requires demonstrating evidence of kidney damage that has been persistent for at least 3 months. Imaging abnormalities may be consistent with kidney damage, but more commonly this is shown by detection of albuminuria or by reductions in the clearance of toxins by the kidney. Albuminuria may be detected in a spot collection of urine and is best when reported as an albumin-to-creatinine ratio (ACR). In general, an ACR of 30 mg/g or greater confirmed on repeat sample and without evidence of urinary infection raises concern for a diagnosis of CKD and warrants additional investigation.

Measurement of clearance of toxins by the kidney is most often estimated as the glomerular filtration rate (eGFR). Initial assessment should be performed using a serum creatinine-based estimating equation. These include the Modification of Diet in Renal Disease (MDRD) Study Equation and the Chronic Kidney Disease Epidemiology Collaboration (CKD-EPI) equation. Each of these has limitations and cautions regarding application of its results, and a detailed overview can be found in the KDIGO 2012 Clinical Practice Guidelines. Another serum biomarker, cystatin C, may be considered and integrated into another estimating equation for patients who have an eGFR 45-59 mL/min/1.73 m^2 and who may not have albuminuria or kidney imaging abnormalities to confirm evidence of CKD.

Once a diagnosis of CKD is established, management goals include (1) prevention of progression of CKD, (2) identifying and treating symptoms and complications of CKD, and (3) preparing patients for renal replacement therapy (RRT) where appropriate.

TREATMENT

Prevention of Progression

In addition to treatment of the specific underlying cause of kidney disease, methods used to slow progression of CKD include optimal control of hypertension, diabetes, and other cardiovascular disease risk factors (i.e., tobacco cessation), use of medications that block the RAAS pathway, diet modifications, avoidance of nephrotoxins, and addressing potentially reversible causes of acute kidney injury in the setting of CKD.

Management of Hypertension and Diabetes

Several controlled trials have conclusively confirmed that treatment of hypertension attenuates the rate of progression of kidney disease. The present recommendation is to target blood pressure to lower than 130/80 mm Hg in patients with diabetes or kidney disease. However, the evidence supporting this recommendation in CKD is limited and there is debate suggesting a higher target may be acceptable. Medications that block the production or effect of angiotensin II prevent the progression of CKD above and beyond control of hypertension in patients with proteinuria. Dihydropyridine calcium-channel blockers have not been shown to be as beneficial as ACE inhibitors or ARBs in slowing CKD progression.

For patients with diabetes mellitus, adequate glycemic control has been shown to prevent progression of CKD. Recommended goal glycosylated hemoglobin (A_{1c}) measures are less than 7% irrespective of a concurrent diagnosis of CKD, although this level of glycemic control warrants caution due to hypoglycemic risk. ACE inhibitors and ARBs may be considered in patients with diabetes and proteinuria, but without hypertension, to slow CKD progression. More recently, use of sodium-glucose cotransporter-2 (SGLT2) inhibitors have shown beneficial effects on kidney outcomes mainly in patients

所致。尿毒症出血通常可以通过冷沉淀、去氨加压素、结合雌激素、治疗贫血和透析来控制。

CKD 患者的体液免疫和细胞免疫系统都存在缺陷。虽然晚期 CKD 患者的白细胞计数正常且对刺激有恰当反应，但患者通常会存在免疫抑制，容易感染。这可能是由于多核白细胞、淋巴细胞和其他细胞的宿主防御功能异常所致。此外，CKD 患者对疫苗接种的免疫反应可能存在差异。

内分泌和代谢紊乱

尿毒症时甲状腺功能检测可能不太可靠。常见的实验室检查结果包括三碘甲状腺原氨酸摄取率增加、外周甲状腺素向三碘甲状腺原氨酸的转化受阻导致三碘甲状腺原氨酸水平较低，以及正常的甲状腺素水平。促甲状腺激素水平通常正常。

垂体－性腺轴紊乱可导致性功能障碍，表现为阳痿、性欲减退、闭经、不孕和子宫出血。患者血浆睾酮、雌激素和孕酮水平降低，促卵泡激素、黄体生成素和催乳素水平正常或升高。在 GFR 低于 30 ml/min 的女性患者中，妊娠的可能性较小。

血脂异常在 CKD 中也很常见，符合Ⅳ型高脂蛋白血症，表现为血浆甘油三酯显著升高，总胆固醇轻度升高。尿毒症时，脂蛋白脂肪酶活性降低，导致极低密度脂蛋白向低密度脂蛋白的转化减少，从而导致高甘油三酯血症。首选的治疗药物是羟甲基戊二酰辅酶 A 还原酶（HMG-CoA）抑制剂类药物，尤其是对于尚未进行维持性透析的 CKD 患者，因为这些药物对炎症和动脉粥样硬化具有多方面的作用。

电解质

CKD 患者会出现高钾血症，主要原因是肾脏对钾的清除能力下降、肾功能衰竭引起的代谢性酸中毒导致钾从细胞内向细胞外转移，以及同时使用 RAAS 阻滞剂等药物。主要的治疗方法是通过饮食减少钾的摄入，也可使用袢利尿剂或钾结合药物。低钾血症在 CKD 中较为少见，但在营养摄入极差或使用大剂量排钾利尿药的情况下也可能发生。

皮肤

尿毒症皮肤色素沉着呈现黄褐色，可能是脂溶性色素如脂色素和类胡萝卜素潴留的结果。尿毒症皮肤色素沉着通常可通过透析、控制甲状旁腺功能亢进、改善钙磷平衡来改善，少数情况下可接受紫外线照射治疗。尿毒症的指甲表现包括半月形指甲，特征为甲床远端呈现红色、粉红色或褐色褪色，指甲苍白以及指甲碎裂出血。其他常见的症状和体征还包括瘙痒和因凝血障碍引起的瘀斑。钙化防御或钙化性尿毒症性小动脉病变会导致痛性皮肤钙化，常见于未控制的甲状旁腺功能亢进症的患者。使用华法林可能是导致这种情况的危险因素。

诊断

肾脏疾病的综合照护包括筛查、诊断和治疗 CKD 及其并发症，以及预防 CKD 的发展和进展。建议对有高危合并症（如糖尿病、高血压、肾脏病家族史）的患者进行 CKD 筛查。慢性肾脏病的诊断需要证实肾脏损伤已持续至少 3 个月。影像学异常可能佐证肾脏损伤，但更常见的是通过检测白蛋白尿或肾脏清除毒素能力下降来证明。白蛋白尿可通过随机尿液标本采集检测，最佳报告方式是白蛋白与肌酐比值（ACR）。一般来说，如果重复采样检测确认 ACR 在 30 mg/g 或以上，且没有泌尿系统感染的证据，则应考虑诊断为慢性肾脏病，并进行进一步检查。

肾脏清除毒素能力通常通过肾小球滤过率（eGFR）来估算。初步评估应使用基于血清肌酐的估算方程，包括肾脏病饮食改良试验（MDRD）方程和慢性肾病流行病学协作组（CKD-EPI）方程。这些方程的应用都有其局限性和注意事项，详细概述可参见《KDIGO 2012 临床实践指南》。对于 eGFR 为 45～59 ml/（min·1.73 m²）且没有白蛋白尿或肾脏影像学异常的患者，可考虑使用另一种血清生物标志物——胱抑素 C 以及将胱抑素 C 纳入 eGFR 估算方程，进一步确认 CKD 诊断。

一旦确诊为 CKD，管理目标包括以下几点：①预防 CKD 进展；②识别和治疗 CKD 的症状和并发症；③在适当的情况下，为患者做好接受肾替代治疗（RRT）的准备。

治疗

预防进展

除了针对导致肾脏疾病的具体病因进行治疗外，延缓 CKD 进展的方法还包括：优化控制高血压、糖尿病和其他心血管疾病风险因素（如戒烟），使用阻断 RAAS 通路的药物，调整饮食，避免使用肾毒性物质，以及解决 CKD 基础上发生急性肾损伤的潜在可逆性原因。

高血压和糖尿病的管理

多项对照研究已经证实，治疗高血压可减缓肾脏疾病的进展速度。目前建议糖尿病或肾病患者应将血压控制于 130/80 mmHg 以下。然而，在 CKD 患者中支持这一建议的证据有限，有学者建议可以接受更高的血压目标值。对于有蛋白尿的患者，阻断血管紧张素Ⅱ生成或作用的药物除了通过降血压延缓 CKD 的进展之外，还有不依赖降压的肾脏保护作用。二氢吡啶类钙通道阻滞剂尚未显示出与 ACE 抑制剂或 ARB 同样有益的延缓 CKD 进展的效果。

对于糖尿病患者，充分的血糖控制可以预防 CKD 的进展。无论是否同时诊断为 CKD，推荐的糖化血红蛋白（A1c）目标值为低于 7%，但需要警惕低血糖风险。对于同时有糖尿病和蛋白尿但无高血压的患者，可考虑使用 ACE 抑制剂和 ARB 以减缓 CKD 的进展。最近，钠-葡萄糖共转运体-2（SGLT2）抑制剂的使用在肾脏

TABLE 8.2 Drug Dosages in Chronic Kidney Disease

Major Dosage Reduction	Minor or No Reduction	Avoid Usage
Antibiotics		
Aminoglycosides	Erythromycin	
Penicillin	Nafcillin	Nitrofurantoin
Cephalosporins	Clindamycin	Nalidixic acid
Sulfonamides	Chloramphenicol	Tetracycline
Vancomycin	Isoniazid, rifampin	
Quinolones	Amphotericin B	
Fluconazole	Aztreonam, tazobactam	
Acyclovir, ganciclovir	Doxycycline	
Foscarnet		
Imipenem		
Others		
Digoxin	Antihypertensives	Aspirin
Procainamide	Benzodiazepines	Sulfonylureas
H_2 antagonists	Quinidine	Lithium carbonate
Meperidine	Lidocaine	Acetazolamide
Codeine	Spironolactone	NSAIDs
Propoxyphene	Triamterene	Phosphate-containing bowel-preparation agents

NSAIDs, Nonsteroidal anti-inflammatory drugs.

with type 2 diabetes and established atherosclerotic cardiovascular disease. Several other studies suggested that treatment with glucagon-like peptide-1 (GLP-1) receptor agonists could also have beneficial effects on kidney outcomes in patients with type 2 diabetes.

Diet

Dietary protein restriction is advocated to slow progression of CKD. Several meta-analyses indicate that reduced protein diets may be modestly beneficial to slow CKD progression, but the largest clinical trial, the MDRD study, did not show a significant benefit. The recommended dietary protein intake in advanced CKD is 0.60 g/kg per day with at least 50% of the protein being of high biologic value. The present consensus is that aggressive dietary management in patients with CKD, with proper restriction of sodium, potassium, phosphorus, and protein intake under the supervision of a dietician, may reduce progression of CKD, albeit to a small extent.

Avoidance of Toxic Drug Effects

Many drugs that are excreted by the kidney should be avoided, or their doses should be reduced, as shown in Table 8.2. Drugs may injure the kidney in many ways, including direct toxicity leading to acute tubular necrosis, induction of interstitial nephritis, or development of urinary crystals that obstruct the kidney. Common classes of medications that injure the kidney include antibiotics, specifically aminoglycosides; nonsteroidal anti-inflammatory drugs, including cyclo-oxygenase-2 (COX-2) inhibitors; and antiretroviral medications. Over-the-counter herbal medications, including aristolochic acids, may cause CKD. Others, such as St. John's Wort, may interact with kidney transplant medications and should be avoided. Iodinated radiocontrast agents can cause acute worsening of kidney function, especially in patients with CKD. Iso-osmolar contrast agents are less toxic than high-osmolar agents. Patients at high risk for contrast-induced kidney injury should receive adequate hydration, and the volume of the contrast should be minimized. The magnetic resonance imaging (MRI) contrast agent gadolinium, has been associated with the severe fibrotic skin condition of nephrogenic systemic fibrosis in patients with advanced CKD.

Reversible Causes of Acute Deterioration in Kidney Function

The rate of decline in GFR for individual patients is generally log linear. Accordingly, plotting 1/serum creatinine against time usually predicts the rate at which a specific patient will reach ESRD. When such a patient suddenly shows acute worsening of kidney function, the differential diagnosis should be considered and investigated, as described in Chapter 7.

Care for the Patient With End-Stage Renal Disease

As CKD progresses to kidney failure, preparation is needed for RRT. Patients with moderate CKD should be referred to a nephrologist for co-management, including evaluation of risk for CKD progression, estimation of timing until initiation of RRT, and education related to RRT. Late referral (<3 months before ESRD) is associated with a higher risk for death after initiation of RRT.

Renal Replacement Therapies

For patients who are suspected to progress to ESRD, discussions to inform patients and their family about available options of RRT should occur early and be paired with an assessment of the expectations and values of the patient. Options include kidney transplantation, dialysis or medical management without dialysis, sometimes referred to as conservative care. In suitable candidates, kidney transplantation is encouraged because it allows a better quality of life, increased survival rate, and greater chance for rehabilitation. In 2016, 87.3% of incident individuals began renal replacement therapy with hemodialysis (HD), 9.7% started with peritoneal dialysis (PD), and 2.8% received a preemptive kidney transplant. Kidney transplants may be from either deceased or living donors. In the United States in 2016, 20,161 kidney transplants were performed, 28% of which were from living donors. There are two types of dialysis, hemodialysis and peritoneal dialysis. The distribution of patients receiving various modalities differs in other countries. Maintenance dialysis is initiated when the patient displays signs of uremia, usually when eGFR is 10 mL per minute or less and there are no apparent reversible causes of kidney failure. However, maintenance dialysis may be started at any time when complications of ESRD, such as volume overload and hyperkalemia, cannot be controlled medically.

表 8.2 慢性肾脏病的药物剂量调整

大幅减量	小幅减量或不减量	避免使用
抗生素		
氨基糖苷类	红霉素	
青霉素	萘呋胺	呋喃妥因
头孢菌素	克林霉素	萘啶酸
磺胺类药物	氯霉素	四环素
万古霉素	异烟肼、利福平	
喹诺酮类	两性霉素 B	
氟康唑	阿奇霉素、他唑巴坦	
阿昔洛韦、更昔洛韦	多西环素（强力霉素）	
膦甲酸钠		
亚胺培南		
其他药物		
地高辛	抗高血压药	阿司匹林
普鲁卡因胺	苯二氮䓬类药物	磺脲类药物
H2 受体拮抗剂	奎尼丁	碳酸锂
美哌啶	利多卡因	乙酰唑胺
可待因	螺内酯	NSAID
丙氧芬	氨苯蝶啶	含磷肠道准备剂

NSAID，非甾体抗炎药。

结局方面显示出有益效果，主要是在患有 2 型糖尿病和已确诊动脉粥样硬化性心血管疾病的患者中。另外几项研究表明，使用胰高血糖素样肽-1（GLP-1）受体激动剂治疗也可能对 2 型糖尿病患者的肾脏结局产生有益影响。

饮食

提倡通过限制饮食蛋白质摄入来延缓 CKD 的进展。几项荟萃分析表明，低蛋白饮食可能对延缓 CKD 的进展有一定益处，但最大的一项临床试验（MDRD 研究）并未显示出显著的益处。晚期 CKD，推荐的每日膳食蛋白质摄入量为 0.60 g/kg，其中至少 50% 的蛋白质应具有较高的生物价值。目前的共识是，在营养师的指导下对 CKD 患者进行积极的饮食管理，适当限制钠、钾、磷和蛋白质的摄入量，可以减缓 CKD 的进展，但程度有限。

避免药物毒性作用

许多经肾排泄的药物应避免使用或减少剂量，如表 8.2 所示。药物可通过多种方式损伤肾脏，包括直接毒性导致急性肾小管坏死、引发间质性肾炎，或形成尿液结晶阻塞肾脏。常见的肾脏损伤药物包括抗生素，特别是氨基糖苷类；非甾体抗炎药［包括环氧化酶-2（COX-2）抑制剂］；以及抗逆转录病毒药物。包括马兜铃酸在内的非处方草药可能会导致 CKD。其他草药如圣约翰草，可能会与肾移植药物发生相互作用，应避免服用。碘造影剂可导致肾功能急性恶化，尤其是在 CKD 患者中。等渗造影剂的毒性低于高渗造影剂。造影剂肾损伤的高危患者应充分水化，并尽量减少造影剂的用量。在晚期 CKD 患者中，磁共振成像（MRI）造影剂钆与肾源性系统性纤维化所致的严重纤维性皮肤病有关。

肾功能急性恶化的可逆原因

对于个体患者，GFR 下降速率一般呈对数线性。因此，将血清肌酐的倒数与时间的关系绘制成图，通常可以预测特定患者达到 ESRD 的速度。当这样的患者突然出现肾功能急性恶化时，应考虑是否存在急性加重原因并进行相关鉴别诊断，详见第 7 章所述。

终末期肾病患者的护理

随着 CKD 进展至肾衰竭，需要为 RRT 做好准备。中度 CKD 患者应转诊至肾脏专科医生处进行共同管理，包括评估 CKD 进展风险、估算启动 RRT 的时间以及进行 RRT 相关教育。转诊过晚（ESRD 前＜3 个月）与开始 RRT 后的较高死亡风险相关。

肾替代治疗

对于可能进展至 ESRD 的患者，应及早与患者及其家人讨论可供选择的 RRT 治疗方案，并同时评估患者的期望和价值观。可供选择的方案包括肾移植、透析或非透析治疗（有时称为保守治疗）。对于合适的候选者，鼓励进行肾移植，因为肾移植可以提高生活质量、提高存活率并增加康复的机会。2016 年美国 87.3% 的新发 ESRD 患者开始接受血液透析（HD）肾替代治疗，9.7% 开始接受腹膜透析（PD），2.8% 未经透析直接接受肾移植。肾移植的捐献者可能来自已故或者活体捐献者。2016 年美国共进行了 20 161 例肾移植，其中 28% 来自活体捐献者。透析分为血液透析和腹膜透析两种。不同国家接受各种方式透析的患者分布情况有所不同。维持性透析一般在患者出现尿毒症症状时开始，通常 eGFR 为 10 ml/min 或更低且无明显肾衰竭可逆因素。当 ESRD 的并发症（如容量超负荷和高钾血症）无法通过药物控制时，也可随时启动维持性透析。

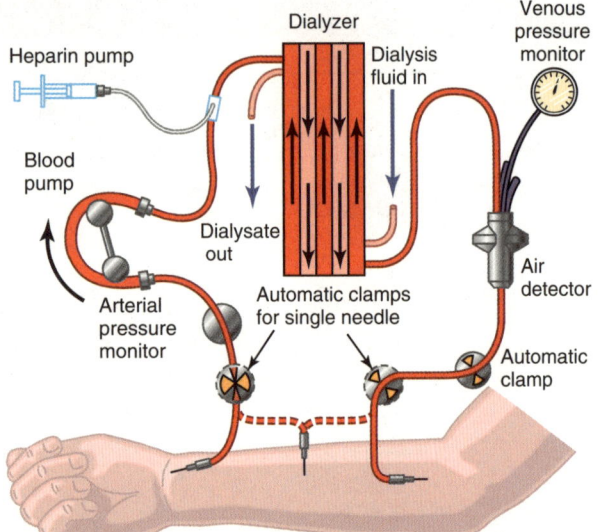

Fig. 8.4 Essential components of a dialysis delivery system that, together with the dialyzer, make up an *artificial kidney*. In isolated ultrafiltration, no dialysis fluid is used (bypass mode). Also shown is the apparatus for using a single needle for inflow and outflow of blood from the patient. (From Keshaviah PR: Hemodialysis monitors and monitoring. In Maher JF [ed]: Replacement of renal function by dialysis, 3rd ed. Boston, Kluwer Academic Publishers, 1989. Reprinted by permission of Kluwer Academic Publishers.)

Hemodialysis

As illustrated in Fig. 8.4, blood is pumped from a vascular access into tubing that leads to a large number of capillaries bundled together in a dialyzer. The capillaries are made up of semisynthetic materials and are semipermeable, capable of allowing exchange of small molecules. Moving in the opposite direction to blood is a dialysate solution that is passing through outside the capillaries, thus allowing countercurrent exchange. This solution contains sodium chloride, bicarbonate, and varying concentrations of potassium. Diffusion through the membrane allows low-molecular-weight substances such as urea and organic acids to move across according to the concentration gradient. Fluid is removed by *ultrafiltration*, which is achieved by applying transmembrane hydrostatic pressure across the dialyzer.

In the setting of ESRD, an average patient undergoing *intermittent* maintenance hemodialysis requires 4 hours of dialysis 3 times a week. Common complications during hemodialysis include hypotension and muscle cramping. Avoiding excessive fluid weight gain can minimize these complications.

Access for hemodialysis. The recommended access for hemodialysis is a permanent access such as an arteriovenous fistula (AVF) or arteriovenous graft (AVG), rather than an indwelling catheter. Although the goal is for more than 70% of prevalent hemodialysis patients to use an AVF or AVG for dialysis access (http://www.healthypeople.gov/2020/), many patients continue to use catheters, especially at the time of initiation of maintenance hemodialysis. Temporary catheters are placed into the internal jugular, subclavian, or femoral veins similar to other central venous lines. Permanent catheters have a cuff around the outer wall of the tubing and tunnel under the chest wall skin for some distance before entering the internal jugular vein. Catheters have higher rates of infection and a higher risk for mortality compared with AVF and AVG.

Peritoneal Dialysis

In peritoneal dialysis, the peritoneal capillaries act as a semipermeable membrane like a hemodialysis dialyzer. This technique has several advantages over hemodialysis because it allows independence from the long time spent in dialysis units, it does not require as stringent dietary restrictions, and more patients return to full-time employment. In continuous ambulatory peritoneal dialysis, dialysate of 2- to 3-L volumes is instilled through a peritoneal catheter into the peritoneal cavity for varying amounts of time and exchanged 4 to 6 times daily. In continuous cyclic peritoneal dialysis, the patient is connected to a machine referred to as a *cycler* that allows inflow of smaller volumes of dialysate with shorter dwell time overnight while the patient sleeps. Modifications in this regimen can be made to fit a patient's lifestyle and still achieve adequate clearance of toxins and removal of fluid. Ultrafiltration is achieved through increasing dextrose concentration in the dialysate. Two major drawbacks of peritoneal dialysis are peritonitis and difficulty in achieving adequate clearances in patients with excess body mass. Peritonitis can be treated with intraperitoneal antibiotics. Additionally, a slow deterioration occurs in the permeability of the peritoneal membrane, especially after one or more peritonitis episodes, leading to inadequate dialysis and, ultimately, the need to change the modality of RRT.

Kidney Transplantation

Kidney transplantation is the preferred modality of RRT. In suitable candidates, it provides patients with superior survival and a better quality of life compared to remaining on maintenance dialysis. It is also a more cost-effective long-term treatment option compared to maintenance dialysis. The variety of available immunosuppressive therapies, including calcineurin inhibitors (cyclosporine and tacrolimus), mammalian target of rapamycin (mTOR) inhibitors (sirolimus and everolimus), mycophenolate mofetil/mycophenolic acid, and novel agents such as belatacept have resulted in excellent short- and long-term graft survival.

Types of kidney transplants. Kidney transplant donors may be deceased or living and, among those living, may be related or unrelated. The majority of deceased donation occurs after brain death but can also occur after cardiac death. Deceased donor 1-year and 5-year graft survival is 93% and 75%, and a living donor is 98% and 85%, respectively.

There is an effort to increase living donation because the deceased donor supply is inadequate, resulting in prolonged waiting times for recipient candidates on the deceased donor waiting list. The advantages and disadvantages of living versus deceased donor transplantation are summarized in Table 8.3. The use of kidney paired donation and/or desensitization allows for transplantation of recipients with potential donors who are blood group or immunologically incompatible. Kidney paired donation utilizes exchange algorithms to bypass incompatibility by matching blood group or human leukocyte antigen (HLA)-incompatible recipient-donor pairs with other incompatible pairs, resulting in each donor donating a kidney to the other person's intended recipient. On the other hand, desensitization utilizes antibody-directed therapy such as plasmapheresis or intravenous immunoglobulin to reduce donor-specific HLA antibodies or blood group antibodies in recipients to prevent acute rejection despite blood group or HLA incompatibility. As a means of expanding the supply of deceased donor kidneys and reducing deceased donor waiting times, kidneys from marginal donors such as those of advanced age or with comorbid conditions such as hypertension and cerebrovascular disease are utilized in selected recipients who would benefit from earlier transplantation. In addition, increased Public Health Service risk donors, such as those who have a history of intravenous drug abuse, are increasingly being utilized. In the setting of negative nucleic acid testing, the absolute risk of transmission of hepatitis C, human immunodeficiency virus, and hepatitis B virus from these donors is less than 1%.

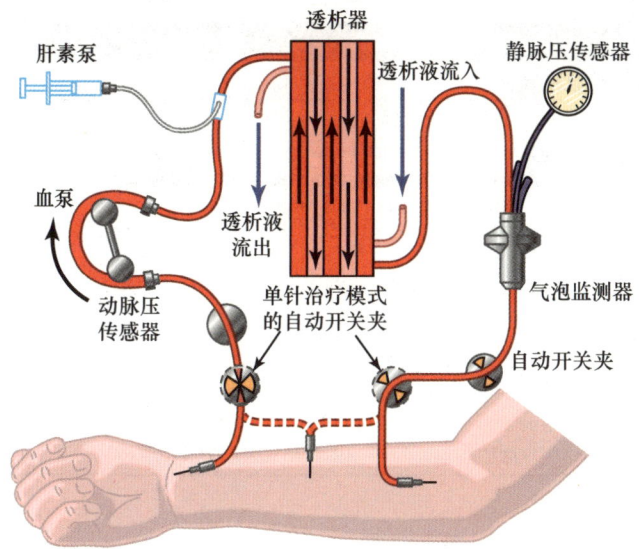

图 8.4 透析输送系统的重要组成部分与透析器一起构成人工肾脏。在单纯超滤过程中，不使用透析液（旁路模式）。图中还显示了使用单针从患者体内输入和流出血液的装置［引自 Keshaviah PR：Hemodialysis monitors and monitoring. In Maher JF（ed）：Replacement of renal function by dialysis，3rd ed. Boston，Kluwer Academic Publishers，1989. Reprinted by permission of Kluwer Academic Publishers.］

血液透析

如图 8.4 所示，血液从血管通路被泵入管道，管道通向一个由大量毛细管束捆绑而成的透析器。这些毛细管由半合成材料制成，具有半渗透性，可允许进行小分子物质交换。透析液与血液逆向流动，透析液从毛细管外通过，从而实现逆流交换。透析液含有氯化钠、碳酸氢盐和不同浓度的钾。通过膜的弥散作用，低分子量物质如尿素和有机酸等可根据浓度梯度跨膜移动。利用超滤原理去除液体，这是通过在透析器上施加跨膜静水压来实现的。

在 ESRD 的情况下，接受间歇性维持性血液透析的患者平均每周需进行 3 次透析，每次持续 4 h。血液透析期间常见的并发症包括低血压和肌肉痉挛。避免液体体重增加过多可最大程度地减少这些并发症。

血液透析的通路 推荐血液透析通路为永久性通路，如动静脉内瘘（AVF）或移植动静脉内瘘（AVG），而不是留置导管。虽然目标是让 70% 以上的血液透析患者使用 AVF 或 AVG 作为透析通路（http://www.healthypeople.gov/2020/），但许多患者仍在使用导管，尤其是在开始维持性血液透析时。类似其他中心静脉导管，临时导管被置入颈内静脉、锁骨下静脉或股静脉。永久性导管的管壁外侧有一个袖套，在胸壁皮肤下穿行一段距离后进入颈内静脉。与 AVF 和 AVG 相比，导管的感染率更高，死亡率也更高。

腹膜透析

在腹膜透析中，腹膜毛细血管类似于血液透析器的半透膜。与血液透析相比，腹膜透析技术有几项优势：不需要长时间留在透析中心，不需要严格的饮食限制，更多患者可以重返全职工作岗位。在持续非卧床腹膜透析模式中，2～3 L 的透析液通过腹膜导管灌入腹腔，停留不同时间后放出，每天交换 4～6 次。在持续循环腹膜透析模式中，患者连接到一台循环控制装置（自动腹膜透析机）上，该机器可在患者夜间睡眠时每次注入较小容量的透析液，并缩短透析液留腹时间，频繁快速交换。腹膜透析处方可以根据患者的生活方式进行调整，达到充分清除毒素和体液的目的。超滤是通过增加透析液中葡萄糖的浓度来实现的。腹膜透析的两个主要缺点是腹膜炎和体重超标的患者难以获得足够的透析充分性。腹膜炎可通过腹腔内给予抗生素治疗。此外，腹膜的通透性会缓慢下降，尤其是在一次或多次腹膜炎发作后，会导致透析不充分，最终需要改变 RRT 方式。

肾移植

肾移植是首选的 RRT 方式。与维持性透析相比，肾移植可以为合适的候选者提供更高的存活率和更好的生活质量，肾移植也是一种更具成本效益的长期治疗方案。现有的各种免疫抑制，包括钙调磷酸酶抑制剂（环孢素和他克莫司）、西罗莫司（雷帕霉素）哺乳动物靶标（mTOR）抑制剂（西罗莫司和依维莫司）、吗替麦考酚酯/麦考酚酸以及新型药物（如贝拉西普），均可显著提高短期和长期移植物存活率。

肾移植的类型 肾移植的供体可以来自尸体供体或活体供体；其中活体供体可以是有血缘关系，也可以是非血缘关系。大部分尸体供体的捐献发生在脑死亡之后，但也可以在心源性死亡之后进行。尸体供体 1 年和 5 年移植物存活率分别为 93% 和 75%，而活体供体的 1 年和 5 年移植物存活率分别为 98% 和 85%。

由于尸体供体量不足，肾移植受体候选人等待时间延长，因此正在努力增加活体捐献。表 8.3 总结了活体与尸体供者移植的优缺点。通过肾脏配对捐献和（或）脱敏疗法，可为血型或免疫不相容的潜在捐献者和受体进行移植。肾脏配对捐献利用交换算法，将一对血型或人类白细胞抗原（HLA）不相容的受者-供者对与另一对不相容的受者-供者对进行匹配，从而绕过不相容性，使一个供者将肾脏捐献给另一个供者的预期受者。另一方面，脱敏疗法是利用针对抗体的治疗方法（如血浆置换或静脉注射免疫球蛋白）以减少受者体内的供者特异性 HLA 抗体或血型抗体，以防止血型或 HLA 不相容情况下的急性排斥反应。为了扩大尸体供肾的供应量、减少等待时间，边缘供者（如高龄或患有高血压和脑血管疾病等共病的供者）的肾脏可用于那些可受益于早期移植的选定受者。此外，公共卫生服务高风险者（如有静脉注射吸毒史者）越来越多地成为供者。在核酸检测呈阴性的情况下，这些供者传播丙型肝炎病毒、人类免疫缺陷病毒和乙型肝炎病毒的绝对风险低于 1%。

TABLE 8.3 Comparison of Donor Sources for Kidney Transplantation

Advantages	Disadvantages
Living Donor	
Waiting time for transplant reduced	Small potential postoperative risks for the donor
Sequelae of long-term dialysis avoided	Small potential long-term risk of kidney function decline in the donor
Elective surgical procedure	Requirement of a willing, medically suitable donor
Better early graft function with shorter hospitalization	
Better short-term and long-term success	
Deceased Donor	
Availability to any recipient	Waiting time variable
Availability of other organs for combined transplants (i.e., kidney-pancreas transplant)	Operation performed urgently
Availability of vascular conduits for complex vascular reconstruction	Higher rates of delayed or slow graft function
	Short-term and long-term success not as good as from a living donor

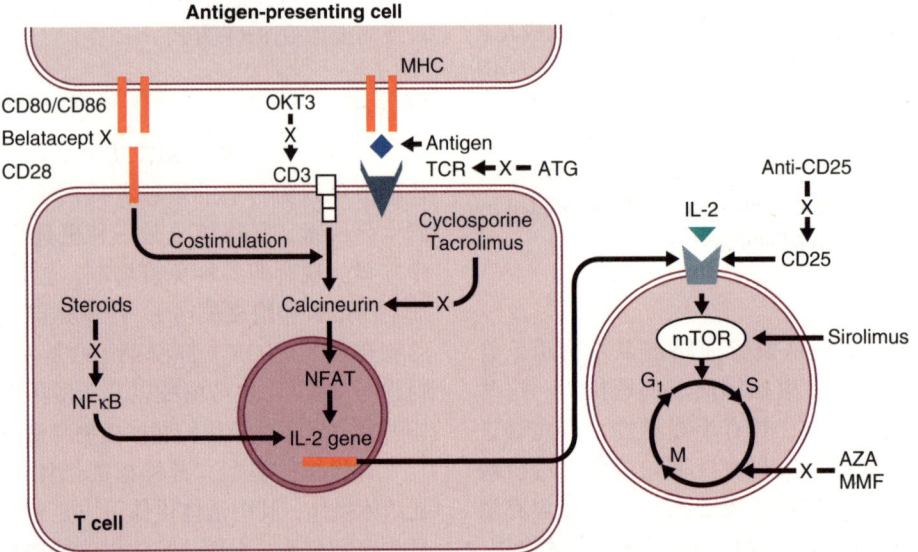

Fig. 8.5 Pathways of T-cell activation and site of action of immunosuppressive agents. *ATG,* Antithymocyte globulin; *AZA,* azathioprine; *IL,* interleukin; *MHC,* major histocompatibility complex; *MMF,* mycoplasma membrane fraction; *MTOR,* mammalian target of rapamycin; *NFAT,* nuclear factor of activated T cells; *TCR,* T-cell receptor.

Immunosuppressant drug therapy. Achieving adequate immunosuppression while minimizing drug toxicity and the risk of infection is at the heart of the success of kidney transplantation. All protocols for immunosuppression aim to inhibit the T lymphocyte, targeting different sites or pathways in the 3-signal model of T-cell activation and proliferation. The mechanisms of action of commonly used immunosuppressants is illustrated in Fig. 8.5. Additionally, antibody-directed therapy is usually employed in those who require desensitization due to preexisting HLA or blood group antibodies.

Induction immunosuppression is administered at the time of transplant and the immediate postoperative period in the form of high-dose steroids, with or without a T lymphocyte–depleting agent such as antithymocyte globulin or a nondepleting agent such as basiliximab (an interleukin-2 inhibitor). *Maintenance immunosuppression* is initiated postoperatively and is composed of at least two drugs, with or without corticosteroids. In the United States, the most common regimen at the time of discharge from the hospital after a transplant is tacrolimus, mycophenolate, and prednisone.

The hepatic cytochrome P-450 system is essential for cyclosporine, tacrolimus, and mTOR inhibitor metabolism. Significant changes in the levels of these drugs may occur when patients start or discontinue taking any of several drugs that can induce or inhibit this system. Therefore, evaluation for drug-drug interactions is critical to prevent toxic or even subtherapeutic effects of either the immunosuppressant drug or the other prescribed therapy. *Cyclosporine* exerts its activity by initially binding to cyclophilin. The cyclosporine-cyclophilin complex subsequently inhibits calcineurin, a calcium-dependent phosphatase that dephosphorylates nuclear factor of activated T cells (NFAT). The inhibition of NFAT dephosphorylation prevents transcription of T-cell activation genes. Side effects of cyclosporine include hypertension, hyperkalemia, hypomagnesemia, exacerbation of gout, dyslipidemia, hypertrichosis, and gingival hypertrophy. *Tacrolimus* has a mechanism of action and side-effect profile like those of cyclosporine. However, it binds to FK-binding protein instead of cyclophilin. It also has additional problems of hyperglycemia and an increased tendency toward neurotoxicity. Rather than causing hypertrichosis, it causes alopecia. Both cyclosporine

表 8.3　肾移植供体来源比较	
优点	缺点
活体供体	
移植等待时间缩短	较小的供体手术潜在风险
避免长期透析的后遗症	较小的供体肾功能下降的潜在长期风险
选择性外科手术	需要自愿且医学上合适的供体
早期移植物功能较好，住院时间较短	
短期和长期成功率较好	
尸体供体	
任何受者可用	等待时间多变
可获得用于联合移植（即肾-胰联合移植）的其他器官	紧急进行手术
可获得用于复杂血管重建的血管导管	移植物功能延迟或缓慢恢复比率较高
	短期和长期成功率不如活体供体

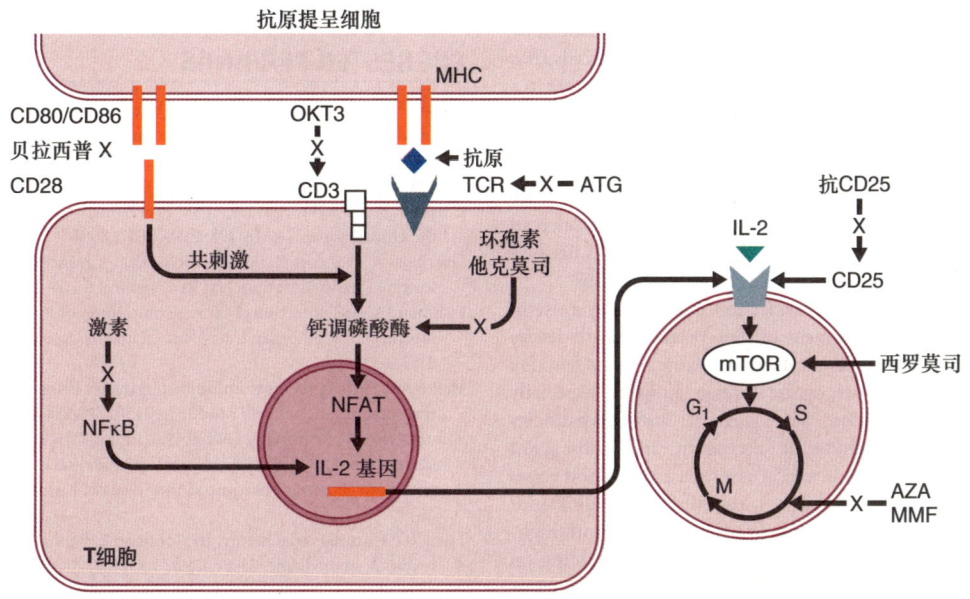

图 8.5　T 细胞活化途径和免疫抑制剂的作用位点。ATG，抗胸腺细胞球蛋白；AZA，硫唑嘌呤；IL，白细胞介素；MHC，主要组织相容性复合体；MMF，吗替麦考酚酯（译者注：原文 mycoplasma membrane fraction 有误）；mTOR，哺乳动物雷帕霉素靶蛋白；NFAT，活化 T 细胞核因子；TCR，T 细胞受体

免疫抑制药物治疗　实现充分的免疫抑制同时最大限度地降低药物毒性和感染风险是肾移植成功的关键。所有免疫抑制方案都旨在抑制 T 淋巴细胞，针对 T 细胞活化和增殖的 3 个信号模型中的不同部位或途径。常用免疫抑制剂的作用机制如图 8.5 所示。此外，针对抗体的疗法通常用于那些由于预先存在 HLA 或血型抗体而需要脱敏治疗的患者。

诱导性免疫抑制治疗是在移植手术时和术后即刻使用的大剂量类固醇激素，可联合或不联合 T 淋巴细胞耗竭剂（如抗胸腺细胞球蛋白）或非耗竭剂（如巴利昔单抗——白细胞介素-2 抑制剂）。维持性免疫抑制治疗从手术后开始，至少由两种药物组成，可包括或不包括皮质类固醇。在美国，移植手术出院时最常用的维持性免疫抑制方案是他克莫司、吗替麦考酚酯和泼尼松。

肝脏的细胞色素 P-450 系统对环孢素、他克莫司和 mTOR 抑制剂的代谢很重要。当患者开始或停止服用任何一种能够诱导或抑制这一系统的药物时，上述这些药物血药浓度可能会发生显著变化。因此，评估药物相互作用对于防止免疫抑制剂或其他处方药物的毒性或低疗效至关重要。环孢素最初是通过与亲环素蛋白结合来发挥其作用的。环孢素-亲环素蛋白复合物抑制钙调磷酸酶，钙调磷酸酶是一种钙依赖性磷酸酶，可使活化 T 细胞核因子（NFAT）去磷酸化。抑制 NFAT 去磷酸化可防止 T 细胞活化基因的转录。环孢素的副作用包括高血压、高钾血症、低镁血症、痛风加重、血脂异常、多毛症和牙龈增生。他克莫司的作用机制和副作用与环孢素相似。不过，他克莫司与 FK 结合蛋白结合，而不是与亲环素蛋白结合。他克莫司还存在升高血糖和神经毒性倾向的问题，而且他克莫司更容易

and tacrolimus can cause calcineurin inhibitor nephrotoxicity, and this is often related to afferent arteriolar vasoconstriction leading to decreased glomerular blood flow. Nephrotoxicity can be acute or chronic and ultimately may contribute to chronic allograft nephropathy and graft loss.

Mycophenolate mofetil or *mycophenolic acid* specifically inhibits T-lymphocyte and B-lymphocyte proliferation by interfering with purine synthesis and thus DNA synthesis. Side effects include leukopenia, anemia, and upper and lower gastrointestinal symptoms.

Sirolimus and *everolimus* bind to FK-binding protein and subsequently inhibit mTOR, thus blocking the phosphorylation of *p70(s6)* kinase and the eukaryotic initiation factor 4E–binding protein, PHAS-I. This action leads to the dampening of cytokine and growth factor activity on T, B, and nonimmune cells. The major side effects are thrombocytopenia, proteinuria, impaired wound healing, and dyslipidemia. mTOR inhibitors can also cause mouth ulcerations, lymphedema, and pneumonitis.

Due to the persistence of episodes of rejection and graft loss over time, novel immunosuppressive agents continue to be developed. Most recently, *belatacept*, a fusion protein that inhibits T-cell activation by blocking the CD80 and CD86 sites on antigen presenting cells, has been shown to confer superior long-term graft function compared to a cyclosporine-based maintenance regimen. This is despite an increased risk of developing early severe acute rejection episodes. Belatacept is administered intravenously and its most serious adverse effect is an increased incidence of post-transplant lymphoproliferative disorder (PTLD) compared to cyclosporine. It is therefore contraindicated in recipients who have not been exposed to Epstein-Barr virus because these patients are at an already higher risk for PTLD at baseline.

Acute rejection. Clinically, acute rejection is detected by a rise in serum creatinine or the development of new proteinuria. In severe cases, graft tenderness and oliguria can occur. *Acute cellular rejection* occurs when T lymphocytes recognize foreign antigens, especially when presented in association with class II histocompatibility antigens. This prompts lymphocyte activation and subsequent invasion of the tubulointerstitium, and in severe cases the blood vessel wall, by activated cytotoxic lymphocytes, resulting in tubulitis and/or endothelialitis. This type of rejection is usually treated with high-dose steroids with or without antithymocyte globulin depending on the severity of the rejection and the initial response to steroid therapy. *Acute humoral rejection* usually occurs in the presence of preexisting or de novo donor-specific HLA antibodies and manifests in the transplanted kidney as microvascular inflammation with or without C4d staining on immunofluorescence. This type of rejection is usually treated with intravenous immune globulin and plasmapheresis, with or without B-cell directed therapy.

Post-transplantation infection. Infection is second only to cardiovascular disease as the leading cause of mortality in kidney transplant recipients. Prophylaxis is used immediately after kidney transplantation to prevent opportunistic infections such as *Pneumocystis jirovecii* pneumonia, cytomegalovirus infection, herpes simplex virus infection, and *Candida* infections. In addition to common community-acquired bacterial and viral infections, kidney transplant recipients are also susceptible to numerous viral, fungal, and other opportunistic infections that normally do not cause severe illness in the immunocompetent host.

Post-transplantation malignant disease. Immunosuppression increases the risk for developing malignant disease. Skin cancer (mostly squamous cell) has the highest incidence in transplant recipients compared with all other types of malignancy. With continuous surveillance and aggressive management, metastasis from skin cancers is rare. Transplant recipients are also at increased risk for developing non-Hodgkin lymphoma and Kaposi sarcoma. In addition to age-appropriate screening, cancer surveillance should be an essential part of post-transplantation care.

PROGNOSIS

The prognosis of CKD varies depending upon the underlying cause, its severity at presentation, and the response to therapy. Yet, it is important to recognize that CKD in general is a significant risk factor for cardiovascular disease and death. Mortality from cardiovascular disease in CKD patients, especially those with stage 3 to 5 disease, is 3.5 times that of an age-matched population and accounts for more than 50% of the deaths in ESRD patients. Research to understand the underlying mechanisms and final pathway, as well as those specific to patients with unique characteristics, will be necessary to advance our efforts to reduce related risks and cure kidney disease.

SUGGESTED READINGS

Abbate M, Remuzzi G: Progression of renal insufficiency: mechanisms. In Massry SG, Glassock RJ, editors: *Massry and Glassock's textbook of nephrology*, 4th ed, Philadelphia, 2001, Lippincott, Williams & Wilkins, pp 1210–1217.

Coresh J, Selvin E, Stevens LA, et al.: Prevalence of chronic kidney disease in the United States, JAMA 298:2038–2047, 2007.

Durrbach A, Francois H, Beaudreuil S, et al.: Advances in immunosuppression for renal transplantation, Nat Rev Nephrol 6:160–167, 2010.

Fishman JA, AST Infectious Disease Community of Practice: Introduction: infection in solid organ transplant recipients, Am J Transplant(Suppl 4)S3–6, 2009.

Halloran PF: Drug therapy: immunosuppressive drugs for kidney transplantation, N Engl J Med 351:2715–2729, 2004.

Kidney Disease: Improving Global Outcomes(KDIGO) CKD Work Group: KDIGO 2012 clinical practice guideline for the evaluation and management of chronic kidney disease, Kidney Inter Suppl 3:1–150, 2013.

Luke RG: Chronic renal failure. In Goldman L, Bennett JC, editors: Cecil textbook of medicine, 21st ed, Philadelphia, 2000, WB Saunders, pp 571–577.

National Kidney Foundation: KDOQI clinical practice guidelines and clinical practice recommendations for diabetes and chronic kidney disease, Am J Kidney Dis 49(2 Suppl 2):S12–S154, 2007.

Sarafidis P, Ferro CJ, Morales E, et al. SGLT-2 inhibitors and GLP-1 receptor agonists for nephroprotection and cardioprotection in patients with diabetes mellitus and chronic kidney disease. A consensus statement by the EURECA-m and the DIABESITY working groups of the ERA-EDTA, Nephrology Dialysis Transplantation 34:208–230, 2019.

Sarnak MJ, Levey AS, Schoolwerth AC, et al.: Kidney disease as a risk factor for development of cardiovascular disease: A statement from the American heart association councils on kidney in cardiovascular disease, high blood pressure research, clinical cardiology, and epidemiology and prevention, Circulation 108:2154–2169, 2003.

U.S. Renal Data System, USRDS 2018 Annual Data Report: Atlas of chronic kidney disease and end-stage renal disease in the United States, National Institutes of Health, Bethesda, MD, 2018, National Institute of Diabetes and Digestive and Kidney Diseases.

Vincenti F, Rostaing L, Grinyo J, et al.: Belatacept and long-term outcomes in kidney transplantation, N Engl J Med 374(4):333–343, 2016.

Voora S, Adey DB: Management of kidney transplant recipients by general nephrologists: core curriculum 2019, Am J Kidney Dis 73(6):866–879, 2019.

导致脱发，而非多毛症。环孢素和他克莫司都可引起钙调磷酸酶抑制剂的肾毒性，这通常与入球小动脉血管收缩导致肾小球血流量减少有关。肾毒性可以是急性的或慢性的，最终可能导致慢性移植肾肾病和移植肾失功。

吗替麦考酚酯或麦考酚酸通过干扰嘌呤合成进而干扰 DNA 合成，特异性地抑制 T 淋巴细胞和 B 淋巴细胞的增殖。副作用包括白细胞减少、贫血及上消化道和下消化道症状。

西罗莫司和依维莫司与 FK 结合蛋白结合，随后抑制 mTOR 活性，从而阻断 p70（s6）激酶和真核细胞启动因子 4E 结合蛋白 PHAS-I 的磷酸化。这种作用会抑制 T、B 和非免疫细胞上的细胞因子和生长因子活性。主要副作用包括血小板减少、蛋白尿、伤口愈合不良和血脂异常。mTOR 抑制剂还可能导致口腔溃疡、淋巴水肿和肺炎。

由于排斥反应和移植物损失的持续存在，新型免疫抑制剂不断被开发出来。最近，一种通过阻断抗原提呈细胞上的 CD80 和 CD86 位点来抑制 T 细胞活化的融合蛋白——贝拉西普（belatacept）显示出与基于环孢素的维持方案相比，具有更优越的维持长期移植肾功能的作用，尽管增加了发生早期严重急性排斥反应的风险。贝拉西普是静脉给药，与环孢素相比，其最严重的不良反应是增加移植后淋巴组织增生性疾病（PTLD）的发病率。因此，对于未暴露于 EB 病毒的受者应禁用该药，因为这些患者本身已经具有更高的 PTLD 风险。

急性排斥反应　临床上，急性排斥反应可通过血清肌酐升高或新发蛋白尿来检测。严重的病例可能会出现移植物触痛和少尿。急性细胞性排斥反应发生在 T 淋巴细胞识别到外来抗原时，尤其是与 II 类组织相容性抗原相关联时。这会促使淋巴细胞活化，随后活化的细胞毒性淋巴细胞侵入肾小管间质，严重情况下还会侵入血管壁，导致肾小管炎和（或）内皮细胞炎。这种类型的排斥反应通常采用大剂量类固醇激素治疗，根据排斥反应的严重程度和对类固醇激素治疗的初步反应，可能会联合抗胸腺细胞球蛋白治疗。急性体液排斥反应通常在预先存在或新形成供者特异性 HLA 抗体的情况下发生，在移植肾中表现为微血管炎症，免疫荧光可有或无 C4d 染色阳性。这种类型的排斥反应通常采用静脉注射免疫球蛋白和血浆置换治疗，伴或不伴 B 细胞的靶向治疗。

移植后感染　感染是仅次于心血管疾病的导致肾移植受者死亡的主要原因。肾移植后应立即进行预防性治疗，以预防机会性感染，如耶氏肺孢子菌肺炎、巨细胞病毒感染、单纯疱疹病毒感染和念珠菌感染。除了常见的社区获得性细菌和病毒感染外，肾移植受者还容易感染多种病毒、真菌和发生其他机会性感染，这些感染通常在免疫功能正常的宿主中不会引起严重疾病。

移植后恶性疾病　免疫抑制剂会增加罹患恶性疾病的风险。所有类型恶性肿瘤中，移植受者中皮肤癌（主要是鳞状细胞癌）的发病率最高。通过持续监测和积极治疗，皮肤癌很少发生转移。移植受者罹患非霍奇金淋巴瘤和卡波西肉瘤的风险也增加。除了进行适龄筛查，癌症监测应成为移植后照护的重要组成部分。

预后

CKD 的预后取决于潜在病因、发病时严重程度以及对治疗的反应。而且要认识到，CKD 是心血管疾病和死亡的重要危险因素。在 CKD 患者中，尤其是 3～5 期患者，心血管疾病的致死率是同龄人群的 3.5 倍，占 ESRD 患者死亡原因的 50% 以上。为了降低 CKD 相关预后风险和治愈肾脏疾病，有必要开展研究以了解潜在机制和最终途径，以及针对特殊表型患者的特定机制。

推荐阅读

Abbate M, Remuzzi G: Progression of renal insufficiency: mechanisms. In Massry SG, Glassock RJ, editors: *Massry and Glassock's textbook of nephrology*, 4th ed, Philadelphia, 2001, Lippincott, Williams & Wilkins, pp 1210–1217.

Coresh J, Selvin E, Stevens LA, et al.: Prevalence of chronic kidney disease in the United States, JAMA 298:2038–2047, 2007.

Durrbach A, Francois H, Beaudreuil L, et al.: Advances in immunosuppression for renal transplantation, Nat Rev Nephrol 6:160–167, 2010.

Fishman JA, AST Infectious Disease Community of Practice: Introduction: infection in solid organ transplant recipients, Am J Transplant(Suppl 4)S3–6, 2009.

Halloran PF: Drug therapy: immunosuppressive drugs for kidney transplantation, *N Engl J Med* 351:2715–2729, 2004.

Kidney Disease: Improving Global Outcomes(KDIGO) CKD Work Group: KDIGO 2012 clinical practice guideline for the evaluation and management of chronic kidney disease, Kidney Inter Suppl 3:1–150, 2013.

Luke RG: Chronic renal failure. In Goldman L, Bennett JC, editors: Cecil textbook of medicine, 21st ed, Philadelphia, 2000, WB Saunders, pp 571–577.

National Kidney Foundation: KDOQI clinical practice guidelines and clinical practice recommendations for diabetes and chronic kidney disease, Am J Kidney Dis 49(2 Suppl 2):S12–S154, 2007.

Sarafidis P, Ferro CJ, Morales E, et al. SGLT-2 inhibitors and GLP-1 receptor agonists for nephroprotection and cardioprotection in patients with diabetes mellitus and chronic kidney disease. A consensus statement by the EURECA-m and the DIABESITY working groups of the ERA-EDTA, Nephrology Dialysis Transplantation 34:208–230, 2019.

Sarnak MJ, Levey AS, Schoolwerth AC, et al.: Kidney disease as a risk factor for development of cardiovascular disease: A statement from the American heart association councils on kidney in cardiovascular disease, high blood pressure research, clinical cardiology, and epidemiology and prevention, Circulation 108:2154–2169, 2003.

U.S. Renal Data System, USRDS 2018 Annual Data Report: Atlas of chronic kidney disease and end-stage renal disease in the United States, National Institutes of Health, Bethesda, MD, 2018, National Institute of Diabetes and Digestive and Kidney Diseases.

Vincenti F, Rostaing L, Grinyo J, et al.: Belatacept and long-term outcomes in kidney transplantation, N Engl J Med 374(4):333–343, 2016.

Voora S, Adey DB: Management of kidney transplant recipients by general nephrologists: core curriculum 2019, Am J Kidney Dis 73(6):866–879, 2019.

索引 Index

A

Acid, gastrointestinal loss of, 58-60
Acid-base disorders, compensation in, 62t
Acidosis
　　potassium losses and, 46
　　renal tubular, 52-54
　　respiratory, 62-64
Acquired cystic kidney disease, 106-108
Acute interstitial nephritis, 98-100, 100t
Acute kidney injury (AKI), 150-168
　　vs. chronic kidney disease, 18
　　approach to patient with, 34-36
　　causes of, 34-36
　　classification of, 152t
　　clinical presentation of, 158-166
　　complications of, 166
　　definition of, 150
　　diagnostic evaluation of, 152-158
　　differential diagnosis of, 158-166
　　end-organ manifestations of, 36
　　epidemiology of, 150
　　etiology of, 150, 154f
　　future tests for, 158
　　hepatorenal syndrome and, 160
　　history and physical examination of, 152
　　in hospitalized patients, diagnostic approach to, 154t
　　intrinsic, 150, 160-166
　　laboratory tests for, 152
　　management of, 158-166
　　outcome and prognosis of, 168
　　postrenal, 150, 166
　　prerenal, 150, 158-160
　　renal imaging for, 156-158
　　risk factors for, 34
　　severity of, 36
　　urinalysis and urine microscopy for, 156, 156t
　　urinary indices and, 156
Acute proliferative glomerulonephritis, 162
Acute tubular injury (ATI), 150
Acute tubular necrosis (ATN), 28f, 36, 150
　　in intrinsic acute injury, 162
　　ischemic, 162
　　nephrotoxic, 162
ADAMTS13
　　in thrombotic thrombocytopenic purpura, 92, 140, 146f
Adenosine triphosphate (ATP), 8
β-Adrenergicagonists, K⁺ shifts and, 44
α1-Adrenergic receptor blockers, for nephrolithiasis, 118
Albumin excretion rate, 24
Albuminuria
　　categories of, in chronic kidney disease, 172t
　　in chronic kidney disease, 22f
　　　　assessment of, 24
Alcoholic ketoacidosis, 58
Aldosterone
　　hypokalemia and, 46
Alkaline therapy, for uric acid stones, 122
Alkalosis
　　metabolic, 58-60
　　　　classification of, 60t
　　respiratory, 60-62

A

胃肠道酸丢失，59-61
酸碱失衡的代偿，63t
酸中毒
　　失钾，47
　　肾小管酸中毒，53-55
　　呼吸性酸中毒，63-65
获得性囊性肾病，107-109
急性间质性肾炎，99-101，101t
急性肾损伤（AKI），151-169
　　vs. 慢性肾脏病，19
　　患者接诊，35-37
　　病因，35-37
　　分类，153t
　　临床表现，159-167
　　并发症，167
　　定义，151
　　诊断性评估，153-159
　　鉴别诊断，159-167
　　影响终末器官的表现，37
　　流行病学，151
　　病因，151，155f
　　未来可用的检查，159
　　肝肾综合征，161
　　病史和体格检查，153
　　（住院）患者的诊断流程，155t
　　（肾）实质性，151，161-167
　　实验室检查，153
　　处理，159-167
　　结果和预后，169
　　肾后性，151，167
　　肾前性，151，159-161
　　肾脏影像学，157-159
　　危险因素，35
　　严重程度，37
　　尿液分析和尿液显微镜检查，157，157t
　　尿液指标，157
急性增殖性肾小球肾炎，163
急性肾小管损伤（ATI），151
急性肾小管坏死（ATN），29f，37，151
　　（肾）实质性急性肾损伤，163
　　缺血性，163
　　肾毒性，163
ADAMTS13
　　血栓性血小板减少性紫癜，93，141，147f
三磷酸腺苷（ATP），9
β受体激动剂，促进K⁺转移，45
α1受体阻滞剂，治疗肾结石，119
白蛋白排泄率，25
白蛋白尿
　　分类，慢性肾脏病，173t
　　慢性肾脏病，23f
　　　　评估，25
酒精性酮症酸中毒，59
醛固酮
　　低钾血症，47
碱化尿液，治疗尿酸结石，123
碱中毒
　　代谢性，59-61
　　　　分类，61t
　　呼吸性，61-63

Page numbers followed by "f" indicate figures, "t" indicate tables, and "b" indicate boxes.

页码数字中，"f"代表"图"，"t"代表"表格"，"b"代表"框"。

A

Allopurinol
    for uric acid stones, 122
Alport syndrome, 92-94, 92f
Amiloride, in hyperkalemia, 48
Amyloidosis, 84-86, 88f, 162
Analgesic nephropathy, 100-102
Anemia
    in chronic kidney disease, 174-176
Angiomyolipomas, in tuberous sclerosis complex, 112
Angioplasty, renal artery
    in atherosclerotic renal artery stenosis, 130
Angiotensin-converting enzyme (ACE) inhibitors
    in chronic kidney disease, 170
        in renal artery stenosis, 126
Angiotensin-receptor blockers (ARBs)
    in chronic kidney disease, 170
Anion gap
    in chronic kidney disease, 170
    metabolic acidosis and, 52-56
Anticoagulation
    in renal vein thrombosis, 148
Antidiuretic hormone (ADH), 12
Antigen-presenting cells, 8
Anti-glomerular basement membrane antibody, glomerulonephritis and, 84, 86f
Antimyeloma therapy, for amyloidosis, 86
Antineutrophil cytoplasmic antibodies (ANCAs)
    vasculitides and, 82-84, 84t
Antiphospholipid antibody syndrome (APS), 146-148
Anxiety-hyperventilation syndrome, respiratory alkalosis and, 62
Aortic dissection, 132-134
Apolipoprotein H, 146
Arcuate arteries, 126
Aristolochic acid, 102, 178
    nephropathy, 102
Arteriography
    renal, in chronic kidney disease, 34
    for renal artery stenosis, 130
Arteriovenous fistula (AVF)
    hemodialysis and, 180
Arteriovenous graft (AVG), hemodialysis and, 180
Aspirin, poisoning from, 58
Asymptomatic microscopic hematuria, 68
Atheroembolic disease, 136
Atherosclerotic renovascular disease, 128-130, 128t
Autosomal dominant polycystic kidney disease (ADPKD), 108-110, 108t-110t
Autosomal dominant tubulointerstitial kidney disease, 112

B

Bacteria, urease-producing, 122t
Balkan endemic nephropathy (BEN), 102
"Beer potomania" syndrome, 38
Belatacept, 184
Bicarbonaturia, 60
Bleeding
    chronic kidney disease and, 174-176
Blood pressure
    aortic dissection and, 134
    in chronic kidney disease, 20
        assessment of, 24
Bosniak renal cyst classification scheme, 106, 108t
Bowman's capsule, 8
Brush border, 8

C

C3 glomerulonephritis, 74-76, 78f
Cadmium, chronic interstitial nephritis from, 102

别嘌呤醇
    尿酸结石，123
Alport综合征，93-95，93f
阿米洛利，治疗高钾血症，49
淀粉样变性，85-87，89f，163
镇痛剂肾病，101-103
贫血
    慢性肾脏病，175-177
血管平滑肌脂肪瘤，见于结节性硬化症，113
血管成形术，肾动脉
    动脉粥样硬化性肾动脉狭窄，131
血管紧张素转换酶（ACE）抑制剂
    慢性肾脏病，171
        肾动脉狭窄，127
血管紧张素受体阻滞剂（ARB）
    慢性肾脏病，171
阴离子间隙
    慢性肾脏病，171
    代谢性酸中毒，53-57
抗凝治疗
    肾静脉血栓形成，149
抗利尿激素（ADH），13
抗原提呈细胞，9
抗肾小球基底膜抗体，肾小球肾炎，85，87f

抗骨髓瘤治疗，治疗淀粉样变性，87
抗中性粒细胞胞质抗体（ANCA）
    血管炎，83-85，85t
抗磷脂综合征（APS），147-149
焦虑-过度通气综合征，呼吸性碱中毒，63
主动脉夹层，133-135
载脂蛋白H，147
弓状动脉，127
马兜铃酸，103，179
    马兜铃酸肾病，103
动脉造影
    肾动脉造影，慢性肾脏病，35
    肾动脉狭窄，131
动静脉内瘘（AVF）
    血液透析，181
移植动静脉内瘘（AVG），血液透析，181
阿司匹林中毒，59
无症状镜下血尿，69
动脉粥样硬化栓塞性疾病，137
动脉粥样硬化性肾血管疾病，129-131，129t
常染色体显性遗传多囊肾病（ADPKD），109-111，109t-111t

常染色体显性肾小管间质性肾病，113

B

产脲酶细菌，123t
巴尔干地方性肾病（BEN），103
"啤酒狂"综合征，39
贝拉西普，185
碳酸氢盐尿，61
出血性疾病
    慢性肾脏病，175-177
血压
    主动脉夹层，135
    慢性肾脏病，21
        评估，25
Bosniak肾囊肿分类法，107，109t
鲍曼囊（肾小囊），9
刷状缘，9

C

C3肾小球肾炎，75-77，79f
镉，慢性间质性肾炎，103

Calcium
　　for hyperkalemia, 50
Calcium channel blockers
　　for nephrolithiasis, 118
Calcium phosphate stones, 120-122
Calcium stones, 120, 120t
Calyces, in kidneys, 4
Captopril, in scleroderma renal crisis, 138-140
Cardiorenal syndrome, in prerenal acute kidney injury, 158-160
Cardiovascular disease (CVD)
　　chronic kidney disease with, 172
Casts, in urine, 32f
Cells, in urine, 26f
Cellular redistribution, hyperkalemia and, 50
Cerebral aneurysms, in autosomal dominant polycystic kidney disease, 110
Cerebral edema
　　hypernatremia correction and, 40
Cerebral salt wasting (CSW), 40
Chest pain
　　aortic dissection and, 132-134
Chinese herb nephropathy (CHN), 102
Cholesterol emboli, 136
Chronic interstitial nephritis, 100-106, 100t
　　conditions associated with, 102t
Chronic kidney disease (CKD), 170-184
　　vs. acute kidney injury, 18
　　acute kidney injury and, 170
　　albuminuria in, 22f, 24
　　approach to patient with, 18-34
　　assessment of kidney function in, 20-24
　　blood pressure in, 24
　　clinical presentation of, 170-176
　　definition of, 18, 170
　　diagnosis of, 176
　　epidemiology of, 170
　　history and examination of, 20
　　hyperkalemia and, 50
　　hypertension and, 176-178
　　hypertensive nephrosclerosis and, 134-136
　　interstitial nephritis and, 100
　　management of
　　　　acute deterioration and, 178
　　　　diabetes in, 176-178
　　　　diet in, 178
　　　　drug toxicities and, 178, 178t
　　　　goals of, 176
　　　　prevention of progression in, 176
　　metabolic disease with, 176
　　microscopic urinalysis in, 24, 26f-32f
　　pathology of, 170
　　prevalence of, 170, 172f
　　prognosis of, 184
　　renal imaging in, 24-34
　　risk factors interacting with, 174f
　　severity of injury of, 36
　　treatment of, 176-184
Chronic Kidney Disease Epidemiology Collaboration (CKD-EPI) equation, 24
Ciliopathies, 108
Citrate, in calcium stone formation, 120
Columns of Bertin, 4
Complex cysts, in kidney, 106
Computed tomography (CT)
　　for acute kidney injury, 158
　　of kidney, 34
　　for renal artery stenosis, 130
Continuous renal replacement therapies (CRRTs), in acute kidney injury, 168
Contrast agents, gadolinium-based, 34
Corticosteroids

钙
　　高钾血症，51
钙通道阻滞剂
　　肾结石，119
磷酸钙结石，121-123
钙结石，121，121t
肾盏，5
卡托普利，治疗硬皮病肾危象，139-141
心肾综合征，见于肾前性急性肾损伤，159-161
心血管疾病（CVD）
　　慢性肾脏病，173
管型，尿液中，33f
细胞，尿液中，27f
细胞内外再分布，高钾血症，51
颅内动脉瘤，见于常染色体显性遗传多囊肾病，111
脑水肿
　　高钠血症纠正，41
脑盐耗（CSW），41
胸痛
　　主动脉夹层，133-135
中草药肾病（CHN），103
胆固醇栓塞，137
慢性间质性肾炎，101-107，101t
　　相关的疾病，103t
慢性肾脏病（CKD），171-185
　　vs. 急性肾损伤，19
　　与急性肾损伤，171
　　白蛋白尿，23f，25
　　患者接诊，19-35
　　肾功能评估，21-25
　　血压，25
　　临床表现，171-177
　　定义，19，171
　　诊断，177
　　流行病学，171
　　病史和检查，21
　　高钾血症，51
　　高血压，177-179
　　高血压性肾硬化症，135-137
　　间质性肾炎，101
　　管理
　　　　急性恶化，179
　　　　糖尿病，177-179
　　　　饮食，179
　　　　药物毒性作用，179，179t
　　　　目标，177
　　　　预防进展，177
　　代谢紊乱，177
　　显微镜检尿液分析，25，27f-33f
　　病理学，171
　　患病率，171，173f
　　预后，185
　　肾脏影像，25-35
　　危险因素，175f
　　损伤严重程度，37
　　治疗，177-185
慢性肾脏病流行病学协作组（CKD-EPI）方程，25
纤毛性疾病，109
枸橼酸盐，见于钙结石形成，121
肾柱，5
复杂性囊肿，肾，107
计算机断层成像（CT）
　　急性肾损伤，159
　　肾CT，35
　　肾动脉狭窄（RAS），131
连续性肾替代治疗（CRRT），见于急性肾损伤，169
钆造影剂，35
皮质类固醇

for focal segmental glomerulosclerosis, 72
for minimal change disease, 70
Cotransporters, 8
Countertransporters, 8
Creatinine, serum
in chronic kidney disease, 170
in kidney function, 20
Crescentic glomerulonephritis, 82, 86f
Cryoglobulinemia, 82, 82t
Cryoglobulinemicglomerulonephritis, 82, 82t
Crystalline nephropathy, in intrinsic acute kidney injury, 164
Crystals, in urine, 30f
Cyclooxygenase-2 (COX-2)
selective, in acute kidney injury, 158
Cyclosporine, 182-184
Cystic kidney diseases, 106-112
acquired, 106-108
Cystine stones, 122
Cystinuria, 122
Cysts, in kidney, 106

D

Dendritic cells, in kidney, 8
Dense deposit disease, 74-76
Deposition disease, 162
Diabetes insipidus
polydipsiain, 42
Diabetes mellitus
chronic kidney disease in, 18, 176-178
nephropathy in, 94-96, 96f
Diabetic ketoacidosis
metabolic acidosis and, 56-58
Diabetic nephropathy, 94-96
Dialysis
pericarditis and, 172
peritoneal, 180
metabolic acidosis and, 54-58
Diet
in chronic kidney disease, 178
hyperkalemia and, 48-50
hyperoxaluria and, 120
hypokalemia and, 46
Distal sodium delivery, primary increase in, 46
Diuretics
for hypercalciuria, 120
in hyperkalemia, 50
hyponatremia and, 40
in metabolic alkalosis, 60
in nephrotic syndrome, 68
D-Lactic acidosis, 56
Drugs
acute interstitial nephritis caused by, 98, 100t
in chronic kidney disease, 178, 178t
Dysproteinemias, 162

E

Eculizumab
in hemolyticuremic syndrome, 90
Effective arterial blood volume (EAV), 40f
Electrolyte disorders, fluid and, 38-64
hyperkalemia, 48-50
hypernatremia, 42-44, 42f
hypokalemia, 44-48
hyponatremia, 38-42, 40f
metabolic acidosis, 50-58, 52f
metabolic alkalosis, 58-60
polydipsia, 42
polyuria, 42, 44f

局灶节段性肾小球硬化，73
微小病变，71
协同转运蛋白，9
反向转运蛋白，9
肌酐（血清）
慢性肾脏病，171
肾功能，21
新月体性肾小球肾炎，83，87f
冷球蛋白血症，83，83t
冷球蛋白血症性肾小球肾炎，83，83t
晶体性肾病，见于肾实质性急性肾损伤，165
晶体，尿液中，31f
环氧合酶-2（COX-2）
选择性COX-2，治疗急性肾损伤，159
环孢素，183-185
囊肿性肾病，107-113
获得性，107-109
胱氨酸结石，123
胱氨酸尿症，123
肾囊肿，107

D

肾树突状细胞，9
致密沉积病，75-77
沉积病，163
尿崩症
烦渴，43
糖尿病
慢性肾脏病，19，177-179
糖尿病肾病，95-97，97f
糖尿病酮症酸中毒
代谢性酸中毒，57-59
糖尿病肾病，95-97
透析
心包炎，173
腹膜透析，181
代谢性酸中毒，55-59
饮食
慢性肾脏病，179
高钾血症，49-51
高草酸尿症，121
低钾血症，47
远端Na$^+$输送，原发性增加，47
利尿剂
高钙尿症，121
高钾血症，51
低钠血症，41
代谢性碱中毒，61
肾病综合征，69
D-乳酸中毒，57
药物
引起急性间质性肾炎，99，101t
慢性肾脏病，179，179t
异常蛋白血症，163

E

依库珠单抗
溶血性尿毒综合征，91
有效动脉血容量（EAV），41f
电解质紊乱，39-65
高钾血症，49-51
高钠血症，43-45，43f
低钾血症，45-49
低钠血症，39-43，41f
代谢性酸中毒，51-59，53f
代谢性碱中毒，59-61
烦渴，43
多尿，43，45f

respiratory acidosis, 62-64
respiratory alkalosis, 60-62
Electrolytes, chronic kidney disease with, 176
Endocrine disease
  chronic kidney disease with, 176
Endogenous nephrotoxins, 34
End-stage renal disease (ESRD)
  atherosclerotic renal artery stenosis and, 130
  care for patient with, 178
  epidemiology of, 170
  β_2-microglobulin in, 172
  prevalence of, 170
Enteric hyperoxaluria, 120
Eosinophilic granulomatosis with polyangiitis (EGPA), 82
Eplerenone
  in hyperkalemia, 50
Erythropoiesis-stimulating agents (ESAs), 16
Erythropoietin (EPO), 16
  chronic kidney disease and, 174-176
Escherichia coli
  hemolytic-uremic syndrome and, 90
  Shiga toxin-producing, 140-142
Ethylene glycol poisoning, 58
Extracellular fluid (ECF)
  volume, 38
Extrarenal potassium losses, 46
Eye, cholesterol embolization to, 136

F

Fabry's disease, 94, 94f
Fanconi syndrome, in interstitial nephritis, 102
Fibrillary glomerulonephritis, 82, 84f, 162
Fibroblasts, in kidneys, 8
Fibrocystin, 110
Fibromuscular dysplasia (FMD), 130-132
  classification of, 132f, 132t
Focal segmental glomerulosclerosis, 70-72, 70f
  causes of, 72t

G

Gadolinium
  in chronic kidney disease, 178
Gadolinium-based contrast agents, 34
Gastrointestinal
  chronic kidney disease with, 172
Giant cellarteritis (GCA), 134
Glomerular basement membrane (GBM), 8
  abnormalities, 92-94
Glomerular diseases, 66-96
  associated with hypocomplementemia, 74t
  clinical presentation of, 66-68
  clinical syndromes, 68
  with glomerular basement membrane abnormalities, 92-94
  glomerulonephritis, associated with HBV infection, 88
  hepatitis B virus infection and, 88
  in intrinsic acute kidney injury, 162
  with nephritic syndrome, 74
  with nephrotic syndrome, 68
  from plasma cell dyscrasias, 84-88
  with rapidly progressive glomerulonephritis, 82
  thrombotic microangiopathies, 88-92
Glomerular filtration rate (GFR), 18
  categories of, 172t
  in chronic kidney disease, 22f
  estimation of, 22
  rate of decline in, 178
Glomerulonephritis, 8
  acute kidney disease in, 150, 154f
  acute proliferative, 162

呼吸性酸中毒，63-65
呼吸性碱中毒，61-63
电解质，慢性肾脏病，177
内分泌紊乱
  慢性肾脏病，177
内源性肾脏毒素，35
终末期肾病（ESRD）
  动脉粥样硬化性肾动脉狭窄，131
  患者护理，179
  流行病学，171
  β_2-微球蛋白，173
  患病率，171
肠源性高草酸尿症，121
嗜酸性肉芽肿性多血管炎（EGPA），83
依普利酮
  高钾血症，51
红细胞生成刺激剂（ESA），17
促红细胞生成素（EPO），17
  慢性肾病，175-177
大肠埃希菌
  溶血性尿毒综合征，91
  产志贺毒素大肠埃希菌，141-143
乙二醇中毒，59
细胞外液（ECF）
  细胞外液体积，39
肾外失钾，47
眼部胆固醇栓塞，137

F

法布里病，95，95f
范科尼综合征，见于间质性肾炎，103
纤维性肾小球肾炎，83，85f，163
成纤维细胞，肾，9
纤维囊蛋白，111
纤维肌发育不良（FMD），131-133
  分类，133f，133t
局灶节段性肾小球硬化，71-73，71f
  病因，73t

G

钆
  慢性肾脏病，179
钆造影剂，35
消化道
  慢性肾脏病，173
巨细胞动脉炎（GCA），135
肾小球基底膜（GBM），9
  异常，93-95
肾小球疾病，67-97
  低补体血症相关，75t
  临床表现，67-69
  临床综合征
  肾小球基底膜异常，93-95
  肾小球肾炎，与HBV感染相关，89
  乙型肝炎病毒感染，89
  肾实质性急性肾损伤，163
  肾炎综合征，75
  肾病综合征，69
  浆细胞病，85-89
  急进性肾小球肾炎，83
  血栓性微血管病，89-93
肾小球滤过率（GFR），19
  分类，173t
  慢性肾脏病，23f
  估算，23
  下降率，179
肾小球肾炎，9
  急性肾脏病，151，155f
  急性增殖性，163

anti-glomerular basement membrane antibody-mediated, 84, 86f
chronic, 68
cryoglobulinemic, 82, 82t
fibrillary, 162
immune-complex, 74-84
infection-related, 74, 76f
membranoproliferative, 74-80, 78f
rapidly progressive, 68
Glomerulosclerosis
diabetic, 96f
focal segmental, 70-72, 70f
causes of, 72t
Glomerulus, 8
injury to, 66
Gluconeogenesis, in kidneys, 12
Glucose
with insulin, in hyperkalemia, 50
Glucose intolerance
hypokalemia and, 48
Goodpasture disease, 84
Granulomatosis with polyangiitis (GPA), 82

H

Heart failure
acute kidney injury and, 158-160
Heavy metals, chronic interstitial nephritis from, 102
Hematologic
chronic kidney disease with, 174-176
Hematuria, IgA nephropathy and, 74
Hemodialysis
access for, 180
in acute kidney injury, 168
for chronic kidney disease, 180, 180f
Hemolytic-uremic syndrome (HUS), 90, 140-144
acute kidney injury and, 162
atypical, 90, 142-144
vs. thrombotic thrombocytopenic purpura, 144t
Hepatitis B
glomerulonephritis and, 88
Hepatorenal syndrome (HRS)
in prerenal acute kidney injury, 160
Herbal medications, in chronic kidney disease, 178
nephropathy in, 88
Hydronephrosis, 166
1α-hydroxylase, 16
Hypercalciuria, 120
Hypercapnia, primary, 62
Hypercapnic encephalopathy, 62-64
Hyperchloremic metabolic acidosis, 52, 56
in chronic kidney disease, 170
Hyperglycemia
hyponatremia and, 38
Hyperkalemia, 48-50
in chronic kidney disease, 176
distal tubular defects and, 50
renal tubular acidosis with, 56t
Hyperkalemic distal renal tubular acidosis, 54
Hypernatremia, 42-44, 42f
Hyperoxaluria, 120
Hyperparathyroidism
chronic kidney disease and, 176
Hyperpolarization, cell, hypokalemia and, 46-48
Hypertension
in chronic kidney disease, 18-20
cryoglobulinemia and, 82
with preeclampsia, 136-138
with renal artery stenosis, 128
renal manifestations of, 134-136
Hypertensive nephrosclerosis, 134-136

抗肾小球基底膜抗体介导的, 85, 87f
慢性, 69
冷球蛋白血症性, 83, 83t
纤维性肾小球病, 163
免疫复合物, 75-85
感染相关性, 75, 77f
膜增生性, 75-81, 79f
急进性, 69
肾小球硬化
糖尿病（肾小球硬化）, 97f
局灶节段性, 71-73, 71f
病因, 73t
肾小球, 9
损伤, 67
糖异生, 肾, 13
葡萄糖
联用胰岛素, 见于高钾血症, 51
糖耐量异常
低钾血症, 49
Goodpasture 病, 85
肉芽肿性多血管炎（GPA）, 83

H

心力衰竭
急性肾损伤, 159-161
重金属, 慢性间质性肾炎, 103
血液系统
慢性肾脏病, 175-177
血尿, IgA 肾病, 75
血液透析
通路, 181
急性肾损伤, 169
慢性肾脏病, 181, 181f
溶血性尿毒综合征（HUS）, 91, 141-145
急性肾损伤, 163
非典型, 91, 143-145
vs. 血栓性血小板减少性紫癜, 145t
乙型肝炎
肾小球肾炎, 89
肝肾综合征（HRS）
肾前性急性肾损伤, 161
草药, 见于慢性肾脏病, 179
肾病, 89
肾积水, 167
1α-羟化酶, 17
高钙尿症, 121
原发性高碳酸血症, 63
高碳酸血症脑病, 63-65
高氯性代谢性酸中毒, 53, 57
慢性肾脏病, 171
高血糖
低钠血症, 39
高钾血症, 49-51
慢性肾脏病, 177
远端肾小管功能缺损, 51
肾小管酸中毒, 57t
高钾血症性远端肾小管酸中毒, 55
高钠血症, 43-45, 43f
高草酸盐尿症, 121
甲状旁腺功能亢进症
慢性肾脏病, 177
细胞超极化, 低钾血症, 47-49
高血压
慢性肾脏病, 19-21
冷球蛋白血症, 83
先兆子痫, 137-139
肾动脉狭窄, 129
肾脏表现, 135-137
高血压性肾硬化症, 135-137

Hypervolemic hypernatremia, 42, 42f
Hypocalcemia
    chronic kidney disease and, 172-174
Hypocapnia, 60-62
Hypocitraturia, 120
Hypocomplementemia, glomerular diseases associated with, 74t
Hypokalemia, 44-48
    approach to patient with, 48f
    cellular potassium shift in, normal total body potassium, 44
    chronic kidney disease and, 176
    clinical presentation of, 46-48
    decreased total body potassium, 44-46
    definition of, 44
    extrarenal potassium losses in, 46
    renal potassium losses in, 46, 46f
    treatment for, 48
Hypokalemic distal renal tubular acidosis, 54
Hypokalemic periodic paralysis, 44
Hyponatremia, 38-42, 40f
Hypotonic hyponatremia, 38
Hypovolemic hypernatremia, 42, 42f

I

Ileal conduits, metabolic acidosis and, 56
Imaging
    renal, for acute kidney injury, 156-158
Immune complex-mediated membranoproliferativeglomerulonephritis, 76, 78f
Immunoglobulin A (IgA), nephropathy, 74, 76f
Immunoglobulin G (IgG), linear deposition of, 68
Immunologic, chronic kidney disease with, 174-176
Immunosuppressive therapy
    chronic kidney disease with, 182-184
    for kidney transplantation, 182f
Immunotactoid glomerulopathy, 82
Infections
    acute kidney injury and, 34-36
    glomerulonephritis and, 74, 76f
    post-transplantation, 184
Inflammation
    acute kidney injury and, 34
Insulin
    K+ level and, 44
Internal K^+ balance, 44
Interstitial disease, in intrinsic acute kidney injury, 164-166
Interstitial nephritis, 8
Interstitium, of kidney, 8
Intravenous pyelography, 34
Intrinsic acute kidney injury, 160-166
Ischemia
    acute kidney injury and, 34
    acute renal, 134
Ischemic acute tubular necrosis, 162
Isovolemic hypernatremia, 42, 42f

J

Juvenile nephronophthisis, 112
Juxtaglomerular apparatus, 8
Juxtamedullary nephrons, 8

K

Kawasaki disease, 134
Kidney
    echogenicity of, 34
    function of, 10-16, 14t
        assessment of, 20-24
        endocrine, 14-16, 14t
        excretory, 10-12, 10f

高容量性高钠血症，43，43f
低钙血症
    慢性肾脏病，173-175
低碳酸血症，61-63
低枸橼酸尿症，121
低补体血症，相关的肾小球疾病，75t
低钾血症，45-49
    患者接诊，49f
    细胞内外的 K^+ 转移，体内总钾量正常时，45
    慢性肾脏病，177
    临床表现，47-49
    体内总钾量减少，45-47
    定义，45
    肾外失钾，47
    肾性失钾，47，47f
    治疗，49
低钾血症性远端肾小管酸中毒，55
低钾性周期性麻痹，45
低钠血症，39-43，41f
低张性低钠血症，39
低容量性高钠血症，43，43f

I

回肠流出道术，代谢性酸中毒，57
影像学
    肾脏影像学，急性肾损伤，157-159
免疫复合物介导的膜增生性肾小球肾炎，77，79f
IgA 肾病，75，77f
IgG 的线样沉积，69
免疫系统，慢性肾脏病，175-177
免疫抑制治疗
    慢性肾脏病，183-185
    肾移植，183f
免疫触须样肾小球病，83
感染
    急性肾损伤，35-37
    肾小球肾炎，75，77f
    移植后感染，185
炎症
    急性肾损伤，35
胰岛素
    K^+水平，45
体内 K^+ 平衡，45
间质性疾病，见于肾实质性急性肾损伤，165-167
间质性肾炎，9
肾间质，9
静脉肾盂造影，35
肾实质性急性肾损伤，161-167
缺血
    急性肾损伤，35
    急性肾缺血，135
缺血性急性肾小管坏死，163
等容量性高钠血症，43，43f

J

少年型肾消耗病，113
球旁器，9
髓旁肾单位，9

K

川崎病，135
肾
    回声，35
    功能，11-17，15t
        评估，21-25
        内分泌，15-17，15t
        排泄，11-13，11f

filtration, 12
integrated models of excretion, 12
metabolic, 14-16
reabsorption, 12, 14t
secretion, 12
nonglomerular disorders of, 98-124
    acquired cystic kidney disease, 106-108
    acute interstitial nephritis, 98-100, 100t
    autosomal recessive polycystic kidney, 110
    chronic interstitial nephritis, 100-106, 100t-102t
    cystic kidney diseases, 106-112
    juvenile nephronophthisis, 112
    medullary sponge kidney, 112
    nephrolithiasis, 116-122
    polycystic kidney disease, 108-112
    tuberous sclerosis, 112
    von Hippel-Lindau disease, 112-114
size of, 18
structure of, 4-10
    circulation in, 4, 6t
    glomerulus, 8
    interstitium, 8
    juxtaglomerular apparatus, 8
    macroscopic anatomy of, 4, 6f
    nephron, 8
    nerves, 4-6
    organelles as mitochondria and endoplasmic reticulum, 8-10
    specialized structures, 8-10
    tubules, 8, 10f
thrombotic microangiopathy of, 140-146, 142f
vascular disorders of, 126-148, 128f
    antiphospholipid antibody syndrome, 146-148
    hemolyticuremic syndrome, 140-144
    renal vein thrombosis, 148
    renovascular disease, 126-140
    thrombotic thrombocytopenic purpura, 140
Kidney disease. *See also* Acute kidney injury; Glomerular diseases; Interstitial nephritis
    cystic, 106-108
Kidney transplantation, 180-184
    acute rejection of, 184
    comparison of donor sources for, 182t
    post-transplantation infection, 184
    types of, 180
Kidney tumors, 114-116, 114t

L

Lactic acidosis, 56, 56t
Lead, chronic interstitial nephritis from, 102
Lenarduzzi-Cacchi-Ricci disease, 112
Light chain deposition disease, 86-88, 90f
Lithium, 104
Lithotripsy, for renal calculi, 118
Lupus nephritis, 80-82
    classification of, 80f, 80t

M

Macula densa, 8
Magnesium sulfate, in preeclampsia, 138
Magnetic resonance angiography (MRA)
    for renal artery stenosis, 130
Magnetic resonance imaging (MRI)
    in chronic kidney disease, 34
Malignant disease, post-transplantation, 184
Masked hypertension, 20
Medications
    in prerenal acute kidney injury, 158
Mediolysis, segmental arterial, 132

滤过，13
排泄的综合模式，13
代谢，15-17
重吸收，13，15t
分泌，13
非肾小球肾脏疾病，99-125
    获得性囊性肾病，107-109
    急性间质性肾炎，99-101，101t
    常染色体隐性遗传多囊肾病，111
    慢性间质性肾炎，101-107，101t-103t
    囊肿性肾病，107-113
    少年型肾消耗病，113
    髓质海绵肾，113
    肾结石，117-123
    多囊肾病，109-113
    结节性硬化症，113
    希佩尔-林道病，113-115
体积，19
结构，5-11
    循环，5，7t
    肾小球，9
    肾间质，9
    球旁器，9
    大体解剖，5，7f
    肾单位，9
    神经，5-7
    细胞器，如线粒体和内质网，9-11
    特殊结构，9-11
    肾小管，9，11f
血栓性微血管病，141-147，143f
血管疾病，127-149，129f
    抗磷脂综合征，147-149
    溶血性尿毒综合征，141-145
    肾静脉血栓形成，149
    肾血管病，127-141
    血栓性血小板减少性紫癜，141
肾病 参见急性肾损伤；肾小球疾病；间质性肾炎
    囊性，107-109
肾移植，181-185
    急性排斥反应，185
    供体来源比较，183t
    移植后感染，185
    类型，181
肾肿瘤，115-117，115t

L

乳酸酸中毒，57，57t
铅，慢性间质性肾炎，103
Lenarduzzi-Cacchi-Ricci 病，113
轻链沉积病，87-89，91f
锂，105
碎石，治疗肾结石，119
狼疮肾炎，81-83
    分类，81f，81t

M

致密斑，9
硫酸镁，见于先兆子痫，139
磁共振血管成像（MRA）
    肾动脉狭窄，131
磁共振成像（MRI）
    慢性肾脏病，35
恶性疾病，移植后，185
隐匿性高血压，21
药物
    肾前性急性肾损伤，159
节段性动脉中膜溶解，133

Medulla, of kidneys, 4
Medullary sponge kidney, 112
Membranoproliferativeglomerulonephritis (MPGN), 74-80, 78f
Membranous nephropathy, 72-74, 72f
Mesangium, 8
Metabolic acidosis, 50-58, 52f
   in acute kidney injury, 166
   anion gap, 56-58
   extrarenal origin of, 54-56
   hyperchloremic. See Hyperchloremic metabolic acidosis
   of renal origin, 52-54, 54f
Metabolic alkalosis, 58-60
   classification of, 60t
   saline resistant, 60, 60t
Methanol poisoning, 58
Microangiopathichemolytic anemia (MAHA), 138
$β_2$-microglobulin
   in end-stage renal disease, 170-172
Microscopic polyangiitis (MPA), 82
Microscopy, urine, for acute kidney injury, 156, 156t
Mineral acidosis, hyperkalemia and, 50
Mineralocorticoid activity
   decrease in, 50
   primary increase in, 46
Minimal change disease, 68-70, 70f
Modification of Diet in Renal Disease (MDRD) equation, 24
Musculoskeletal system
   chronic kidney disease with, 172-174
Mycophenolatemofetil, 184
Mycophenolic acid, 184
Myopathy(ies), 46-48

N

Neonates, autosomal recessive polycystic kidney disease in, 110
Nephritic sediment, 162
Nephritic syndrome, 68
   glomerular diseases with, 74
Nephritis, interstitial, 164-166
Nephrolithiasis, 116-122
   medications associated with, 116t
   treatment for, 118t
   types of, 118-122
   urinalysis and radiographic findings in, 118t
Nephrolithotomy, for renal calculi, 118
Nephron, 8
Nephronophthisis, juvenile, 112
Nephropathy
   crystalline, in intrinsic acute kidney injury, 164
   diabetic, 18
   HIV-associated, 88
   immunoglobulin A (IgA), 74, 76f
   obstructive, 166
   osmotic, in intrinsic acute kidney injury, 164
   pigment, in intrinsic acute kidney injury, 162-164
Nephrosclerosis, hypertensive, 18
Nephrotic syndrome, 24, 68
   glomerular diseases with, 68
   renal vein thrombosis and, 148
Nephrotoxic acute tubular necrosis, 162
Nephrotoxins, acute kidney injury and, 34
Neurologic
   chronic kidney disease with, 172
Nonsteroidal anti-inflammatory drugs (NSAIDs)
   in acute kidney injury, 158
Nuclear imaging, for renal artery stenosis, 130

O

Obstructive nephropathy, 104, 106t, 166
Obstructive uropathy, 166

肾髓质，5
海绵肾，113
膜增生性肾小球肾炎（MPGN），75-81，79f
膜性肾病，73-75，73f
系膜，9
代谢性酸中毒，51-59，53f
   急性肾损伤，167
   阴离子间隙，57-59
   肾外源性，55-57
   高氯性 参见高氯性代谢性酸中毒
   肾源性，53-55，55f
代谢性碱中毒，59-61
   分类，61t
   生理盐水抵抗性，61，61t
甲醇中毒，59
微血管病性溶血性贫血（MAHA），139
$β_2$-微球蛋白
   终末期肾病，171-173
显微镜下多血管炎（MPA），83
尿液显微镜检查，针对急性肾损伤，157，157t
矿物性酸中毒，高钾血症，51
盐皮质激素活性
   降低，51
   原发性升高，47
微小病变，69-71，71f
肾脏病饮食改良试验（MDRD）公式，25
肌肉骨骼
   慢性肾脏病，173-175
吗替麦考酚酯，185
麦考酚酸，185
肌病，47-49

N

新生儿常染色体隐性遗传多囊肾病，111
肾炎性尿沉渣，163
肾病综合征，69
   肾小球疾病，75
肾炎，间质性，165-167
肾结石，117-123
   相关的药物，117t
   治疗，119t
   类型，119-123
   尿液分析和影像学表现，119t
肾镜取石术，治疗肾结石，119
肾单位，9
肾消耗病，少年型，113
肾病
   晶体性，见于肾实质性急性肾损伤，165
   糖尿病（肾病），19
   HIV 相关性，89
   免疫球蛋白 A（IgA），75，77f
   梗阻性，167
   渗透性，见于肾实质性急性肾损伤，165
   色素（肾病），见于肾实质性急性肾损伤，163-165
肾硬化症，高血压性，19
肾病综合征，25，69
   肾小球疾病，69
   肾静脉血栓形成，149
肾毒性急性肾小管坏死，163
肾毒素，急性肾损伤，35
神经系统
   慢性肾脏病，173
非甾体抗炎药（NSAID）
   急性肾损伤，159
核成像，针对肾动脉狭窄，131

O

梗阻性肾病，105，107t，167
梗阻性尿路病，167

Organelles, as mitochondria and endoplasmic reticulum, 8-10
Organic acidosis, hyperkalemia and, 50
Osmolality, 38
Osmolar gap, 38
Osmoregulation, sensors and effectors in, 40t
Osmotic diuresis, 42
Osmotic nephropathy, in intrinsic acute kidney injury, 164
Osteomalacia, 54
Osteopenia, 54
Oxalate nephropathy, acute, 164

P

Paralysis, flaccid, hypokalemia and, 46-48
Percutaneous nephrolithotomy, for renal calculi, 118
Pericarditis
 in dialysis patients, 172
Peritoneal dialysis, 180
Peritubular capillaries, 4
Phosphate
 chronic kidney disease and, 172-174
Pigment nephropathy, in intrinsic acute kidney injury, 162-164
Plasma
 tonicity of, 38
Plasma cell dyscrasias, glomerular diseases from, 84-88
Plasminogen activator receptor, soluble urokinase-type, 70
Podocytes, 8
Podocytopathies, primary, 68-74
Polyarteritis nodosa (PAN), 132
Polycystic kidney disease (PKD), 108-112
Polydipsia, primary, 38
Polyuria, 42, 44f
Postrenal acute kidney injury, 150, 166
Poststreptococcal glomerulonephritis (PSGN), 74
Potassium chloride (KCl) salt, 48
Potassium citrate, for calcium stones, 120
Potassium ions (K$^+$)
 decrease in, 44-46
 excessive dietary intake of, 48-50
 losses, 46, 46f-48f
 renal excretion of, 50
Preeclampsia, 136-138
Pregnancy
 chronic kidney disease and, 176
Prerenal acute kidney injury, 150, 158-160
Protein
 dietary restriction of, in chronic kidney disease, 178
Proteinuria, glomerular, 66-68
Pseudohyperkalemia, 48
Pseudohyponatremia, 38
Pseudotumor cerebri, 62-64
Pure water loss, 42
Pyramids, in kidneys, 4
Pyroglutamic acidosis, 58

R

Radiation nephritis, 102-104
Radiographic findings, on renal calculi, 118t
Radionuclide imaging
 in chronic kidney disease, 34
Rapidly progressive glomerulonephritis (RPGN), 68, 68f
 glomerular diseases with, 82
Renal arteries, anatomy of, 126
Renal artery stenosis, 126
 anatomy of, 128f
Renal biopsy
 for acute kidney injury, 158
 preeclampsia and, 136-138
 in scleroderma renal crisis, 138

细胞器，如线粒体和内质网，9-11
有机酸中毒，高钾血症，51
渗透压，39
渗透压间隙，39
渗透压调节，感受器和效应器，41t
渗透性利尿，43
渗透性肾病，见于急性肾损伤，165
骨软化症，55
骨量减少，55
草酸盐肾病，急性，165

P

弛缓性麻痹，低钾血症，47-49
经皮肾镜取石术，治疗肾结石，119
心包炎
 透析患者，173
腹膜透析，181
肾小管管周毛细血管，5
磷
 慢性肾病，173-175
色素肾病，见于肾实质性急性肾损伤，163-165
血浆
 张力，39
浆细胞病，引起的肾小球疾病，85-89
纤溶酶原激活物受体，可溶性尿激酶型，71
足细胞，9
足细胞病，原发性，69-75
结节性多动脉炎（PAN），133
多囊肾病（PKD），109-113
原发性烦渴，39
多尿，43，45f
肾后性急性肾损伤，151，167
链球菌感染后肾小球肾炎（PSGN），75
氯化钾（KCl）盐，49
枸橼酸钾，治疗钙结石，121
钾离子（K$^+$）
 减少，45-47
 饮食摄入过量，49-51
 失钾，47，47f-49f
 肾脏排钾，51
先兆子痫，137-139
妊娠
 慢性肾脏病，177
肾前性急性肾损伤，151，159-161
蛋白质
 饮食限制，见于慢性肾脏病，179
蛋白尿，肾小球性，67-69
假性高钾血症，49
假性低钠血症，39
假性脑瘤，63-65
纯水丢失，43
肾锥体，5
焦谷氨酸酸中毒，59

R

放射性肾炎，103-105
影像学表现，肾结石，119t
放射性核素成像
 慢性肾脏病，35
急进性肾小球肾炎（RPGN），69，69f
 肾小球疾病，83
肾动脉，解剖，127
肾动脉狭窄，127
 解剖，129f
肾活检
 急性肾损伤，159
 先兆子痫，137-139
 硬皮病肾危象，139

Renal cell carcinoma
    TNM staging system of, 114, 114t
Renal colic, 104
Renal cysts, 106
Renal disease
    approach to patient with, 18-36
        acute kidney injury, 34-36
        chronic kidney disease, 18-34
Renal failure, 4
    acute, nephrotic syndrome and, 68
Renal imaging, 24-34
Renal infarction, 134
Renal insufficiency
    renal tubular acidosis of, 54
Renal potassium losses, 46, 46f-48f
Renal replacement therapies, 178-184
    hospital-based, 168
Renal tubular acidosis
    proximal, 52-54
    of renal insufficiency, 54
Renal vascular, anatomy of, 126
Renal vein, anatomy of, 126
Renal vein thrombosis, 148
    nephrotic syndrome and, 68
Renal venography, in renal vein thrombosis, 148
Renin, 14-16
Renin-angiotensin-aldosterone system (RAAS)
    activation of, 126
        scleroderma renal crisis and, 138-140
    kidneys and, 12
Renovascular disease, 126-140
Respiratory acidosis, 62-64
Respiratory alkalosis, 60-62
Retrograde pyelography, 34
Rituximab
    for membranous nephropathy, 74
    for minimal change disease, 70

S

Salicylate poisoning, 58
Sarcoidosis, 102
Scleroderma renal crisis (SRC), 138-140
Sclerosis, systemic, 138
Segmental arterial mediolysis, 132
Sexual dysfunction
    chronic kidney disease and, 176
Shiga toxin-producing *Escherichia coli* (STEC)
    hemolyticuremic syndrome and, 144t
Shiga-like toxin, hemolyticuremic syndrome and, 90
Shockwave lithotripsy, for renal calculi, 118
Sickle cell disease
    chronic interstitial nephritis and, 104
Simple cysts, in kidney, 106
Skin, chronic kidney disease with, 176
Slit diaphragms, 8
Sodium, dietary, intake of, assessment of, 24
Sodium ions (Na^+)
    decrease in, 38
    distal delivery of, primary increase in, 46
Soluble endoglin (sENG), 138
Soluble FMS-related tyrosine kinase 1 (sFLT1), 138
Soluble urokinase-type plasminogen activator receptor (suPAR), 70
Spironolactone
    in hyperkalemia, 50
Sporadic hemolyticuremic syndrome, 90
Stenting
    in atherosclerotic renal artery stenosis, 130
Steroid therapy
    for tubulointerstitial nephritis, 102

肾细胞癌
    TNM（分期）系统，115，115t
肾绞痛，105
肾囊肿，107
肾脏疾病
    患者接诊，19-37
        急性肾损伤，35-37
        慢性肾脏病，19-35
肾衰竭，5
    急性，肾病综合征，69
肾脏影像，25-35
肾梗死，135
肾功能不全
    肾小管酸中毒，55
肾性失钾，47，47f-49f
肾替代治疗，179-185
    住院，169
肾小管酸中毒
    近端，53-55
    肾功能不全性，55
肾血管，解剖，127
肾静脉，解剖，127
肾静脉血栓形成，149
    肾病综合征，69
肾静脉造影，见于肾静脉血栓形成，149
肾素，15-17
肾素-血管紧张素-醛固酮系统（RAAS）
    激活，127
        硬皮病肾危象，139-141
    肾和RAAS，13
肾血管病，127-141
呼吸性酸中毒，63-65
呼吸性碱中毒，61-63
逆行肾盂造影，35
利妥昔单抗
    膜性肾病，75
    微小病变，71

S

水杨酸中毒，59
结节病，103
硬皮病肾危象（SRC），139-141
硬化症，系统性，139
节段性动脉中膜溶解，133
性功能障碍
    慢性肾脏病，177
产志贺毒素大肠埃希菌（STEC）
    溶血性尿毒综合征，145t
志贺样毒素，溶血性尿毒综合征，91
冲击波碎石，治疗肾结石，119
镰状细胞病
    慢性间质性肾炎，105
单纯性囊肿，肾，107
皮肤，慢性肾脏病，177
裂隙膜，9
膳食钠，摄入量，评估，25
钠离子（Na^+）
    减少，39
    远端Na^+输送，原发性增加，47
可溶性内皮糖蛋白（sENG），139
可溶性FMS相关酪氨酸激酶1（sFLT1），139
可溶性尿激酶型纤溶酶原激活物受体（suPAR），71
螺内酯
    高钾血症，51
散发性溶血性尿毒综合征，91
支架植入
    动脉粥样硬化性肾动脉狭窄，131
类固醇治疗
    肾小管间质性肾炎，103

Struvite stones, 122, 122t
Superficial nephrons, 8
Sweat, potassium losses and, 46
Syndrome of inappropriate antidiuretic hormone (SIADH), 40
Systemic arterial emboli, 134
Systemic vasculitides, 134

T

Tacrolimus, 182-184
Takayasu's arteritis, 134
Thiazide diuretics
　for hypercalciuria, 120
　hyponatremia and, 40
Thin glomerular basement membrane nephropathy, 94, 94f
Thromboembolic disease, 134
Thrombolytic therapy
　acute kidney injury and, 160
Thrombotic microangiopathy, 88-92, 92f
　disorders associated with, 144t
　of kidney, 140-146, 142f
　malignancy-associated, 144
　pregnancy-related, 144-146
Thrombotic thrombocytopenic purpura (TTP), 92, 144t
　vs. hemolyticuremic syndrome, 144t
　acute kidney injury and, 162
Tight junctions, 8
Tonicity, 38
Total body potassium, decrease, 44-46
Total body water, 38
Transesophageal echocardiography (TEE)
　in aortic dissection, 134
Transforming growth factor-β (TGF-β), in chronic kidney disease, 170
Triamterene, in hyperkalemia, 50
Triglycerides
　chronic kidney disease and, 176
Trimethoprim, in hyperkalemia, 50
Triple phosphate stones, 122
Tuberous sclerosis complex (TSC), 112
Tubular cells, in urine, 28f
Tubular disease, in intrinsic acute kidney injury, 162-164
Tubules, 8, 10f
　reabsorption in, 12
Tubulitis, 164
Tumor-node-metastasis (TNM) criteria, for renal cell carcinoma, 114-116, 114t

U

Ultrafiltration, 180
Ultrasonography
　for acute kidney injury, 166
　in chronic kidney disease, 24
Urea
　in chronic kidney disease, 22
Uremic acidosis, 54
Uremic syndrome
　general features of, 170-172, 174f
Uric acid
　crystals, 36
Uric acid stones, 122
Urinalysis
　for acute kidney injury, 156, 156t
　microscopic, in chronic kidney disease, 24, 26f-32f
　in renal calculi, 118t
Urinary total protein excretion, 66
Urinary tract obstruction, interstitial nephritis in, 104-106, 106t
Urine
　acidic, 116
　indices of, 156

磷酸铵镁结石，123，123t
浅表肾单位，9
出汗，失钾，47
抗利尿激素分泌失调综合征（SIADH），41
系统性动脉栓子，135
系统性血管炎，135

T

他克莫司，183-185
大动脉炎，135
噻嗪类利尿剂
　高钙尿症，121
　低钠血症，41
薄基底膜肾病，95，95f
血栓栓塞性疾病，135
溶栓治疗
　急性肾损伤，161
血栓性微血管病（TMA），89-93，93f
　相关疾病，145t
　肾脏的，141-147，143f
　恶性肿瘤相关，145
　妊娠相关，145-147
血栓性血小板减少性紫癜（TTP），93，145t
　vs. 溶血性尿毒综合征，145t
　急性肾损伤，163
紧密连接，9
张力，39
体内总钾量减少，45-47
体内总水量，39
经食管超声心动图（TEE）
　主动脉夹层，135
转化生长因子-β（TGF-β），治疗慢性肾脏病，171
氨苯蝶啶，见于高钾血症，51
甘油三酯
　慢性肾脏病，177
甲氧苄啶，见于高钾血症，51
三磷酸盐结石，123
结节性硬化症（TSC），113
肾小管细胞，尿液中，29f
肾小管疾病，见于肾实质性急性肾损伤，163-165
肾小管，9，11f
　重吸收，13
肾小管炎，165
肿瘤-淋巴结-转移（TNM）标准，肾细胞癌，115-117，115t

U

超滤，181
超声检查
　急性肾损伤，167
　慢性肾脏病，25
尿素
　慢性肾脏病，23
尿毒症性酸中毒，55
尿毒症综合征
　一般特征，171-173，175f
尿酸
　结晶，37
尿酸结石，123
尿液分析
　急性肾损伤，157，157t
　显微镜检，慢性肾脏病，25，27f-33f
　肾结石，119t
尿总蛋白排泄量，67
尿路梗阻，间质性肾炎，105-107，107t
尿液
　酸性，117
　指标，157

Urine anion gap (UAG), 52
Urine osmolality, 42
Uropathy, obstructive, 166

V

Vasa recta
    in kidney, 4
    renal, 126
Vascular disease
    in intrinsic acute kidney injury, 160
Vasculitides
    antineutrophil cytoplasmic antibody-associated, 82-84, 84t
    systemic, 134
Vasculitis
    acute kidney injury from, 160
Venography, in renal vein thrombosis, 148
Vessel vasculitis, large and medium-sized, 134
Vitamin D, 16
    chronic kidney disease and, 172-174
Volume depletion, in prerenal acute kidney injury, 158
Volume homeostasis, normal, 38
Volume regulation, sensors and effectors in, 40t
von Hippel-Lindau disease, 112-114
von Willebrand factor (VWF)
    thrombotic thrombocytopenic purpura and, 92

W

Warfarin
    in antiphospholipid antibody syndrome, 148
Water
    decrease in distal delivery of, 50
    pure loss of, 42
    total body, 38
Water deficit, 42-44
Water diuresis, 42
White coat hypertension, 20

尿阴离子间隙（UAG），53
尿渗透压，43
梗阻性尿路病，167

V

直小血管
    肾，5
    肾，127
血管疾病
    肾实质性急性肾损伤，161
血管炎
    抗中性粒细胞胞质抗体相关，83-85，85t
    系统性，135
血管炎
    急性肾损伤，161
静脉造影，见于肾静脉血栓形成，149
大血管和中血管血管炎，135
维生素D，17
    慢性肾脏病，173-175
容量不足，见于肾前性急性肾损伤，159
容量稳态，正常，39
容量调节，感受器和效应器，41t
希佩尔-林道病，113-115
血管性血友病因子（vWF）
    血栓性血小板减少性紫癜，93

W

华法林
    抗磷脂综合征，149
水
    远端输送减少，51
    纯水丢失，43
    体内总水量，39
缺水，43-45
水利尿，43
白大衣高血压，21